Language and Deafness

Third Edition

Peter V. Paul
Ohio State University

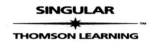

SINGULAR

TM

THOMSON LEARNING

Language and Deafness, Third Edition
by Peter V. Paul, Ph.D.

Business Unit Director:
William Brottmiller

Acquisitions Editor:
Marie Linvill

Developmental Editor:
Kristin Banach

Executive Marketing Manager:
Dawn Gerrain

Channel Manager:
Kathryn Bamberger

Executive Production Editor:
Barbara Bullock

Production Editor:
Brad Bielawski

Library of Congress Cataloging-in-Publication Data
Peter V. Paul
Language and deafness/ Peter V. Paul.—3rd ed.
p. ; cm.
Includes bibliographical references and index.
ISBN 1-56593-999-9 (pbk. : alk. paper)
1. Deaf—Education 2. Deaf children—language 3. Deaf—Means of communication.
4. Deaf—Education—United States. I. Title
1.
HV2471.Q52 2000
371.91'2—dc21   00-061214

PREFACE TO THE FIRST EDITION

The present state of the education of deaf children can be characterized as one of creative confusion. Creative is an appropriate term because the present ferment in the field seems likely to lead to significant changes, which might also be significant advances. Confusion is also an appropriate term since no strongly research-supported directions for educational practice have yet emerged from the ferment. Most of the ferment centers around the languages and the communication modes that should be used initially with deaf infants and children. This book attempts to define the problems and prospects of those languages and communication modes, to discuss elements of the present creative ferment in these areas, to present and discuss much of the data-based research findings pertaining to them, to synthesize the findings and those from other areas (such as bilingualism and English as a second language [ESL]), and to present some conclusions.

The book is seen as being useful to anyone seeking an in-depth introduction to language development in deaf children, but particularly to student teachers and clinicians and practicing teachers and clinicians who bear most of the responsibility for fostering that development both directly and in their training and counseling of parents. The book has much more detail on language than is common in beginner texts, but that is because the authors believe that teachers and clinicians must have a great deal of detailed knowledge about language and communication to promote, through naturally oriented practices, the initial language development of deaf children; and to direct, through analytically oriented practices, more structured development at later ages if the naturally oriented practices do not produce adequate language development. As Russell, Quigley, and Power (1976) have claimed: "It is probably a fair analogy to state that teachers of deaf children should be expected to know as much about language as a teacher of chemistry is expected to know about chemistry" (p. xi). This is not so that teachers can teach language didactically but in order that they have the knowledge and skills to structure situations and construct materials that will allow language to develop in a natural manner or, when necessary, in a more structured manner.

Both natural and structured approaches are seen as playing a role in the language development of deaf children. The preferred approach is the natural approach, in which language is acquired (or absorbed) unconsciously by the child through fluent communicative interaction with the parents in infancy and early childhood and later with teachers. Unfortunately, this early natural development does not always take place (in fact, it rarely takes place), and at some point many teachers feel the need to use more structured approaches to language development. It follows from this, that teachers and clinicians must be familiar with both approaches and know when to use each.

The statement that early language development requires fluent communicative interaction between child and parents and child and teacher raises immediately the question of communication modes, the form in which parent, teacher, and child will communicate. Here again, as with language approaches, no absolute position is taken in the book. All major approaches are described and explored. It is recognized and stated that it is not possible to examine the language development of deaf children apart from the specific communication mode through which it was developed. With hearing children, language is acquired through speech, and spoken language is the primary language on which the secondary language forms of reading and writing are based. Individual variations in IQ, socioeconomic status, educational opportunities, and other factors might alter the degree of language mastery by individual hearing children, but they will not alter the form. All variations are variations on the same basic form, spoken language.

With deaf children the situation is quite different. Any of several communication modes or forms might be used early with them, and language development can be discussed only in relation to the particular form used. That approach is followed here, particularly in Chapter 3 on Primary Language Development and in the concluding chapter. The major communication forms that can be used with deaf children are referred to throughout the book as oral English (OE), manually coded English (MCE), and American Sign Language (ASL). These are described in Chapter 1 on Definitions and Historical Perspectives. Pidgin sign English (PSE) is categorized here as a form of MCE, but it can be regarded also as a separate form. MCE systems are contrived systems (contrived usually by hearing people) which attempt in various ways to conform signs and finger spelling to the structure of English. PSE is a linguistically natural language form developed from interaction or interfacing of the visual ASL with the oral OE.

As with language approaches, it follows from the variety of communication modes and the present support that exists for each, that teachers and clinicians who work with deaf children need to be conversant with, and fluent in, all of them. And since the secondary language forms of reading and writing, at least in our present state of knowledge, have to be related to the child's primary language, teachers and clinicians need to understand the implications of each primary language form (OE, MCE, ASL) for the development of reading and written language. If OE is used exclusively with a deaf child, then perhaps the methods of teaching reading to hearing children (which assume the existence of a spoken language) can be used with that child; but if ASL is the child's primary language, then it is likely that other methods of teaching reading must be sought.

In addition to being skilled in the various language approaches (natural and structured) and the various communication forms (OE, MCE, ASL) that are used with deaf children, teachers and clinicians need to be highly knowledgeable in the language and communication development of hearing children. It is important also that they be familiar with the special problems and techniques used in language development with certain other special populations, especially problems and techniques in bilingualism and the teaching of English as a second language (ESL). All of this amounts to a great deal of knowledge and skill in a large number of areas, but it is difficult to see how a teacher of deaf children can be fully competent without all of it.

This book treats, though only to limited extents, each of these areas of knowledge and skill. References are provided throughout where the reader can obtain more detailed information on the major topic discussed in each chapter. In most chapters, the topic of the chapter (e.g., reading) is discussed first in relation to the hearing population. This is in accord with the stated position that the language development of deaf children can best be examined and understood in the context of language development in general. Each chapter topic is then discussed in relation to deaf children as defined in Chapter 1 and some conclusions and possible applications are presented.

Chapter 1 provides definitions of important terms and historical perspectives on important issues and topics. One of the most neglected issues in the education of deaf children is the differentiation of children who are deaf (visually oriented for purposes of communication even with the best amplification) from those who are hard of hearing (at least partially auditorily oriented). An attempt is made to do this in Chapter 1. In that chapter also, definitions are provided for the various language and communication approaches used with deaf children. Then the historical paths of the various language and communication approaches are traced in an effort to show that most of the present approaches (with the exception of such relatively recent technological advances as amplification) have very long histories. This should not be surprising. The formal teaching and tutoring of deaf children has almost a 400-year history and has involved many very intelligent people. In that lengthy period, it is likely that every conceivable approach has been tried. The fact that none has prevailed, and dissension still reigns, indicates that there is as yet no one "true path" in the education of deaf children.

Chapter 2 deals with language and cognition. Again the topic is discussed in terms of hearing individuals and then in relation to deaf individuals. The position is taken that language is a subset of cognitive abilities and that adequate language development requires adequate cognitive development. It is also accepted that soon after language begins to develop, language and cognition become almost inseparable. Symbolic mediation is discussed in this chapter; the forms of internalized language used by hearing and by deaf individuals as mediators of thought and of the secondary language forms of reading and writing.

Chapter 3 presents current theories of language and traces the development of primary language in hearing and in deaf individuals. As previously stated, the language development of deaf children must be examined in relation to the communication form through which it was developed and given expression. This is done in Chapter 3, with development being discussed within the communication forms of OE, MCE, and ASL. Some implications of the various forms for the later development of reading and written language are discussed. The lack of research based data is stressed.

Chapter 4 presents considerable information on the reading of hearing and of deaf children; Chapter 5 similarly treats written language. The original intent had been to treat these two topics in a single chapter to emphasize their close relationship and the primacy of reading, but the large amount of material available dictated separate chapters. It is recognized, and expounded in the book, that skilled development of reading and written language requires adequate development of a primary language, which in turn is dependent on early fluent communication between parent and child. But the development of literacy is the road to learning and is the primary responsibility of teachers, clinicians, and the schools. Other aspects of the deaf child's development certainly are important. But the failure to develop literacy cannot be compensated for by the promotion of cultural identity or the development of a positive self-image, important as those might be. In fact, it is doubtful that an adult who is semiliterate or illiterate for all practical purposes can have a very positive self-image or find much satisfaction or reward in cultural identity.

Chapter 6 deals with the processes and problems, theories and practices, of bilingualism and the development of English as a second language with minority-culture hearing children, and relates these areas analogically to the language development of deaf children. This is likely to be an area for much fruitful exploration and research with deaf children during the decade of the 1980s. Some of the problems and some of the possible programs and procedures that could be tried with deaf children, based on research with minority-culture hearing children, are discussed. It is emphasized that successful bilingual and ESL programs seem to require that the child come to the program with at least one language already reasonably well established. That, of course, is not the case with many deaf children who often enter school and preschool programs without any well-developed first language. (Some deaf children of ASL-using deaf parents might be exceptions to this.) This reinforces the importance of the family, or some substitute, providing the deaf child with a primary language in infancy and early childhood through some fluent form of communication.

Chapter 7 treats language assessment and some of the major methods used in language development and instruction. Some material in these areas is also presented, where appropriate, in other chapters and much of the other material could have been similarly treated. It was considered convenient for students and teachers, however, to have a separate chapter on these important areas. The material on instructional approaches is related back to the historical treatment of earlier approaches in Chapter 1.

In the final chapter (8), some general summation of the book's topics is provided and some implications for present and future educational practices with deaf children are discussed. If there is a general focus, or unifying theme to the book, it is provided by Chapter 8 and this Preface. The theme is simply that there is as yet no data-based justification for any communication and language approach as the sole means of developing language in deaf children. The teacher and the clinician must master a variety of language approaches (from natural to analytic) and communication forms (e.g., OE, MCE, ASL) to function effectively with a range of deaf children. Fortunately, teachers and clinicians are usually more eclectic and more pragmatic than many textbook writers. They are usually willing to try new approaches on the basis of logical and theoretical arguments, but are also ready to abandon them if they do not seem to work.

A companion text to the present book, *Reading and Deafness*, by Cynthia M. King and Stephen P. Quigley, will be published soon by the same publisher. The topics of the two books, language and reading, are obviously closely related, and the use of a single publisher allows for some overlap of content without the authors having to go through a frustrating rewriting exercise to say the same thing in different words in two different books so as not to violate copyrights held by two different publishers. A major difference between the two texts is that *Reading and Deafness* will provide both a knowledge base and instructional techniques on its topic whereas *Language and Deafness* deals primarily with a knowledge base and treats instructional techniques only generally. This is because the wider scope of the present book makes inclusion of detailed material on instruction impractical. A special chapter on assessment and instruction has been provided for the present book by Barry W. Jones, and a related text on instructional processes and techniques in language development is tentatively planned.

The authors are indebted to many persons for assistance in the preparation of this book. A major debt is acknowledged to the many teachers, clinicians, researchers, and thinkers who provided most of the material on which the book is based. Some, but certainly not all, of this debt is acknowledged by appropriate citation and referencing of the more than 500 authors whose work was used in preparation of the text. Grateful acknowledgment is also made to the graduate students who aided in locating and abstracting the works of those many authors: Jean Andrews, Cheryl Bolebruch, Cynthia King, John-Allen Payne, Stephanie Quigley, Lou Reeves, Marilyn Salter, and Pam Stuckey. And finally, the major and indispensable assistance provided by Ruth Quigley in all phases of the planning, preparation, and completion of the manuscript is gratefully acknowledged and lovingly appreciated.

PREFACE TO THE SECOND EDITION

All intelligent thoughts have already been thought;
what is necessary is only to try to think them again.
(*Johann Wolfgang von Goethe,* in Beck, 1980, p. 397)*

The quote above captures in a nutshell the major intention of the second edition of *Language and Deafness*. With a few exceptions, the second edition adheres to the conceptual framework established by the first edition as described in the first Preface. There are, of course, some notable differences. As much as possible, we have updated the theories and research in a number of areas in almost every chapter. This new source of information did not radically change our original conclusions stated in the first edition. However, it did lead to a refinement of some issues, particularly concerning the interrelationships among language, cognition, and literacy.

This refinement led us to hypothesize that the development of English literacy skills might not be a realistic goal for some, perhaps many, students with severe to profound hearing impairment. We express this concern in our first edition; however, we have become more convinced of this situation. Similar to other scholars, we firmly believe that it is important to develop a first language at as early an age as possible. Unfortunately, we have made little progress since our first edition; that is, there is still not enough evidence on which a firm decision can be based.

Another major change in the second edition is the concept of metatheory—the driving, conceptual framework which influences the construction of theories, the undertaking of research, the use of specific methods, and, most importantly, the interpretation of results. There should be sufficient background on this concept so that the reader can understand why it is difficult for oral proponents to "agree" with TC proponents, or why each group can offer a different interpretation of the same data. In essence, the notion of metatheory was discussed relative to language acquisition and perspectives on deafness.

As stated in the first edition, this text is useful for preservice personnel and inservice professionals, for example, students, teachers, and clinicians in programs for deaf individuals. As will be seen, there is a much heavier emphasis on the knowledge base of language development. This necessitated the elimination of some information that can be found in other texts. This change

---

*Beck, E. (Ed.). (1980). *John Bartlett's familiar quotations: A collection of passages, phrases, and proverbs traced to their sources in ancient and modern literature*. Boston: Little, Brown.

is in keeping with the growing movement of teachers-as-scholars (or, clinicians-as-scholars). In essence, teachers or clinicians can no longer be viewed as the personnel who only apply knowledge. They are being encouraged, in some cases, required, to evaluate and provide "support" for their techniques and materials. Teachers and clinicians probably realize that there is, or should be, strong inter-relations among theories, research, instruction, curricula, and assessments.

Chapter 1 of the second edition provides an overview of the broad domains of language and deafness. This chapter presents more background information than the first chapter of the first edition on the functions and structure of language. Although both editions provided descriptions of deafness and communication modes, the second edition elaborates on these issues and discusses the metatheoretical framework of clinical and cultural perspectives.

Chapter 2 is a new chapter that contains both old and new information. The old information involves basically the same theoretical frameworks as discussed in the first edition. It is our hope, however, that the new information provides a better understanding of the foundations of these theories—that is, the metatheoretical foundations. As stated in the chapter, one of the functions of metatheorizing is to understand extant theory. This tool enables us to discuss, in one sense, the "levels" of theoretical adequacy, proposed by Chomsky. More important, the reader should obtain a sense of the growing tension in the field between "child language researchers" (mostly, psycholinguists and psychologists) and "language researchers" (primarily linguists). The information in this chapter should shed more light on the theories and research in the subsequent chapters.

In many ways, Chapter 3 of the second edition is similar to Chapter 2 of the first edition. However, there is additional information on the relationship between language and thought, as can be seen in the discussion of language-based and cognitive-based hypotheses. The new information concerns what can be labeled a fourth stage of intelligence tests—the process paradigm. We also feel that the chapter offers a more efficient framework for understanding the relationships among language, cognition, and intelligence. In fact, this framework builds on the well-stated information in an earlier text (Quigley & Kretschmer, 1982). For example, there is sufficient information to make some strong inferences about the short-term working memory capacity of deaf individuals and about the relationship between short-term working memory and literacy skills. We also felt that there was sufficient information to address the controversial long-standing question: Is there a psychology of deafness? Obviously, there is no simple yes or no answer.

Chapter 4 of the second edition is very similar to Chapter 3 of the first edition. Unfortunately, this is a reflection of the little research that continues to be undertaken in this area, relative to deafness. Nevertheless, we have improved somewhat in our understanding of the manually coded English systems, especially in relation to the representation of English. There is much more research on American Sign Language (ASL) than there was 10 years ago, and this research has started to unravel some of the mysteries surrounding the development of this language. There is still some debate on the nature of its syntax and nonmanual aspects and its use among deaf people.

Chapter 5 fulfills our original intention of the first edition. That is, we decided to treat the two topics, reading and writing, in a single chapter because of their similar underlying processes. In this chapter, we tried to show that the development of English literacy skills is heavily dependent upon existing conversational language skills in English. This reciprocal relationship is discussed within the framework of interactive theories of reading. In the section on writing, we not only provided a conceptual framework for the consideration of writing, but also included some of the more recent studies on writing as a process approach. As will be seen, viewing writing as a process approach does not mean excluding important lower-level skills such as spelling and grammar. Similar to the process of reading, it is important for the writer to have automatic lower-level skills so that they can engage in the higher-level composition activities such as organization and intent.

Chapter 6 of the second edition contains a great deal of new information, reflecting not only the growing developments in second-language learning, but also the influence of first-language theories on understanding second-language development. The exemplar is the influence of interactive theories of reading, which have essentially replaced the linear bottom-up and top-down models (e.g., Bernhardt, 1991; Grabe, 1988). In the first edition, we predicted that bilingualism would become a major theoretical and research activity in the field of deafness. Our prediction was only partly confirmed. On the one hand, there has been a growth in the development of bilingual education models. However, many of these models are not based on theory and research; at least, the description of the theoretical and research foundation is not always explicit. We have proposed a bilingual model based on our critical reflections. This model has evolved somewhat since its original appearance (e.g., Paul & Quigley, 1987b, in press). Although much more theorizing and modeling need to occur, there is also a need for empirical research, which, to our surprise, has been very limited. In addition, some of the more recent investigations seem to be heavily influenced by earlier research.

Chapter 7 provides definitional and historical background for the major language-teaching approaches in the education of deaf children and adolescents. The new information concerns our treatment of what is becoming "the great debate" relative to language acquisition: the learnability/teachability dichotomy. The outcome of this debate has important implications for future research and instruction in language and deafness. Other new additions include examples of instructional strategies or lessons based on the social-cognitive interactive perspective of language comprehension.

As in the first edition, Chapter 8 covers language assessment, including a discussion of some language tests. The second edition of the chapter, however, offers more basic information on language and assessment, for example, types and purposes, and a more detailed discussion on validity. The second edition also offers some insights into the issues of assessment and bilingualism. This information is important if there are attempts to establish bilingual education programs for deaf students. The focus of this chapter is on the knowledge base of language, particularly language assessment, which is critical for the "teacher-as-scholar" movement discussed previously.

In Chapter 9, we present our reflections regarding the development of language and literacy in deaf individuals. This chapter is organized around two questions, based on the ones proposed by King (1981): (1) How do deaf children learn both (a) the conversational forms of English and American Sign Language and (b) the written form of English? If we have done our work in the earlier chapters, the reader will be able to anticipate our conclusions. In addition, we hope our provocative remarks regarding the development of literate thought stimulate additional theorizing and research in this area. Similar to the first edition, we still firmly believe that there is no "true path" in the language development of deaf students; however, it is critical to develop a first language at as early an age as possible.

The authors are indebted to the many scholars who provided most of the theoretical and research thinking on which this text is based. We want to state also that some of the information in Chapters 7 and 8 was based on the framework and the work of the late Barry W. Jones in the first edition. With our brand of "metatheorizing," we hope that we have not only articulated the major findings but also have added to the knowledge base.

As usual, we thank our wives, Mary Beth Pilewski Paul and Ruth Quigley, for putting up with us and putting up without us.

PREFACE TO THE THIRD EDITION

A little learning is a dang'rous thing;
Drink deep, or taste not the Pierian spring.
There shallow draughts intoxicate the brain,
And drinking largely sobers us again.
   by Alexander Pope (Essay on Criticism, *p. 38)**

In the preface to the first edition of this text (1984), it was remarked that the present state of the education of deaf and hard-of-hearing children and adolescents can be characterized as one of creative confusion, much of which concerns the languages and communication modes that should be used initially with these individuals. Since that time, there have been attempts to clarify the confusion. Nevertheless, keeping in mind Alexander Pope's message in the earlier passage, there is still a great need for further development of theory and research. With this current edition, it is hoped that readers will obtain a better and deeper understanding of the issues.

To assist readers, this edition contains an update on theories and research with respect to the development of language in deaf and hard-of-hearing children and adolescents. There is additional information on the structures and functions of language, the instruction and assessment of language, the development of English literacy skills, and the use of English in bilingual or second language programs. This edition also includes separate chapters on oral English (orality) and Total Communication (signed systems), and there is a chapter devoted to the structure and development of American Sign Language.

The major focus is still on children and adolescents with severe to profound hearing impairment. However, there is some discussion of the language acquisition of individuals with less severe hearing losses (i.e., hard-of-hearing individuals), particularly in the chapter on the development of oral English skills. In essence, the perceptions of educators and scholars on the effects of hearing impairment are bound to be affected dramatically by the advance of technology involving cochlear implants and other aids (e.g., tactile aids).

The current text has continued to develop an idea that was introduced in the previous edition—literate thought. Readers are exposed to this concept in the first two chapters, and a fairly comprehensive discussion is undertaken in the concluding chapter. It is hoped that the discussion of literate thought enables readers to understand on a basic introductory level the intricate, complex

---

*Kronenberger, L (Ed.). (1951). *Alexander Pope: Selected works.* New York: Random House.

relations among cognition, language, and literacy. It has become increasingly clear that the development of a first language at as early an age as possible is critical for the subsequent academic achievement of individuals, including those who are deaf and hard of hearing.

To acquire a first language, deaf and hard-of-hearing children need to be exposed to a fluent, intelligible, complete communication system—a point that was made in the first edition. There seems to be growing evidence that the litmus test for any language/communication system is how well it represents the phonology of a language because phonology is considered the building block. In addition, deaf and hard-of-hearing students need to acquire an understanding of the other language components such as morphology, syntax, semantics, and pragmatics. Nevertheless, the internalization of the rules of the other components might be facilitated by access to the fundamental building block of phonology. This is true for all languages whether phonology is based on sound mechanisms, as is the case for English, or on visual-gestural mechanisms, as is the case for American Sign Language.

I am indebted to all the researchers and scholars who contributed the findings on which this book is based. I thank Dr. Erik Drasgow, University of South Carolina, for providing valuable comments on earlier versions of the manuscript. In addition, I thank both Ms. Jennifer Wolf, a doctoral student at Ohio State University, for being the model for several pictures in the text and Mr. Brian Chipman (B&T AlleyCat Productions, P.L.L.; http://www.btacprod.com) for his work with the photography. I appreciate the assistance of the staff at Singular Publishing Group/Thomson Learning—Candice Janco and Kristin Banach. I also thank Cecelia Musselman of Argosy Publishing for her guidance during the copyediting process. My wife, Mary Beth, has been very supportive throughout this arduous process, and our son, Peter Ben, has helped me to keep things in perspective.

Dr. Stephen Quigley, who collaborated on the previous two editions, was unable to participate in the current work due to being heavily involved in preparing the third edition of *Reading Milestones*, the extensive reading series for students with hearing impairment and for other exceptional learners. I have been extremely fortunate to have the opportunity to work and publish with Dr. Quigley, first as a doctoral student and subsequently as a colleague. Under his guidance, I have learned the importance of being meticulous, comprehensive, and balanced. The third edition of *Language and Deafness* is dedicated to him.

TABLE OF CONTENTS

Introduction to Language and Deafness

Why does language provide such a fascinating object-of-study? Perhaps because of its unique role in capturing the breadth of human thought and endeavor. We look around us, and are awed by the variety of several thousand languages and dialects expressing a multiplicity of world views, literatures, and ways of life. We look back at the thoughts of our predecessors, and find we can see only as far as language lets us see. We look forward in time, and find we can plan only through language. We look outward in space, and send symbols of communication along with our spacecraft, to explain who we are, in case there is anyone there who wants to know. (Crystal, 1997, p. 1)

In the education of deaf and hard-of-hearing children and adolescents, there are a number of controversies, issues, and ongoing debates that revolve around the concept of language. From one perspective, it seems that educators have devoted a disproportionate amount of attention and energy to language acquisition that they may have forgotten that education involves, at least, the acquisition of knowledge from other subjects such as mathematics, science, and history. Nevertheless, language should be at the center of our educational endeavors because it is doubtful that a substantial amount of reflective understanding of the other subjects is really possible without it.

This is one point that can be inferred from the passage at the beginning of this chapter. There seems to be a strong belief that language is paramount, based on our current understanding of the intricate, complex interrelations between language and other areas that fall under the rubric of cognition, psychosocial development, and literacy—to name just a few. A quick perusal of the vast—and growing—literature on language also supports its prestigious position in the education of deaf and hard-of-hearing students.

To the novice and even to many experienced educators (and, of course, parents) in the United States, it must be truly perplexing, frustrating, and mindboggling to learn that many students with hearing impairment have difficulty acquiring a level of proficiency in the English language that is commensurate with that of their typical hearing peers. This is the case, at least during the formative years and the compulsory education period, that is, from preschool to graduation from high school, and even extending into the postsecondary education time frame. As with all other complex entities, there is no simple, all-encompassing reason why the development of English, indeed most spoken languages and especially phonetic languages, is problematic for many deaf and hard-of-hearing students (see Allen, 1986; King & Quigley, 1985; Paul, 1998a).

With the advent and proliferation of the use of signed systems along with the legitimacy and use of sign languages, our understanding of language has been enriched and has grown exponentially. In addition, the debate on language for deaf and hard-of-hearing students in the United States entails not only what language—English or American Sign Language (ASL)—but also what form of the language—oral English or signed English. Within the arena of form, there are additional micro skirmishes on which type is best or most effective—for example, cued speech, verbotonal method, signing exact English, seeing essential English, and so on. Of course, not to be neglected are the issues for children who reside in homes in which neither English nor ASL is the first language (e.g., Spanish or German). To complicate matters further, the scholarly debate is also fueled by whether language can be taught, either as a first or second communicative symbol system, or whether it can only be caught—that is, acquired in naturally occurring, meaningful milieus with a minimal amount of direct instruction or intervention.

It would be shortsighted to categorize all of the most important battles on language and deafness as scholarly, scientific, or educational with noble goals such as the advancement of knowledge and the improvement of communication and thinking skills. The study of language is also political, as indicated by the debates within the purviews of language policy or language choice. With respect to deaf and hard-of-hearing individuals, questions such as what should be the first language for young children and who should make this decision are not easily answered by the so-called empirical, scientific approaches. One might suspect that the answers should depend, at least, on both the home culture of the children and the majority culture of the country in which they live. As is discussed later in this text, many different kinds of arguments, mostly controversial, are proffered.

Political battles, of course, can lead to legal entanglements. These legal ramifications surely must be confusing to parents and significant others who, for the most part, have good intentions for their children. Consider this: There has been some discussion that parents (or caregivers) should be charged with mental abuse if they refuse to learn and use a natural language with their deaf and hard-of-hearing children, namely, a sign language such as American Sign Language, in this country. The assumption is that a sign language such as ASL is easily learnable—much easier than a spoken one such as English—and that parents would be denying a basic right of the child by not using this sign communication system. This assumption is based on one that was presented previously—language is paramount. Denying a child his or her rightful exposure to a bona fide, complete, easily learned language is said to cause irreparable damage to other psychological functions. In effect, this is denying the child the right to grow up into a productive, healthy, contributing member of society.

With these introductory remarks, it is hoped that the reader has obtained a sense of what is covered within the pages of this text. It should be clear that the range of topics and issues and the breadth and depth of the discussion are influenced pervasively by the author's biases, which are based on cumulative, ongoing effects from education, philosophical and theoretical persuasions, personal experiences, and so on. Nevertheless, the intent is to represent a variety of voices with the hope of creating a fairly balanced, comprehensive, and accessible text.

The intent of this introductory chapter is to provide a brief overview of some of the major issues involving the development or instruction of language in deaf and hard-of-hearing students. The chapter introduces readers to terminology and perspectives regarding deafness and language. The three major sections are: "Acquisition and Instructional Issues," "Philosophical Perspectives," and "Metatheory, Paradigm, and Language." The section on acquisition and instructional issues demonstrates the importance of understanding differences between the following—often misunderstood—pairs: acquisition and instruction, competence and performance, and signed system and sign language. Next, two major philosophical perspectives on deafness are discussed: clinical and cultural. These perspectives and their variations have had a marked influence on theory, research, and practice in language development and deafness. Finally, there is a brief discussion of perspectives on language in which the reader is exposed to concepts such as metatheory and paradigm. The attempt is to show that adherence to a particular metatheory or paradigm drives the development and interpretation of specific theories, research, and practices.

ACQUISITION AND INSTRUCTIONAL ISSUES

In any discussion of language and deafness, there is bound to be considerable confusion when readers encounter words such as *acquisition* and *instruction* (see discussions in Quigley & Kretschmer, 1982; Quigley & Paul, 1994). Adding to the confusion are related terms such as *use, representation, exposure,* and *communication form.* Concepts such as use, representation, and exposure are critical because of the various combinations of spoken and/or sign communication forms that may be used with many deaf and some hard-of-hearing children and adolescents.

Educators, researchers, and theorists are often interested in language acquisition for different reasons. Language acquisition is synonymous with language development, and the focus is on how children acquire or develop language. The details of the how are influenced by the various language development or acquisition models, which also entail descriptions of the nature of language (e.g., see discussions in Cairns, 1996; Owens, 1996).

It might be thought that once the language acquisition process is understood, it should be possible to teach language, especially to children who seem to have difficulty acquiring it. However, for a number of theorists and researchers, language instruction is not related necessarily to language acquisition. In fact, it is sometimes argued that language cannot be taught, especially through the use of direct instruction techniques; it can only be acquired in natural, meaningful situations. This situation is often referred to as the *learnability/teachability dichotomy.* With respect to deaf and hard-of-hearing students, language instruction often reflects the use of specific methods that are used in the classroom, based on adaptations or variations of traditional approaches such as the Fitzgerald Key (Fitzgerald, 1949), the Barry Five Slate System (Barry, 1899), and the Natural Method (Groht, 1958). Language-teaching methods can be classified as structural or natural or some eclectic combination (see discussions in King, 1984; Kretschmer & Kretschmer, 1978; Luetke-Stahlman, 1998, 1999; McAnally, Rose, & Quigley, 1994). The details of some of these methods, including research on their effectiveness, are discussed in Chapter 10 of this text.

Exposure, Use, and Representation

Perhaps the bulk of the confusion in language and deafness is due to the remaining terms of interest here: *exposure, use,* and *representation.* These concepts are complex and have multiple interpretations. Only a limited discussion is presented here, and this discussion is based on the implications of the following passage from Quigley and Kretschmer (1982): "The primary issue in the education of deaf children is the form of language and communication that should be used by and with the children in school and in their infant and early childhood years in the home" (p. 9).

Quigley and Kretschmer (1982) asserted that there are two language forms—American Sign Language and English—and two communication modes—oral and manual. ASL and English are two different languages, each with its own grammar and culture. The oral communication form refers to the use of speech in the expression of information, whereas the sign communication form refers to the use of manual or hand movements in signed systems and both manual and nonmanual movements (e.g., eyebrows and cheeks) in sign languages. It is possible to use some combination of oral and manual forms as in specific signed systems such as signed English (Bornstein, Saulnier, & Hamilton, 1983) and signing exact English (Gustason, Pfetzing, & Zawolkow, 1980). Table 1-1 depicts the languages, modes, and forms involved; additional details on these areas can be found in Chapters 5 to 7.

It should be noted that the focus on only two languages—American Sign Language and English—seems to overlook the fact that there are other languages

TABLE 1-1 Languages, Modes, and Approaches

Language and Communication Issues

Languages	English		American Sign Language
Modes	Oral	Oral/manual (sign)	Manual and nonmanual cues
Approaches	Oral education	Total Communication	Bilingual-bicultural

Examples

Primarily auditory [Aural-oral, etc.]	*English signing/fingerspelling* [e.g., Contact Signing, Conceptually Accurate Signed English (CASE), Pidgin Sign English (archaic); etc.]	
Multisensory [Auditory-Visual-Tactile] [Cued speech]	*Signed or manual systems* [Signed English] [Signing Exact English] [Seeing Essential English] [Rochester Method]	

and cultures such as Spanish and German that are reflective of the home environments of a number of deaf and hard-of-hearing children and adolescents. The focus on English in the United States is probably understandable, especially with respect to English as the majority language of mainstream society. However, the reasons for the focus on ASL as the minority sign language are complex and controversial and are influenced by the fact that ASL is the predominant sign language used by Deaf individuals in the Northern Hemisphere (i.e., United States and Canada) and one of the most widely studied sign languages in the world (Lane, Hoffmeister, & Bahan, 1996).

The terms *exposure, use*, and *representation* are sometimes confused with language instruction. In addition, a better understanding of these terms contributes to a deeper understanding of the learnability/teachability issue, mentioned previously. Despite the lack of widespread agreement on the descriptions of these concepts, there seems to be some understanding that the relationships between and among them are extremely complicated and in need of extensive research.

As noted previously, language instruction refers to the specific language-teaching methods or approaches that have been attempted in education and deafness. Exposure to a communication system such as signing exact English or cued speech/language by itself does not necessarily constitute instruction in language, even within the so-called natural approaches. Furthermore, what is meant by exposure can also be difficult to explain or understand. Under reasonable circumstances, one can argue that most typical children who are hearing and are exposed to their native spoken language (or languages) in natural, meaningful situations will acquire or learn that language (or languages) with relative ease within a brief period of time—say, 2 to 3 years. No one—not even their parents—actually teaches them the language. Without specifying too much detail here, one may posit that children are born with an innate capacity to learn a language and need a reasonable, meaningful linguistic environment, which includes reasonable exposure to that language. The use of the word *reasonable* is deliberate here because children do not need to be exposed to all examples of linguistic usage.

What is probably most interesting about the exposure issue is that many native language users can produce and understand utterances that they have never heard or read previously. Intuitively (not in a formal knowledge sense), language users understand that their language system is finite (i.e., has a finite set of rules governing usage). In other words (Baker & Cokely, 1980):

> *All languages are composed of a limited number of units that are related or connected to each other in specific ways. For example, spoken languages use sound units as their basic building blocks. Each spoken lan-*

guage uses a particular set of these building blocks (i.e., sounds) and combines them in specific ways to form words. These words are then combined in specific ways to form sentences. Sentences, then, can be combined in specific ways to form speeches, stories, poems, conversations, and so on. (p. 33)

Thus, with the acquisition of the building blocks and an intuitive understanding of the rules for combining them, language users are able to produce and understand a wide variety of grammatically acceptable expressions, many of which they have not uttered or been exposed to previously.

The exposure situation is quite different for many children with severe to profound hearing impairment. It seems that many of these children are exposed to either the oral, manual, or combined (oral and manual) forms of English (or, perhaps, other spoken languages) in the homes and in school yet do not approach mastery or understanding or even approach the ability of their peers, who are typically hearing, on graduation from high school. As discussed later in this text, one of the central arguments is that these children are not exposed to language building blocks that are clear, unambiguous, and complete. This can lead to a number of questions, some of which are addressed in this text. The most basic question for the author is: Why is exposure to a spoken language such as English different for many deaf and some hard-of-hearing individuals; that is, why is it different from that of individuals who are hearing peers?

There have been at least two salient lines of research on this question. One line has examined the nature of the representation of English—either orally or manually or some combination of these two modes. This text examines and presents research on several queries within this research framework: (a) What does it mean to represent English?; (b) how much of English needs to be represented?; and (c) can English be represented completely or adequately via the use of present communication systems? Perhaps, as suggested by Quigley and Paul (1994):

The notion of representation should be applied only to TC [Total Communication] methods (and possibly cued speech) because oral-aural methods attempt to improve the reception and production of speech, which functions both as a medium and a manifestation of spoken language. (p. 269)

It is possible that an understanding of the issue of representation might shed more light on the exposure issue; however, any discussion on representation inevitably leads to one on use—which has been a second line of research. That is, is there a relationship between representation and use? Or, is there a relationship between representation and performance on language or reading achievement measures? Unfortunately, much of the empirical research on these questions—despite the intense interest in the outcomes—has been too narrow and, in some cases, an oversimplification. In general, the results have not been favorable and seem to call into dispute the learnability of the various signed systems (see research syntheses in Drasgow & Paul, 1995; Paul & Drasgow, 1998). In addition, there seems to be much doubt that English can really be represented completely or adequately, and even if it can (as some have argued for cued speech; Fleetwood & Metzger, 1998), it still might not be learnable due to the unnaturalness of the representation or other factors (e.g., the lack of a reasonably rich linguistic environment). In any case, the point here is that there is no simple linear relationship between representation and use despite the fanatical desires of some researchers (and educators and parents).

If the hope is to improve the English acquisition process of deaf and hard-of-hearing individuals, then more attention needs to be devoted to the interrelationships among exposure, representation, and use. It could be argued that part of the reason for the rise of or call for the establishment and implementation of ASL/English bilingual-bicultural programs is due to researchers' difficulty in resolving or understanding these interrelationships. There are, of course, other important reasons. In any case, the ASL/English issue is also not above practical or theoretical concerns (see discussions in Mayer & Akamatsu, 1999; Paul, 1998a). Controversies notwithstanding, there are critical lessons to be learned from this push for bilingual/bicultural programs in education and deafness.

Acquisition of More Than One Language

One of the most controversial topics in recent years has been the application of bilingualism and multiculuralism principles in the education of deaf and hard-of-hearing students. There seems to be little doubt that some—indeed a sizable minority of—deaf and hard-of-hearing students are reared in homes in which English is neither the first language nor the home language. Many of the controversies in the larger field of bilingualism, multiculturalism, and children with typical hearing are also applicable here. However, there are some very interesting differences—at least on the surface level. For example, most hearing minority-language children are born into and have assimilated (i.e., acquired in a relatively natural manner) the culture(s) and language(s) of their parents. Although some deaf and hard-of-hearing students are also born into similar situations (e.g., ASL or some other foreign language), the overwhelming majority of students with severe to profound hearing impairment are born into English-speaking homes, especially to hearing parents in the United States. Nevertheless, many proponents of bilingualism/biculturalism espouse ASL/English bilingual/bicultural programs for these students, indeed for all or most deaf and hard-of-hearing students due to, in part, the accessibility and ease of acquiring a first language such as American Sign Language and the assumption that Deaf culture is or will be the majority culture for these students as they become mature adults (see Lane et al., 1996; Livingston, 1997; Mason & Ewoldt, 1996). There is the assumption (with some empirical data) that these deaf (and some hard-of-hearing) students do not readily acquire the spoken home language and much of the culture that is available or transmitted via the use of a bona fide linguistic system. Indeed, these two concepts, ASL and Deaf culture, are so pervasive and powerful that the application of them to all or most deaf and hard-of-hearing children seems either to ignore or downplay the existing languages (typically, spoken) and cultures of the home environments of these children. An understanding of this phenomenon is only possible when the focus is on the predominant amount of research that documents the marked benefits of acquiring a first language at as early an age as possible. The acquisition of a first language, particularly a spoken language, is extremely difficult for most students with severe to profound hearing impairment, and this situation has pervasive effects on the development of other areas such as cognition, psychosocial aspects, and script literacy (i.e., reading and writing) skills.

Another major difference between bilingualism/biculturalism for hearing children and that for deaf and hard-of-hearing students—one that has been discussed in detail elsewhere (Paul, 1998a)—is the argument on the most efficient or best way to develop English literacy in bilingual or second-language literacy programs. There have been several misinterpretations of this issue, which has been complicated by the fact that American Sign Language does not have a script literacy system (e.g., written language system) similar to that found in chirographic (i.e., handwriting) or typographic (i.e., print) cultures. That is, individuals do not read or write, in the traditional sense, in the language of American Sign Language. From one perspective, ASL, similar to other sign languages, can be compared to predominant oral cultures, including preliterate cultures (e.g., see Olson, 1989, 1994); however, ASL and its users coexist in a culture that is heavily steeped in the use of chirographic (writing) and typographic (print) media. The complexity of traditional oral cultures should not be underestimated, and no denigration is intended here by comparing it to ASL and Deaf culture. Nevertheless, it might be an advantage to understand some aspects of these cultures to develop educational programs that suit the needs of many deaf and, perhaps, hard-of-hearing children. In addition to the need for developing a bona fide first language as early as possible, another critical implication is that the real goal of education should be the development of literate thought—that is, the ability to think creatively, logically, reflectively, and rationally. Literate thought might be mode independent—that is, it might not be dependent on a particular mode for delivering or receiving information such as script literacy via reading and writing skills. This issue will be returned to later in this text.

Table 1-2 presents some of the major highlights of the discussion on acquisition and instructional issues.

PHILOSOPHICAL PERSPECTIVES ON DEAFNESS

Any discussion on theory, research, and intervention/practice is incomplete until it is accompanied by a rendition of the various perspectives held by professionals in the field. It is becoming clear that language theories, research, and practices are influenced by philosophical perspectives on deafness, for example, how deafness is viewed or defined. In addition, interpretations of theories, research, or practices are not really possible or even understandable unless one can refer to the underlying frameworks. To paraphrase a popular statement, there is no God's eye view of deafness.

With respect to deaf and hard-of-hearing children and adolescents, there are two broad perspectives, clinical and cultural, that have been described in the literature (Baker, & Cokely, 1980; Lane, 1992; Paul & Jackson, 1993). In one sense, these perspectives are similar to the notions of metatheory and paradigm, discussed in the next section of this chapter. Hitherto, the clinical view has dominated the thinking of metatheorists, theorists, researchers, and practitioners in disciplines that have focused on the study of deafness (Lane, 1992; Lane et al., 1996; Paul, 1998a; Paul & Jackson, 1993).

In reading the following descriptions of the two broad viewpoints, the reader should keep several major points in mind. The descriptions represent extreme bipolar positions. There are a number of variations on a continuum between these two extreme views. Research and program models have been influenced by variations that combine tenets from both perspectives (Liedel & Paul, 1991; Paul, 1990, 1991), although some scholars have argued that these two bipolar views are incompatible (Crittenden, 1993; Lane, 1988, 1992; Reagan, 1990). In addition, there seems to be a growing belief that it is unrealistic or problematic to adopt one particular perspective. In fact, the real world of humans seems to require an individualized, situation-bound, problem-solving solution; that is, there might be no real need for overarching models, theories,

TABLE 1-2 Major Highlights of Acquisition and Instructional Issues

- A clear understanding is needed of the similarities and differences among acquisition, instruction, use, representation, exposure, and communication form to improve the English acquisition process of deaf and hard-of-hearing individuals.

- Language instruction is not related necessarily to language acquisition.

- There are two language forms—American Sign Language (ASL) and English—and two communication modes—oral and manual—that account for most of the communication approaches in education and deafness.

- Exposure to a language/communication system does not necessarily constitute instruction in language.

- It is important to research the issue of exposure. One possible question: Why is exposure to a spoken language such as English different for many deaf and some hard-of-hearing individuals; that is, why is it different from that of individuals who are hearing peers?

- Many of the controversies in the larger field of bilingualism, multiculturalism, and children with typical hearing are applicable to some children who are deaf and hard of hearing.

- Although a sizeable minority of deaf and hard-of-hearing children are born into minority language/culture homes, the overwhelming majority are born into English-speaking homes, especially to hearing parents in the United States.

- There is evidence that many deaf and some hard-of-hearing students do not readily acquire the spoken home language and much of the culture that is available or transmitted via the use of a bona fide linguistic system. This situation has pervasive effects on the development of other areas such as cognition, psychosocial aspects, and script literacy skills.

- There is a great deal of controversy on the most efficient or best way to develop English literacy in bilingual or second-language literacy programs for deaf students. This is due, in part, to the fact that ASL does not have a script literacy system (i.e., written language system) similar to that found in cultures that have writing systems.

or perspectives because each person is unique and is surrounded by varying sets of circumstances and experiences. This last issue is examined periodically throughout the text; indeed, it has become a prevalent concern in descriptions of language development that emphasize individual differences (Shore, 1995).

It has been argued that if the two bipolar perspectives are indeed incompatible, they are products of different underlying paradigms (or metatheories) (Paul & Jackson, 1993). If this is true, then the perspectives must be accepted as different worldviews—that is, each represents a broad lens that adherents wear for interpreting and understanding the world. This assertion has critical implications, especially for parents and educators who are dogmatic and inclined to favor one view over the other. The crux is this: It is not possible to determine by using the scientific method which lens provides the better description of reality. In essence, one perspective is not true or false; it is simply one way of viewing the world or, in this case, one way of viewing the condition of deafness.

Paradoxically, there will always be a number of perspectives in any given scientific field. If a perspective attains the status of a paradigm or metatheory, it is feasible to refine or improve theories, research, and practices within that particular viewpoint. It should be emphasized that the perception of incompatibility itself is a perspective (i.e., a point of view). It is possible—and has been done—to combine principles from two purportedly incompatible viewpoints and create a new or slightly different viewpoint that seems to have a life of its own (Ritzer, 1991, 1992).

Clinical Description of Deafness

Relative to deafness, the clinical view has been labeled as a *medical* or *pathological* view (Baker & Cokely, 1980; Lane, 1988, 1992; Reagan, 1990). However, most of the descriptions of this view have a negative or pejorative tone, implying that the view is wrong or inappropriate. As discussed previously, it is possible to have an opinion about a view, but views or lenses by themselves are not right or wrong; they simply are ways of seeing the world. Perhaps a better description of the clinical view is to label it as a *mainstream* perspective (Gliedman & Roth, 1980). In other words, deaf children are described relative to the characteristics of or goals for typical children (i.e., normally hearing children) in mainstream society (e.g., schools, businesses, and so on). Some pertinent differences between the two broad, amorphous groups—deaf and hearing—are the ability to use speech, hearing, and English language skills.

Clinical proponents study the impact of deafness on cognitive, linguistic, and psychosocial developments, typically within the purview of mainstream theories and research on children without disabilities. The focus is on remedying the deficiencies or improving the skills of deaf and hard-of-hearing children and adolescents. One of the main goals is to enable deaf and hard-of-hearing individuals to participate in mainstream society on social, political, and economic levels. For example, the prevention or cure of deficiencies associated with deafness and perhaps even deafness itself might lead to an improvement in the low academic achievement levels that have been documented since the inception of formal standardized achievement tests (Quigley & Paul, 1986).

Clinical or mainstream theories should not be applied indiscriminately to children with disabilities (Gliedman & Roth, 1980). Nevertheless, they may be sufficient starting points, especially in the absence of other established theories (Paul & Jackson, 1993). Adequate clinical research on deaf individuals requires the documentation of salient, long-standing demographics and characteristics that have affected the development of English language skills. These include degree of impairment, age at onset, etiology (cause), location of the impairment, parental hearing status, and the status of additional disabilities (Myklebust, 1964; Quigley & Kretschmer, 1982).

Dimensions of Hearing Impairment

Dimensions of hearing impairment include degree, age at onset, etiology, and location. Age at onset is a linguistic dimension, whereas the others are audiological in nature. The focus here is on two of the major dimensions—degree and age at onset—particularly in relation to the development of spoken language.

Hearing impairment is a general audiological term that pertains to all degrees of losses, regardless of etiology and location. Hearing acuity is measured in decibels across a range of frequencies, typically from 125 to 8000 hertz, or cycles per second (for a complete description of the measurement and types of hearing losses, see H. Davis, 1978; Meyerhoff, 1986). The acuity is reported as the average threshold level of pure audiometric tones (pure tone average or PTA) in the better unaided ear across the speech frequencies, that is, 500, 1000, and 2000 hertz. Table 1-3 illustrates an example of computed PTAs.

There are five audiological categories that correspond to degrees of hearing impairment (Acoustical Society of America, 1982). There is some debate on what should constitute the slight category (Ross, 1986, 1990). In essence, the main argument is that the lower end should be fewer than 27 decibels (dB) because of the documented effects on language ability. The five categories are as follows: slight (27 dB to 40 dB), mild (41 dB to 55 dB), marked or moderate (56 dB to 70 dB), and extreme or profound (91 dB or greater). The educational implications of groups of students with these characteristics

TABLE 1-3 Examples of Pure Tone Average (PTA)

decibels	Frequency					
	125	250	500	1000	2000	4000
−10						
0						
10						
20						
30						
40						
50			X			
60				X		
70					X	
80			O	O		
90						
100						
110					O	

Note: **X** *PTA for Left Ear = 60 dB (i.e., average of 50 dB, 60 dB, 70 dB).*
O *PTA for Right Ear = 90 dB (i.e., average of 80 dB, 80 dB, 110 dB).*
PTA for Better Unaided Ear = 60 dB (based on the score for Left Ear).

have been reported in a number of sources (Moores, 1987, 1996; Paul & Quigley, 1990; Quigley & Kretschmer, 1982).

Traditionally, students with slight to moderate hearing impairment have been classified as hard-of-hearing individuals. One of the most robust findings in the research literature on these groups of students is that even a slight impairment can negatively affect language, literacy, and academic achievement (Paul & Quigley, 1987a, 1989; Ross, Brackett, & Maxon, 1982). With early intervention and an adequate management program that includes a comprehensive array of support services, most students with slight to moderate losses can achieve a high level of competence in English language skills (see discussions in Ross, 1990; Ross et al., 1982). The overwhelming majority of these students, many of whom are not identified, are enrolled full time in general education programs.

Students with severe impairment have constituted a gray area. That is, some of these students perform in a manner similar to that of traditional hard-of-hearing students. However, others may have difficulties similar to those of students with extreme or profound impairment. It has been argued that poor classroom management conditions have led to the underdevelopment of these students' academic skills (e.g., Ross, 1986; Ross et al., 1982). In addition, placing these students in Total Communication programs (discussed later in this text) or labeling them as *deaf* has resulted in an exposure to a lower quality of oral communication aspects such as training in speech, speechreading, and the use of residual hearing (e.g., Ross & Calvert, 1984).

In the author's view, students in the extreme or profound category are the only ones who should receive the label *deaf*. That is, deaf refers to individuals who, with or without amplification, are either receiving a fragmented, incomplete auditory message or no message at all. Most—but not all—of these students are connected to a world of vision in which they are dependent on some form of signing to receive and express information. Some students with profound hearing impairment use their eyes (and other skills) to receive information by speechreading a speaker's lips. However, these students are essentially connected to a world of audition, although they may not hear the sounds adequately (Paul & Jackson, 1993; Ross, 1990). There are also a few students in this category who are able to use their residual hearing along with their speechreading skills to achieve high levels of both speech and language development (Connor, 1986; Ling, 1984, 1989).

A better understanding of the language achievement levels of students with hearing losses can be obtained when degree of loss is considered in conjunction with the age-at-onset factor. *Age at onset* refers to the age at which the hearing impairment occurred. The time of occurrence of the impairment has a pervasive effect on the development of spoken language.

Because of this notion, age at onset is a linguistic factor. In this conceptual framework, the hearing impairment may be prelinguistic or postlinguistic. A prelinguistic impairment occurs prior to or at the age of 2 years, whereas a postlinguistic impairment occurs after the age of 2 years. Birth to 2 years is considered an important period for prelinguistic development; however, a severe to profound hearing impairment disrupts this process, especially for children who have hearing parents and are attempting to learn or acquire a spoken language (Moores, 1987, 1996; Paul & Jackson, 1993; Rodda & Grove, 1987).

Given the growing knowledge and understanding of the prelinguistic period of language development (see Chapter 4), there has been some discussion that the prelinguistic period—that is, the most important part of this period—should be restricted to birth to 1 year of age when describing this condition for children with hearing impairment.

Considering both degree and age at onset of impairment together, researchers have reported significant impacts on the development of language and literacy skills (see reviews in Moores, 1996; Paul, 1998a; Quigley & Kretschmer, 1982; Webster, 1986). For example, a student with a postlinguistic severe hearing impairment may have a higher English language achievement level than a student with a prelinguistic severe hearing impairment. The more severe the impairment and the earlier the age at onset, the more significant the impact on language and literacy acquisition.

Degree and age at onset of hearing impairment are highlighted here because of their combined effects. It is also important for researchers to consider other factors such as etiology, location of impairment, and the presence of additional disabilities. For example, it has been reported that about one-third of students with hearing impairment have additional disabilities (Wolff & Harkins, 1986). That these additional disabilities affect academic achievement is not in doubt. However, it is still difficult to detect the presence of some disabilities such as learning disabilities, although there has been some recent effort and success in this area (e.g., Elliott & Powers, 1988; Powers, Elliott, & Funderburg, 1987; Samar, Parasnis, & Berent, 1998).

One of the most widely researched and controversial factors is parental hearing status (see discussion in Drasgow, 1998). This factor pertains to the hearing acuity of the parents/caregivers, that is, whether the parents/caregivers have normal or impaired hearing. A number of studies have compared the achievement of deaf children of deaf parents (dcdp) with that of deaf children of hearing parents (dchp). It should be clear that parental hearing status, similar to socioeconomic status, is not a causative factor. That is, hearing status by itself is not the major reason for the differences in achievement in children. Other variables associated with this factor, for example, level of acceptance and quality and form of communication, should be considered (Paul & Jackson, 1993). More important, parental hearing status is just one factor to consider in light of evolving views and influences of family system theory.

Cultural Description of Deafness

At the other end of the spectrum is what can be described as a cultural perspective of deafness (Baker & Cokely, 1980; Lane, 1988, 1992; Paul & Jackson,

1993). Only a few remarks are made here. A more detailed discussion of this entity can be found elsewhere (Gannon, 1981; Lane et al., 1996; Neisser, 1983; Padden & Humphries, 1988). Although there are several ways to interpret the word *cultural* (e.g., alternative, individualistic, and humanistic), especially when it is being contrasted with clinical, the focus here is on the view that some deaf and hard-of-hearing individuals are members of a distinct, ethnic, sociological group.

In general, cultural proponents view deafness as a natural condition, not as a disease or disability that needs to be cured or prevented. It is argued that Deaf individuals do not want to be like individuals who have typical or normal hearing. That is, the ability to speak and hear are not desirable goals; in fact, these skills are considered to be unrealistic goals for most Deaf people (Lane, 1992; Lane et al., 1996). In essence, the role models for deaf and hard-of-hearing children and adolescents are Deaf adults, especially those individuals who use ASL and are members of the Deaf culture.

An eloquent anecdote that illustrates the feelings of culturally Deaf individuals is as follows:

> *A short time ago some members of Congress discussed the establishment of a research institute to identify deafness early and to prevent and cure it. Several deaf activists protested that because they are an ethnic group, the government shouldn't seek to cure their ethnicity. "If I had a bulldozer and a gun," a Gallaudet student leader was quoted as saying, "I would destroy all scientific experiments to cure deafness. If I could hear, I would probably take a pencil and poke myself to be deaf again." (Kisor, 1990, p. 259)*

The depathologizing of deafness and the emergence of Deaf culture proceeded in tandem with the growing recognition of ASL as a bona fide language. In addition, it was argued that the use of ASL is not a compensatory endeavor as implied by Myklebust (1964) and other scholars, who seemed to be influenced by the basic tenets of the clinical perspective. Rather, ASL, similar to any other language, is used to express many functions of Deaf individuals. For example, one of the most important language functions is identity—personal, social, and political.

The use of a sign language such as ASL is thought to be a reflection of Deaf individuals' predisposition toward the acquisition of a visual language. As noted by Neisser (1983), this predisposition is different from the one for hearing individuals, who possess the ability to acquire and use a spoken language:

The hearing world is deeply biased toward its own oral language, and always prefers to deal with deaf people who can speak. But speech is always difficult for the deaf, never natural, never automatic, never without stress. It violates their integrity; they have a deep biological bias for the language of signs. (p. 281)

One of the most powerful influences of the cultural perspective is the passionate call for the establishment and implementation of ASL/English bilingual-bicultural programs. Some of the support for this educational approach has come from extant theories and research on second-language learning; however, much of the impetus seems to come from the tenets of critical theory with a strong emphasis on concepts such as empowerment, oppression, and values—which includes the following question among others: Whose interests/values are being served? The strong bias against the use of anything that is associated with sound—speech, speechreading, and residual hearing—has led to a misinterpretation of some theories, notably, those of Cummins and Vygotsky (see Mayer & Akamatsu, 1999; Mayer & Wells, 1996; Paul, 1998a), and has led to an oversight of the importance and effects of the alphabetic system for the development of reading and writing skills (Adams, 1990, 1994; Snow, Burns, & Griffin, 1998). Nevertheless, one of the most important points made by ASL/English proponents is the need for a developed bona fide language as early as possible in the childhood years. Essentially, these proponents attempt to make the case that ASL is a natural language for all deaf and hard-of-hearing children and thus should be the first language of these individuals.

This is only a brief discussion of the concept of culture as it relates to Deaf individuals. For a number of individuals, including educators in the field of education and deafness, it might be difficult to understand how deafness can be considered a natural condition rather than a type of disability. It does not seem to fit the mainstream views of culture involving ethnic and minority groups. Nevertheless, there have been a number of published works that have gone to great pains to illustrate these differences and to argue for a cultural view of deafness as being the most productive and fair perspective. Consider the words of one of the strongest proponents of the cultural view, Harlan Lane (1992):

To apply a cultural model to a group is to invoke quite a different conceptual framework. Implicit in this posture are issues such as: What are the interdependent values, mores, art forms, traditions, organizations, and language that characterize this culture? How is it influenced by the physical and social environment in which it is embedded? Such questions are, in principle, value neutral, although of course some people are ill-disposed to cultural diversity, while others prize it. The institutions invoked by a cultural model of a group include the social sciences; professions in a mediating role between cultures, such as simultaneous interpretation; and the schools, an important locus of cultural transmission.

I maintain that the vocabulary and conceptual framework our society has customarily used with regard to deaf people, based as it is on infirmity, serves us and the members of the deaf community less well than a vocabulary and framework of cultural relativity. I want to replace the normativeness of medicine with the curiosity of ethnography. (pp. 18–19)

Table 1-4 presents highlights and a few implications of the discussion on philosophical perspectives.

TABLE 1-4 Major Highlights of Philosophical Perspectives

- Language theories, research, and practice are influenced by philosophical perspectives on deafness—that is, how deafness is viewed or defined.

- There are two broad perspectives, clinical and cultural, that have been described in the literature.

- Although research and programs have been influenced by combinations of principles from both perspectives, the clinical view has dominated much of the activity in the education of deaf and hard-of-hearing students.

- Clinical proponents study the impact of deafness on cognitive, linguistic, and psychosocial developments, typically within the purview of mainstream theories and research on children without disabilities. The focus is on remedying the deficiencies or improving the skills of deaf and hard-of-hearing children and adolescents.

- Adequate clinical research requires the documentation of variables such as degree of hearing impairment, age at onset of the impairment, etiology (cause), location of the impairment, parental hearing status, and the presence

(continues)

Table 1-4 (continued)

of additional disabilities. Two of the most important variables seem to be degree and age at onset of the hearing impairment.

- In the cultural perspective, the focus is on the view that some deaf and hard-of-hearing individuals are members of a distinct, ethnic, sociological group.

- Cultural proponents view deafness as a natural condition, not as a disease or disability that needs to be cured or prevented. The role models for deaf and hard-of-hearing children and adolescents are Deaf adults, especially those individuals who use American Sign Language (ASL) and are members of the Deaf culture.

- One of the most powerful influences of the cultural perspectives is the call for the establishment and implementation of ASL/English bilingual-bicultural programs.

METATHEORY, PARADIGM, AND LANGUAGE: A BRIEF INTRODUCTION

Similar to the earlier discussion on views of deafness, there are ongoing debates and controversies on perspectives of language. How to approach, investigate, and describe language, language acquisition, and language development and how to decide whether entities such as language, acquisition, and development even exist are markedly influenced by certain underlying frameworks, belief systems, or philosophies. As such, some of the confusion in language and deafness might be due to the lack of or poor articulation of these frameworks—which will be called here, for simplistic's sake, *metatheories* and *paradigms.*

Admittedly, metatheories and paradigms have been influenced by long-standing philosophical debates in the areas of metaphysics (e.g., mind–body problems) and epistemology (e.g., absolute vs. relative knowledge). Nevertheless, some understanding of these issues is required if practitioners desire to make sense of the ongoing arguments on effective or best instructional practices for the development of language. Indeed, questions such as what is language, can language be taught, and how should language be measured are undergirded by metaphysical and epistemological concerns. Theorists, researchers, and practitioners have to wonder whether there is a correct or true way (i.e., The way) of perceiving these issues or whether one's understanding is influenced by the selection or existence of a particular mental framework, which seems to suggest a relativistic, pragmatic approach (i.e., an individualized approach that varies from child to child).

Whether the reality of language (or knowledge, etc.) is a product of rationalism or empiricism, objectivism or subjectivism, or absolutism or relativism and whether one can find this out by breaking it up into smaller parts for study and then putting them back together again for a conclusion (i.e., reductionism) or perusing the entity as a whole or system because the whole is greater than the sum of its parts (i.e., constructivism) depends on one's worldview (see Table 1-5 for additional descriptions of terms). This worldview is often called a *paradigm*—a word that has been misused, abused, and so on—or a *philosophy*—another ambiguous term. Perhaps it is best to discuss a worldview with respect to the notion of metatheory, which can be related to and is somewhat similar to paradigm. It should become clear that the following discussion of metatheory and paradigm is based on the author's perspectives.

TABLE 1-5 A Few Metaphysical and Epistemological Concepts

Concept	Description
Absolutism	This refers to the notion of an ultimate reality or principle that is perfect and complete. If knowledge is absolute, then there is an ultimate objective reality that is independent of the observer and capable of being discovered and shared.
Constructivism	This is a theory of knowledge that asserts that reality is not objective or independent of the observer but is constructed or developed by the observer. The constructions vary across people via social interactions and are influenced by culture and history. This term refers to both cognitive constructivism, influenced by Piaget, and social constructivism, influenced by Vygotsky. However, Piaget's notion assumes an objective reality that is understood by individuals via the development of cognitive structures.
Empiricism	This is a philosophical position that asserts that experience is the source of all knowledge. That is, knowledge is obtained via the use of direct observations of phenomena and from introspections. The strong position avers that there are no innate ideas, concepts, or structures. Weaker versions assert that although not all ideas or concepts are causally associated with experience, they must be verified

(continues)

Table 1-5 (continued)

	or justified via the test of experience as in the scientific method or approach.
Objectivism	This is related to the concepts of absolutism and empiricism. Objectivism assumes that there is a separation between the individual (i.e., subject having an experience) and the perception/experience of the individual (i.e., object that is experienced). With objectivism, it is believed that the object has specific inherent qualities that shape or determine the experiences of the observer. It is assumed that these experiences can be accurately perceived by the observer and shared by other observers. Thus, there is such an entity as objective knowledge, independent of observer's bias and prejudice and open to public inspection and verification.
Rationalism	This philosophical position is often contrasted with empiricism. It asserts that reason is the path to the obtainment of knowledge, not direct experience or observation. In one sense, rationalism is the opposite of empiricism. However, it is often accepted that scientific knowledge is the result of observations or experiences interpreted by rational thought. In this sense, rational thought is considered to be separate or different from nonrational thought sources such as personal intuition or supernatural revelation. From another perspective, personal intuition or judgment is considered to be rational and acceptable, especially within a philosophy such as constructivism—notably, social constructivism.
Reductionism	This is a view that assumes that the best way to understand a phenomenon is to reduce it into smaller components or parts. An analysis of the parts yields an understanding of the whole—that is, the phenomenon. For example, the behaviorist is likely to reduce phenomenon to stimulus and response terms. With reductionism, there is the belief that ultimate reality (or all systems) can be reduced to a unifying or unitary principle, law, or substance. In one sense, reductionism is the opposite of constructivism, which can also be interpreted as the whole is greater than the sum of its parts. Reductionism has been

the traditional hallmark of the scientific method but has encountered difficulty, especially in addressing complex issues such as language acquisition and consciousness.

Relativism | This concept is the opposite of absolutism, particularly in philosophy. Thus, there is no absolute knowledge, values, or truths. The understanding of reality is based on the personal and historical perspectives of an individual via interactions in culture. Relativism is a major component of constructivism, especially social constructivism. There are several types of relativism. For example, pertinent to deafness, one can speak of cultural relativism in which customs, mores, and belief systems should be evaluated or understood within the context of a particular culture such as Deaf culture. This is a major concept for understanding the multicultural movement.

Subjectivism | This notion is often contrasted with objectivism and considers the perceptions of the subject to be paramount in understanding reality. That is, the perceptions or views of an individual are responsible for interpreting or understanding an experience (or an object that is being experienced). The so-called inherent qualities of the object are interpreted or judged from the framework of the individual. In essence, there are no objective qualities—only subjective interpretations. These qualities are supplied by the individual's mind.

Note: For additional discussions of the terms in the table and related terms, readers are encouraged to consult the following accessible sources:
Chaplin, J. (1975). Dictionary of psychology. *New York: Dell Publishing Co.*
Guttenplan, S. (Ed.). (1994). A companion to the philosophy of mind. *Cambridge, MA: Blackwell.*
Norton, A-L. (Ed.). (1994). Dictionary of ideas. *Oxford, England: Helicon.*
Rohmann, C. (1999). A world of ideas: A dictionary of important theories, concepts, beliefs, and thinkers. *New York: Ballantine.*

Metatheory

Without oversimplifying, a metatheory is a framework or perspective that determines the manner in which one should do science or conduct scholarly inquiries (Ritzer, 1991, 1992). From one perspective, it is a theory about theories. It can be a theory about scholarly disciplines as a whole and about their internal parts as well. In addition, a metatheory might define what constitutes a discipline, its internal parts, its boundaries, and the manner (i.e., method of inquiry) in which everything should be investigated. On the macro level, there might be an overarching perspective (i.e., The metatheory); on the micro level, the focus might be on certain areas, methods, practice, and so on within a field.

The word *meta* has several meanings; one meaning that is applicable here is: "more comprehensive: transcending—used with the name of a discipline to designate a new but related discipline designed to deal critically with the original one" (*Webster's New Collegiate Dictionary,* 1979, p. 715). Thus, one can have terms such as *metalinguistics, metapsychology, metaphilosophy* (strange but true!), and even *metaeducation.* There are even micro-metaanalyses within a field. For example, in the field of language (and reading), there are terms such as *metalanguage, metalinguistic, metacognition, metamemory,* and *metacomprehension,* and the results are theories or metatheories about language, cognition, memory, and comprehension. To complicate matters, theories (i.e., general or abstract principles or laws illustrating and explaining relationships among entities) can function as metatheories and vice versa.

A metatheory can also focus on whether a particular discipline is a science or not. For example, there have been ongoing debates on whether psychology belongs to the sciences or to the humanities (Bunge & Ardila, 1987). Although the term *metatheory* is related to others such as *paradigm* (Kuhn, 1970) and *philosophy* (Baars, 1986; Bunge & Ardila, 1987; Ritzer, 1991), these terms are not synonymous.

Most important, within a scholarly field, a metatheory directs the composition of theories and the types of research methodologies. Theories are tested and refined, and the ones that are the most predictive (or aesthetic!) survive the test of time. Thus, a metatheory can be an overarching framework for the scholarly activities within a particular discipline (Ritzer, 1991).

Because of its nature, it is not possible to evaluate an overarching metatheory as accurate or inaccurate. It is also difficult to compare one overarching metatheory with another overarching metatheory. This situation is somewhat similar to the evaluation of paradigms, as discussed by Kuhn (1970) and mentioned in the previous section on philosophical perspectives on deafness. Some eloquent statements from Regis (1987) are borrowed to explicate this issue:

> *For example, if a given scientific community accepts the idea that nature is alive, the notion that there's an* elan vital *at work in the universe, then those scientists will be inclined to interpret natural phenomena teleologically. They'll see events happening for purposes, and view them*

as if they're all part of a master plan. But another group, one which holds to a philosophy of mechanism (according to which events occur in strict "billiard ball" cause-and-effect sequences), those scientists will perceive the world quite antithetically. As to whose picture of reality is correct, well . . . that's not a question we ask, Kuhn said. At least we don't ask such a question as scientists. (p. 213)

Paradigm

As mentioned previously, metatheory is often confused with the concept *paradigm*, which—albeit related—is not the same entity. Paradigms have become as ambiguous as philosophies—especially when the latter refers to a philosophy or perspective of life or of school and so on. The concept *paradigm* should be considered as a belief system or perspective within a field. In this sense, it is argued that the two philosophical perspectives, clinical and cultural, discussed previously, can be labeled as *paradigms*. There is the tendency to consider a paradigm as a viewpoint for the whole field—similar to a metatheory, but in most cases, there are numerous paradigms within a scholarly discipline. One apt description of paradigm was provided by Ritzer (1991):

> *A paradigm is a fundamental image of the subject matter within a science. It serves to define what should be studied, what questions should be asked, how they should be asked, and what rules should be followed in interpreting the answer obtained. A paradigm is the broadest unit of consensus within a science and serves to differentiate one scientific community (or subcommunity) from another. It subsumes, defines, and interrelates the exemplars, theories, and methods and instruments that exist within it. (p. 120)*

It is possible to argue that paradigms are similar to metatheories, but there seems to be the sense that metatheories are more developed and certainly more apt to reveal explanatory adequacy (i.e., the reason or explanation for the relations or parts within an entity or for the entity itself). It should be clear that paradigm analysis is a form of metaanalysis and can result from metatheorizing as well. For present purposes, the word *paradigm* refers to the broadest consensus of a perspective regarding theory, research, and practice. For example, an individual might favor the overarching metatheory of behaviorism (discussed later in this text) and adhere to the use of a research paradigm that espouses positivism, namely, the use of the experimental approach involving quantitative or single-subject designs.

Utility of Metatheorizing and Paradigm Analysis

It might be asked: What do metatheory and paradigm have to do with language and deafness? Should this discussion be best left to those academic metatheorists and theorists and thus not having much to do with the daily concerns of educators, teachers, and other practitioners? It is believed here that these questions and others are based on a misunderstanding of the influences of the complex concepts of metatheory and paradigm (including philosophical perspective). This animosity toward metatheory (or metatheorizing) and paradigm (or paradigm analysis) might be quite prevalent in the field of deafness, and it might evoke comments such as "armchair theorizing" or the pejorative "navel gazing."

The major problem is that individuals do not always recognize that they adhere to some underlying metatheory or paradigm, implicitly or explicitly, and also do not recognize that this influences the way they think or operate. In addition, the author believes that this results in numerous misunderstandings and tensions between and among professionals. Furthermore, it is extremely difficult to resolve differences—at least, scientifically or logically—when these differences flow from different underlying metatheories or paradigms (or perspectives). For example, if individuals adhere strongly to a cultural perspective (paradigm) of deafness, they are not likely to develop (or even support) theories or conduct research that focus on the improvement of speech and hearing variables. These proponents are likely to view the development of theories and research on, for example, cochlear implants, as a waste of time and resources or, even worse, unethical or wrong.

The influences of metatheories and paradigms are demonstrated throughout the rest of this text. The next two chapters relate these influences to the discussion of the components and functions of language (Chapter 2) and to the development of language acquisition models (Chapter 3). That there are a variety of metatheories and paradigms is not difficult to imagine or accept. However, addressing conflicts that arise from these differences seems to be, in many professionals' eyes, insurmountable.

Of course, there are no easy answers. Paul and Ward (1996) suggested that:

> *The first step in improving communication or in managing these conflicts is for individuals to articulate their paradigmatic underpinnings. A clear articulation and acknowledgment of a paradigm should lead to an improvement of theories, research, and practices within that paradigm. There also needs to be respect and recognition for individuals who ascribe to a different paradigm. Similar to other either-or situa-*

tions (e.g., nature-nurture, reductionism-constructivism, quantitative-qualitative), additional efforts should be devoted to the development of new *paradigms that incorporate the best, and perhaps, common features of those views on both ends of a bipolar continuum. (p. 10)*

Table 1-6 presents a summary of major points on the discussion of metatheories and paradigms.

FINAL REMARKS

The intent of this chapter is to provide an overview of a few of the salient topics associated with deafness and language that are elaborated on in the rest of this text. The goal is to present a variety of voices with respect to philosophy, theory, research, and practice/intervention. The intention was not to be balanced for balance's sake; however, a multiple-perspective approach is necessary because there is no God's eye view of language and deafness. And, it is highly unlikely that there will ever be one all-encompassing perspective

---

TABLE 1-6 A Few Major Highlights on Metatheory and Paradigm

Metatheory and Paradigm

- A metatheory is a framework or perspective that determines the manner in which one should do science or conduct scholarly inquiries. It might define what constitutes a discipline, its internal parts, its boundaries, and the manner in which everything should be investigated. In a sense, a metatheory is a theory about theories.

- On the macro level, there might be an overarching perspective (i.e., the metatheory); on the micro level, the focus might be on certain areas, methods, and practices.

- In general, there are theories within a metatheory, although it is possible for a theory to function as a metatheory and vice versa.

- Paradigm refers to the broadest consensus of a perspective regarding theory, research, and practice. A paradigm is a belief system or perspective within a particular field or discipline. Examples of paradigms are the clinical and cultural perspectives.

- To minimize misunderstandings and misinterpretations, it is important for individuals to articulate their paradigmatic underpinnings.

---

that will resolve all educational issues in the development of language with deaf and hard-of-hearing children.

The use of the phrase *deaf and hard-of-hearing* is adopted here mainly because it seems to be appearing in the major journals associated with deafness. To minimize the repetitive use of this phrase, the phrase *students with hearing impairment* is also employed in this text, which is still useful and necessary. Most important, the reader will know when either deaf or hard-of-hearing individuals or both are being referred to with respect to specific audiological information. As much as possible, it is still crucial to provide characteristics such as degree of hearing impairment, age at onset, and so on, especially when discussing the results of salient empirical research studies. Of course, cultural characteristics are included where applicable and available for studies that focus on the sociological phenomenon of deafness. Nevertheless, with respect to the clinical variables and even to the cultural ones, it is not possible to make generalizations or even to establish policy without some reference points that typically represent subgroups of the deaf and hard-of-hearing populations. Even when making a generalization or forming a policy is not the major goal, such information still provides a context for understanding theory, research, and practice/intervention. In any case, the bulk of the information in this text concerns individuals with severe to profound hearing impairment with some applications to individuals with hearing impairment from slight to moderate.

This introductory chapter organizes information into three major sections, "Acquisition and Instructional Issues," "Philosophical Perspectives," and "Metatheory, Paradigm, and Language." A brief summary of some of the salient highlights is as follows.

Acquisition and Instructional Issues

- A clear understanding and in-depth research on concepts such as use, representation, and exposure—and their interrelationships—are important to improve one's knowledge of the various language-communication modes used with deaf and hard-of-hearing children.

- Exposure to a communication system is not the same as language instruction. Language instruction refers to the specific language-teaching methods or approaches that have been used in education and deafness.

- Many of the controversies in the larger field of bilingualism, multiculturalism, and children with typical hearing are applicable to the situations for deaf and hard-of-hearing children. There are, of course, some major differences, especially for children for whom ASL is a first language or for other children with severe to profound impairment who are limited speakers of their home languages.

- There are ongoing arguments and disagreements on the most efficient or best way to develop English literacy in bilingual or second-language literacy programs.

Philosophical Perspectives

- There are two major philosophical perspectives, clinical and cultural, that have been described in the literature. There are also variations of these major perspectives. Because of the so-called incompatibility of the two major perspectives, it is possible to view them as different paradigms.

- The clinical perspective has dominated the thinking of professionals, theorists, and researchers in the education of deaf and hard-of-hearing children. The focus is on remedying the deficiencies or improving the skills of deaf and hard-of-hearing individuals and adolescents with the model for comparison being children and adolescents with typical hearing.

- In the cultural perspective, proponents view deafness as a natural condition, not as a disease or disability that needs to be cured or prevented. The role models for deaf and many hard-of-hearing individuals are Deaf adults, especially those individuals who use ASL and are members of the Deaf culture.

Metatheory, Paradigm, and Language

- A metatheory is a framework or perspective that determines the manner in which one should do science or conduct scholarly inquiries. In general, it is a theory about theories; however, it is based on metaanalyses of a variety of products such as theories, research, and practices.

- A paradigm is a belief system or a perspective within a scholarly field. In this sense, it covers less ground than a metatheory. It is the broadest unit of consensus within a field and serves to differentiate one scholarly community from another one.

- Misunderstandings about metatheories and paradigms have led to unproductive scholarly debates and professional disagreements. It seems to be difficult for professionals to accept the fact that metatheories and paradigms cannot be proven to be true or false. They represent viewpoints, which are based on reflections and interpretations and cannot be resolved by the use of the scientific method.

In sum, there is no question that language development is serious business with educational, psychological, social, economical, and political implications. But before one can decide whether language can or needs to be taught, one should have some background on the nature of language or language development. What is the nature of this phenomenon that some scholars continue to call magic or mysterious? In the next chapter, the focus is on the structures and functions of language.

INTRODUCTION TO LANGUAGE AND DEAFNESS COMPREHENSION QUESTIONS

1. There seems to be some confusion surrounding the interpretations of terms such as *acquisition, instruction, use, representation, exposure,* and *communication form*. Describe each term (and create examples, if possible). Are these terms related to each other? How? Which terms seem to cause the most confusion? Why?

2. With respect to exposure, the author remarked that the most basic question is: Why is exposure to a spoken language such as English different for many deaf and some hard-of-hearing individuals; that is, why is it different from that of individuals who are hearing peers? According to the author, how has this question been investigated? That is, what is/are the focus/foci of research endeavors?

3. Many of the controversies in the larger fields of bilingualism, multiculturalism, and children with typical hearing are also applicable to children who are deaf and hard of hearing. However, there are some differences. Discuss these differences. (For further discussion, you might want to propose other differences, based on your understanding of the issues.)

4. The chapter discussed two broad philosophical perspectives on deafness: clinical and cultural. Describe each view. Are these the only perspectives? Is it possible to label these perspectives metatheories or paradigms? Why or why not? According to the author, is it possible

to evaluate a particular perspective as right or wrong? Why or why not?

5. Briefly describe the five audiological categories that correspond to degree of hearing impairment. Relate the terms *hard of hearing* and *deaf* to these categories. With respect to degree of impairment, what is the "gray area"? Why has this been problematic?

6. Describe the variable of age at onset. What does it mean to say that age at onset is a linguistic factor? List and discuss other factors that have often been used to describe deafness clinically.

7. Reread the quote by Harlan Lane on the cultural view. Do you think Lane's remarks indicate that there is only one right view? Is it clear from this passage that the cultural view should apply to all individuals who are deaf and hard of hearing?

8. Describe the terms *metatheory* and *paradigm* (provide as much information as possible). Are they similar or different? Why does the author think that an adequate understanding of these terms is important not only for theorists and researchers but also for educators and practitioners?

9. Questions such as what is language, can language be taught, and how should language be measured are undergirded by metaphysical and epistemological concerns. Given the information in the chapter, what does the author mean?

CHALLENGE QUESTIONS

(Note: Complete answers are not in the text. Additional research is required.)

1. In the beginning of the chapter, there were two questions posed: What should be the first language for young children (who are deaf and hard-of-hearing) and who should make this decision. It was stated that the answers to these questions are not easily answered by the so-called empirical, scientific approaches. What does this mean? What other approaches might be necessary to answer these questions? What are your answers? On what did you base your answers?

2. Should hearing parents be charged with mental abuse if they do not learn to sign to their deaf children? Why or why not? How about if

they do not learn to use ASL with their children? Why or why not? Is it fair or possible for agencies, institutions, courts, and so on to evaluate the type of communication mode used by parents with their children to determine if parents are fit to be parents? Is type of communication mode the major issue only? What are some others, if any?

3. It has often been remarked that there is no God's eye view of deafness. What does this statement mean? Do you agree or disagree? Why? Do you think that this statement applies to all aspects of deafness, for example, language acquisition, literacy development, and so on? Why or why not?

4. One of the most controversial debates in the field of deafness is the selection of a philosophical perspective, clinical or cultural. Here are some questions for you to consider:

   • Should this issue be construed as an either-or choice? That is, must educators/parents choose one or the other? Why or why not?

   • Who decides the interpretation of either the clinical or cultural view? Who should decide?

   • Can the clinical view be espoused by a deaf or Deaf (i.e., culturally Deaf) person? Why or why not? Can the cultural view be supported by a hearing person? Why or why not? Are there other combinations? Discuss them.

FURTHER READINGS

Bloom, L. (1978). *Readings in language development.* New York: John Wiley.

Chomsky, N. (1986). *Knowledge of language: Its nature, origin, and use.* New York: Praeger.

Harley, T. (1996). *The psychology of language: From data to theory.* Hillsdale, NJ: Lawrence Erlbaum.

Lang, H., & Lang, B. (1996). *Deaf persons in the arts and sciences: A biographical dictionary.* Westport, CT: Greenwood.

Ogden, P. (1996). *The silent garden: Raising your deaf child.* Washington, DC: Gallaudet University Press.

CHAPTER

2

Language Functions and Structures

The question *"Why do we use language?" seems hardly to require an answer. But, as is often the way with linguistic questions, our everyday familiarity with speech and writing can make it difficult to appreciate the complexity of the skills we have learned. This is particularly so when we try to define the range of functions to which language can be put. (Crystal, 1997, p. 10)*

The structure of language is something most of us take completely for granted. We are so used to speaking and understanding our mother tongue with unselfconscious ease that we do not notice the complex linguistic architecture that underlies almost every sentence. We forget the years we expended in mastering this skill, so that when we encounter the structural complexity of a foreign language as an adult, we are often amazed at the level of difficulty involved. Similarly, when we hear of people whose ability to control the structures of their language has broken down . . . we can be surprised at the amount of structural planning involved in the linguistic analysis and treatment of their handicap. Such instances suggest the central importance of the field of linguistic structure, not only to such specialists as teachers or therapists, but to all who wish to further their understanding of the phenomenon of language. (Crystal, 1997, p. 81)

One of the debates in the education of students with hearing impairment concerns the amount or kind of knowledge teachers should have about language.

This is a pertinent issue with respect to whether teachers and other professionals intend to teach a language or remedy language difficulties. The author strongly agrees with Russell, Quigley, and Power (1976) who asserted that: "It is probably a fair analogy to state that teachers of deaf children should be expected to know as much about language as a teacher of chemistry is expected to know about chemistry" (p. xi). Schoolteachers are not expected to teach about language theories or metatheories or even about specific types of noun or verb phrases. However, an in-depth knowledge of language by teachers seems to be necessary to accomplish some of the purposes cited in the earlier passages with respect to acquisition and development. Obviously, this in-depth knowledge also helps to appreciate the complex phenomenon of language.

As indicated in Chapter 1, any discussion about a complex topic such as language is influenced markedly by a person's mental framework, based on his or her interpretation of extant theories and research. Admittedly, the author has been heavily affected by and strongly favors the theoretical persuasion of Chomsky and his followers. Some of this influence can be seen in the discussion of syntax in this chapter. Although the author favors the notion of explanatory adequacy and other new terms, especially via the framework of transformational generative grammar, the judicious use and descriptions of traditional terms such as *noun, pronoun, adjective*, and so on within the domain of word classes (i.e., traditionally, parts of speech) have not been abandoned. This chapter attempts to reflect a representative variety of voices with respect to discussions of the functions and structures of language. The array of representative views might be most noticeable in Chapter 3 on language acquisition.

As can be inferred from the earlier discussion, there are two major sections in this brief chapter: "Language Functions" and "Language Structures." The intent is to provide a broad overview of these two concepts. Readers are referred elsewhere for more details (see accessible accounts in Crystal, 1995, 1997; Dale, 1976; Russell et al., 1976). The first section provides information on the general functions of language. It should be clear that although the most common function of language is the communication of ideas, there are other major important functions, several of which are transparent and not easily recognizable. In addition, social interactionists, with their emphasis on pragmatics or the use of language (see Chapter 3), argue that children learn language in social intercourse due to the influences of the interactions and the functions of the language. In this sense, language acquisition is functional and social.

Whereas the first section of the chapters presents general, overall functions of language, the second section provides a discussion of language structures, including a brief description of the area that governs language use—that is, pragmatics. In essence, pragmaticists argue that specific communicative, pragmatic functions (e.g., requesting information and asking for clarification) shape, support, and drive the acquisition and development of a language, especially in children. To avoid confusion, the reader should remember that one of the goals of the second section is to provide a brief discussion of pragmatics and other language structures. Strictly speaking, pragmatics is not considered to be a language structure; however, this topic is placed in the second section because pragmatics is considered a component of language. Furthermore, a better understanding of pragmatics can be obtained from its juxtaposition with language structures such as phonology, morphology, syntax, and semantics.

To understand the information in this chapter, it might also be beneficial for readers to consider three common terms often used to describe language: *form, meaning,* and *use* (Bloom & Lahey, 1978). Form refers to phonology, morphology, and syntax; meaning to semantics; and use to pragmatics. In essence, an understanding of a language means an understanding and simultaneous integration of form, meaning, and use. Any framework that is used is actually arbitrarily selected for discussion purposes; there is no best framework for analyzing and discussing language. Nevertheless, a framework is necessary to assist in the understanding of the phenomenon of language and to teach or develop it, if necessary.

It should be reemphasized that the intent of this chapter is to provide an overview of the functions and structures of language and not to overwhelm readers with a litany of language facts. Due to space constraints, the discussion of the various language aspects is notoriously brief but should provide enough detail for the reader to obtain a basic understanding. This understanding should assist the reader in interpreting information on language development and deafness in this text. For an in-depth, lucid discussion of the functions and structure of language, including the English language, the author recommends the works of Crystal (1995, 1997).

LANGUAGE FUNCTIONS

Language can be used to perform a number of general functions that contribute to the impetus for and process of acquisition or development. The most conspicuous recognized functions seem to be the communication of ideas, especially during social intercourses, and to think—that is, the use of language as a tool for thought (Cairns, 1996; Cromer, 1988a, 1988b, 1994; Crystal, 1997; Owens, 1996). Other language usages—some of them transparent or not always apparent—include the expression of emotions, the control of reality, the expression of identity, and the recording of information.

Communication of Ideas

Perhaps the best way to illustrate the communication of ideas function is to state the classic definition provided by Bloom and Lahey (1978): "Language is described as a code whereby *ideas* about the world are represented by a conventional system of signals for *communication* [italics added]" (p. 4).

This is actually a useful, succinct definition that highlights several other related general functions often associated with language: referential, propositional, and ideational (Cairns, 1996; Crystal, 1997; Owens, 1996). To communicate, both the receiver and the sender need to understand the parameters (i.e., rule-governed principles) of the code represented by an agreed-on conventional system of signals (e.g., string of sounds to represent specific spoken languages or a string of signs for specific sign languages). This communication involves any spoken, signed, or written interaction between the participants in which there is an exchange of ideas, opinions, facts, and other types of information. As is discussed repeatedly throughout this text, access to the code does not guarantee understanding or interpretation of the message, but access is a necessary first step.

To simplify, communicating and thinking about ideas can occur in two broad contexts. One context entails everyday, communicative, or real-time interactions, which can be conducted face-to-face or through the use of electronic media such as telephones and other two-way communication devices and involve what can be called the *performance* mode of the language (i.e., typically speech and/or signs). This type of context is considered natural (i.e., typical manner for receiving and expressing information) and redundant (i.e., the use of overlapping cues—verbal and nonverbal—to minimize misunderstandings). The information itself might also be learned—that is, involving the understanding and use of topic-specific or selection-specific vocabulary such as the terminology associated with physics, law, or education.

The second type of context can be labeled *decontextualized*. Decontextualized situations refer to the delivery of information that has been captured, recorded, or preserved (Denny, 1991; Feldman, 1991; Olson, 1989, 1994). In decontextualized contexts, the information is essentially removed from real-time or live contexts; thus, there are no face-to-face or live interactions between authors/speakers and readers/listeners. Typically, the interactions involve participants (e.g., teachers, students, and readers) who have read, listened to, or viewed the text (i.e., captured information) and are requested to perform some function for a purpose such as taking a test, recalling major points, answering questions, relating the information to other similar or personal situations, and so on. It is possible to capture, record, or preserve discussions, debates, or lectures that occur in education, business, law, and government. This can be accomplished via print (similar to captions on television or just the script without the video) or through the use of electronic media (videotape, audiotape, compact discs, etc.). All of these texts (again, examples of captured information) require that the participants be familiar with the specialized language, jargon, or lingo of the specific topic to participate in an informed, intelligent manner. To reiterate, the capture of information, whether in print or by electronic media, renders this information as decontextualized—in this case, removed from the present context. Captured, decontextualized information lends itself to study and reflection, processes that are often associated with the thought and consciousness of Western civilization (Olson, 1989, 1994). Traditionally, the medium for capturing information has been the use of typographic (e.g., print) or chirographic (e.g., writing) forms. Nevertheless, there should be similar effects for information that has been captured electronically. There are, of course, some differences, and these are discussed later in this text.

This basic—albeit simplified— distinction between contextualization and decontextualization of information is a critical issue with respect to the development of overall language comprehension ability. To access captured, decontextualized information, particularly learned information, it has been argued that individuals need to learn or to acquire specific skills that are unique to the code of the medium. For example, to access English print (words on paper), some scholars believe that it is critical to have a working knowledge of the alphabetic principle—that is, knowledge of consonants and vowels and sound/letter or phoneme/grapheme correspondences (Adams, 1990; Paul, 1998a). Interestingly, an individual's performance in decontextualized situations might not be a good index of his or her conversational language ability—that is, the ability to use speech and/or signs for everyday purposes, basic needs, and so on. This distinction between contextualization and decontextualization is related somewhat to Cummins' notions (1979, 1980, 1984) of communicative proficiency (i.e., contexualized language) and academic proficiency, which have been used to explain the development of language proficiency in bilingual and/or second-language learning academic environments. In essence, these two contexts demand different levels and types of language proficiency. It might be assumed that decontextualized situations require, at the very least, the ability to engage in communicative proficiency.

On the basic of the earlier discussion, it is useful to delineate, again, the three broad media for the expression and reception of information: performance, performance literacy, and script literacy. Only a few brief comments on these concepts are presented in this section to illustrate and clarify some previous points.

The term *performance*, as mentioned earlier, simply refers to the reception and expression of information in contextualized, face-to-face, or real-time interactions. Traditionally, this refers to the conversational form of the language that has or can have several renditions, for example, speech, cued speech, signed systems, and sign language. There are other situations, such as the use of communication boards (e.g., bliss symbols, etc.). However, much of the attention is focused on information that is expressed through oral, manual (hand), or combination (i.e., simultaneous use of oral and manual) performance forms.

Information that has been captured, recorded, or preserved can be labeled as examples of literacy. A distinction was made briefly between performance literacy and script literacy. Performance literacy refers to the face-to-face, through-the-air, or real-time interactions and monologues that have been captured by the electronic media. Examples include conversations, plays, and lectures in various settings. These instances are decontextualized (separated by time and context) and can be subjected to further reflection and study. When information is captured typographically or chirographically, this can be labeled as examples of script literacy.

Whether an individual encounters decontexualized information in the performance literacy mode or in the script literacy mode, she or he will need to possess certain skills for accessing the information in the particular mode. It could be argued that there are major differences between performance literacy and script literacy. However, many of these mode differences are related to type of genre and, indeed, may be arbitrary. In some cases, the distinction between the two modes may be blurred, as in the case for talking books for individuals who are visually impaired. In essence, it is more accurate to say that there are or might be salient differences between information that has not been captured or preserved and information that has and that these differences are dependent on the use of a specific genre or other factors such as the sophistication and attention of the audience/receivers.

The crux of the brief foregoing discussion is to inquire and investigate whether literate thought is mode specific or mode independent. The interest is in the nature of the ability to think logically, creatively, rationally, and reflectively about information either in contextualized or decontextualized situations.

Much of the focus has been on decontextualized information, particularly information that has been captured in print. Chapter 12 takes the position that in general, the development of literate thought is mode independent—that is, it is not dependent on a specific mode of captured information (performance literacy or script literacy). It might be dependent on the study and reflection of captured information; however, there is not widespread agreement on this issue either (see Olson, 1994). In any case, the outcomes of these debates have pervasive implications for developing the language and cognitive skills of deaf and hard-of-hearing students.

At the very least, literate thought requires the development of a bona fide language (as early as possible) and the skills for accessing decontextualized information, which includes the understanding and inferential use of a meta-language (i.e., specialized language or terminology). To use a crude analogy: The skills for performance literacy include listening/watching aspects, similar to the word identification skills for accessing English script literacy. Similar to what is required for script literacy, individuals also need prior knowledge and metacognitive skills, often called comprehension or top-down skills, to make inferences, draw conclusions, and so on with respect to the information in the performance literacy mode. It cannot be overemphasized that access to the captured information does not guarantee an understanding or a meaningful interpretation of it.

A summary of major points discussed in this section is provided in Table 2-1.

TABLE 2-1 Summary of Major Points for the Communication Function of Language

---

- Communicating and thinking about ideas can occur in two broad contexts, contextualized and decontextualized.

- Contextualization entails everyday real-time interactions conducted face-to-face or through the use of electronic media such as telephones and other two-way communication devices. This type of context is considered natural and redundant.

- Decontextualization refers to the delivery of information that has been captured, recorded, or preserved. The information is removed from real-time or live contexts.

(continues)

(Table 2-1 continued)

- Captured decontextualized information lends itself to study and reflection, processes often associated with the thought and consciousness of Western civilization.

- To access captured decontextualized information, an individual needs to learn or acquire skills that are unique to the code of the medium (i.e., of the captured information).

- Performance refers to the reception or expression of information in contextualized interactions. In this text, this refers to the conversational form of a language—either spoken and/or signed.

- Information that has been captured, recorded, or preserved can be labeled as examples of literacy.

- Performance literacy refers to the face-to-face, through-the-air, or real-time interactions and monologues that have been captured by the electronic media.

- Script literacy refers to information that has been captured typographically (print) or chirographically (written).

- It is possible that literate thought is mode independent—that is, it is not dependent on a specific mode of captured information. It might be dependent on the study and reflection of captured information.

Social Interactions

It is safe to conclude that humans are social creatures. The social interaction (or social) function of language pertains to the use of words or phrases to establish and maintain a rapport between language users (Cairns, 1996; Crystal, 1997; Owens, 1996). In some cultures, for example, English-speaking cultures, certain stereotypical automatic phrases are used as conversational openers or conversational fillers. Examples include "How are you?," "Good Morning," "Hello," "Is it hot enough for you today?," and "Bless you" (after someone sneezes). The main intent of these phrases is not to communicate ideas or to exchange information. Rather, the intent is to signal friendship or a non-threatening or comfortable encounter.

Interestingly, the lack of acknowledgment (e.g., being silent after meeting someone for the first time or after someone sneezes) may be interpreted as aloofness, alienation, or a threat. For instance, there are cases where individuals do not desire to engage in any social intercourse for a number of reasons. Consider the various—perhaps uncomfortable—times when one has walked on the sidewalk and has encountered other individuals who have, for example, stared straight ahead or looked down to avoid eye contact and, possibly, verbal exchanges. Even more uncomfortable are cases where individuals might cross the sidewalk to the other side of the street, for whatever reasons, to avoid eye or other communicative contacts.

Identity and Language

Language can also be used to express the identity of the language user (Crystal, 1997; Goodluck, 1991; Muma, 1986; Whitehead, 1990). Individuals have multiple identities, for example, personal, social, and political. The language that speakers/signers use can reveal information about their background, education, vocation, age, gender, geographical location, belief systems, and other personal characteristics. In fact, identity is also associated with or influenced by factors that also affect dialects (e.g., variations across language users as in pronunciation and grammar) and registers (e.g., variations within a language user as in the use of informal and formal expressions).

A good illustration of political identity can be seen in the following example: In the 1992 presidential primaries, Jerry Brown, a Democratic candidate, took his place on the podium. Before he could speak, several individuals from the audience shouted one of his favorite slogans: "We must take back America!" Hearing these words brought a smile to Mr. Brown's face.

Rather than communicate ideas, these words reflect the individuals' sense of political identity. One can pick up almost any newspaper and find numerous examples, or slogans, often associated with political candidates, especially during election periods, or for social issues such as medicare, social welfare, and education. Consider phrases such as "a thousand points of lights," "it's the economy, stupid," and "it's the right thing to do."

It is not difficult to find examples of expressions of social identity, particularly with the use of language that unites a group. These include the shoutings or roars that occur at sporting events, the bursts of affirmation that accompany religious sermons, and the appreciative sounds from family members on seeing a Thanksgiving turkey dinner. These remarks represent "the signalling of who we are and where we 'belong'" (Crystal, 1997, p. 13).

The expression of identity is important for understanding a movement that can be labeled as the *depathologizing of deafness* (Lane, 1988; Padden &

Humphries, 1988; Reagan, 1990). This movement has been fueled by the establishment of American Sign Language as a bona fide linguistic system and the recognition of Deaf culture as a legitimate sociological phenomenon rather than a compensatory reaction to deafness. The expression of social, political, and personal identities are evident in statements such as "Deaf is Beautiful," "Deaf Power," and the "Use of Sign Language Is the Native Right of All Deaf Children." The call for the establishment of bilingual/bicultural education programs for deaf and hard-of-hearing students has also been motivated, in part, by the use of language in the expression of identity.

Table 2-2 contains part of a poem that exemplifies the social and personal identities of some members of Deaf culture with an emphasis on the importance of using signs or ASL for communication purposes.

LANGUAGE STRUCTURES

In this section, the intent is to discuss briefly the various components of language such as phonology, morphology, syntax, semantics, and pragmatics. Additional details on these areas are presented in the tables.

TABLE 2-2 Examples of Social and Personal Identities of Language

---

The Deaf: "By Their Fruits Ye Shall Know Them"

Nature hates force. Just as the flowing stream seeks the easiest path, so the mind seeks the way of least resistance. The sign language offers to the deaf a broad and smooth avenue for the inflow and outflow of thought, and there is no other avenue for them unto it. —G. M. Teegarden

You Have to be Deaf to Understand

What is it like to comprehend
Some nimble fingers that paint the scene,
And make you smile and feel serene
With the "spoken word" of the moving hand
That makes you part of the world at large?
You have to be deaf to understand.—Willard J. Madsen

Source: Adapted from Gannon (1981).

In discussing the structures of language, one is faced with the decision of the type of terminology to use. Most readers might be familiar with traditional terms such as *nouns, verbs,* and *adjectives* as opposed to recent terms, due to the influence of transformation generative grammar, such as *noun phrase, verb phrase,* and *determiners.* To provide an anchor point for the discussion of the various language structures in this chapter, it is important to discuss the concept of word classes as a starting point. These structures are integral parts of noun phrases and verb phrases. For example, a noun phrase (NP) might contain elements such as nouns, determiners (e.g., articles such as *a, an,* and *the*), and verbs.

Word Classes

It is possible to categorize words into word classes, traditionally known as parts of speech. Although there are disagreements among linguists, many of them agree that there are at least eight categories or classes of words, for example, nouns, pronouns, adjectives, verbs, prepositions, conjunctions, adverbs, and interjections.

The sounds of the letters in words are discussed in phonology (see "Phonology"). The variations of words and the formations of new words fall within the domain of morphology (see "Morphology"). The order of words within sentences is discussed in syntax (see "Syntax"). The nuances and meanings of words are discussed in semantics (see "Semantics"). The use of words is discussed in pragmatics (see "Pragmatics").

With respect to the notion of word classes, it is difficult to provide definitions of the classes as was the case in traditional grammarian approaches. For example, one might encounter the description that a noun is the name of a living substance or being or lifeless thing. Thus, examples of nouns include: *boy, girl, newspaper, Jeremy, Marianne, horse, New York,* and *courage.* These definition attempts have been criticized as being vague or incomplete. Linguists started asking questions such as is courage a thing? The recent focus has been on describing the manner in which the structural features of words behave in a particular sentence. Thus, articles (in the adjective class) such as *a, an,* and *the* (i.e., determiners) indicate that the next word is a noun, as in the following items: *a car, the newspaper,* and *an apple.* The notion of word class is useful if it is clear that all words within the particular class behave in the same way. For example, all words in the noun class should behave similarly. Any grammatical operation (e.g., plurality, possessive, etc.) performed on one word within the class could also be performed on the other words. It might also be useful to categorize further the words in each class. For example, in the noun class, we can discuss common nouns (e.g., *parent, teacher, cow, plant,* and *courage*), proper nouns (e.g., *Chicago, Shakespeare,* and *Sunday*), common nouns that can be used as proper nouns (e.g., *Life* is funny), and proper nouns that can be used as common nouns (e.g., He is an *Einstein*). Nevertheless, the recent focus for scholars of English is typically on distinctions such as masculine/feminine and human/nonhuman. For example, the pronoun *he* can be classified as masculine and human.

Keep in mind, it is sometimes difficult to identify the form class of words in isolation. Consider the following items for *run* and variations of this word.

1. I run every hour.
2. There is a run in my stocking.
3. Running is good exercise.
4. The woman is running toward the gate.
5. Sosa hit 7 homeruns yesterday!
6. She runs 5 miles a day.

Thus, in these examples, it can be seen that a number of words in one class may have a function in another class, particularly when they are inflected or may be derivatives (see the section on Morphology next).

For the purpose of convenience, definitions are avoided and examples simply provided in the broad word classes in Table 2-3.

For detailed discussions of word classes and traditional parts of speech categories, see Crystal (1997) and Curme (1947).

TABLE 2-3 Examples of Word Classes

Examples of Words That Can Function as Nouns

apple, baseball, beauty, Capitol, cat, courage, development, [the] drive, education, elephant, foolishness, herd, honesty, Kleenex, metatheory, nation, newspaper, Ohio, [the] plant, [the] project, theory, truth, virtue, White House, woman, running, walking, wisdom, writing, youth

Examples of Words That Can Function as Pronouns

I, me, thou, he, she, it, we, us, they, them, myself, ourselves, yourself, yourselves, himself, herself, itself, themselves, each other, one another, that, which, who, whom, whose, whatever, whichever, whoever, whomever, anybody, anyone, anything, nobody, nothing, somebody, someone, something, somewhat

Examples of Words That Can Function as Adjectives

a, an, the, this, that, these, those, runny [nose], broken [car], up-to-date [book], sick, tired, exhausted, dying [man], hopeful, childish, cold-blooded, my, his, her, their, your, first, second, last, another, few, several, [a] Yale [supporter], American [universities]

Examples of Words That Can Function as Verbs

love, kiss, hug, squeeze, hit, struck, is kissing, is hitting, act, do [it], bark [at], chase [the car], drive, dream, am, is, are, become, was, were, will, should, need, seem, look, see, feel, get, jump, skip, hop, ride, go, precede, proceed, follow, take, think, metatheorize, educate, teach, instruct

Examples of Words That Can Function as Prepositions

after, around, at, before [dinner], behind, by, for, from, in, into, of, over, under, with, within

Examples of Words That Can Function as Conjunctions

and, because, but, if, for, or, both—and, as well as, either-or, neither-nor, not only—but or but also, too (for a relative discussion of this topic for deafness, see "Syntax").

Examples of Words That Can Function as Adverbs

almost, around, fast, firstly, happily, here, how [did she do that?], immediately, lovingly, now, often, once, so, soon, then, there, twice, undoubtedly [a smart woman], very, well, when [will we eat?], yesterday

Examples of Words That Can Function as Interjections

alas, gosh, oh, Ouch!, Why!

Note: For additional information, see Curme (1947) and Crystal (1995).

Phonology

Phonology pertains to the building blocks of a particular language. For spoken languages, this concerns elements of the sound system, whereas for signed languages, this concerns elements of manual and nonmanual movements (e.g., see Chapter 7 on ASL). With respect to spoken languages, "phonology is the aspect of language concerned with the rules governing the structure, distribution, and sequencing of speech sounds and the shape of syllables" (Owens, 1996, p. 21). Humans are capable of producing a range of sounds with their vocal apparatus; however, only a small arbitrary sample of those sounds is meaningful for a particular language user. The sound system of English refers to the use of approximately 45 phonemes (more or less due to dialectical variations). A *phoneme* is an abstract concept, which actually refers to a family of distinctive, similar sounds and guides the pronunciation of words. A phoneme is the smallest linguistic unit of sound that can signal a difference in meaning. *Allophones* refer to the individual members of a phoneme family, which are slightly different from each other but not different enough to warrant a member of a different phoneme family and to modify the meaning of a particular word. Another term that should be mentioned is *phonetics*, which is concerned with the production and description of speech sounds. Table 2-4 presents a list of selected phonemes (i.e., consonants and vowels) in English.

Here is a brief illustration of the concepts of phoneme and allophone. For example, the consonant (or sound) *b* can be represented by /b/ as in *bat, baseball, bean,* and so on. /b/ is different from /p/ (as in *pop, paste,* etc.). If you repeat the /b/ sound successively for about seven times, each production will sound slightly different or will vary due to a number of physiological and psychological reasons (e.g., length of airstream, motivation, and context). Nevertheless, these slight variations do not alter the meaning of the sound or the word containing that sound. Due to coarticulation (i.e., surrounding sounds in a word), it is possible to detect differences in the production of /b/ in words such as *bat, baseball,* or *beat,* yet these differences are similar enough to belong in one family or group. The crux is that the differences in the earlier examples constitute the concept of allophone and that these allophones are all members of one family—that is, of one phoneme. Thus, /b/ constitutes one distinct English phoneme that contains several allophones. The classification of phonemes is based on entities such as acoustic or sound properties, production (i.e., modification of the air stream), and place of articulation or production (i.e., placement along the vocal tract). It is also possible to discuss the phonology of soundless languages such as sign languages (Liddell, 1980; Wilbur, 1987), and this is covered in Chapter 7. A more detailed discussion of the anatomy and physiology of speech sounds can be found elsewhere (Menn & Stoel-Gammon, 1993; Owens, 1996).

The phonological system also consists of prosodic features such as stress, intonation, and rhythm, which are critical for the perception of speech (Crystal, 1997; Goodluck, 1991). These features are considered as suprasegmental phe-

TABLE 2-4 List of Selected Consonants and Vowels of English

Consonants	Vowels
/b/ as in bat	/a/ as in mass
/d/ as in dunk	/e/ as in mate
/dz/ as in jet	/i/ as in beat
/f/ as in fish	/I/ as in hit
/g/ as in give	/u/ as in mood
/h/ as in hat	/U/ as in book
/k/ as in cat	/o/ as in boat
/l/ as in lake	
/m/ as in moon	
/n/ as in noon	
/p/ as in pet	
/r/ as in bar	
/s/ as in some	
/t/ as in time	
/v/ as in van	
/w/ as in wad	
/wh/ as in what	
/z/ as in zip	

Source: Adapted from Creaghead and Newman (1985) and Ling (1976).

nomena. Rules associated with the construct of stress enable listeners to perceive a particular syllable that is emphasized over the others. An adequate knowledge of the phonological system of English includes an intuitive knowledge of rules relating to the production of both segmental (phonemes) and suprasegmental aspects. As discussed later in this text, both segmental and suprasegmental knowledge seem to be important for the development of adequate, high-level literacy skills, especially if such skills assist in an understanding of phonics—the relationships between phonemes and their representations in print (Adams, 1990, 1994; Liberman, Shankweiler, & Liberman, 1989; Stanovich, 1991, 1992).

Morphology

Morphology is the study of morphemes, which can be described as the smallest segment of speech that carries meaning (Goodluck, 1991; Matthews, 1991). In this sense, morphology is related to phonology and is concerned with the structure of words. To put it another related way: Phonemes are the building blocks of a language and are combined to produce morphemes. Morphology is also influenced by and related to syntax, the order of words; for example, the use of tense (past or future) or number (plural) might be affected by the surrounding words or phrases (Brown, 1973; Crystal, 1997; deVilliers & deVilliers, 1978; Russell et al., 1976). Consider the following sentences:

1. The boy *win/won* the prize yesterday. (Past tense, *won*, is dictated by the word *yesterday*.)

2. The boy *win/wins* the prize! (The singular form of *win* is dictated by the noun phrase.)

Similar to phonology, morphology is concerned with the internal structure, or parts of words; however, in this case, the concern is with a minimal unit of meaning. For example, consider the following words that can be divided into meaningful parts:

unmoved	*un- move d*
walking	*walk ing*
girls	*girl s*
blueberry	*blue berry*
lovable	*lov[e] able*

With respect to these words, meanings can be assigned to all the parts, for example, *girl* (a female) and to *-s* (plurality; more than one).

With respect to morphology, there are a number of concepts to describe. The ones included in this section are allomorph, inflectional, and derivational morphemes; the traditional terms of *affix*, *prefix*, and *suffix*; bound and free morphemes; and word family.

Allomorph

Previously, the term *allophone* was mentioned in the discussion of phonology. There are also *allomorphs*, which refers to the variant forms of a morpheme and complicates this business of understanding morphology. For example, a morpheme (e.g., the plural morpheme) may assume variant shapes with respect to the words to which they are attached. These different shapes are called allomorphs of the morpheme. The plural morphological structure can be expressed as: *-s* as in *girls*, *-es* as in *boxes*, *-en* as in *oxen*, *-ren* as in *children*, and change of internal vowel as in *men*, *women*. Because of the influence of phonology, morphophonology is the study of the manner in which allomorphs are selected and represented in conventional orthography. Another common example is the pronunciation and expression of the past tense morpheme as in words such as *walked*, *rated*, and *jumped*.

The most interesting example is the phonetic forms associated with the past-tense morpheme such as *-ed* . This is of interest because, as will be seen in Chapter 6 on signed systems, the past-tense morphemes (and others) have caused considerable debate on how these variations (especially for irregular verbs) should be represented by the use of the so-called sign markers. The situation here is this: The past-tense morpheme *-ed* has three different pronunciations; *id* as in *wanted* because the preceding sound is /t / or /d/; *t* as in *balked* because the preceding sound is voiceless; and *d* as in *bowled* because the preceding sound is voiced. Should each example be represented by a different sign (i.e., sign marker)? Or should the same sign marker be used for all examples? What is the rationale for this decision? These have been and still are critical questions for the developers of the various signed systems.

Inflectional and Derivational Morphemes

The research discussed in this text on deaf and hard-of-hearing students is concerned mostly with two major divisions of morphology, inflectional and derivational. Inflectional morphology focuses on the manner in which words can vary (or be inflected) for grammatical purposes. Examples include plurality (singular/plural) and tense (past/present/future). In traditional grammar terminology, this was referred to as *accidence* (Curme, 1947). Within this framework, it was possible to talk about the inflection of nouns (*girl* to *girls*; The man is giving *his boy* a car), pronouns (as in reflexive pronouns such as *myself* and *himself*), adjectives (as in I bought a *black one*), verbs (as in voice: active [*I hit the ball*] and passive [*The ball was hit by me*]; and tense: I *walk, I walked, I have walked, I had walked,* etc.), and adverbs (as in *beautifully*). The word classes that are not inflected include prepositions, conjunctions, and interjections (see Table 2-3).

Derivational morphology addresses the manner in which words become new words as in the following examples: *lovable* from *love*, *development* from *develop*, *disengage* from *engage*, and *rewrite* from *write*. Derivational morphology plays a major role in reading programs that emphasize the use of structural analysis as a component of the word identification process. Typically, the focus might be on affixes, prefixes, suffixes, compound words (e.g., *baseball, ice cream, hot dog,* and *sidewalk*), and contractions (e.g., *don't, won't,* and *shouldn't*). With respect to the focus here, there are several ways in which new words can be constructed from already existing words. The examples below are taken from Crystal (1997).

- *prefixation*: an affix is placed before the base of the word, e.g., *disobey.*

- *suffixation*: an affix is placed after the base of the word, e.g., *kindness.*

- *conversion*: a word changes its class without any change of form, e.g., (the) *carpet* (noun) becomes (to) *carpet* (verb).

- *compounding*: two base forms are added together, e.g., *blackbird.*

- *reduplication*: a type of compound in which both elements are the same, or only sightly different, e.g., *goody-goody, wishy-washy, teeny-weeny.*

- *clippings*: an informal shortening of a word, often to a single syllable, e.g., *ad, gents, flu, telly.*

- *acronyms*: words formed from the initial letters of the words that make up a name, e.g., *NATO, UNESCO, radar* (= radio detection and ranging); a sub-type is an alphabetism, in which the different letters are pronounced, e.g., *VIP, DJ.*

- *blends*: two words merge into each other, e.g., *brunch* (from "breakfast" + "lunch"), *telex* ("teleprinter" + "exchange"). (p. 90)

Affix, Prefix, and Suffix

The reader has already been introduced to these terms as part of derivational morphology. A few additional remarks are made here. It should be clear that an affix is a morpheme that is added to the base or root word (e.g., a free morpheme—see following discussion), which results in a change of meaning.

A prefix is a type of affix that is attached to the beginning or to the left of a root or word part (typically, a free morpheme). Deighton (1959) constructed a list of about 70 commonly used prefixes, some of which have invariant meanings (i.e., only one meaning) and others with variant meanings (i.e., more than one meaning). Johnson and Pearson (1984) compiled a number of these prefixes that should be part of classroom instruction with respect to the ability level of students. For example, Johnson and Pearson (1984) recommended instruction (i.e., creative and meaningful) that focus on the following prefixes:

Invariant Prefixes

apo-	apoplexy, apogee
circum-	circumnavigate, circumvent
equi-	equidistant, equilibrium
extra-	extracurricular, extrasensory
intra-	intravenous, intramural
intro-	introspection, introvert
mal-	maladjusted, malapropism
non-	nonentity, nonprofit
syn-	synagogue, synapse, synonym

Variant (more than one meaning) but Common Prefixes

bi-	bicycle, biannual
de-	dethrone, deactivate
fore-	forewarn, forecast
in-	inept (irresponsible, illegal, immaterial), indoors
pre-	preschool, preadolescent, precaution, prearrange
pro-	pro-war, pro-life, proceed, project
semi-	semicircle, semiannual, semiabstract, semiautomatic
re-	redraw, rearrest, recall, reaction
un-	unable, unbecoming, unlock, untie (pp. 129–130)

A suffix is a type of affix that is attached at the end or the right of the root or word part. Banking on the work of Deighton (1959), suffixes can indicate the word class (part of speech) of words to which they are attached and/or provide additional clues to the meaning of a word. Some common noun suffixes include -*ance* as in *tolerance*, -*ence* as in *violence*, -*ation* (-*tion* and -*ion*) as in *motivation*, -*ism* as in *behaviorism*, -*dom* as in *kingdom*, -*ery* as in *drudgery*, -*mony* as in *harmony*, and -*ment* as in *development*. Some common adjective suffixes include -*est* as in *fastest*, -*fold* as in *tenfold*, -*scopic* as in *microscopic*, -*less* as in *helpless*, -*able* (-*ible* and -*ble*) as in *lovable*, -*like* as in *lifelike*, -*ous* as in *joyous*, and -*ful* as in *playful*. Again, it is recommended that the teacher include the common suffixes listed earlier and others as part of their vocabulary and reading instruction. One of the goals is to provide students with a tool for figuring out the meanings of unknown or slightly known words. The merits of this type of instruction, also known as structural analysis, is discussed briefly in Chapter 8 of this text.

Bound and Free Morphemes

Bound morphemes are morphemes that cannot occur alone or in isolation but need to be combined with at least one other morpheme (free or bound) in the formation of a word. Typically, bound morphemes are affixes such as prefixes (e.g., *in-* and *un-*) and suffixes (e.g., *-ly, -ment,* and *-ness*) and inflections (e.g., *-s, -ing,* and *-ed*). Thus, bound morphemes can be derivational or inflectional in nature. Many of the difficult words of English are combinations of free and bound morphemes. Consider the following examples: *disinfectant* (*dis-* + *infect* + *ant*), *deodorant* (*de-* + *odor* + *ant*), and *reinvestment* (*re-* + *invest* + *ment*). And, there are also words that contain only bound morphemes. Consider the word *irrevocable*, which has four morphemes. Three of the morphemes are affixes—two prefixes (*ir-* and *-re-*) and one suffix (*-able*). One morpheme is considered the root (*-voc-*).

Succinctly stated, a free morpheme represents the minimum notion of a word. For example, words that cannot be divided further into morphemes include *book, boy, cat, girl, no,* and *yes*. Some complex words contain both free morphemes and bound morphemes or bound morphemes and a root, as in the previous discussion of bound morphemes. In essence, the reader should now recognize that the discussion of bound and free morphemes is similar to a discussion of the use of terms such as affixes (prefix and suffix) and root or base words or word stems (see next section).

Word Family

The placement of words in a family is based on the root form of a word, for example, *bio* (life), *geo* (earth), *sect* (cut), *dict* (speak), *micro* (small), and *struct* (build). It is also often considered an effective teaching strategy that assists students in remembering words and in figuring out what a word could possibly mean. One scholar who has focused intensely on the development and instruction of this strategy is O'Rourke (1974), from which the following two examples are taken.

> Knowing the Greek root phil *(love) as in* philosopher *(lover of wisdom) helps the student generalize or remember the meaning of other* phil *words such as* philanthropist *(lover of mankind). Thus a* philatelist *"loves" stamps. People who "love" harmony or good music may listen to* philharmonic orchestra. *A flower that "loves" the shade is the* philodendron—

from Greek dendron—tree (i.e., tree-loving). Phil*adelphia is called the "city of brotherly love," from* phil *(love)* + adelphos *(brother). The transfer potential is great. The list may go on—*Anglophile, Francophile, philology, philogeny, philander, *etc. (O'Rourke, 1974, p. 101)*

The next example involves words with the root *gyn* meaning woman. As might be guessed, the list is practically endless: misogyny, philogyny, gynandrous, gynogenesis, gynecology, gynephobia, monogyny, gynecoid, gynospore, gynecocentric, gynocracy, polygyny, gynophore, gyniatrics, and gynarchy (O'Rourke, 1974).

The examples on word family should provide insights into the argument offered by some scholars that knowledge of morphology (i.e., via structural analysis) might assist in developing rapid word identification skills and in expanding knowledge of word and word parts for readers and writers. For example, with this type of knowledge in hand, it is suspected that students would use a wide variety and more creative words in their written language productions. There is still a great deal of controversy surrounding these assertions. It is still not clear just how much knowledge a reader and writer needs with respect to morphology.

Controversy notwithstanding, it seems that a little knowledge can go a long way. In fact, O'Rourke (1974) argued that students become more sensitive to the idea of word parts and even begin to speculate on "words that could be words, but may not be real words" (i.e., made-up words that do not violate phonological or morphological principles). With a little practice (and some courage), it is possible for students to benefit from a basic understanding of word families. Consider one last example of this idea: The root *cred* means believe and contributes to the meaning of the following words (O'Rourke, 1974):

> *cred* it
> *cred* o
> *cred* itor
> *cred* ence
> ac*cred* it
> *cred* entials
> *cred* ibility
> *cred* itable
> *cred* ulity
> in*cred* ulous
> dis*cred* it (p. 67)

And a Little More About Morphemes

Some words that cannot be divided further into meaningful parts (i.e., have no internal grammatical structure) include: *cat, boy, no, yes,* and *beet.* These words are free morphemes, as discussed previously. It is possible to analyze the various sounds of the words in this list; however, none of the sounds has a meaning by itself or in isolation. Linguists are still debating what to do with words (e.g., irregular nouns and verbs) that seem to have internal parts but defy the use of traditional methods for identifying the parts; for example, consider words such as *feet, women, deer* (plural use), and so on.

In one sense, an understanding of morphology (or even phonology, syntax, or semantics) might not really be complete without a good understanding of what a word is. However, questions such as what is a word, what is a word meaning, and even what is a meaning have been the topics of ongoing linguistic, philosophical debates, which—albeit interesting and important—are beyond the scope of this text. As mentioned previously, the study of morphology is important for understanding the development of the English signed systems (e.g., signed English and signing exact English) used with deaf and hard-of-hearing children. The various signed systems are purportedly based on the morphosyntactic properties of standard written English; however, the developers have had to make some difficult decisions, some of which do not seem to be supported by current understanding of morphology and some of which are not really consistent with the so-called rules associated with the various systems. Nevertheless, the reason for the existence of several signed systems is due to the fact that the systems have different rules for executing signs, including the use of inflectional signs as well as the construction of new signs via sign markers (similar to derivational morphemes) (Wilbur, 1987). It is also critical to stress that the morphology of the signed systems is different from that of ASL. More important, the differences across the signed systems seem to be arbitrary (i.e., based on the perceptions of their creators) and are not reflective of dialectical differences that are often associated with a language. (The exception here is the use of cued speech, which is not a signed system, but does use hand signals. However, these hand signals, plus facial positions, deal with the phonological system, and the execution can vary according to dialects. See discussion of cued speech/language in Chapter 5).

Additional discussion and examples on morphology can be located in the following sources: Deighton (1959), Johnson and Pearson (1984), O'Rourke (1974), and Russell et al. (1976). Table 2-5 provides some major highlights discussed in this section on morphology.

TABLE 2-5 Highlights of Morphology

- Morphology is the study of morphemes—the smallest segment of speech that carries meaning.

- Morphology is concerned with the internal structure or parts of words.

- Allomorph refers to the possible phonetic forms of a morpheme. As an example, the English possessive ending, spelled *s,* has three allomorphs: /s/, /z/, and /əz/. The particular allomorph that is used depends on the final sound of the word.

- Inflectional morphology is the study of word variations or inflections such as plurality (*girl, girls*) and tense (*walk*—present; *walked*—past). Thus, inflections refer to changes in the root or base word (i.e., uninflected, citation form) to express syntactic functions and relationships. These changes do not affect the meaning of the root or base word.

- Derivational morphology deals with the construction of new words, typically via additions of specific morphemes (e.g., *in-, re-, -ment,* and *-ness*). Derivational morphemes may change the meaning of a word as in *clear* and *unclear* or indicate the part of speech (form class) of a word, for example, noun suffixes such as *-ance* in *tolerance* and *-dom* in *freedom.* It should be clear that these are examples of different words, each with its own grammatical properties or aspects.

- Affix is considered a bound morpheme; that is, a morpheme that cannot occur alone or in isolation. A prefix is a type of affix that is attached to the beginning or to the left of a word stem as in *re*ice, *un*happy, and *in*complete. A suffix is attached to the right of the word stem as in judg*ment*, lov*able*, and like*ness*.

- Free morpheme represents the minimal notion of a word. Examples of free morphemes are *cat, dog,* and *box.*

- Word family refers to the grouping of words based on the root form of a word. The root form *cred* leads to the grouping of words such as *credit, credence, credentials*, and *credibility.*

Note: For additional information, see Deighton (1959), O'Rourke (1974), and Johnson & Pearson (1984).

Syntax

Syntax refers to rules that governed the order or arrangement of words. This arrangement reveals meaningful relationships within and between sentences— that is, the arrangement concerns word order, sentence organization, relationships between words, and so on. Similar to the issue of word, it is difficult to define a sentence with respect to traditional terminology such as subject (i.e., topic) and predicate (i.e., what is said about the topic). Obviously, this is not a problem for some sentences such as: *I am happy* and *Mary is an intelligent woman.* It is difficult, however, to use these traditional notions for sentences such as: *It's raining* and *It's a wonderful life!* In addition, the topic may not really be clear in sentences with the following construction: *Erik asked Peter for a computer.* It is possible to argue that there are three topics, *Erik, Peter,* and the *computer!*

Perhaps a better way, albeit still not perfectly clear, to describe a sentence is that it must contain at least a noun phrase (NP) and a verb phrase (VP). A noun phrase contains at least a noun with the option of one or more determiners (e.g., adjectives). The NP may also contain an embedded sentence and other NPs, as well as VPs, within the framework of transformational generative grammar. A VP consists of an auxiliary (e.g., modal, tense, or aspect: see "Verbs") and a verb and may contain noun phrases, embedded sentences, and prepositional phrases.

Consider the following examples.

1. The young boy runs fast.
2. That color is ugly for a car.

In Sentence 1, the NP contains two determiners [*The* and *young*] that describe the quality of the noun—*boy.* In Sentence 2, there are actually two NPs: *That color* and *a car.* In the first NP, *that* is a determiner describing the noun *color.* The second NP (*a car*) is part of the VP *is ugly for a car.* The word *a* is the determiner and *car* is the noun. In this sentence, the VP contains a preposition (*for*) and a NP (*a car*). In the first sentence, the VP is *runs fast,* which contains a verb and auxiliary (*runs; run + s*), and an adverb (*fast*).

With respect to sentences, syntax rules specify the word combinations that are acceptable or grammatical and also which combinations are not. For example, in the following sentences, 1 is grammatically acceptable, whereas 2 is not.

1. The storyteller told a story.
2. Storyteller The story told a.

As mentioned previously, each sentence must contain a noun phrase and verb phrase, and the rules of syntax specify the elements (i.e., word classes, etc.)

as well as the relationships between the two phrases. In Sentence 1, *The storyteller* is the noun phrase and *told a story* is the verb phrase.

Most syntactic investigations have focused on the relations expressed at the sentence level (i.e., sentence comprehension). This is "where the most important grammatical relationships are expressed" (Crystal, 1997, p. 94).

Linear and Hierarchical Categories

For the purposes of this text, it is useful to divide syntactic relations into two major categories: linear and hierarchical. Although descriptions of these terms vary (Crystal, 1997), linear structures are defined here as being fairly simple constructions that can be interpreted in a left-to-right fashion, for example, subject-verb-object (SVO), as exemplified in the following sentences:

3. The boy hit the ball.
4. Mary read a book.
5. John gave Mary a rose.
6. The man smoked a pipe.
7. The woman drove a truck.

Hierarchical structures are complex and cannot be interpreted in a simple SVO fashion. Consider the following sentences as examples:

8. The boy who kissed the girl ran away.
9. The light on the blue police car turned.
10. The girl was mauled by the pit bull.
11. Visiting professors can be boring.
12. That the man was sad was perceived by the woman.

The competent language user understands that the subjects of Sentences 8 and 9 are *The boy who kissed the girl* and *The light on the blue police car*, respectively. These subjects are also noun phrases. In Sentence 10, *the pit bull* is the performer of an action, whereas *the girl* is the recipient. Sentence 11 is ambiguous; that is, there are at least two interpretations: *Professors who visit* can be boring and [The act of] *visiting professors* can be boring. There is also a third interpretation that is analogous to the academic position visiting scholar or visiting professor. In other words, a person who is a faculty member from one university and who has been invited to another different university to teach classes and so on might receive the title *visiting scholar* or *visiting professor.* Thus, these *visiting professors* can be boring. In Sentence 12, *the woman* is the person who performs the act of perception. In addition, it is clear to the native user of English that it is not *sadness* or *the man* that is perceived; rather, it is *the sadness of the man.*

The issue of noun phrase and verb phrase can become quite complicated in hierarchical embedded sentences if one ascribes to the notion of transformation generative grammar. Consider the following example: The man who is beating the drum plays the violin.

In this sentence, there is a main NP and a main VP as follows: NP = *The man who is beating the drum* and VP = *plays the violin.*

According to transformational grammar, the relative clause *who is beating the drum* is part of an embedded sentence structure representing: *The man is beating the drum.* Thus, before applying the transformation (i.e., the relative clause transformation), there are two additional NPs: NP = *The man* (referring to "who") and NP = *the drum.*

Also within the embedded sentence there is a VP—*is beating the drum.* This VP contains a verb plus auxiliary (*is beating*) and a NP (*the drum*), mentioned previously. The main VP, after the main NP, contains a verb (*plays*) and a NP (*the violin*). Now that the reader has become somewhat skilled in NPs and VPs, perhaps she or he can explain (i.e., parsed, etc.) the following grammatical sentence (for fun, of course): It must have appeared to them that I was incompetent although I thought that I have tried really hard to disprove that notion.

As discussed later in the text, many deaf and some hard-of-hearing students have had enormous difficulty comprehending hierarchical sentences, especially on a sentential level (see review in Russell et al., 1976). Much of the research on syntax and deafness has been conducted by Quigley and his collaborators and has involved major syntactic structures such as negation, conjunction, disjunction and alternation, question formation, pronominalization, reflexivization, verbs, complementation, relativization, and nominalization (see Table 2-6 for examples of these structures).

In general, as discussed in Chapter 8, deaf children's and adolescents' difficulty with these structures seems to stem from the fact that they apply, indiscriminately, a subject-verb-object strategy to interpret the sentences. Consider the following two sentences:

1. The boy who kissed the girl ran away.
2. The light on the blue car turned.

In these sentences, it is not uncommon for students to state that it was the girl who ran away (Sentence 1) and that it was the car that turned (Sentence 2).

The Influence of Syntax

Chomsky (1957, 1965, 1975, 1988) revolutionized the field of linguistics with his study of the syntactic component of a language. Chomsky's notion of

TABLE 2-6 A Few Examples of Syntactic Structures

Structure	Examples
Negation	The woman can *not* go to the opera.
	The girl did *not* see the movie.
	The man does *not* have any money.
Conjunction	*John and Mary* ran a marathon.
	The boy *caught and cleaned* the fish.
	The day is *dark and gloomy*.
	I *write books and play the flute*.
	The man likes *ice cream and cookies*.
	The soldiers move *quickly and quietly*.
Disjunction and alternation	I read the book, *but* you did not.
	The food was delicious *but* cold.
	He is *either* crazy *or* intelligent.
	Either Mary Beth *or* I will play the piano.
Question formation	Do you like to drink coffee?
	Were you at the movies yesterday?
	Where is my pipe?
	What are you talking about?
	You ate the cookie, didn't you?
	The boy doesn't look happy, does he?
Pronominalization	Jerry is my friend and *he* lost some books.
	He is my friend and Jerry lost some books.
	The man who saw Mary kissed *her*. (ambiguous!)
Reflexivization	I think the woman shot *herself* in the foot.
	You should have faith in *yourself*.
	I did this *myself*.
Verb processes (e.g., passive voice)	The dog was washed by the boy.
	The dog was bit by the cat.
	The window was broken.
Complementation	*That Mary was happy* disappointed Stephanie.
	It disappointed Stephanie *that Mary was happy*.
	For Jean to be happy is highly unusual.
	It is highly unusual *for Jean to be happy*.
	Erik knows *Peter is a hard worker*.

(continues)

Relativization	I saw the boy *who jumped*.
	The boy *who kissed the girl* ran away.
	The man *whom the woman hit* was unhappy.
	I saw the boy *whom the girl kissed*.
Nominalization	*The sound of the siren* shocked the little boy.
	The boy's laughter was heard for miles.
	The people heard *the screams of the little girl*.

Note: For additional information, see Russell, Quigley, and Power (1976) and Quigley, Steinkamp, Power, and Jones (1978).

transformational generative grammar, which has gone through several revisions (Cairns, 1996; Cook & Newson, 1996; Culicover, 1997), is typically a syntax-based grammar. In other words, Chomsky asserted that syntax plays a major role in explaining the grammar of a language and most specifically in understanding the mind of the language user. Details on Chomsky's contributions are presented in Chapter 3. Cairns (1996) offered an eloquent synopsis of these contributions:

> *The papers he wrote in the early 1960s claimed that language is not simply a collection of speech sounds organized into words and phrases; nor is it a complex chain of speech behaviors shaped in the infant; nor can it vary without limit. He said that human language comprises a complex set of rules that are known by speakers of a language and used by them to construct and perceive sentences in that language. Chomsky argued that linguistics should be thought of as theoretical psychology, and that psychology should be considered a theory of mind rather than of behavior. Further, he claimed, there is a fundamental similarity among all human languages, and that similarity is rooted in human biology. Children are not taught language by reward and nonreward, but acquire it naturally through an interaction between inborn structures and experience with the language of the child's environment.* (p. 17)

Reactions to Chomsky's view of syntax per se have catapulted two other components of language, semantics and pragmatics, into the limelight. These two components have captured the attention of a number of psycholinguists and other researchers who are interested in understanding how a child develops language, especially within a social-interactive milieu. Semantics and pragmatics are considered to be two different language components; however, as is discussed next, there seems to be some overlap between these two domains.

Semantics

One of the classic texts on language development provides a framework that focuses on three broad concepts, mentioned previously, form, content, and use (Bloom & Lahey, 1978). Thus far, this section of the chapter has briefly covered the form of the language, that is, phonology, morphology, and syntax. Language content pertains to semantics, and language use refers to pragmatics. Semantics is the study of meaning in language (Crystal, 1997; Lyons, 1995; Pustejovsky & Boguraev, 1996). To simplify, meaning can occur at several levels: word (or word parts), phrase, sentence, and beyond the sentence. It could be argued that comprehension, whether of speech, print, or other media, is essentially the construction of meaning or the construction of reality.

Meaning, of course, is difficult to define and just as difficult to assess. There seems to be no question that meaning is critical to understand language acquisition; yet it might be surprising to most readers that linguists have only recently seriously considered the role of meaning in language.

Chapter 3 illustrates how general linguistic theories of semantics have been influenced by the thinking of philosophers, logicians, and cognitive psychologists (Baars, 1986; Crystal, 1997; Goodluck, 1991; Steinberg, 1982). In essence, semantic theorists argue that semantics is primary and syntax secondary; that is, semantics determines syntactic representation. Steinberg (1982) provided an early, classic description of semantics theorists' objections to Chomsky's notion of generative grammar. Semantic theorists:

> *argue that syntax cannot be done independently of semantics. Furthermore, they see little need for two levels of syntax. They advocate abandonment of Deep Structure and Base rules, holding that what a grammar must do is to relate the semantic level of structure . . . to a syntactic level of structure, Surface Structure. They posit that this be done with a set of transformational rules and a lexicon. Transformational rules might usefully be regarded as constituting the "syntactic" component of their grammar. The Transformational rules and the Lexicon are viewed as continually interacting so as to produce a final structure, Surface Structure. This view sharply contrasts with that of Chomsky where lexical items are inserted all at once into an already completed tree structure (Deep Structure). (pp. 48–49)*

As implied here, one of the most interesting areas within semantics is how children acquire word meanings—that is, the development of their lexicons. This has been an area of intense research (Pustejovsky & Boguraev, 1996) and considerable controversy and has focused on the notions of semantic features and selection restrictions. Semantic features refer to the aspects of meaning that define or characterize the word. For example, the semantic features of *father* include *parent* and *male*. One of these two features (*parent*) is shared with the word *mother* and the other with *man*. In this example, neither word, *father* and *mother*, shares both features, and, of course, there needs to be unshared features to have different words. Selection restrictions refer to features (often formulated as rules or conventions) that prohibit certain word combinations due to the meaningless or even redundancy of these combinations. It is not difficult to create examples: female mother, male father, or—a favorite commercial slogan—"kill roaches dead."

The notion of semantic features has become operationized in the field of literacy, as can be seen in the widespread classroom use of semantic elaboration techniques such as word maps, semantic maps, semantic feature analysis, word webs, and semantic webs (see lucid examples in Heimlich & Pittelman, 1986; Pearson & Johnson, 1978). It is sometimes forgotten that features is also important for understanding other instructional notions such as synonyms, antonyms, analogies, and categorization/classification (see Table 2-7 for additional discussions and examples of these terms).

TABLE 2-7 A Sample of Semantic Aspects

Term	Description/Examples
Synonyms	Words that have similar but not identical meanings Examples of pairs of synonyms include: *happy—glad, unhappy—sad, large—big, smart—intelligent*
Antonyms	Words that are opposite or nearly opposite in meaning Examples of pairs of antonyms include: *hot—cold, dull—sharp, big—small, smart—dumb, night—day*
Analogies	Problem-solving activities requiring judgments about the relationships among two pairs of words Examples from Johnson and Pearson (1984) include: 1. Characteristics: *Rain* is to *wet* as *sun* is to *dry.* 2. Part/Whole: *Leaf* is to *tree* as *feather* is to *bird.* 3. Whole/Part: *Cup* is to *handle* as *clock* is to *hands.* 4. Location: *Teacher* is to *classroom* as *sailor* is to *ship.* 5. Action/Object: *Run* is to *track* as *swim* is to *pool.* 6. Agent-action or Object: *Teacher* is to *students* as *doctor* is to *patients.* 7. Class or Synonym: *Smell* is to *sniff* as *see* is to *look.*

8. Familial: *Uncle* is to *nephew* as *aunt* is to *niece*.
9. Grammatical: *Hear* is to *heard* as *look* is to *looked*.
10. Temporal or Sequential: *Fifth* is to *first* as *twenty-fifth* is to *fifth*.
11. Antonyms: *Smile* is to *happy* as *frown* is to *sad*. (p. 47)

Classification	Arrangements of words, ideas, pictures, or objects into groups or categories based on specific (predetermined) criteria Examples include:

Class/Example

food:	*carrot, milk, hamburger, potatoes, bread*
vehicles:	*car, bus, train, bicycle, truck*
mammals:	*cats, bats, horses, pigs, humans*

Word/Feature

car:	*tire, window, door, hood, engine*
elephant:	*trunk, tusks, tail, legs, ears*
computer:	*monitor, keyboard, mouse*

Note: Other types of semantic aspects include word maps, semantic maps, and semantic feature analysis. See D. Johnson and Pearson (1984) for more details.

There has been some research in the field of deafness on vocabulary development, including the acquisition of words with multiple meanings (polysemy) (see Paul, 1998a). Although this line of research has contributed to the understanding of semantic development as well as to the importance of vocabulary knowledge for reading comprehension, future researchers need to be concerned with determining how words—lexemes or lexical items—are processed, organized, and retrieved from the mind (see readable accounts in Aitchison, 1994; Crystal, 1997; for research review, see Balota, Flores D'Arcais, & Rayner, 1990). Aside from contributing to the understanding of general language acquisition, further developments in this area should increase researchers' knowledge of word identification in literacy. As discussed in Chapter 8 (also see Paul, 1998a), there seems to be some confusion between word identification skills (phonics, structural analysis, etc.) and lexical access processes, although there might be a relation between these two entities. Specifically, it is the nature of children's lexical access processes that have determined the importance of phonemic awareness in English reading and has led to the debate on how and if phonemic awareness can and should be taught. This debate is also applicable to deaf and hard-of-hearing children, and it might offer a compelling argument for the difficulty that many children have in learning to read and write well.

In essence, research on lexical access has been concerned with, at least, the nature of the retrieval routes for accessing words from memory. A number of hypotheses have been proffered, for example, phonological, morphological, semantic, visual (or orthographic), and dual (typically, phonological and visual). For several reasons, the semantic and the orthographic hypotheses are deemed appropriate for deaf and hard-of-hearing children due to their difficulty in using the sound system—that is, phonology. Ironically, orthography (representation of sounds via printed symbols; dealing with spelling and letters) is influenced or assisted by and is related to phonology. In any case, good readers and writers need to be aware of more than just the semantic features of words to develop rapid, automatic, word identification skills. Ehri (1991) provided an eloquent description of lexical access for reading purposes:

> *Speakers of a language possess a* lexicon—*that is, a store of words held in memory. When people read words by sight or lexical access, they utilize information that is remembered about the words from previous experiences reading these words. Upon seeing the spellings, readers access the identities of the words in memory. These identities include the word's pronunciation, its meaning, its syntactic identity (i.e., its typical grammatical role in sentences), and its orthographic identity (i.e., information remembered about its conventional spelling). (p. 384)*

There are wide-reaching influences associated with the study of semantics. For example, in psychology, there are a number of memory models involving the use of notions such as networks, frames, and scripts (see discussions in Johnson-Laird, 1988; Rumelhart, McClelland, & the PDP Research Group, 1986; Shadbolt, 1988). These knowledge or memory models have had a tremendous influence on theories of reading acquisition (Samuels & Kamil, 1984) and on the thought/language debate in language acquisition (see Chapter 3). Semantics is also a major aspect in many theories of cognitive development. In fact, there is considerable overlap between cognitive and semantic developments in the early language acquisition of children (e.g., see Chapter 4 of this text).

Table 2-8 provides a summary of highlights for this section on semantics with some additional information relevant to this domain.

Pragmatics

Pragmatics is the study of the use of language, particularly within a communicative situation, milieu, or context (see readable discussions in Crystal, 1997; Owens, 1996). Two philosophers who have played an influential role in the understanding of pragmatics are Austin and Searle. Austin (1962), a British

TABLE 2-8 A Few Highlights on Semantics

- Semantics is the study of meaning in language.

- Meaning is not an entity separate from language. Thus, modern linguists analyzed the manner in which words and sentences are used in specific contexts.

- Semantics is not directly concerned with the study of the external world or its conceptualization.

- Semantic models have influenced the understanding of reading acquisition, including metacognitive development.

- Much attention in this field has been devoted to the acquisition of word or vocabulary knowledge. However, recently, there has been a focus on the analysis of sentences or "at least, of those aspects of sentence meaning that cannot be predicted from the 'sum' of the individual lexemes" (Crystal, 1997).

Examples of Sentence Meaning (Crystal, 1997)

Prosodic meaning. The way a sentence is said, using the prosody of the language, can radically alter the meaning. Each of these sentences carries a different implication, as the stress (indicated by capitals) moves:

John's bought a red CAR (not a red bicycle).

John's bought a RED *car* (not a green one).

JOHN'S *bought a red car* (not Michael).

The prosody informs us of what information in the sentence can be taken for granted (is "given") and what is of special significance (is "new").

Grammatical meaning. The categories that are established by grammatical analysis can also be analysed from a semantic point of view. A sentence such as *John read a book yesterday* consists of Subject + Verb + Object + Adverbial; but it can also be analysed as an "actor" performing an "action" on a "goal" at a certain "time." There is a great deal to be said about the "semantic roles" played by syntactic elements—an area of study that falls uneasily between semantics and grammar.

Pragmatic meaning. The function performed by the sentence in a discourse needs to be considered. The meaning of the sentence—*There's some chalk*

(continues)

(Table 2-8 continued)

on the floor—seems plain enough; but in some situations it would be interpreted as a statement of fact ("Have you seen any chalk?") and in others as a veiled command (as when a teacher might point out the chalk to a child in class).

Social meaning. The choice of a sentence may directly affect the social relationships between the participants. We may convey such impressions as politeness, rudeness, competence, or distance, and this will affect our status and role within a community. "What do you mean by talking to me like that?" is a question that raises larger issues than the meaning of the individual lexemes and sentences that have been used.

Propositional meaning. Perhaps the most important trend in modern semantics is the investigation of sentence meaning using ideas derived from philosophy and logic. In this kind of approach, a careful distinction is drawn between sentences and propositions. A proposition is the unit of meaning that identifies the subject matter of a statement; it describes some state of affairs, and takes the form of a declarative sentence, e.g., *Mary loves Michael.* In such theories as "truth-conditional semantics," sentences are analysed in terms of the underlying propositions they express, and these propositions are then tested to see whether they would be true or false in relation to the real world. (p. 107)

---

philosopher, was one of the first scholars to focus attention on functions of speech utterances (known as *speech acts*) in social interactions. These utterances are considered actions (i.e., performatives). Examples include statements that contain the words, *I believe, I promise,* and *I apologize.*

For a speech act to be valid (or meaningful), certain conditions must be met or satisfied. For example, if a child utters "Help me," there needs to be a situation in which she or he needs help and there needs to be a person who can help. The importance of pragmatics becomes painfully obvious in many children with language disorders—especially children with autism, who may not have developed a framework for understanding language use in social interactions.

Not all utterances are performatives. Consider statements such as the following:

1. Mary should apologize for that stupid remark!

2. John ought to give back some of his riches.

In these examples, Sentence 1 does not make an apology, and Sentence 2 does not mean that John will give back some of his money. These statements are merely opinions.

Searle (1976) studied extensively the effects of speech utterances on the behaviors of both speakers and listeners. His theory of speech acts, particularly his classification of illocutionary acts (the act performed after the speaker's utterances), has influenced a long line of research on pragmatics, especially in children who attempt to deal with language ambiguity by asking for clarification (see discussion in Ninio & Snow, 1996). Although there are a number of possible illocutionary acts, there have been attempts to develop a small number of categories. Searle (1976) delineated five basic types: representatives, directives, commissives, expressives, and declarations (see Table 2-9 for further explanations).

As discussed in Chapters 3 and especially 4, a number of scholars have argued that the social function of language (i.e., pragmatics) is so critical in determining the form of the utterances. Clearly, any description of language needs to include a discussion of pragmatics. Indeed, it has been argued that language only develops as a consequent of social and communicative interactions.

In addition to investigating purposive and intentional communicative interactions, researchers have focused on how children learn to adapt to listener's knowledge and perspectives with strategies such as asking for clarification or requesting information (see review in Ninio & Snow, 1996). This is critical for repairing what is often called communicative breakdowns. A number of pragmatics behaviors have been identified in the communicative interactions of young children, for example, requesting, showing off, labeling, repeating, negating, and so on (Thompson, Biro, Vethivelu, Pious, & Hatfield, 1987). Descriptions of some of these behaviors are as follows (Thompson et al., 1987):

Requesting: *Solicitation of a service from a listener.*

Repeating: *Repetition of part or all of previous adult utterance. Child does not wait for a response.*

Negating: *Denial, resistance to, or rejection by child of adult statement, request, or question. (pp. 11, 13)*

Owens (1996) provided a good readable description of the range of research in the area of pragmatics, especially with respect to the maintenance and repair of communicative interactions:

Pragmatic rules govern a number of conversational interactions: sequential organization and coherence of conversations, repair of errors, role, and speech acts. . . . Organization and coherence of conversations include taking turns; opening, maintaining, and closing a conversation;

*establishing and maintaining a topic; and making relevant contribu-
tions to the conversation. Repair includes giving and receiving feedback and correcting conversational errors. The listener attempts to keep
the speaker informed of the status of the communication. If the listener
doesn't understand or is confused, he might assume a quizzical expression or say, "Huh?" Role skills include establishing and maintaining a
role and switching linguistic codes for each role. In some conversations
you are dominant, as with a small child, and in others you are not,
as with your parents, and you adjust your language accordingly. Finally,
speech acts include coding of intentions relative to the communicative
context. (p. 25)*

There seems to be some overlap between pragmatics and other language
components or areas of language inquiry. For example, both pragmatics and
semantics are concerned with the intentions of the language user and the
background knowledge about the world of both speakers and listeners as they
interact. There are also overlaps between pragmatics and areas such as psycholinguistics and discourse analysis (Crystal, 1997). The analysis of conversations, for example, is within the purview of both pragmatics and discourse
analysis (also see Table 2-9 for additional information on the overlapping areas).

In sum, pragmatics is not considered a part of language structure (or form)
in the same way as phonology, morphology, syntax, and semantics. A good
illustration of this assertion can be seen in the fact that pragmatics errors do
not affect the rules of these other language components. Nevertheless, pragmatics is intricately connected to the other language domains. As is discussed
in Chapter 4, pragmatics is essential for language development. Researchers
still do not have a clear picture of the nature and extent of this constantly
evolving and growing language domain. According to Crystal (1997):

*Pragmatics is not at present a coherent field of study. A large number
of factors govern our choice of language in social interaction, and it
is not yet clear what they all are, how they are best interrelated, and
how best to distinguish them from other recognized areas of linguistic
enquiry. (p. 120)*

Table 2-9 provides a summary of major highlights of pragmatics and
includes other pertinent information related to this language domain.

FINAL REMARKS

How much should language teachers know about language? What is it that
they should know? Is knowledge about language similar to knowledge about

TABLE 2-9 A Few Highlights on Pragmatics

- Pragmatics is the study of the use of language, particularly with.. a communicative situation, milieu, or context.

- Pragmatics guides the use of language during social interactions, specifically the use and selection of words, sentence constructions, and content of messages.

- Pragmatics has been influenced by the theory of speech acts (Searle, 1976). In analyzing speech acts, there is typically a threefold process. First, the analyst recognizes the existence of the locutionary act; that is, a communication act has taken place—something has been uttered and/or performed. Next, the analyst examines the effects of the communicative act. What action is performed as a result of the utterance or communicative act? If saying = doing (e.g., promising, warning), then this is classified as an illocutionary act. Finally, the analyst examines the effects of the speaker's utterance on the listener or receiver. The eliciting of the effects—laughing, crying, performing, and so on—is referred to as the perlocutionary act. There might be a discrepancy between the illocutionary act and the perlocutionary action. For example, you might provide sound advice on a business deal (illocutionary), but the advice is ignored (perlocutionary).

- Searle (1976) identified five basic types of illocutionary acts (although there are literally numbers of them). These are described as follows:

  1. *Representatives.* The speaker/presenter is committed in varying degrees to the truthfulness of a proposition. For example, the speaker/presenter might affirm, warn, document, or deny something.

  2. *Directives.* The speaker/presenter attempts to persuade a listener/receiver to perform an act. For example, the speaker/presenter might render a request, demand, or challenge.

  3. *Commissives.* The speaker/presenter is committed in varying degrees to performing a particular act or course of action. For example, the speaker/presenter might guarantee, vow, or promise.

  4. *Expressives.* The speaker/presenter expresses an attitude about a particular state of affairs. For example, the speaker/presenter might use language to express an apology or gratitude (thanks), to welcome or congratulate someone, or to express regret or disgust.

(continues)

(Table 2-9 continued)

5. *Declarations.* The speaker/presenter alters or modifies the current situation (i.e., status or condition) solely by making an utterance such as *I resign* or *I quit, I declare you to be. . .* , or *You're promoted!*

- According to Crystal (1997), there are several areas of overlap with pragmatics as follows:

Semantics. Pragmatics and semantics both take into account such notions as the intentions of the speaker, the effects of an utterance on listeners, the implications that follow from expressing something in a certain way, and the knowledge, beliefs, and presuppositions about the world upon which speakers and listeners rely when they interact.

Stylistics and sociolinguistics. These fields overlap with pragmatics in their study of the social relationships which exist between participants, and of the way extralinguistics setting, activity, and subject-matter can constrain the choice of linguistic features and varieties.

Psycholinguistics. Pragmatics and psycholinguistics both investigate the psychological states and abilities of the participants that will have a major effect upon their performance—such factors as attention, memory, and personality.

Discourse analysis. Both discourse analysis and pragmatics are centrally concerned with the analysis of conversation, and share several of the philosophical and linguistic notions that have been developed to handle this topic (such as the way information is distributed within a sentence, deictic forms [e.g., use of pronouns and time markers] or the notion of conversation "maxims" [e.g., see Grice, 1975]). (p. 120)

- Dialects and registers. Dialects refer to spoken variations of a language. These variations are influenced by several factors, for example, geography (i.e., regional dialects) or personal characteristics such as education, age, gender, race, and class (social dialects). By definition, dialects are understandable by speakers of the language despite differences in pronunciations, grammar, or lexicon. Registers refer to variations within the speaker/user according to the demands/requirements of specific social and communicative situations. For example, informal language (use of colloquialisms) may be used in the home, whereas more formal language (more sophisticated syntax) might be used in lecture halls of universities.

Note: For additional information on these and other issues, see Crystal (1997).

other so-called rigorous content areas such as chemistry, physics, or mathematics? Or is it comparable to knowledge in areas such as psychology, sociology, and anthropology? What about the contributions of philosophy? Do the answers to these questions—or the nature of the questions themselves—impact the manner in which language courses should be taught in university-level education or training programs?

These questions and others are still controversial in the education of deaf and hard-of-hearing students and even in teacher education programs at the university level. The issue becomes even more complex when consideration is given to the fact that English might need to be taught as a first or second language to many of these deaf and hard-of-hearing students in public schools, assuming that English—or any other language—can be taught at all. Indeed, perspectives on whether a language can be taught also influence what it is that teachers should know about a language as well as how they should proceed with the teaching of it in classroom settings.

Historically, teachers of deaf and hard-of-hearing students have always considered themselves mainly as teachers of language. However, this perspective might be changing due to the need for qualified teachers of other content areas such as reading, writing, science, and mathematics. In any case, within the purview of teachers of language, it is still not clear what teachers should know and how they should teach language.

This chapter's intention is to expose readers to a general overview of the functions and structures of language. The text is selective and brief because it is too easy to become overwhelmed by the wealth of information available on this topic. Indeed, it was difficult to make choices, but hopefully the information is sufficient for readers to obtain a basic understanding.

The chapter has two major sections: functions and structures. Summaries of major points are provided throughout the chapter. Here is an overall synopsis.

Language Functions

- The most obvious language function is communication; however, there are several other critical functions that entail personal, social, and political identities. A number of factors influence the nature of these identities—for example, geographical location, age, gender, education, vocation, sexual orientation, race/ethnicity, and so on. Not to be forgotten in the area of language functions is the fact that language is a tool for thought.

- Within the communication function, the chapter delineates two types of contexts: contextualized and decontextualized. Contextualization refers to live, through-the-air exchanges, whereas decontextualization refers to the capture of exchanges or information either in print (script literacy) or electronically (videotapes, audiotapes, and compact discs).

- Literate thought—the ability to think reflectively, logically, rationally, and creatively—seems to be independent of mode of information (i.e., contextualized or decontextualized). However, a learned level of literate thought—associated with Western culture—requires the ability to deal with decontextualized captured information.

Language Structures

- This section provides information on the following language structures: phonology, morphology, syntax, semantics, and pragmatics.

- Phonology is concerned with the building blocks of a language. For spoken language, this entails elements of the sound system, whereas for signed languages, this involves elements of manual and nonmanual movements. If students cannot access these building blocks, it is hypothesized that they will not develop or internalize the structure of language. Knowledge of phonology seems to be crucial for understanding the alphabet writing system of English.

- Morphology is concerned with minimal meaning elements, labeled *morphemes*. The focus is on words and their internal parts. Along with phonology, morphology seems to be crucial for the understanding of orthography (i.e., the arrangement of letters on the page; graphemes). This knowledge enables readers/writers to become proficient in conventional spelling of words. The concept of morphology has played a major, albeit controversial, role in the development of the English signed systems.

- Syntax refers to the order or arrangement of words in a sentence. The linguist/philosopher Chomsky revolutionized the thinking on the importance of syntax. Two categories of syntax were discussed: linear and hierarchical. Linear structures are fairly simple constructions that can be interpreted in a left-to-right fashion using a subject-verb-object strategy. Hierarchical structures contained embedded structures such as phrases, clauses, and sentences and cannot be interpreted in a SVO fashion. Deaf students have enormous difficulty with hierarchical structures due to their persistent use of a SVO strategy (as well as other reasons).

- Semantics is the study of meaning in language. The area of semantics has had wide-reaching influences in a number of disciplines or scholarly fields such as reading, writing, cognitive development, language-thought debates, and the domain of pragmatics. Traditionally, much of the focus in semantics has been on lexical development—that is, the acquisition of words and their meanings. However, the recent ongoing focus seems to be on an analysis of meaning in sentences. This type of analysis has become quite complex due to the need for understanding aspects of logic and philosophy.

- Pragmatics is the study of language use. It has been argued that an understanding of pragmatics is necessary for understanding the acquisition of language, including the use and development of language structures. This is a strong social-interactionist view of language development. There seems to be overlap between the domain of pragmatics and other areas such as semantics, psycholinguistics, sociolinguistics, and discourse analysis. As a result, pragmatics does not seem to be a coherent field of study at present; nevertheless, it has the potential to become a dominant and influential language component in the study of language development.

Even with this brief introduction to the functions and structures of language, no doubt readers will agree that language is indeed a complex phenomenon. There is of course much more to this phenomenon, as will become evident in the next chapter on language acquisition with the focus on theories and models as well as the relationship between language and cognition.

LANGUAGE FUNCTIONS AND STRUCTURES COMPREHENSION QUESTIONS

1. What is the most commonly recognized general function of a language? List and describe at least five other general language functions.

2. With the "Communication of Ideas" issue, the author discussed two broad contexts—contextualized and decontextualized. Describe each type of context. Why is the distinction between each type so important?

3. What is meant by the following terms:
   a. performance
   b. performance literacy
   c. script literacy

4. What is literate thought? What does it mean to say that it is mode independent? What are the requisites (requirements) for literate thought? (These questions will be asked again for Chapter 12.)

5. The chapters discussed five major components of language: phonology, morphology, syntax, semantics, and pragmatics. Describe briefly each language component.

6. Describe the following terms:
   a. inflectional morphology
   b. derivational morphology
   c. allophones
   d. allomorphs
   e. phonemes
   f. morphemes
   g. bound morphemes
   h. free morphemes
   i. affix
   j. word family

7. List the prosodic features associated with the phonological system of a spoken language. Why are these features important?

8. Describe and provide examples of the two major categories of syntactic relations: linear and hierarchical.

9. Within the domain of semantics, there have been several (perhaps many!) interesting lines of research. One is on children's development of word meanings. Discuss some of the findings/issues associated with this line of research (including research on deaf and hard-of-hearing students).

10. In some sense, pragmatics is an exciting, incoherent, perhaps dynamic field of inquiry. Briefly discuss Searle's contributions to the understanding of pragmatics and his influences on research in this area. Describe the range of research foci in the area of pragmatics.

CHALLENGE QUESTIONS

(Note: Complete answers are not in the text. Additional research is required.)

1. Consider the quote by Russell, Quigley, and Power (1976) in the chapter: "It is probably a fair analogy to state that teachers of deaf chil-

dren should be expected to know as much about language as a teacher of chemistry is expected to know about chemistry." Is this quote applicable to the information that was discussed in the chapter? In what way? Is it possible for a teacher (or anyone else for that matter) to have knowledge of language that is as reliable and valid as the knowledge that a teacher may have about chemistry or physics? Why or why not?

2. The chapter states that "an understanding of a language means an understanding and simultaneous integration of form, meaning, and use." What does this statement mean? How might it be useful for a teacher or a researcher? Does this mean that it is not practical or useful to learn about the components of language—that is, phonology, morphology, syntax, semantics, and pragmatics? Why or why not?

3. Consider the assertion that literate thought is mode independent. What are the implications of this assertion for the use of proficiency exams or any other kind of test that relies predominantly on script literacy for measuring academic achievement? Can this be construed as an oppression issue? Why or why not? (Literate thought is discussed again in some detail in Chapter 12.)

4. There is an ongoing debate on whether language should be taught or caught. What does this mean? What is your opinion (so far!) on this issue? If you feel language can be taught, how should one do it? If you feel language should be caught, how should one implement this idea? Should this debate be construed as an either-or phenomenon? Why or why not?

FURTHER READINGS

Bailey, C-J. (1973). *Variation and linguistic theory*. Arlington, VA: Center for Applied Linguistics.

Chase, S. (1938). *The tyranny of words*. London: Methuen.

Crystal, D. (1969). *Prosodic systems and intonation in English*. Cambridge, UK: Cambridge University Press.

Fry, D. (1979). *The physics of speech*. Cambridge, UK: Cambridge University Press.

Keyser, S., & Postal, P. (1976). *Beginning English grammar*. New York: Harper & Row.

Premack, D., & Premack, A. (1983). *The mind of an ape*. New York: Norton.

Language Acquisition: A Brief Overview of Perspectives

Theorizing language [title of the book] can be dangerous. Or, on the other hand, illuminating. It may be spelled with an "s" instead of a "z." Or it might be just the last book you ever read on the theory of language. We can be sure that no matter how theorizing language is to be characterized—whether as dangerously misleading, therapeutically illuminating, crassly misspelled, or boring and over-priced—all will depend on how it (that is, theorizing language and/or its characterization) is integrated into the circumstances of its occurrence. Under one set of circumstances, theorizing language will appear as a kind of discourse (compare: "political language"), under a second as a metalinguistic activity (compare: "studying language"), under a third as a matter of contested norms (cf., "skepticism" vs. "scepticism"), and under a fourth as a cultural-commercial artifact (viz., that which you are holding in your hands). In other words, from one set of circumstances to another, everything changes. Still, in the end, merely recognizing that it (theorizing language and/or its characterization) can appear under any of various different aspects may be what turns out to have been the most valuable part of the whole experience. Or that was how it seemed to me. (Taylor, 1997, p. 1)

The emergence of language had pervasive implications for the social and cognitive development of humans. The study of language—particularly how it is acquired, what is acquired, and the time frame in which it is acquired—has intrigued scholars for centuries. A number of current language scholars have stated that the remarkable achievement of language acquisition is part of the general puzzle of human knowledge acquisition. In essence, the acquisition of language occurs within a relatively short period of time, and this, as well as other issues, has caused considerable debate among metatheorists, theorists, and researchers. The pursuit of explanatory adequacy, or some other similar activity, is important for both theoretical and practical reasons. For example, a complete theoretical understanding of language might lead to the development of practice for improving acquisition for individuals who are experiencing much difficulty.

This chapter discusses a few of the highlights of the major theories of language acquisition and some of their general aspects such as innateness, maturation, functionalism, and competence/performance. Most current language theories are essentially mental models due to the influence of the cognitive revolution. However, some theorists, notably Searle (1992), have questioned the notion of building and testing mental models for language or other cognitive activities. Nevertheless, relative to language theories, a better understanding of the models requires an adequate description of their metatheoretical foundations. Thus, the chapter begins with brief descriptions of the major mental frameworks (i.e., metatheories) that have influenced language acquisition theories, research, and practices (see Chapter 1 for a brief discussion of metatheory and paradigm).

The last section of the chapter provides a few remarks on the relationship between language and thought and relates this to deaf and hard-of-hearing children and adolescents. The language/thought phenomenon has also been influenced by the underlying metatheories (i.e., mental frameworks) and by theories of both language acquisition and cognitive development. The language/thought relationship has marked implications for the development of language as well as for the development of cognition. For example, if language and thought are mutually exclusive domains, language deficits cannot be attributed to cognitive deficits or even to cognitive development. The converse is also true; that is, cognitive deficits are not related to language deficits or to language development.

One of the most persistent questions in the research on deafness has been whether there are quantitative or qualitative differences in both language and cognition between individuals with severe to profound hearing impairment and those with typical hearing acuity. In light of a relationship between language and thought, the resolution of this issue provides insights into the acquisition of English language and literacy by deaf and hard-of-hearing individuals. That is, if certain differences do exist, they might indicate limitations on deaf persons' abilities to acquire particular skills (e.g., reading and writing) that are acquired fairly readily by individuals with typical hearing or they might dictate that to acquire those skills, different developmental and teaching approaches need to be used with deaf children than are used with children who are typically hearing.

In presenting an overview of the current thinking on the language/thought relationship, it is important to investigate whether a high-level development of language is dependent on a high-level development of thought or vice versa. As might be expected, there does not seem to be an unambiguous, straightforward, agreed-on answer. Nevertheless, there does seem to be a consensus that it is important to learn a language at as early an age as possible for the further development of literate thought.

THE INFLUENCES OF MENTAL FRAMEWORKS ON LANGUAGE

The theories of language development discussed in this chapter have been influenced by several broad metatheories in psychology—introspectionism, behaviorism, and cognitive science—and by sociocultural perspectives from sociology and anthropology (i.e., mostly social theories such as those espoused by Durkheim and Weber and later by those of Vygotsky and Luria). Each metatheory is distinguished by its approach to the study of the mind, or what is commonly known as the oldest, enduring problem in philosophy—the mind/body problem (Baars, 1986; Eacker, 1975; also see Bunge & Ardila, 1987, and Priest, 1991, for in-depth discussions of the various perspectives on the mind/body problem). The mind/body problem has played an important role in a branch of philosophy known as *metaphysics*, which is defined as the study of the nature and meaning of the universe or what lies beyond the physical dimension (Taylor, 1983). However, the mind/body phenomenon has also exerted its influence in other branches of philosophy as well, notably epistemology, the study of the nature and extent of knowledge. It is important to emphasize that the broad metatheories discussed here are based on the author's interpretation of a few conceptual frameworks synthesized from several publications (i.e., Baars, 1986; Case, 1996; Olson, 1994). There might be variations of these major concepts, which are beyond the scope of this chapter.

INTROSPECTIONISM

Introspectionism can be defined as the process of examining one's mind, specifically the contents, thought processes, or sensory experiences. It is related somewhat to the notion of metacognition (Baker & Brown, 1984) and to that of mentalism (see discussions in Baars, 1986; Steinberg, 1982). According to introspectionism, psychologists (and related scholars) should focus on conscious human experiences. The systematic investigations of human consciousness should lead to a complete understanding of humanity (i.e., human behavior or conduct). The research methodology can be described as systematic or analytic self-observation. It was hypothesized that thoughts could be analyzed or, rather, reduced to substructures or elements (Baars, 1986; Medin & Ross, 1992).

The appeal of this approach to the study of the mind can be seen in the following passage:

> *It would seem that we are all potential experts on how the mind works because we have a lot of firsthand experience with our own thoughts and other people's behavior. We often make inferences about other people's beliefs, desires, and intentions and we seem to have privileged, direct access to our own thoughts. Therefore, what better source of information about the mind than introspection? (Medin & Ross, 1992, p. 23)*

The use of systematic or analytic self-observation has provided data for the development of some linguistic theories, particularly those influenced by the mentalistic, rationalistic thinking of Chomsky (1957, 1975). There have been other applications of or influences by this mode of thought. Consider, for example, the development of Freud's thought and subsequent influences (Fine, 1973) and the evolution of critical theory, especially with the use of self-reflective analyses and deconstruction techniques (Geuss, 1981; Gibson, 1986; Horkheimer, 1995; Morton, 1993). Nevertheless, one major reason that introspectionism as a metatheory is not in vogue (or widely espoused) is due in part to the influences of the unconsciousness on human behavior, which was not considered, for the most part, in the traditional introspectionist framework (Medin & Ross, 1992).

The notions of consciousness, unconsciousness, and other concepts such as intentionality and mental framework have engendered a great deal of controversy and debate in the philosophy-of-mind academic arena. Given the amount of confusion that surrounds this debate, it is easy to see why some scholars, most notably behaviorists, believe that this is a misguided, misfocused discussion. This will become clear in the next section on behaviorism.

BEHAVIORISM

As a metatheory, behaviorism was a reaction to the notion of introspectionism (Baars, 1986; Medin & Ross, 1992). In general, behaviorists asserted that psychology should focus on the study of observable behavior. Influenced by the work of John B. Watson, behaviorism dominated the field of psychology, particularly experimental psychology, in the United States from about the early 1910s to the late 1940s (Baars, 1986; Medin & Ross, 1992). In contrast, European psychologists were influenced by movements such as Gestalt psychology, psychoanalysis, and Piagetian theory. Watson, who is considered to be the father of behaviorism

> *argued that behavior is objective and observable and that the agenda for psychology consists of formulating laws relating stimulus conditions to behavior. Consciousness, introspection, and the mind were to play no role in this science of behavior. His views were reinforced by the logical positivist movement in philosophy. Logical positivism emphasized operational definitions tied to specific operations or observations. (Medin & Ross, 1992, p. 24)*

The views of Watson and other radical behaviorists, notably B. F. Skinner, represented the most extreme antimentalist position relative to the mind/body problem (Baars, 1986; Priest, 1991; Steinberg, 1982). Several behaviorist positions on the mind/body phenomenon have been delineated (J. Cooper, Heward, & Heron, 1987; Steinberg, 1982). Regardless of the differences among the positions, the common area of agreement was that the focus of investigation should be on the body (i.e., observable behaviors). In one sense, this was interpreted to mean that psychology is not fundamentally different from physiology.

The decline of behaviorism began during the late 1940s. Although behaviorism has declined tremendously since the late 1950s, especially after a scathing review by Chomsky (1959), it still exerts a considerable influence in clinical and animal psychology and in some areas of special education. Perhaps much of the influence in special education is due to the usefulness of single-subject research methodology and in the application of direct teaching techniques such as precision teaching. In addition, it is possible to see some influence of behaviorism on current language theories, especially those that emphasize the importance of the language user's performance aspect (e.g., spoken or sign utterances) and the role of the social environment.

To understand this influence, it is important to present the general tenets of behavioristic views of language learning. As is discussed later, the focus is on the model of Skinner (1957), who attempted to describe language learning in terms of reinforcement principles within the framework of operant conditioning. At present, the general principle of behaviorism is thought to have a small role in the language acquisition process (Medin & Ross, 1992; Owens, 1996; Steinberg, 1982). Perhaps the best explanation for this situation is "behaviorism . . . never got very far in accounting for complex learning" (Medin & Ross, 1992, p. 25).

COGNITIVISM

It is difficult to label the cognitive revolution; in psychology, it could be labeled as *cognitive psychology* (Baars, 1986; Medin & Ross, 1992). However, because the revolution has influenced research and thinking in other fields, notably linguistics, computer science, and philosophy, it could be labeled as *cognitive science*.

Relative to psychology, one common rendition of the cognitive metatheory asserts

> *that psychologists observe behavior in order to make inferences about underlying factors that can explain the behavior. They agree with behaviorists that the data of psychology must be public, but the purpose of gathering this data is to generate theories about unobservable constructs, such as "purposes" and "ideas," which can summarize, predict, and explain the data. In particular, cognitive psychologists often talk about the* representations *that organisms can have of themselves and of their world, and about the transformations that these representations undergo. "Transforming representations" is sometimes called* information processing. *Using this kind of theoretical metaphor, cognitive psychologists can interpret commonsense psychological terms in a rather straightforward way. Thought, language, knowledge, meaning, purpose, imagery, motives, even consciousness and emotion—all the commonsense vocabulary inherited from our culture becomes scientifically useful again. (Baars, 1986, pp. 7–8)*

As indicated by this passage, the grand aims of cognitive science seem to focus on resolving long-standing, controversial epistemological issues, namely, those that deal with the nature, extent, and development of knowledge (Baars, 1986; Shadbolt, 1988). One of the most controversial areas is the nature of mental representation. That is, knowledge is represented by symbols, which are in turn manipulated (e.g., organized, etc.) by an information-processing system. As discussed later, Chomsky attempted to address mental representation by analysis of the structure of syntax in language.

From another perspective, the concept of mental representation has become operationalized as a computer metaphor. That is, there have been numerous attempts to explain the functions of the brain (including the mind) with respect to the framework of a computer. This perspective has dominated the research on deafness until quite recently; indeed, it has dominated much of the theorizing about the reading process until quite recently (see Samuels & Kamil, 1984; also see discussions in Ruddell, Ruddell, & Singer, 1994). However, it seems that the computer metaphor has lost or is losing favor. The unsuccessful attempts with models and theories have led some scholars to inquire: Is the concept of mental representation really necessary?

Searle (1992, 1995) argued that it is not and proposed that any understanding of the mind cannot proceed without a discussion of consciousness and intentionality. In developing his hypothesis on the manner in which the mind works, Searle focused on resolving the famous mind/body problem, which has baffled philosophers for centuries (Priest, 1991). In essence, Searle's position is that there is no need for developing mental models or models that explain how the brain processes information. This proposal is a reaction against the thinking of Chomsky in particular and other cognitive information-processing models in general. For example, Searle argued that there is no psychological reality for the notion of universal grammar (see discussion of this concept in the section on "Linguistic Theories"). In addition, there is no rule following and no language of thought in the brain. Searle (1992, 1995) reasoned that mental events are features of the brain in the same way that liquidity is a feature of water. Researchers should focus on understanding the parameters of consciousness and intentionality. This perspective has pervasive implications for theory, research, and instruction relative to language acquisition. For example, it might be debatable whether language can be taught via the presentation of a natural order of structures based on a mental model of how language is acquired. In sum, the development of mental models is, in Searle's view, a misguided, dead-end endeavor.

It seems that Searle's thinking is an extension of his views on speech acts relative to a social-interactionist view of language development (discussed later). Searle's remarks seem to be influenced somewhat by the introspectionist metatheory with the addition of a strong neurobiological component. A sample of Searle's (1992) argument is as follows:

> The brain, as far as its intrinsic operations are concerned, does no information processing. It is a specific biological organ and its specific neurobiological processes cause specific forms of intentionality. In the brain, intrinsically, there are neurobiological processes and sometimes they cause consciousness. But that is the end of the story. All other mental attributions are either dispositional, as when we ascribe unconscious states to the agent, or they are observer relative, as when we assign a computational interpretation to his brain processes. (p. 226)

In addition to the information-processing framework, the cognitive perspective of language development has been influenced pervasively by the work of Piaget. Piaget's (1952, 1971) model is based on biology and is focused on the internal hardware of the developing organism. In essence, Piaget proposed a developmental model in which cognitive structures provide the underpinnings for the growth of knowledge in areas such as language and mathematics. Growth in understanding is a reflection of the cognitive growth of the individual. This growth has been referred to as cognitive constructionism (or constructivism) and has influenced a group of language models known as cognitive interactionist, discussed later.

SOCIOCULTURAL FRAMEWORKS

There is also a social component to the cognitive or cognitive science mental framework, and the salient underpinnings of this aspect can be traced, for the most part, to the work of Vygotsky (1962, 1978) and the thinking of others in social literary criticism, sociolinguistic, and sociocultural fields. The group of language models influenced by this perspective has been called *social-interactionist* (Bohannon, 1993; Owens, 1996). Thus, the interactionist framework has both a strong cognitive component (Piaget) and a strong social component (Vygotsky).

To obtain a good understanding of the social features of these models, it is necessary to discuss briefly the cognitive view of social theorists. For example, social theorists argue that social changes (e.g., urbanization, deinstitutionalization, social Darwinism, etc.) produce changes in cognition, individually and collectively. As noted by Olson (1994), the early development of theories of modern thought (i.e., cognitive theories) were proffered by social theorists, namely, early pioneers such as Durkheim, Weber, Vygotsky, and Luria. In essence, only the sociological aspects of these early thinkers (i.e., mostly Durkheim and Weber) have remained influential, especially in fields such as sociology and anthropology.

The works of both Vygotsky and Luria, however, have had a marked impact on not only social-interactionist language models but also on current views on the relationship between language and thought (discussed briefly later), including the development of process-oriented cognitive tests (Luria), which have replaced traditional intelligence tests (e.g., tests based on psychometric aspects or cluster analyses of factors such as the work of Binet, Terman, and Thurstone) (see discussion in Paul & Jackson, 1993). In addition, both Vygotsky and Luria seemed to emphasize that literacy (i.e., reading and writing skills) has contributed greatly to the development of Western thought. As argued by Olson (1994):

> *Both [Vygotsky and Luria] adopted the view that the "higher mental processes" always involve the use of socially invented signs such as lan-*

*guage, writing, numerals, and depictions which are culturally diverse, and which . . . have a history. The means by which these cultural resources come to be psychological is described as "internalization."
. . . They offered specific proposals as to just how writing and literacy could influence cognitive operations and activities and offered these proposals as candidate explanations of the development from primitive to modern forms of thinking, a development they both associate with literacy. (pp. 26–27)*

This brief discussion of cognitive and sociocultural underpinnings does not capture the entire story. The views of both Piaget and Vygotsky have undergone a number of reinterpretations by their followers and have influenced several lines of research on language acquisition. Muma (1998) provided an eloquent synthesis of some major philosophical views and theoretical perspectives in the field of language development and acquisition. With respect to constructivism—from Piaget—and the work of Vygotsky, Muma remarked that:

Constructionism *is the view that an individual actively constructs possible worlds or situated minds by virtue of living in the world. Early constructions are evidently derived from embodiment . . . whereby schemas may be established. Such schemas are rudimentary notions of one's situated place in scripts and formats and they constitute early versions of event representations . . . or procedural knowledge. . . . The essence of constructionism is that an individual from infancy throughout adulthood is an active learner in constructing possible worlds or a situated mind.*

Social mediation is the neo-Vygotskian view that cognition is inherently social and cultural in nature. The implication is that cognition and language are not entities unto themselves; rather, they are products of a socially and culturally situated mind. (p. 17)

Table 3-1 presents a summary of the major tenets of the broad metatheories or mental frameworks.

THEORIZING LANGUAGE: A GLIMPSE OF THE VISION

The influences of the mental frameworks discussed earlier will become evident in the brief, broad, ensuing discussion of language theories. Practitioners are almost always interested in the applications of theories, especially if they produce successful outcomes, assuming that there is a consensus on the nature

TABLE 3-1 A Few Major Points on the Broad Metatheories/ Mental Frameworks

Introspectionism

- Defined as the process of examining one's mind, specifically the contents, thought processes, or sensory experiences. It is hypothesized that thoughts can be analyzed or reduced to substructures or elements.

- Focus is on conscious human experiences, which should lead to a complete understanding of human behavior or conduct.

- Research methodology is systematic or analytic self-observation.

- This view is not widely espoused at present because of its inability to address the influences of or to explain concepts such as consciousness or intentionality. In the traditional framework, the role of unconsciousness on behavior caused problems.

Behaviorism

- Focus is on the study of observable behavior in the environment (i.e., empiricism). The most radical form espouses what is called an antimentalist position—that is, there is no need to study the mind and its attributes to understand human behavior.

- Psychology is not fundamentally different from physiology. Observable behavior can be reduced to simpler components, which can be analyzed (i.e., reductionism).

- Language learning is described in terms of reinforcement principles.

Cognitivism

- Main reason for observing behavior is to make inferences about underlying factors that can explain the behavior.

- Focus on resolving long-standing, controversial epistemological issues, namely those that deal with the nature, extent, and development of knowledge.

- One of the most controversial areas is the nature of mental representation— that is, models of how the mind works.

- There are several variations—some focus on biology and maturation; others on neurophysiology; still others on using the computer as a metaphor. There are also combinations of these variations—for example, Piaget's model with information processing (computer).

Socioculturalism

- Cognition and language have social and cultural underpinnings.

- Social and cultural forces are mainly responsible for the development of cognition and language, indeed, for all of human behavior.

- Cognition is not an entity unto itself; it is a product of a socially and culturally situated mind. The same is true for language. In fact, neither can be understood separate from cultural and historical contexts.

- Two major aspects of this view seem to be constructionism and social mediation. Constructionism asserts that individuals construct reality (e.g., situated minds) by virtue of living in the world. Social mediation maintains that cognition and language are not entities by themselves—they are the products of a socially and culturally situated mind.

Note: Adapted from Baars (1986), Muma (1998), and Shadbolt (1988).

of success and the nature of outcome. Despite the difficulties of proceeding from theory to practice, one important question that needs to be raised is: Is there indeed a coherent theory of language acquisition? If not, will there ever be a coherent theory? Can this theory account for individual differences? (see Shore, 1995). Thus far, despite advances in understanding, the pursuit of a comprehensive, coherent theory is still fruitless, and this, no doubt, presents enormous challenges for language-intervention/teaching/faciliatative endeavors. Many language scholars are still mystified by the language acquisition process and seem to still agree with the process being characterized as magic or as mysterious (see discussions in Bohannon, 1993; Crystal, 1987, 1997). This is surely no small comfort to educators, parents, and interested others attempting to improve the language acquisition process of many children who are deaf and hard of hearing.

Why is it so difficult? Perhaps one reason is that any general theory needs to connect what is known within the various components such as phonology, morphology, syntax, semantics, and pragmatics. It is difficult to find principles that are common within these language domains, much less those that are common across them. There seems to be a great deal of confusion that has resulted from contradictory research findings. This has compelled researchers to focus on narrow problems within each language component rather than working on the big picture of language acquisition. Ironically, there seems to be a greater need for metaanalysis, particularly metatheorizing, to obtain some understanding of these broader issues, especially given the wide range of thought and research paradigms.

Perhaps another—hopefully manageable—way to conceptualize language theorizing is to relate it to Marr's levels hypothesis (1982). Marr (1982) posited three level accounts. Level 1 account can be considered the computational level. At this level, researchers/scholars specify what it is they are attempting to solve (i.e., goals such as letter recognition, syntactic knowledge, etc.), why they are solving it (i.e., appropriateness of the goal), and how they expect to arrive at a goal of computation (i.e., strategy). Level 2 account deals with the implementation of Level 1. Specifically, this concerns the representation of input/output phenomena and the algorithm (i.e., step-by-step procedures) for the transformation process, that is, the transformation of the sensory data to representations (e.g., mental representations). Level 3 account involves the hardware implementation. It describes the intricate apparatus of the physical structure or device (e.g., the brain) in which the aspects of Level 2 are housed.

Each level has a role to play in contributing to a comprehensive, complete explanation of the cognitive process. Relative to language development, Chomsky (1975) argued that Marr's Level 3 account is not important for developing a comprehensive theory of human language acquisition or for any aspect of human behavior such as cognition or psychosocial development. For example, understanding the physiological processes (e.g., theory of neurons and brain-mapping techniques) of the language area of the brain will not explain the language competence (i.e., intuitive knowledge) of the language user.

This is not to deny the importance of physiology such as the brain-mapping techniques or the neurophysiological models of language that are under consideration (for a brief, accessible discussion of issues, see Cairns, 1996; Owens, 1996). In fact, some of this research has offered some insights into the localization functions of the brain and to the question of whether there is a critical period (i.e., age) for language acquisition (see discussions on critical period in Lenneberg, 1967; Rymer, 1992). Nevertheless, at this point, it is not believed that physiology—albeit helpful—is sufficient to solve all or even most psychological issues relative to either language acquisition or even language development. Of course, this view could be mistaken by future developments. Nevertheless, the author agrees with Bandura (1997), who remarked:

The fact that cognition is a cerebral occurrence does not mean that the laws expressing functional relations in psychological theory are reducible to those in neurophysiological theory. One must distinguish between how cerebral systems function and the personal and social means by which they can be orchestrated to produce courses of action that serve different purposes. . . . Knowledge of the brain circuitry involved in learning does not tell one much about how to provide incentives to get people to attend to, process, and organize relevant information; in what modes to present information; and whether learning is better achieved independently, cooperatively, or competitively. The optimal conditions must be specified by psychological principles. Nor does understanding how the brain works furnish rules on how to create efficacious parents, teachers, or politicians. . . . Were one to embark on the road to reductionism, the journey would traverse biology and chemistry and would eventually end in atomic particles, with neither the intermediate locales nor the final stop supplying the psychological laws of human behavior. (p. 4)

In any case, with respect to Marr's (1982) hypothesis, most of the theories in this chapter can be labeled predominantly a Level 1 account with the goal of attaining a Level 2 account (of course, some theorists think that they have already attained a Level 2 account!). Whether a Level 3 (physiological) account is necessary or even possible, as discussed briefly, remains open to question.

The next section provides a brief discussion of the major tenets of three broad groups of language theories: behaviorism, linguistic, and interactionism. To assist the reader in understanding the information, Table 3-2 illustrates, in general, the background and organization of these groups of theories, including a discussion of a few major similarities and differences with respect to dichotomies such as functionalism-structuralism, performance-competence, and empiricism-nativism. Some of these dichotomies are discussed in the ensuing sections on language theories. At the end of the discussion of each theoretical group, additional, specific information is presented in a summary table.

BEHAVIORIST THEORIES

Behaviorist theories have been influenced by the behaviorism metatheory, which posits that only the body (i.e., observable behaviors) of the mind/body phenomenon is capable of being studied and, consequently, measured. The intent here is to discuss the general tenets of behavioristic theories, specifically those that relate to language development. Because of the emphasis on observable data, behaviorists are interested in the associations or connections between

TABLE 3-2 Background and Organization of Language Theories

One feasible way to view the three broad groups of language theories (behaviorism, linguistic, and interactionist) is to show how they relate to the following dichotomies: functionalism-structuralism, performance-competence, and empiricism-nativism.

Dichotomies

- Functionalism proponents examine relationships between environmental variables and language development—that is, the pragmatic use of speech sounds (or other building blocks), words, and sentences. Most of the emphasis is on the social communicative contexts or situations in which language is used.

- Structuralism focuses on invariant processes and mechanisms that undergird observable language data. The form or organization of language behavior that is common across individuals and situations is important. Structuralists use formal language or symbolism to describe language data.

- Performance refers to the various instances (words and sentences) of the language users. That is, this refers to the performance (spoken and signed) utterances of language users.

- Competence refers to the knowledge of the language users (i.e., abstract knowledge) or to the underlying rule system based on data from theoretically possible language usage (e.g., grammatical usage) as opposed to only the error-prone data from the actual performance of the language users. Performance data are considered but only in light of competence models.

- Empiricism emphasizes the influence of the environment in fostering the acquisition of language. Proponents argue that language behaviors are not much different from other types of learned behaviors or skills. A complete model of how language is acquired can be developed by observing the use of language in social interactions. That is, all of language is learned.

- Nativism asserts that language is too complex and is acquired in a short period of time. Although language needs an environment in which to flourish, the environment, including any known methods, is not essentially responsible for language development. It seems that some critical components of language must be innate (i.e., inborn) to permit its rapid development with minimal, reasonable exposure. This explains why language users can understand and produce utterances to which they have never been exposed.

Application to Language Theories

- It should be remembered that many theories within the three broad groups cannot be placed solely at one end of the continuum of the various dichotomies. The ensuing discussion should be considered as examples. It is safe to say that a particular theory is predominantly at one end of the dichotomies (i.e., representative) rather than to pigeonhole it.

- Both behaviorism and most of linguistic theory ascribe predominantly to structuralism, although their research approaches differ. However, they differ dramatically with respect to the other dichotomies. Behaviorism espouses the notion of performance and empiricism, whereas linguistic theory favors competence and nativism.

- Some of the differences or variations within linguistic theory center on the argument between the supremacy of syntax versus semantics. There is still an emphasis on structuralism, competence, and nativism. However, some semanticists argue that knowledge structures in the mind should be described with respect to cognitive attributes—using terms such as *propositions* or *schemas*, which are semantic, or meaning structures, as opposed to syntactic structures. Other semanticists, who are more oriented toward pragmatics, tend to espouse the importance of performance data and a functionalist approach.

- Interactionists represent a rather broad group with several factions, depending on the nature and extent of reactions against both behaviorism and linguistic theory—as influenced by Chomsky. It has been argued that interactionism is a balance between behaviorism and linguistic theory—however, the nature of this balance depends on the focus. In general, interactionists acknowledge interactions among a number of variables such as cognitive, social, linguistic, biological, physiological, and environmental. Cognitive-interactionists may emphasize the predominant importance of cognitive or biological factors (i.e., structuralism), which influence their interpretations of nativism (i.e., as biological development rather than innate language structures). Social-interactionists focus mostly on social factors (e.g., pragmatics, communicative interactions, and environment) to explain

(continues)

(Table 3-2 continued)

(i.e., functionalism) the acquisition of language. Some interactionists, notably information processing, utilize a computer metaphor to explain acquisition, whereas others focus on neurophysiological components of the brain to account for language development. In general, it is possible to remark that interactionism oscillates between the bipolar continua of the three dichotomies.

environmental stimuli (empiricism) and the language behaviors of the child (performance).

Two general processes describe these associations or connections: classical conditioning and operant conditioning (Skinner, 1957). Typically, language (mostly vocabulary) and an additional learning principle, that is, operant conditioning, account for productive speech. These two processes assume that all behaviors are learned and that there is little or no need for the concept of innate structures.

Classical or Respondent Conditioning

One of the most well-known examples of classical conditioning (also known as respondent conditioning) is the experiment of the Russian physiologist, Pavlov. In this experiment, the sound of a bell by itself was a neutral stimulus, which did not elicit the salivation of a dog. After the bell was associated with presentation of food several times, it became a conditioned stimulus (CS). Consequently, the ringing of the bell alone elicited the salivation of the dog (see accessible account in Cooper et al., 1987). The dog had learned (or had been conditioned) to salivate by responding to a new stimulus—the ringing bell.

This example refers to the first type of behavior, termed *respondent behavior.* Cooper et al. (1987) remarked:

> *Respondents are behaviors that are elicited, or brought out, by stimuli that precede the behavior. Reflexes such as pupil constriction in bright light and the patellar tendon reflex (knee jerk) are examples of respondent behaviors. Respondent behaviors are essentially involuntary and occur whenever the eliciting stimulus is presented. (p. 10)*

There have been attempts to relate this type of behavior to the early language learning behaviors of infants in response to words uttered by significant others, particularly mothers. Bohannon (1993) provided an example that focuses on an infant's learning to respond to the word *milk*, which became a conditioned stimulus when associated with the substance milk.

Milk (UCS [unconditioned stimulus]) fed to a hungry infant usually results in physiological responses in the infant (UCR [unconditioned response]). When the infant's mother says the word milk prior to or during feeding, this word (CS [conditioned stimulus]) becomes associated with the primary stimulus of the milk and gradually acquires the power to elicit a response (CR [conditioned response]) in the child that is similar to the response to the milk itself.

Once a CS (a word) has come to elicit CR, it can then be used as a UCS to modify the response to another CS. For example, if a new CS, such as the word, bottle *, frequently occurs with the word* milk, *it may come to elicit a CR similar to the response to* milk. *The associations formed between several stimuli (CSs) and a single response lead to the formation of associations between the stimuli themselves. Thus, not only may arbitrary verbal CSs be associated with specific internal meanings (CRs), but the words themselves may be connected by stimulus-stimulus associations. In this way, classical conditioning is used to account for the interrelationship of words and word meanings. (p. 246)*

Operant Behavior and Operant Conditioning

Whether the description by Bohannon (1993) of respondent behavior (i.e., stimulus-response (S-R), or respondent, paradigm) and classical conditioning is accurate is debatable. Skinner (1957) argued that most human behaviors cannot be accounted for or explained by the stimulus-response (S-R) paradigm; rather, what is needed is an analysis of operant behavior and operant conditioning. According to Skinner, operant behaviors are not elicited by preceding stimuli; they are influenced by stimuli that follow the behavior.

To account for the child's production of speech, the principle of operant conditioning entails the notions of imitation and reinforcement used by parents. The parents provide a language model for the child. The child is rewarded after a successful imitation of the model, moving from simple sounds to more complex speech. This process is called *shaping*, which results in the acquisition of the desirable behaviors.

Bohannon (1993) offered an eloquent description of operant conditioning (also see Moerk, 1983) and argued that the basic processes of learning, that is, classical and operant conditioning, are responsible for the development of the child's verbal behavior. With respect to operant conditioning, Bohannon (1993) remarked that:

> *Operant conditioning concerns the changes in voluntary, nonreflexive behavior that arise due to environmental consequences contingent upon that behavior. Simply put, behaviors that most frequently result in rewards tend to be repeated, whereas behaviors that result in punishment do not tend to recur. All behavioristic accounts of language acquisition assume that children's productive speech is shaped by differential reinforcers and punishments supplied by environmental agents (e.g., parents). Behaviorists assume that children's speech that more closely approximates adult speech will be rewarded, while meaningless or inappropriate speech will be ignored or punished. Gradually, the response unit will change from simple sounds to whole words as the parents change their reinforcement practices, eventually restricting rewards to only those utterances that are meaningful and adultlike. (p. 246)*

Criticisms of Behaviorism

As with any group of language theories, it is not difficult to find criticisms, and even setting aside the infamous Skinner-Chomsky debate, there have been many attacks on behaviorism. Only a few remarks are made here. In light of current prevailing thinking on language development, the notions of imitation and reinforcement play a very small role in the child's production of language. The imitation and reinforcement paradigm does not account for the child's playing with the language, that is, the child's inventiveness, even when the child seems to know the meaning of a word. Interestingly, parents only reinforce a small portion of what their young children say, and much of the focus is on the truthfulness of the utterances. In addition, the notion of children's errors needs to be considered in another light. Consider the classic examples of *All gone cookie* and *He goed.* At first glance, these examples are ungrammatical and are not spoken (or reinforced) by typical parents or adult users of the language. These utterances, and others, are understood better with respect to children's progress toward linguistic maturity. That is, these statements represent intermediate steps (e.g., hypothesis testing) in children's acquisition of the grammar of mature language users.

Perhaps the biggest criticism of behaviorism is the fact that there seems to be almost no consideration for what the child brings to the language-learning task (i.e., the child as thinker or as a knowledgeable person) (Olson & Bruner, 1996). This seems to favor a theory of learning in which the child is viewed as a doer or knower. As a doer, the child needs to use his or her—roughly speaking—imitation skills to become a skilled performer, that is, to know how to do things, in this case, speak a language. Practice and drill are part of the regimen of obtaining the know-how or procedural knowledge (Olson & Bruner, 1996). As a knower, the child needs to be taught that or know that, which is described as propositional knowledge. In this instance, the teacher (or parent) is viewed as the expert, and knowledge is imparted from expert to learner, often in a didactic, one-sided fashion. In essence, the child is viewed as a passive learner with a tabula rasa (blank tablet) for receiving and accumulating information.

Despite the proliferation of a new wave of learning theories based on constructivist principles (e.g., thinker, interpreter, or constructor of meaning), it would be shortsighted to dismiss behaviorism entirely. At the very least, there might be an occasional need for the use of doer and knower principles, especially within a framework such as direct teaching or precision teaching. To put it naively and simplistically, the question is: What happens when the child does not seem to make progress? Is some form of sequencing or arranging or prescribing critical (and even acceptable) in the overall language learning process? The chapter on language instruction (Chapter 10) argues that setting this up as an either-or phenomenon (to teach or not to teach, natural or structural, etc.) might not benefit all or even most deaf and hard-of-hearing children. Of course, whether using these direct teaching approaches really result in the acquisition of language is debatable; nevertheless, it seems that behaviorism itself does not offer an adequate explanation for language development.

TABLE 3-3 A Few Major Points of Behaviorist Theories

- Behaviorists are interested in the associations or connections between environmental stimuli (empiricism) and the language behaviors of the child (performance).

- Two general processes characterize the associations or connections: classical and operant conditioning.

- Classical conditioning is also known as respondent conditioning. The use of classical conditioning has also been referred to as stimulus-response (S-R), or respondent, paradigm.

(continues)

(Table 3-3 continued)

- It has been argued that most human behaviors cannot be accounted for or explained by the S-R paradigm—what is needed is an analysis of operant behavior and operant conditioning.

- Operant conditioning entails both reinforcement and punishment. Operant conditioning is concerned with voluntary, nonreflexive behavior. Cooper, Heward, and Heron (1987) stated that "if a behavior is followed by an event that increases the probability of that behavior occurring again in the future, reinforcement has taken place. Conversely, if a behavior is followed by an event that decreases the probability of that behavior's future occurrence, punishment has taken place" (p. 24).

- The two general processes, classical and operant conditioning, assume that all behaviors are learned and that there is little or no need for the concept of innate structures.

- There have been many criticisms of behaviorism. Perhaps the biggest criticism is the fact that there seems to be almost no consideration for what the child brings to the language-learning process.

Table 3-3 presents some of the major highlights of behaviorism, discussed in this section.

LINGUISTIC THEORIES

Prior to the recognition of the work of Chomsky, the behaviorist metatheory as well as the logical positivist movement in philosophy exerted a marked influence on linguistic theorists (Baars, 1986; Cairns, 1996; Medin & Ross, 1992; Owens, 1996; Whitehead, 1990). This was most evident in the works of structural linguists, including those who focused mainly on the phonological component of languages although some structuralists were concerned with syntax or sentence structure. With the focus on linguistic description, one of the major shortcomings of structural linguistics was its difficulty (or, rather, inability) to explain how language users understand the ambiguity of sentences, for example: *The chicken is ready to eat* and *Visiting linguists can be dangerous*. Using traditional methods (e.g., diagramming sentences), it was impossible to demonstrate adequately the various meanings of these ambiguous sentences. Furthermore, structural linguists found it difficult to explain the manner in which language users arrived at an understanding of such ambiguity.

Despite their differences, many current linguistic theories have been influenced by the cognitive metatheory and the views of Chomsky (1957, 1965, 1975, 1980, 1988, 1991; also see Bohannon, 1993; Cook & Newson, 1996; Owens, 1996). Chomsky (1975) asserted

> *that by studying language we may discover abstract principles that govern its structure and use, principles that are universal by biological necessity and not mere historical accident, that derive from mental characteristics of the species. A human language is a system of remarkable complexity. To come to know a human language would be an extraordinary intellectual achievement for a creature not specifically designed to accomplish this task. A normal child acquires this knowledge on relatively slight exposure and without specific training. . . . For the conscious mind, not specially designed for the purpose, it remains a distant goal to reconstruct and comprehend what the child has done intuitively and with minimal effort. Thus language is a mirror of mind in a deep and significant sense. It is a product of human intelligence, created anew in each individual by operations that lie far beyond the reach of will or consciousness. (p. 4)*

The information in this passage provides the background for the discussion of a few of Chomsky's major principles: theoretical adequacy, innate capacity, and the notion of competence.

Theoretical Adequacy

Chomsky (1957, 1965, 1988, 1991) proposed that the road to theoretical adequacy consists of answering three broad questions: What constitutes knowledge of language?, How is such knowledge acquired?, and How is such knowledge put to use? The linguist needs to describe (or catalog) all behaviors that are a part of language. These language behaviors must be distinguished from nonlanguage behaviors. To reach the next level of adequacy, the linguist needs to identify a finite number of connective principles that account for (and predict) the appearance of the language behaviors. In other words, the linguist needs to describe what individuals know about language, how they acquire this knowledge, and how they use it. In Chomsky's view, a complete theory of language development must account for both the language behaviors and the processes and mechanisms used by children during the entire language development period. Chomsky's (1975) central concept is Universal Grammar (UG) described as: "the system of principles, conditions, and rules that are elements or properties of all human languages not merely by accident, but by necessity . . . the essence of human language" (p. 29).

Innateness

Because of the limited, albeit adequate, exposure to language and the time frame in which language is acquired, Chomsky championed the idea of innate knowledge (i.e., an innate predisposition to acquiring knowledge principles). In general, Chomsky believed that humans are born with minds that contain an innate proclivity for a number of different areas (Chomsky, 1975; also see Cairns, 1996; Cook & Newson, 1996; Steinberg, 1982). The faculties of mind are argued to be independent of one another. Thus, the faculty containing an innate predisposition for language is independent of that containing an innate predisposition for mathematics. In essence, the language innate device is responsible alone for the development of language; knowledge of mathematics or logic is not necessary. It should be clear that Chomsky's theory is a theory of knowledge, not of behavior. This theory is concerned with the internal structure of the human mind.

The foregoing remarks also influenced the work of Fodor (1983), who proffered his modularity hypothesis, which was motivated by the notion of Universal Grammar (i.e., Chomsky's theory of language knowledge) and influenced a line of research itself. The modularity hypothesis also influenced the thinking of scholars in the area of deafness (see Marschark, Siple, Lillo-Martin, Campbell, & Everhart, 1997). Fodor's view is that the brain is organized in a vertical manner with separate modules to deal with specific localized information in a set of modules. Initially, these modules do not communicate with other areas of the brain, but communication does occur later in development. Despite the influence of this model, it has been criticized because of its inability to deal with the complex operations of the brain such as self-awareness and memory.

Interestingly, one of the most vociferous debates has been the modularity-connectionist one. Connectionist models have been influenced by the work of McClelland, Rumelhart, and the PDP Research Group (1986) and are essentially interactionist (information-processing) models. This is discussed in the next section. The connectionist model has influenced much research in the area of reading, particularly interactive (i.e., schema-interactive) theories with their focus on parallel processing capacities.

Returning to Universal Grammar and Chomsky, it should be highlighted that innate knowledge has been labeled the LAD, or the Language Acquisition Device (see readable discussion in Cairns, 1996). This knowledge becomes functional or operational when it interacts with the linguistic environment. In Chomsky's view, the environment does not shape linguistic knowledge; rather, it activates the innate linguistic knowledge. This business of what humans bring to the task of learning (i.e., language learning) seems to provide a perspective on Bertrand Russell's (1948) question: "How comes it that human beings, whose contacts with the world are brief and personal and limited, are nevertheless able to know as much as they do know?" (p. 5). Chomsky (1975) offered a compelling, illuminating response:

> *We can know so much because in a sense we already knew it, though the data of sense were necessary to evoke and elicit this knowledge. Or to put it less paradoxically, our systems of belief are those that the mind, as a biological structure, is designed to construct. We interpret experience as we do because of our special mental design. We attain knowledge when the "inward ideas of the mind itself" and the structures it creates conform to the nature of things. (p. 8)*

Competence

It can be inferred that linguistic theories of language are theories of language competence (Cairns, 1996; Cook & Newson, 1996; Stevenson, 1988). These theories attempt to describe the abstract system of rules that account for a person's knowledge of language. This rule system must be sufficient enough to explain a native language user's production and comprehension of a myriad of sentences, many of which she or he has not heard or read previously. According to Chomsky (1957, 1965, 1975, 1988; also see Cairns, 1996; Cook & Newson, 1996; Culicover, 1997), this knowledge is not completely evident in the speaker's performance, that is, the speaker's utterances. For example, the utterances of speakers are subjected to memory lapses, false starts, and parsimony. Although many speakers can produce and understand complex sentences of unlimited lengths, they choose to produce shorter sentences. A theory of grammar should describe speakers' knowledge of all possible, permissible sentences, not only sentences that they utter. Only by appealing to speakers' intuitions can linguists arrive at a theory of grammar. Thus, a competence theory "is designed to account for our ability to decide whether or not a sentence is grammatical" (Stevenson, 1988, p. 8). Essentially, it can be stated that all linguistic approaches assume that language contains a fixed structure that is basically independent of language use. This accounts for how a finite set of rules can be used to generate an infinite number of utterances, including novel utterances, which can be understood easily by the native listener.

Culicover (1997) provided a perspective on the notion of competence, including the methodology for developing linguistic theory that is based on the language user's competence:

The mind is not subject to direct examination. Thus, indirect methods must be found to investigate the nature of linguistic knowledge and how language is acquired by the mind. The methodology that has proven most productive in the development of linguistic theory has been to examine closely selected sentences and phrases that native speakers of a language judge to be possible, impossible, and marginal. By studying these external manifestations of linguistic knowledge, we seek to arrive, indirectly, at an understanding of the mental apparatus that gives rise to them.

Application of this methodology may give the incorrect impression that the objective . . . is to provide complete descriptions of human languages, conceived of as sets of linguistic expressions (i.e., words, phrases, and sentences). But these expressions are simply the data that are used in the investigation, and are not themselves the object of the theory. The overriding concern on this approach is not with what a speaker or group of speakers say . . . but with the character of what is in the human mind that accounts for our ability to acquire, speak, and understand language. . . . (pp. 1–2)

Evolution of Linguistic Theory

Linguistic theory has evolved significantly since the beginning of transformational generative grammar (TGG). The evolution of the theory has proceeded from standard theory to extended standard theory to government-binding theory (Chomsky, 1988; Cook & Newson, 1996; Goodluck, 1991; Stevenson, 1988). Chomsky felt the phrase *government-binding* was misleading; thus, *principles and parameters* has become a popular replacement (Cook & Newson, 1996; Culicover, 1997). A readable introductory account of the main tenets of the latest syntactic theory can be found in Cook and Newson (1996) and Culicover (1997).

As discussed earlier, Chomsky based his notions of innate faculties and the competence/performance distinction on the study of syntactic structures. Many linguists accept the major features of these notions; however, most of the objections (or differences) are due to the emphasis on a syntax-based grammar, which seems to be only remotely related to meaning and even use (Bohannon, 1993; Lyons, 1995; Owens, 1996; Steinberg, 1982). A number of scholars criticized the fact that Chomsky's early model could generate syntactically acceptable sentences that did not make sense, as in the following example: *Curious green dreams sleep furiously.* These theorists objected to the primary role being assigned to syntax with a secondary role assigned to semantics. This has led to the development of several competing generative grammars as well as to the few grammars based on semantics (see discussions in Lyons, 1995; Pustejovsky & Boguraev, 1996).

The Influence of Semantics

These and related difficulties of Chomsky's early TGG resulted in the beginning of a strong semantic movement with the publication of Lois Bloom's work (1970) based on her analysis of children's language in both linguistic and nonlinguistic contexts. The analysis is called a *rich interpretation* because it proceeds beyond the analysis of words only, which is considered necessary to understand the child's intention (or meaning) (see review in Bloom & Lahey, 1978). For example, depending on the analysis of the context in which the phrase is uttered by the child, the words *Daddy shoe* could have a number of meanings. The child could say this as she was picking up Daddy's shoe or as Daddy was putting her (the child's) shoe on her foot and so on (see discussions and examples in Bloom & Lahey, 1978). This is an example of different meanings for the same surface structure or utterance, which cannot be understood by an analysis of syntax alone. Arguments for the semantic basis in language have fueled the development of models by a number of scholars (Brown, 1973; Chafe, 1970; Greenfield & Smith, 1976; Lyons, 1995).

In general, semantic theorists argue that semantics is primary and syntax is secondary. It should be reemphasized here that semantics refers to meaning in language—however, it might be necessary to examine the context in which the sentence is uttered (especially for young children). The most prominent semantic movements were those associated with the notions of generative semantics, case grammar, and relational grammarians (see discussions in Cann, 1993; Lyons, 1995; Steinberg, 1982; Steinberg & Jakobovits, 1971). Essentially, semantic theorists argue that semantic structures can be specified independently of syntactic structures and that syntax depends on or is guided by semantic underpinnings. Semanticists assert that it is the development of semantics, not innate structures, that reflect or represent a general organization and pattern of cognitive development. As is discussed later, this has become the driving force for one type of interactionist view (i.e., cognitive interactionist) and has influenced cognitive-dominates-language perspectives in the thought-language debates (discussed later in this chapter).

A Few Salient Aspects of Semantic Theory

Drawing on the work of Kempson (1977), Cann (1993) reiterated a few salient concerns (and included an additional one) that might be adopted as criteria for determining the explanatory adequacy of semantic theories. Cann (1993) remarked that:

(1)   A semantic theory must:

1. capture for any language the nature of the meaning of words, phrases, and sentences and explain the nature of the relation between them;

2. be able to predict the ambiguities in the expressions of a language;

3. characterize and explain the systematic meaning relations between the words, the phrases, and the sentences of a language.

(2)   A semantic theory must provide an account of the relation between linguistic expressions and the things that they can be used to talk about. (p. 1)

Semantics, particularly generative semantics, has had a checkered history, with most linguists accepting the fact that generative semantics does not have a strong theoretical foundation (Huck & Goldsmith, 1995). However, the case is not closed because (a) some of the central tenets of generative semantics are still in vogue and (b) there are existing, unresolved questions concerning the relationship between syntax and semantics. It seems that generative semantics is just as tenable as interpretative semantics, which was advanced and developed by Chomsky (Huck & Goldsmith, 1995).

Competence versus Performance

A heavy emphasis on the notion that language has a grammar that is separate from or independent of its use plus a different perspective on the notion of nativism (e.g., constructionist, within interactionist perspectives) have created what can be described as "two distinct fields of language acquisition" (Ingram, 1989, p. 27). As discussed by Wasow (as cited in Ingram, 1989):

There has been, for some years now, a fairly sharp split in the field of developmental psycholinguistics between what I will call researchers in "child language" versus those in "language acquisition." Child language research is concerned primarily with what children say; that is, it focuses on the data. The central concern of most child language research is on data collection and classification, with correspondingly close attention to data collection techniques, and relatively little concern for abstract theoretical issues. Language acquisition specialists . . . regard child language as interesting only to the extent that it bears on questions of linguistic theory. (p. 27)

Relative to this discussion, most language acquisition specialists are linguists, that is, they have received their formal training in linguistics. In contrast, most child language researchers are psychologists who have received their formal training in psychology with an emphasis on language development (Ingram, 1989). These individuals are also known as psycholinguists. Language acquisition specialists begin with linguistic theory (i.e., competence model) and then focus on the problems of language acquisition (i.e., performance data). On the other hand, child language researchers tend to engage in what can be called inductive theorizing, that is, hypotheses are generated from the patterns observed in the performance data of children.

In sum, there are a number of scholars who believe that a complete theory of language acquisition needs to consider both competence and performance (Cairns, 1996; Ingram, 1989; Pinker, 1984; Stevenson, 1988). Many child language researchers disagree with linguists on the notion of nativism and the role of the social environment. In fact, a number of child language researchers belong to a third group called *interactionist* (Bohannon, 1993) and have also been influenced by what is now called *sociolinguistic theory* (Owens, 1996), which focuses on the pragmatics component (i.e., use) of language.

Table 3-4 presents some of the major highlights of the linguistic theories.

TABLE 3-4 A Few Major Points of Linguistic Theories

- Most linguistic theories have been influenced by the views of Noam Chomsky and by the cognitive metatheory.

- Linguistic theories are theories of language competence with a mostly structuralist framework. For the most part, these theories attempt to address the internal structure of the human mind. Variations of the theories are based on the support of or reactions against Chomsky's major themes involving concepts such as the language acquisition device, universal grammar, competence, and innate structures. Some of the variations result from a shift from syntax to semantics as being paramount for understanding language acquisition.

- Linguistic theories, with a focus on syntax, have evolved from standard theory to extended standard theory to government and binding, also known as principles and parameters.

(continues)

(Table 3-4 continued)

• The most prominent semantic movements (i.e., reactions against syntax) were those associated with the notions of generative semantics, case grammar, and relational grammar.

• Some semanticists assert that it is the development of semantics, not innate structures, that reflect or represent a general organization and pattern of cognitive development—that is, the structure of the mind.

• The debate on the competence-performance dichotomy engendered the development of two broad types of language scholars/researchers. One group of researchers—child language researchers—is concerned primarily with what children say—that is, there is a focus on performance data. The other group—language acquisition scholars—is concerned with linguistic or competence theory, using only performance data when they relate to the development of models.

• Despite these variations, there seems to be a growing consensus that any complete model of language acquisition needs to consider both competence and performance.

INTERACTIONISM

The interactionist theory (perhaps, a micro-metatheory) incorporates tenets from both behavioristic and linguistic approaches. The term *interactionism* implies that there are a number of factors—for example, cognitive, linguistic, and social—that are critical for the development of an individual. It is important to emphasize the interactive influences of these factors. For example, language factors influence the development of cognitive and social development. As another example, cognitive and social factors affect the acquisition of language. The interactionist framework has had a marked influence on the thinking of the relationship(s) between thought and language (Bohannon, 1993; Cromer, 1981, 1988a, 1988b, 1994).

Within the interactionist framework, there are several major approaches (Bohannon, 1993; Owens, 1996; Whitehead, 1990). One approach, labeled *cognitive-interactionist*, is concerned primarily with the relationship between cognition and language development. This approach, also called a *cognitive approach* (e.g. Whitehead, 1990), has engendered several cognitively based thought/language hypotheses.

The second group of approaches has been influenced by the information-processing paradigm, as exemplified by the use of a computer metaphor. One of the major models has been the PDP, or parallel distributed processors, developed by McClelland, Rumelhart, and the PDP Research Group (1986), and is also known as the connectionist model. The notion of parallel processing has replaced the linear or serial processing models, which were quite prominent in early extant reading theories (i.e., as bottom-up and top-down models) until about the late 1970s. PDP has engendered other models, most notably Bates and MacWhinney's (1987) competition model (for an update, see Fletcher & MacWhinney, 1995).

The third major approach, labeled *social-interactionist*, focuses primarily on the relationship between social development and language acquisition. Although this approach has also contributed to the thinking of the relationship between cognition and language, one of its major influences seems to be on theories and research on pragmatics, that is, factors that govern language choices during social intercourse (Bohannon, 1993; Crystal, 1987, 1997; Ninio & Snow, 1996; Owens, 1996). A few basic tenets of each group are presented in the ensuing paragraphs.

Cognitive-Interactionist

The major impetus for the cognitive-interactionist position is the work of Jean Piaget on the development of cognition (see readable discussions of Piaget's work in Flavell, 1985, and Phillips, 1981). Piaget's thinking highlights two important differences—mentioned previously—between the cognitive-interactionist and linguistic positions: competence/performance and nature/nurture (or rather, a different interpretation of the innate principle).

Similar to the linguistic advocates, cognitive-interactionists recognize the distinction between competence and performance. However, cognitive-interactionists believe that performance data can provide useful information on the language acquisition process of children (Bohannon, 1993; Ingram, 1989; Stevenson, 1988). It is argued that the cognitive capacity of children is both qualitatively and quantitatively different from that of the mature adult language user. By observing the performances of children, it is possible to provide a more complete understanding of the road to mature linguistic development. Cognitive-interactionists also believe that the cognitive processes that underlie children's linguistic performance are also the same processes that account for children's linguistic competence.

The innate principle was one of the major topics of a debate by Chomsky and Piaget (Ingram, 1989; Piattelli-Palmarini, 1980, 1994). Chomsky's views on the innate principle discussed previously (i.e., LAD or Universal Grammar) have been labeled as *maturationism*. Succinctly stated, the maturationist position of innateness posits that linguistic knowledge is innate and becomes functional or operational when the individual interacts with the environment (Cook & Newson, 1996; Ingram, 1989; Steinberg, 1982). Thus, environmental stimuli activate this innate knowledge; they do not shape or modify it.

Piaget's views on the innate principle have been labeled as constructivism. The constructivist position assumes that "the complex structures of language might be neither innate nor learned. Instead, these structures emerge as a result of the continuing interaction between the child's current level of cognitive functioning and his current linguistic, and nonlinguistic, environment." (Bohannon & Warren-Leubecker, 1985, p. 189).

In this view, language development (as well as other kinds of development) is said to be a part of the overall cognitive development of individuals. Language development may be an independent system; however, its growth depends on the development of cognitive underpinnings. This approach is somewhat compatible with Vygotsky's (1962) notion of inner speech (i.e., symbolic speech) in which thinking dominates or regulates language processes. However, Vygotsky believed that social forces contribute to the existence and growth of cognition, language, and other characteristics of humans (see discussion in "Social-Interactionist").

Information-Processing Models

As discussed previously, one of the most common metaphors of the information-processing paradigm is the computer. The stage-of-processing model seems to be most commonly used in the research on deafness (see Paul & Jackson, 1993); however, there is a trend toward the use of other models (e.g., connectionist and modularity), particularly for understanding the relationship between language and cognition in deaf children, and especially for deaf children who use sign (see discussion in Marschark et al., 1997). Within the stage-of-processing model, there are three major components: sensory register, short-term memory, and long-term memory (see Table 3-5 for a brief discussion of these terms). Much of the research in this area has focused on the organization and representation of knowledge and the retrieval of that information for application purposes. One of the most common themes is that the processing of children is qualitatively similar to that of adults. In essence, children are developing from novice users to skilled users of information, particularly, for the purposes here, linguistic information. One robust line of research has been that on the relationship between short-term (i.e., working) memory and reading comprehension (discussed in Chapter 8 of this text).

The critical aspect of the information-processing approach, especially the model by McClelland, Rumelhart, and the PDP Research Group (1986), is that

---

TABLE 3-5 A Few Terms Associated with the Stage-of-Processing Model

---

Information Processing: Stage-of-Processing Model

Sensory Register

• This is also known as sensory store or sensory memory.

• There is purported to be a sensory register for each of the senses. In relation to language and reading, much attention has been devoted to the stores for vision and audition.

• Despite the hypothetical large capacity of the sensory register, it can only take in unanalyzed information for about one second. This information will disappear unless it receives focused attention and is transferred to the second stage—short-term (or working) memory.

Short-term Memory (STM)

• Information can remain in STM for about 30 seconds.

• This is a temporary storage, and the amount of information that can be held is about seven, plus or minus two units. A unit is considered to be a chunk of information and is influenced by the third stage—long-term memory (LTM).

• Research on deafness has been influenced by a model of working memory (WM) proposed by Baddeley (1990). In this view, WM is considered to be a component of STM. Research has revealed five types of coding strategies in WM for deaf students—sign, dactylic (fingerspelling), visual (shape of letters or words), phonological (mental representations of the auditory-articulatory processes), and multiple (combinations of these). Albeit a controversial finding, it has been shown that deaf students who use predominantly a phonological-based code in WM tend to be better readers than other deaf students who use predominantly a nonphonological-based code (also see Chapter 8 of this text).

Long-term Memory (LTM)

• The strength and efficiency of the relationship between STM and LTM is markedly influenced by the development of a well-established social-conventional language.

(continues)

(Table 3-5 continued)

- The manner in which information is represented or organized in LTM and retrieved from LTM is a major focus of the bulk of research in cognitive science.

- The LTM of an individual contains that person's knowledge about the world, including knowledge about language and reading/writing. This stored information enables the individual to interpret, understand, and store new experiences.

Note: Additional information can be found in the following sources—Hanson (1989), Medin & Ross (1992), Miller (1956), and Shadbolt (1988).

of parallel processing. Unlike serial or sequential processing in which there is a single operation performed one at a time in a linear manner, parallel processing involves the use of multiple operations in a simultaneous fashion. There have been several descriptions of this complex model; however, the following passage by Bohannon (1993) was found to be most helpful, albeit a little challenging:

> *In parallel processing, networks of processors are mutually linked or connected such that many operations or decisions may proceed concurrently. These networks have come to be called* parallel distributed processors, *or PDPs for short. . . . PDP models consist of a series of processing units, called* activation nodes. *These are meant to resemble or model individual neurons or assemblies of neurons in the brain. Each unit is connected to other units by pathways that vary in the "strength" of their connections. These pathways are meant to model the dendrites and axons that connect neurons in the brain. The strength of the connections is seen as reflecting the extent of a neural connection, the number of axon terminals, dendritic spines, etc. Activation nodes, like neurons, are decision mechanisms. They receive input from other nodes across pathways of varying strength, weigh the input, and "decide" whether or not to activate. This is seen as similar to the process by which neurons sum all incoming signals and "fire" or not depending upon the amount of stimulation. If sufficient input has occurred across the pathways, the unit may activate itself, thus sending activating information out its own output pathways to other nodes. (p. 267)*

The connectionist model has been used to explain the word identification process in reading and to address the learning of language items such as past tense and other grammatical aspects. As discussed in Chapter 8 on literacy, this cognitive model is considered to be more productive than the other serial, linear reading models associated with bottom-up and top-down processing. With the focus on connections and nodes, it is clear this view is quite different from that of Fodor (1983), who argued for an independent module for language development and processing. In addition, the notion of parallel processing is different from what has been argued for the linguistic approach, motivated by Chomsky. For example, Pinker (1989) stated that the linguistic approach is primarily serial. One example is that the linguists (i.e., those influenced by Chomsky's thinking) attempted to formulate the deep structure relations prior to demonstrating the application of transformations such as questions, relativization, pronominalization, and so on, which are also performed in a certain serial order (examples of these syntactic structures were provided in Chapter 2).

Social-Interactionist

Perhaps the compromise between behaviorist and linguistic approaches is most evident in the social-interactionist framework. In describing this framework, Whitehead (1990) remarked that many developmental psychologists, who were interested in human (i.e., adult-child) interactions, began to pay more attention to and to reaffirm the roles that these interactions play in the learning process. In particular, there was an emphasis on language interactions. It was argued that the language-learning process is facilitated by the critical functions of language—for example, for social-communication interactions and making sense of the world in which one lives. Thus, developmental psychologists began to support the concepts associated with the linguistic theory of pragmatics. Additional support for the social-interactionist view can be gleaned from the research on the social activity and sensitivity of infants, including the newborn.

Similar to linguistic proponents, social interactionists assert that language has a unique, rule-governed structure. However, they argue that these structures develop (i.e., emerge or result) from the social functions of language as evident in human interactions. The development of more mature linguistic functions permits the growth of more sophisticated human interactions. Social-interactionists view language acquisition as a complex, reciprocal, dynamic interplay between the child and the social-linguistic environment.

A better understanding of this dynamic interplay may be seen in the following discussion. Consider that linguists view children as active processors of language. Because of language's specialized nature, children's development is guided by maturation (Bohannon, 1993; Ingram, 1989; Whitehead, 1990). The input of significant others is important because this input triggers (sets in motion) the innate structures.

On the other hand, behaviorists view children as passive processors of language information. Children's development is guided mainly by the stimuli and actions (e.g., reinforcement) of significant others, particularly parents. In essence, the input and actions of significant others are totally responsible for children's language development.

By focusing on turn-taking and other pragmatics functions (e.g., those associated with speech acts), social-interactionists assert that children's utterances elicit a response from parents (particularly mothers) and vice versa. The social interaction is dynamic and enriching because parents provide language stimuli necessary for children's language growth. Relative to the competence/performance issue, social-interactionists believe the linguistic competence of children can only be understood by their performance (i.e., understanding and use) within a social context.

It can be inferred from the foregoing discussion that social-interactionists believe that both nature and nurture factors contribute to the child's acquisition of language. Social-interactionists assert that some experience and training are necessary for children's language to develop. It is also argued that the innate mechanism by itself cannot explain children's mastery of language. The following passage exemplifies this position:

> *Social interactive approach assumes that language development is the result of acquiring grammatical rules. The child is also assumed to bring a number of innate predispositions to the language learning situation that constrain children in their search for linguistically relevant distinctions. On the other hand, the environment is believed to be almost as constrained as the children, in order to supply children with the types of language experience necessary for development. Language development is viewed as an orderly, although complex, interactive process where social interaction assists language acquisition and the acquisition of language allows more mature social interaction. (Bohannon, 1993, pp. 276–277)*

Table 3-6 provides a summary of the major points of the interactionist language theories.

LANGUAGE AND THOUGHT

This section of the chapter discusses a few issues on the relationship between language and thought and provides a brief overview of this relationship to

---

TABLE 3-6 **A Few Major Points of Interactionist Theories**

- In general, these theories incorporate tenets from both behavioristic and linguistic approaches. This is considered to be a balanced perspective; however, the nature of the balance depends on the specific focus of models.

- In contrast to modularity, interactionists maintain that there are a number of factors—for example, biological, cognitive, linguistic, environmental, and social—that interact and are critical for the development of an individual.

- Within the interactionist framework, there are three broad approaches—cognitive-interactionist, information processing, and social-interactionist.

- The cognitive-interactionist approach is concerned with the relationship between language and thought and has been influenced mostly by the work of Piaget. Cognitive-interactionists believe that the cognitive processes that underlie children's linguistic performance are also the same processes that account for children's linguistic competence. In essence, this view asserts that language development is part of the overall cognitive development of individuals.

- One of the most common metaphors of the information-processing paradigm is the computer. A great deal of research on deafness has been influenced by the stage-of-processing model with three major components—sensory register, short-term memory, and long-term memory. Much of the focus of research in the information-processing paradigm has been on processes, including memory and attention span.

- Some scholars argued that the real balance between behavioristic and linguistic approaches is most evident in the third major interactionist paradigm—social-interactionist. Social-interactionists assert that language has a unique, rule-governed structure; however, these structures develop (i.e., emerge or result) from the social functions of language, as evident in human interactions. Language acquisition is said to be a complex, reciprocal, dynamic interplay between the child and the social-linguistic environment. It is argued that both nature and nurture factors contribute to the child's acquisition of language.

---

the study of deafness. Any discussion regarding the relationship of thought and language is not an exercise in futility or merely an academic debate. If researchers move away from an emphasis on the global comparison of the two entities to a focus on the relationship of specific features of each domain, a better understanding of this relationship might surface, and it might even be possible to proffer some sound educational implications (see Cromer, 1981, 1988a, 1988b, 1994; for a perspective on deafness and signing, see Marschark et al., 1997; also see Marschark, 1993). For example, researchers' knowledge of the reading difficulties of students with hearing impairment has progressed because of studies on the relationship between the processes of short-term memory (specific aspect of cognition) and comprehension of sentences, particularly syntactic constructions (specific aspect of language). This line of research has underscored the importance of using a phonological code in short-term memory (STM) because of the increasing importance of the relationship between phonemic awareness and reading achievement during the early years (Adams, 1990; also see Chapter 8 of this text). This is controversial and problematic for individuals with severe to profound hearing impairment (Hanson, 1989; Paul, 1998a; Paul & Jackson, 1993).

In essence, there might not be one relationship between language and thought; in fact, it might be that there are several or many relations. Some of these relations might be relevant to specific domains or categories of language or to specific domains or categories of cognition (Bates, Bretherton, & Snyder, 1988; Karmiloff-Smith, 1989). The single-directional influences and their variations (e.g., strong and weak cognitive hypotheses to be discussed later) might not be as useful or productive as the notion that the relations between language and cognition vary across the course of the individual's development within and across specific domains such as literacy and psychosocial development.

The goal in this section is not to present a comprehensive review of the various thought-language models. Rather, the focus is on providing some basic tenets. More important, the section emphasizes the eventual interactive effects of thought and language. The author's reflections on the findings of the interactive effects have led to the conclusion that high-level performance in one domain is dependent on a high-level development in the other domain. In addition, it can be argued that some knowledge is domain specific and does not always depend on a corresponding level of knowledge in the other domain. For example, the understanding of a relative clause is predominantly a language-specific behavior that does not depend on cognitive prerequisites, other than a basic level of developmental maturity.

Language-specific knowledge has been influenced by the notion of constraints, especially within a modularity hypothesis (see Fodor, 1983), which has been motivated by Chomsky's concept of innate structures or the language acquisition device (Chomsky, 1975; Fodor, 1983; also see Cairns, 1996; Cook & Newson, 1996). The works of pioneers such as Piaget, Vygotsky, and Luria have also influenced the development of language models. The cognitive-interactionist view is based on Piaget's model of cognition, whereas the social-interactionist view is based in part on Vygotsky's model.

Both cognitive theorists and language theorists, for example, Chomsky, Sapir, and Whorf, have influenced the various models concerning the relationship between thought and language (see Byrnes & Gelman, 1991). Both groups of theorists view language as a window into the intricate operations of the mind. Some language theorists are interested in the linguistic underpinnings of the development of language, whereas some cognitive theorists focus on the cognitive underpinnings. These single-directional emphases represent what are considered strong views of the thought-language relationships (Cromer, 1981, 1988a, 1988b, 1994). There is also evidence for weak views of this relationship, which seem to include the framework of an interactive relationship (see discussions in Bohannon, 1993; Paul & Jackson, 1993). From one perspective, it is feasible to consider nearly all views, except the independent modularity one, as versions of an interactive perspective with qualifications on the strength, direction, and extent of the interaction. However, interactionist accounts seem to be biased toward cognition due to the fact that there is much discussion on the influences of cognitive development on language acquisition.

Without oversimplifying, it is possible and feasible to describe the overall views of the relations between cognition and language. What is often called single-directional approaches, which are characterized as cognition-dominates-language (i.e., cognition influences language) or language-dominates-cognition (i.e., language influences cognition) view, have been mentioned. There are strong and weak versions of the single-directional approaches. The weak versions seem to be influenced by the relative lack of substantial empirical support for the strong versions and by the notion of an interactive reciprocity between language and cognition. However, even in the weak versions, there seems to be a bias toward the cognitive domains, as mentioned previously. There is also the concept that language and thought are independent of each other. This view has been proffered by Chomsky and developed even further by Fodor (1983) with his modularity hypothesis.

The one view that is not discussed in detail is the language-equals-thought perspective. This has been another aspect of the behaviorist metatheory, which is not widely accepted by most psychologists or philosophers. It seems to be clear that individuals without a bona fide symbol system are capable of thought. Just how far and deep thought can be developed (as in the concept of literate thought) without a language and whether it is equivalent to individuals with a language is the subject of debate, especially with respect to some deaf children and adolescents (e.g., see Marschark, 1993; Marschark et al., 1997).

Thought-based Hypotheses

The basic premise of thought-based hypotheses is that thought (cognition) influences or accounts for the development of language (Byrnes & Gelman, 1991; Cromer, 1988a, 1988b; Snyder, 1984). That is, language grows out of cognition, or language is a mapping out of cognitive skills. Variations among the hypotheses are related to the interpretation of the strength of the influence of thought on language development.

The strong forms of thought-based hypotheses assert that language is not possible without cognitive underpinnings. This is a unidirectional model in which the direction of influence is from cognition to language. In these versions, the development of language is equal to but does not exceed cognitive development. This implies a one-to-one, or perfect, correlation between thought and language development.

The strong forms of thought-based hypotheses have been influenced pervasively by the work of Piaget (1980; also see Flavell, 1985; Phillips, 1981). Piaget asserted that language has only a modest, albeit important, role in the development of thought. Nevertheless, the role of language has called into question the basic tenets of the strong views. Relative to research on cognition and deafness, some scholars (Kusche & Greenberg, 1991) have argued that discrepancies between individuals who are hearing and those who are hearing impaired on high-level, abstract cognitive tasks might be due predominantly to the effects of an inadequate development of a language in the individuals with hearing impairment.

The thinking of Cromer (1974, 1976, 1981) has influenced the weak versions of thought-based hypotheses. Weak versions assert that thought does not completely account for the development of language. It is acknowledged that some linguistic knowledge is dependent on language-specific skills. Language development is equal to or less than but does not exceed the development of thought. Evidence for the weak thought-based hypotheses has been reported in a number of investigations (see reviews in Cromer, 1988a, 1988b; Johnston, 1985; Slobin, 1979; also see a readable account in Owens, 1996).

Other variations of thought-based hypotheses can be found elsewhere (see discussions in Gelman & Byrnes, 1991; Snyder, 1984). Harris (1992) proffered some compelling data against the strong thought-based hypotheses. This scholar argued that one possible implication of the strong view is that older second-language learners' acquisition of a language should be qualitatively different from that of first-language learners. For example, the older learners should know concepts (i.e., aspects of thought) that are not known by younger first-language learners. Harris concluded that research has not confirmed this argument. In fact, there is ample research showing that the language acquisition patterns of both first- and second-language learners (of English) are qualitatively similar, at least from a global, overall perspective. That is, both groups proceed through similar stages, make the same errors, and use congruent strategies in the acquisition of a language (McLaughlin, 1984, 1985).

Language-based Hypotheses

Similar to the thought-based hypotheses, there are strong and weak versions of language-based hypotheses and variations of these views. The strongest version asserts that language determines thought (i.e., linguistic determinism) (Sapir, 1958; Whorf, 1956). Within this framework, there is a perfect, one-to-one correspondence between linguistic and cognitive aspects. However, in this case, the direction of the influence flows from language underpinnings to thought structures. This position is exemplified by the linguist Sapir (1958) who remarked that:

> *It is quite an illusion to imagine that one adjusts to reality without the use of language and that language is merely an incidental means of solving specific problems of communication or reflections . . . we see and hear and otherwise experience as we do because the language habits of our community predispose certain choices of interpretation. (p. 162)*

Although the evidence on the strong version is equivocal (see Bloom, 1981, for affirmative data and Au, 1988, for contrary evidence; also see a readable account in Owens, 1996), it is not a widely accepted hypothesis. The focus seems to be on weak variations or on language-specific hypotheses that take into consideration the notion of innate structure and one of its major implications—constraints. One view that seems to be gaining proponents is the learnability hypothesis (see discussion in Pinker, 1989).

Table 3-7 presents a few major highlights based on this brief discussion of cognitive and language-based hypotheses.

TABLE 3-7 A Few Principles of Thought/Language-Based Hypotheses

---

General Principles

- Traditional basic premise is that one domain influences or accounts for the development of the other domain.

- Variations among the hypotheses are related to the interpretation of the strength of the influence of one domain on the other.

(continues)

(Table 3-7 continued)

- Two major theoretical influences are modularity (Fodor, 1983) and connectionism (McClelland, Rumelhart, & the PDP Research Group, 1986).

Thought Hypotheses

Strong Versions

- Language is not possible without cognitive underpinnings.

- Direction of influence is from thought to language.

- Development of language is equal to but does not exceed cognitive development.

- There is a one-to-one correlation between language and thought.

Weak Versions

- Thought does not completely account for the development of language.

- Language development is equal to or less than but does not exceed the development of thought.

Other Perspectives

- Thought and language share common underpinnings.

- Relationships between language and thought are influenced by social and cultural factors.

- There are many relations between thought and language that vary across the individual's life span.

Strong Versions

- Language determines thought, as in linguistic determinism.

- There is a perfect one-to-one correspondence between linguistic and cognitive aspects.

- The direction of influence is from language to thought.

Other Versions (Modularity)

- Most of these versions consider the notion of innate structure and one of its major aspects, constraints.

- Although language receives important input from cognitive and social forces, its main development is contained within or influenced by its own module or faculty and operates on maturation principles.

Reflections and Other Perspectives

There seems to be growing evidence that the relationship between thought and language is bidirectional and interactive. In some variations of this view, language plays an influential role, and in others, cognition plays an influential role. It might be also that the so-called interactions between language and cognition can be explained by other factors, indicating that neither language nor cognition is in the dominant, driver position. From another perspective, it could be argued that culture determines or influences both language and cognition (which leads to various views on the similarity of language and cognition). This possibility was alluded to in the brief discussion of the sociocultural framework earlier in this chapter (which might also be known as the sociocultural-historical framework). This view, influenced pervasively by social theories or the predominance of social and cultural influences as discussed in the thinking of Vygotsky and others, acknowledges the critical contributions of environmental or experiential factors to the development of both language and cognition. In essence, language and cognition grow as a part of the influences of the culture or environment. These influences can include the emotions and interactions from the family and significant others as well as cultural values associated with families and groups (for an interesting perspective on this issue and deafness, see Clark, 1993). Marschark and Everhart (1997) summarized this view briefly and eloquently: "The common root of cognitive and linguistic growth might not be in the child at all but may be inherent in the structure of the world and/or the phylogeny of human beings" (p. 11).

LANGUAGE, COGNITION, AND DEAFNESS: A BRIEF OVERVIEW

This section presents a brief discussion of the implications of the thought/language debate for deaf and hard-of-hearing individuals. This discussion is

118 ■ LANGUAGE AND DEAFNESS

selective; a few salient theoretical aspects and research findings are related to an understanding of the importance of language development as indicated by the previous discussion of thought-language relationships. Much of the research on deafness has been based on the models of Piaget, Vygotsky, and information processing, known as a stage-of-processing model. A more detailed discussion of these models as well as good reviews of the cognitive research on deafness can be found elsewhere (Greenberg & Kusche, 1989; Marschark, 1993; Marschark et al., 1997; Martin, 1991; Moores & Meadow-Orlans, 1990; Paul & Jackson, 1993).

During much of the 19th century, most researchers on deafness seemed to have been influenced by a version of the language-dominates-thought hypothesis, ranging from the strong version to the weak and interactive ones. For example, both Pintner (Pintner & Paterson, 1917; Pintner & Reamer, 1920) and Myklebust (1964) argued that the intellectual deficits of many deaf individuals as determined by the IQ tests (or some variation of these tests) were due primarily and predominantly to language deficiencies. Myklebust went further and argued that due to the lack of a bona fide language, many deaf individuals perceived the world differently because they were compelled to rely on their other intact senses for interpreting information. Myklebust did not recognize a language of signs. In essence, the language-deficit hypothesis still has some strong proponents today. Moores (1987) categorized the influential works of Pintner and Myklebust as reflective of two major stages of research on intelligence and deafness labeled *Deaf as Inferior* and *Deaf as Concrete*, respectively.

During the latter part of the 1900s, the cognition-dominates-language hypothesis and the cognition-and-language independent hypothesis influenced the thinking of scholars on the intellectual development of deaf individuals. This resulted in the third major stage of research on intelligence and deafness, which Moores (1987) labeled the *Deaf as Intellectually Normal*.

Table 3-8 provides the salient principles and findings of all three stages of intelligence and deafness.

Until the publication of texts on the language status of American Sign Language (Klima & Bellugi, 1979; Liddell, 1980; Wilbur, 1987) and the existence of other sign languages, some scholars assumed that many deaf individuals (i.e., those with severe to profound impairment) did not have a command of a social-conventional language in any modality or form, for example, a spoken language such as English. Thus, by studying these individuals, it was assumed that this would shed light on how cognition could grow in the absence of a well-developed bona fide linguistic system. This line of thinking has been influenced by the cognition-dominates-language position or, more

TABLE 3-8 Research on Intelligence and Deafness

Stages of Intellectual Development and Deafness

Tenets of Stage 1

• The first stage was labeled *The Deaf as Inferior.*

• Most of the tests used with deaf individuals were developed for and normed on individuals with normal hearing ability.

• It was argued that deafness leads to intellectual deficiency.

• Most of deaf students' difficulty was attributed to the lack of an internalized verbal symbol system, such as a language, and its associated representations of experiences.

• Findings were interpreted within a language-dominated-thought paradigm.

Tenets of Stage 2

• This stage was labeled *The Deaf as Concrete.*

• There were qualitative differences between deaf and hearing individuals relative to tasks that require abstract thinking.

• Mykebust's organismic shift hypothesis asserted that deprivation of the hearing sense leads to a different organization of experiences by the other senses.

• The proffering of unique qualitative differences between deaf and hearing individuals led to the notion that there is a psychology of deafness.

• Findings were interpreted within a language-dominated-thought paradigm.

Tenets of Stage 3

• This stage has been labeled *The Deaf as Intellectually Normal.*

• Deaf individuals are considered to be intellectually and cognitively similar to hearing individuals in all important abilities.

• Differences that still exist between deaf and hearing individuals are assumed to be due to linguistic, cultural, environmental, and task factors rather than to the condition of deafness.

• Findings were interpreted within a thought-dominated-language paradigm.

Note: Adapted from Moores (1987) and Paul and Jackson (1993).

commonly, by the cognition-and-language-independent position, mentioned previously. The work of Furth (1966) is illustrative. Furth attempted to determine whether language is critical for the development of Piagetian structures in deaf individuals (see Table 3-9 for a discussion of Piaget's stages).

Piaget identified three time periods at which language might play an important—albeit modest—role in the development of thought. These three time periods are transitions from one stage to the next—for example, from sensorimotor to preoperation, from preoperation to concrete operation, and from concrete operation to formal operation (Byrnes & Gelman, 1991). Piaget also divided the development of children's language into two broad stages. The first stage includes egocentric speech that emerges from noncommunicative thought. This involves monologues and language play where the child repeats simply for the pleasure of talking. The second stage involves socialized speech that develops to include eventually all the forms required for social communication such as information, criticism, commands, requests, questions, and so forth.

It should be underscored that Piaget only assigned a modest role for language in the development of thought. As stated in the following passage:

Language is thus a necessary but not a sufficient condition for the construction of logical operations. It is necessary because without the system of symbolic expression which constitutes language the operations would remain at the stage of successive actions without ever being integrated into simultaneous systems or simultaneously encompassing a set of interdependent transformations. Without language the operations would remain personal and would consequently not be regulated by interpersonal exchange and cooperation. It is in this dual sense of symbolic condensation and social regulation that language is indispensable to the elaboration of thought. (Piaget, 1968, p. 98)

With respect to deaf individuals, Furth's (1966) conclusions are similar to those of Piaget; that is, language does not play a major role in the development of cognitive structures. Nevertheless, Furth did maintain that language was important, specifically when it comes to addressing abstract concepts—concepts that need to be represented by linguistic symbols. Despite the role of language, Furth concluded that the cognitive level of deaf individuals is roughly commensurate with that of their hearing counterparts.

Others have viewed this situation from different perspectives. For example, most interpretations of the performances of deaf children and adolescents on Piagetian tasks are related to the nature and administration of the tasks. Some scholars (notably, Rodda & Grove, 1987) remarked that the inferior

TABLE 3-9 Major Principles of Piaget's Stages of Cognition

Sensorimotor Stage

- This stage covers the period from birth to about 2 years of age.
- Six substages have been identified.
- Child perceives and reacts to sensory data as related to basic needs and begins to organize and integrate these data into schemas.

Preoperational Stage

- This stage extends from about 2 to 7 years of age.
- There is an ability to think in a logical manner.
- Egocentrism prevents the child from separating the personal perspective from that of others, as manifested in the social interactions of the child.

Concrete Operational Stage

- This stage extends from 7 to about 11 years of age.
- The child is now able to distinguish personal self from others.
- The child is now able to perform mental operations on objects that are physically present.

Formal Operational Stage

- This stage is the final stage and extends from about age 11 to about age 15 years.
- The stage is characterized primarily by abstract thinking and a shift from the need for concrete objects and experiences.
- The individual can engage in metalinguistic and metacognitive activities, that is, she or he can think about language or about thinking.

Note: Adapted from Flavell (1985) and Phillips (1981).

performances of deaf children and adolescents are the result of social and psychological factors such as reduced stimulation, restricted educational access, and inadequate social and communicative interactions. This is an experiential hypothesis, which might also include language deprivation.

The effects of language on cognition cannot be overemphasized relative to the current thinking on the thought-language relationship. The interactive effects of language and cognition might have influenced the performances of deaf children on many tasks in the concrete and formal operational stages (also see the discussions of various perspectives in Greenberg & Kusche, 1989; Marschark, 1993; Paul & Jackson, 1993). The lack of language or a poorly developed language can affect the way information is organized, stored, and retrieved. It has even been speculated that this language deprivation prevents a transfer of function from the right hemisphere to the left hemisphere of the brain, which deals with processes that require a highly organized descriptive system or code (e.g., language) (see a readable account in Sacks, 1989).

Relative to deaf individuals' performances on Piagetian tasks, this view has also been stated by Greenberg and Kusche (1989). Greenberg and Kusche (1989) acknowledged the role of visual-spatial ability for progress through the sensorimotor and much of the peroperational stages. In addition, these researchers asserted that:

> *Although Furth . . . has interpreted the literature as evidence that language does not affect thinking, we believe that language has a strong effect on concrete and formal operational modes of thinking, while it has relatively less influence on sensorimotor and preoperational thought. . . . With regard to abstract-proportional (or formal operational) thought, it may be that episodic memories which are encoded linguistically and/or symbolically (in speech or in signs) in the hippocampal areas . . . perhaps through the use of verbal/sign mediation, are more easily translated into propositional concepts or schemes in the association area of the cortex . . . than are visually encoded memories or images. (p. 101)*

There is still quite a bit of work to do on the complex relationship between language and cognition given the existence of contradictory evidence. As stated previously, the author's bias is that there is an interactive, reciprocal relationship between language and thought. Language is critical for the development of higher aspects of thought (e.g., literate thought) and vice versa. A language problem does not always reflect an underlying deficit in cognitive development, and the opposite is also true. To put it another way, there might be deficits in specific processes that are unique to either language or cognition. Stating it yet another way, Cromer (1981, 1988a, 1988b, 1994) suggested that the presence of language difficulties may be reflective of problems in processes such as short-term memory, auditory processing, auditory storage, and hierarchical planning. The interrelationships among these variables are not completely understood, even in the voluminous research that has been conducted on language-disordered children (see brief discussion in Snow et al., 1998).

In sum, there are theoretical and practical reasons for continuing the theorizing, research, and debate on the nature of the relationships between language and thought. With respect to deafness, there are numerous important issues on which to reflect and examine, many of which have been discussed in other sources (Marschark, 1993; Marschark et al., 1997; Moores & Meadow-Orlans, 1990; Paul & Jackson, 1993). The few selected issues highlighted here are not the only ones that are important; however, these issues are examined in the ensuing chapters of this text. For example, the language-thought debate (as well as related aspects of it) might offer insights into the development of concrete and abstract reasoning abilities; the effects, if any, of exposure to the various oral and manual communication systems on the development of language and thinking (including perceptual) skills; the effects of acquiring a language later in life (say, early or late adolescence) versus acquiring one during the typical time frame; the development of categorical knowledge and hierarchical organization (critical for literacy, for example); and of course, whether there are indeed quantitative or qualitative similarities or differences between deaf and hearing individuals. The most interesting and far-reaching revelations for the teaching-learning situations in schools would be a better understanding and implications of the language-cognition-experiential (i.e., sociocultural-historical) paradigm.

FINAL REMARKS

This chapter presents basic information on metatheories and theories of language acquisition. Theorizing about language has been a difficult endeavor, and at present, there does not seem to be a widely accepted view of the language acquisition process. This makes it difficult to proffer suggestions for the improvement of language in deaf and hard-of-hearing children and adolescents.

This chapter also describes a few broad perspectives on the relationships between language and cognition. The nature of this relationship is so complex that it has become counterproductive to assume that there might be one all-encompassing view that seeks to determine which one is dominant or basic or to assume that there is only one type of relationship. There seems to be a growing consensus that there are many relations that occur during the developmental cycle of humans. The influences of a cultural paradigm (i.e., sociocultural-historical paradigm) on the language-thought relations seems to be a promising area for further theorizing and research.

Summaries of major points have been presented throughout the chapter; here are only a few general points, which are organized within three headings: Metatheories, Language Theories, and Language-Thought Debates.

Metatheories

- Theories of language development have been influenced by several broad metatheories in psychology—introspectionism, behaviorism, cognitivism, and socioculturalism. Each metatheory is distinguished by its approach to the study of the mind.

- The influences of both introspectionism and behaviorism are not widespread; it is safe to say that most of the current thinking on language and thought adheres to salient principles of cognitivism and socioculturalism and variations of these concepts.

- There is a growing consensus that any adequate metatheory needs to consider a wide array of factors or conditions that interact within and outside of individuals (e.g., biological, cognitive, environmental, social, neurophysiological, etc.).

Language Theories

- At present, there is no comprehensive, coherent theory of language development.

- It is not clear if a complete theory of language needs to include both psychological (e.g., learning principles, laws) and physiological (e.g., brain-mapping) components.

- There are essentially three groups of language models—behaviorism, linguistic, and interactionist—with variations within each group.

- Many of the current prominent language theories have been influenced mainly by the work of Chomsky. That is, there are either variations of Chomsky's thinking or negative reactions to it.

- There seems to be a growing consensus that any complete model of language acquisition needs to consider what Bloom and Lahey (1978) labeled as *form* (e.g., phonology, morphology, and syntax), *content* (e.g., semantics), and *use* (e.g., pragmatics).

Language-Thought Debates

- Traditionally, there have been discussions of cognition-dominates-language models or language-dominates-cognition models with strong or weak variations.

- There is some consensus that the traditional language-thought models are incomplete or inadequate due to the focus on single-directional influences.

- One emerging view is that there might be several or many relations between language and thought. Some of these relations might be relevant to specific domains or categories of language or to specific domains or categories of cognition. It needs to be kept in mind that relations between language and cognition vary across the course of an individual's development.

- With respect to deafness, the language-thought debates might eventually offer insights into, for example, the development of concrete and abstract reasoning abilities; the effects, if any, of exposure to the various oral and manual communication systems on the development of conceptual and perceptual skills; the effects of acquiring a language later in life; the development of categorical knowledge and hierarchical organization (e.g., critical literacy); and whether there are quantitative or qualitative similarities or differences between deaf and hearing individuals.

Research on the qualitative-quantitative issue, mentioned earlier, should provide some perspectives on the development of a first language in students who are deaf and hard of hearing at as early an age as possible. In addition, the question of whether English, or any spoken language, is a feasible language for students with severe to profound impairment is a possible area of debate that could be gleaned from the discussion of language theories or the language-thought debates. Finally, the outcomes of these lines of theoretical and research debates should provide some insights into the question of whether mainstream theories of language can be applicable to deaf and hard-of-hearing students.

Before proceeding further, there needs to be a discussion of the typical development of language in children, and this is the topic of the next chapter.

LANGUAGE ACQUISITION:
A BRIEF OVERVIEW OF PERSPECTIVES
COMPREHENSION QUESTIONS

1. Describe briefly the broad metatheories in psychology that have influenced theories of language development (e.g., discuss a few basic tenets of each metatheory. How do they differ from each other?). Each metatheory is distinguished by its approach to the study of _____, or what is commonly known as the oldest, enduring problem in philosophy:_____.

2. Discuss the major tenets of the following language theories:
   a. behavioristic theories
   b. linguistic theories (e.g., Chomsky's work and the semanticists)
   c. interactionist theories (e.g., cognitive, information processing, and social)

   What are some major criticisms of behavoristic and linguistic theories (especially, the work of Chomsky)?

3. Describe the following terms/phrases:
   a. Chomsky's road to theoretical adequacy
   b. performance/competence of speakers
   c. classical conditioning
   d. operant conditioning
   e. Universal Grammar
   f. innate structures or knowledge

4. According to Wasow (as cited in Ingram, 1989), what is the difference between child language research and language acquisition research? How did this distinction (two distinct fields) come about?

5. According to the author, why is the discussion on the relationship between language and thought important on both a theoretical level and a practical application level?

6. Discuss the various perspectives on the relations between language and thought (e.g., consider the strong, weak, and interactive aspects of thought-based positions and language-based positions).

7. List and briefly describe the major highlights and research findings of the three stages of research on intelligence and deafness. To which stage can one attribute the phrase *psychology of deafness,* particularly as it relates to qualitative differences in language and cognition?

8. Much of the research on cognition and deafness has been conducted using the paradigm of Piaget's work. Describe Piaget's four stages of cognition. What was Piaget's position on the influence of language on cognition?

9. In addition to the effects on intelligence and deafness, the chapter focused on other implications of the thought/language debate for deaf and hard-of-hearing individuals. What are some implications/effects of this debate? (You might want to discuss the influences of positions such as language dominates thought, thought dominates language, cognition and language are separate, and interactive views. You might also mention views on language development and deafness and interpretations of the results on Piagetian tasks.)

CHALLENGE QUESTIONS
(Note: Complete answers are not in the text. Additional research is required.)

1. The chapter provided information on the broad metatheories of psychology that have influenced theories and research on language development. Describe the influences of these metatheories on other content areas such as reading, writing, and mathematics (i.e., discuss the various theories, research paradigms, and instructional approaches). (Some information on literacy [reading and writing] may be gleaned from Chapter 8 of this text.)

2. In this chapter, it was argued that there is no comprehensive, coherent theory of language acquisition. Do you agree or disagree? Why or why not? Can you support your convictions with a review of the literature (i.e., can you find research to support your views)? Do you think a comprehensive, coherent theory of language acquisition is necessary for establishing effective language intervention or language-teaching programs? Why or why not? What does it mean to develop a comprehensive, coherent theory? That is, what would one expect from such a theory?

3. Consider each broad group of language theories. What are some possible instructional and clinical implications? For example, how would each group address the teaching of language or communication? What does each group have to say about teacher education or, specifically, the teacher of language or communication?

4. Do you think that a deep understanding of the relationships between language and thought is important for teachers and other practitioners? Why or why not? What are some possible instructional or clinical applications or implications of understanding this relationship (e.g., consider issues such as instructional strategies, types of academic tests, the development of a language as early as possible, and the subsequent development of other skills)?

5. There has been much debate (e.g., interpretations and research) on the question of whether there is a psychology of deafness. What are the various interpretations of this question? Is the question important? Why or why not? Does the answer have implications for understanding language and deafness? The development of English reading/writing skills?

FURTHER READINGS

Chomsky, N. (1995). *The minimalist program*. Cambridge, MA: M.I.T. Press.

Feldman, L. (Ed.). (1995). *Morphological aspects of language processing*. Hillsdale, NJ: Lawrence Erlbaum.

Green, G. (1996). *Pragmatics and natural language understanding* (2nd ed.). Hillsdale, NJ: Lawrence Erlbaum.

Jackendoff, R. (1990). *Semantic structures*. Cambridge, MA: M.I.T. Press.

Nelson, K. (1996). *Language in cognitive development*. New York: Cambridge University Press.

Rice, M. (Ed.). (1996). *Toward a genetics of language*. Hillsdale, NJ: Lawrence Erlbaum.

CHAPTER 4

Primary Language Development: Perspectives and Issues

Why do we study language development? This phenomenal yet basically universal human achievement poses some of the most challenging theoretical and practical questions of our times: How and why do young children acquire complex grammar? What if no one spoke to them—would children invent language by themselves? Are humans unique, or could language be taught to higher primates? Are there theories or models that can adequately account for language development? Is language a separate capacity, or is it simply one facet of our general cognitive ability? What is it that individuals actually must know in order to have full adult competence in language, and to what extent is the development of those skills representative of universal processes? What about individual differences? What happens when language develops atypically, and is there anything we can do about it? What happens to language skills as one grows older—what is acquired, and what is lost? (Gleason, 1993, p. 2)

As discussed in Chapter 3, the acquisition of a first language (indeed any language) seems to be impossible or magical. With little difficulty, most hearing children learn the languages of their society, that is, the ones to which they are exposed. This process appears effortless and relatively simple; however, an in-depth analysis reveals its complex and intricate nature. Hearing children's ability to understand and produce the spoken message is limited primarily by the extent of their linguistic and cognitive development (Cairns, 1996; Goodluck, 1991; Ingram, 1989).

There is still much controversy surrounding theory and research on the acquisition of language by children. There are disagreements regarding methodologies for gathering data, interpretation or categorization of data within the various linguistic components (e.g., morphology and semantics), and the construction of grammars or theories that achieve explanatory adequacy or that best fit the data. These debates seem to have resurrected the traditional arguments regarding the philosophical notions of rationalism (e.g., use of reason to discover knowledge) and empiricism (e.g., experience as the source of knowledge), which were discussed in Chapter 3 (also see Demopoulos, 1989; R. Matthews, 1989).

With respect to this chapter, it should be emphasized that it is difficult to interpret the language performance of children, especially in the early stages of development. One major controversy is the extent to which nonlinguistic data (e.g., context cues) should be used as an adjunct to linguistic data in descriptions of language development. Another area of difficulty is the relationship between comprehension and production (Cairns, 1996; Ingram, 1989; Schlesinger, 1982). These controversies and others have sometimes placed in question the psychological reality (e.g., truthfulness) of the various linguistic terminologies (e.g., the semantic relation categories) used in describing child language development (Schlesinger, 1982).

Despite these problems and controversies, it is possible to provide a general description of child language development that can be referred to in attempting to understand the language development of deaf and hard-of-hearing students. The focus here is on the acquisition of a spoken language by children with typical hearing. The conceptual framework for charting the development of typical hearing children entails two broad time periods, prelinguistic and linguistic, and provides some general developmental information within the major components of language, as discussed in Chapter 2 (e.g., phonology, syntax, semantics, and pragmatics). As might be expected (at least from Chapter 3), there are a number of theories associated with each domain. Discussing these theories in detail is avoided because this distracts from the intent to provide an overall general description of language development (for details on these theories, see Crystal, 1995; Lightfoot, 1999).

The first section of this chapter concerns the period of prelinguistic language development. For the prelinguistic period, the chapter discusses what are considered precursors for the various language components, for example, phonology, morphology and syntax, semantics, and pragmatics. The discussion of precursors includes an overview of the production and perception abilities of infants with respect to the development of segmental (e.g., speech sounds such as vowels and consonants) and suprasegmental (e.g., stress, intonation, and rhythm) aspects. In the domains of semantics and pragmatics, one salient topic of interest is the expression of communicative intents (i.e., prior to the emergence of the first words). It has been suggested that the desire to communicate or the expression of intentions is a major force behind the acquisition of language, at least during the early formative years.

The second section of the chapter focuses on the period of linguistic development, which commences with the emergence of the first words. Several models/views are presented on the development within the major language components during the first-word stage and beyond. For example, despite conflicting perspectives, there is a consensus that children's perception of speech proceeds from larger units (sentences and phrases) to smaller units (words) and eventually to the segmental units (e.g., phonemes). In learning the meanings of words, children engage in processes that are often described as overextension and underextension. The discussion of syntax, particularly grammar, begins with the emergence of the two-word stage, although there are syntactic precursors. The continual development of purposive and intentional behaviors is covered in the section on pragmatics. Prior to discussing the three-word stage and beyond, the reader is introduced to a few aspects of the comprehension-production debate, that is, whether comprehension of speech precedes production or vice versa.

Within the linguistic period, information is presented on what is called *linguistic maturity*—the three-word stage and beyond. There is no question that the period from birth to the three-word stage is very important for language development. In fact, it is quite awesome to take stock of what children have accomplished during this period and how fast they do it. The phrase *linguistic maturity* is apt for what occurs during and beyond the three-word stage. Children start to utter and understand very complex linguistic structures. They begin to utilize some of the major transformations (e.g., question forms, relative pronouns) and indicate that they are acquiring (i.e., tacitly or intuitively) the mature adult rules of language. Another interesting topic discussed for this period is metacognitive development, a very critical skill for learning to read, write, and think well. Of course, metacognitive development is also important for the continual development of literate thought—the ability to think reflectively, logically, rationally, and creatively.

The last section of the chapter provides a few brief remarks on descriptions of the primary language development of deaf and hard-of-hearing children. The reader should see the difficulty and complexity of attempts to describe or chart the development of the performance aspects (i.e., speech and/or signs) of this population. Readers are introduced to this concept, which is elaborated on during the next three chapters of this text (Chapters 5, 6, and 7).

PRELINGUISTIC LANGUAGE DEVELOPMENT

It is a gross understatement to assert that the first few years of life are the most critical for language development. However, the study of the prelinguistic or preverbal period has been a relatively recent phenomenon (Jakobson, 1968). *Prelinguistic* or *preverbal* refers to the period prior to the emergence of the first words (spoken or signed). In the past, most researchers viewed this era as uninteresting albeit important to the later linguistic development of the child.

There are a number of reasons why there is a renewed interest in this area. The development and use of new technology (e.g., tape recorder and computers) and faster, more convenient data analysis programs (e.g., software for coding and tabulating data) have made it easier and more convenient for collecting and analyzing a voluminous amount of data. Another contributing factor is the notion that the subsequent development of an individual is pervasively dependent on the presence of linguistic and cognitive precursors. Perhaps one of the most influential factors is the recent and continuing focus on the functional aspects of language (e.g., pragmatics and communicative intent) as opposed to the long-standing emphasis on categorizing and understanding the structural aspects such as phonology and syntax (Callanan, 1991; Gleason, 1993; Menyuk, 1977).

The ensuing paragraphs attempt to describe this prelinguistic development with respect to language components such as phonology, morphology, syntax, semantics, and pragmatics. It should be kept in mind that these developments are occurring simultaneously. The child is not working on one domain separately from the others. Interestingly, during this prelinguistic period, the early behaviors of infants are meaningful and informational but are not considered intentional. Nevertheless, mothers/caregivers (in the United States) consider or treat these behaviors as intentional. For example, the mother/caregiver

> *does this by fitting her verbalizations and/or vocalizations in between those of her baby and constructing them so that they imply that her baby's vocalizations, vegetative noises (burps, wheezes, and so on), and actions were intended as contributions to the conversation. (Holzman, 1983, p. 25)*

Thus, infants do learn from their mothers/caregivers what their particular signaling behaviors are taken to mean. Extending the arms in the direction of an object has taken on the meaning that the infant or child wants the object.

This meaning has been constructed within the interactions of significant others and caregivers.

Development of Form, Content, and Use

Phonological development can be discussed relative to two aspects of speech: segmentals and suprasegmentals (Cruttenden, 1979; Crystal, 1987, 1997). The segmental aspect refers to the sounds of speech (i.e., vowels and consonants), whereas the suprasegmental aspect refers to factors such as intonation, stress, and rhythm. To understand these features of speech, it is important to discuss the speech production and perception capabilities of infants during this period. A good theoretical and research review of speech production and perception as well as the emergence of other prelinguistic behaviors can be found elsewhere (Ingram, 1989; Menn & Stoel-Gammon, 1993; Sachs, 1993).

Segmental Aspects: Production

A number of frameworks have been used to discuss the prelinguistic development of infants. The one proposed by Kaplan and Kaplan (as cited in Quigley & Paul, 1990) for speech production is useful for the purposes here (for a finer distinction of stages, see Menn & Stoel-Gammon, 1993). Kaplan and Kaplan delineated four broad stages of prelinguistic development. Stage 1 represents the crying behaviors. During Stage 2, the infant produces other vocalizations and cooing behaviors. Stage 3 is the babbling period, and Stage 4 is the transitional period between babbling and the emergence of the first words (also see Petitto & Marentette, 1991, for research on deaf infants). It should be kept in mind that these stages are not distinct or mutually exclusive but, rather, are continuous. In addition, not all children proceed through them in a similar manner or at the same time.

The development from Stage 1 through Stage 4 is quite remarkable. In the beginning, the newborn baby has a repertoire of what can be termed *survival,* adaptive behaviors. In one sense, these behaviors are similar to the innate repertoires of behaviors of other animal species. Here, the concern is with the repertoire of language behaviors during the prelinguistic period, for example, crying, cooing, smiling, and movements—mostly from arms and legs. This repertoire is effective (for the most part) in eliciting responses from the mother or some other significant caregiver. The cries and arm movements can be observed immediately after birth, whereas the smiling and cooing (i.e., comfort sounds) emerge within a few weeks (or the first month) of life. During the prelinguistic period, the infant's signaling responses change in part because of maturational or growth changes. And, the vocalizations are influenced by the verbal and social interactions between infants and their caregivers. The precise nature and extent of this social dance is, of course, a continual source of debate.

The production and perception of sounds are pervasively influenced by the developmental growth of the infant during the first year. There is change in the growth of the larynx and speech articulators and in the control mechanisms necessary for speech (see the brief discussion in Chapter 5 of these structures). There is also an explosion of neural pathways in the area of the left hemisphere of the brain, which is responsible for the motor control of speech (and for language development).

The beginning of the babbling stage occurs around the third or fourth month (Cruttenden, 1979; Crystal, 1987, 1997; Ingram, 1989). This stage is characterized by two salient events: (a) the emergence of pulmonic-lingual sounds and (b) the infant's pleasure in producing such sounds. *Pulmonic-lingual* sounds refers to those sounds produced as air is interrupted when passing through the tongue along with vowel-like, or vocalic, sounds. During this period, the infant realizes that producing sounds is pleasurable. In fact, this activity may occur with or without the presence of an adult/caregiver. In producing the segmental aspect of speech, the infant is beginning to coordinate his or her articulators, specifically, the tongue, lips, and teeth.

When the coos and other vocalizations progress into the babbling stage, it is typically referred to as *syllabic babbling*. The babbling sequences are comprised of nonsense utterances (or words); nevertheless, the structures of these utterances resemble the phonetic segments (e.g., open vowels and simple stops) and prosody of simple sentences. These strings of babbled utterances sound like sentences with intonation, stress, and rhythm. These sentences, however, have no meaning per se. The babbled consonants and vowels exhibit a phonetic resemblance to those that actually occur in the infant's home language. Nevertheless, they are different acoustically (e.g., the stop consonants) due to the nature and development of the infant's speech mechanisms (e.g., vocal and laryngeal control for producing adult-like stop consonants such as /p/ and /b/).

In general, it seems that the production of consonants moves from the back of the mouth to the front. Another observed pattern concerns the structure of the babbling syllables. That is, vocalic sounds occur initially followed by consonant-vowel (C-V) combinations. Next to occur are the vowel-consonant-vowel (V-C-V) combinations, then the vowel-consonant (V-C) combinations, and finally the reduplication of C-V combinations (Cruttenden, 1979; Crystal, 1987, 1997; Goodluck, 1991; Menyuk, 1977).

It should be noted that when infants babble, they seem to play with sounds almost as much as they play with some of their body parts such as fingers and toes. There has been considerable debate on the relationship between babbling and talking, particularly on whether these are distinct stages. There seems to be a consensus that babbling blends into early speech and might also continue even after the appearance of words that are recognizable or understandable (Blake & Boysson-Bardies, 1992). Thus, the relationship between babbling and speech might best be viewed within a continuity framework (Menn & Stoel-Gammon, 1993). Babbling in sign, particularly American Sign Language, is discussed in Chapter 7. Additional details on the production of speech sounds during the babbling stage can also be found elsewhere (see the accessible description in Menn & Stoel-Gammon, 1993).

Segmental Aspects: Perception

One of the most interesting areas of research during this prelinguistic period has been the measurement of infants' speech perception or discrimination abilities. Discrimination is not similar to recognition or comprehension. With infants, *discrimination* refers to the ability to differentiate between two stimuli (i.e., the second stimulus is different from the first one). Researchers have had to be creative with their techniques for observing infants' responses (e.g., physiological or behavior) to a wide variety of auditory and speech stimuli. Menn and Stoel-Gammon (1993) described a successful method, known as high amplitude sucking, used with infants.

> *In this method, the infant is given a pacifier to suck on that is connected to a sound generating system. Each suck causes a noise to be generated and the infant learns quickly that sucking brings about the noise. At first, babies suck frequently and the noise occurs often; then, gradually, they lose interest in hearing repetitions of the same noise and begin to suck less frequently. At this point, the experimenter changes the sound that is being generated. If the babies renew vigorous sucking, it can be inferred that they have discriminated the sound change and are sucking more, in response to their interest in a new and different sound. (p. 78)*

Using this technique (or similar ones), it has been demonstrated that infants can discriminate between speech sounds during the first few months of life. For example, the investigations of Eimas, Siqueland, Jusczyk, and Vigorito (1971) and Morse (1974) showed that infants as young as 1 month are responsive to speech stimuli and are able to perceive differences between voiceless /p/ and voiced /b/ phonemes produced by an adult. In addition, infants between the ages of 2 and 7 months, inclusive, have been observed to possess crude localization abilities for sound, as evidenced by these infants turning their heads in the direction of a particular sound. By the age of 3 months, infants respond differently to their mother's voice compared to those of other adult females. In fact, it appears that 3-day-old infants can identify their own mothers' voices from an array of women's voices (DeCasper & Fifer, 1980). Even more interesting, these young infants prefer to listen to their mothers' voices than to other women's voices. The discrimination skills of these days-old infants are most likely related to their perception of prosodic cues in the spoken utterances than of the phonetic features of sounds in the utterances. It is assumed that prosodic cues can be perceived by fetuses in their mother's uterus (see discussion in Menn & Stoel-Gammon, 1993).

In general, the infant's ability to discriminate between speech contrasts is superior to his or her ability to discriminate between nonspeech contrasts. This finding implies that sensitivity to speech or speech-like sounds may be unique to human infants during this period (see discussion in Cairns, 1996). Thus, it seems that infants either have an innate (i.e., built-in) capacity to make these distinctions (e.g., similar to Chomsky's idea for syntax discussed in Chapter 3) or they learn to perform these tasks very early and quickly. The most interesting findings on these issues have come from studies from different cultures. It has been argued that infants have an innate capacity to discriminate phonetic contrasts in any language of the world. However, with exposure to the specific language of their culture, they become adept with those contrasts that are found in their language (Werker & Lalonde, 1988). The decline in infants' ability to perceive contrasts outside their own language is due to the similarity of the foreign contrasts to those in their own language. Thus, infants have difficulty discriminating sounds from a foreign language that are phonetically similar to those in their home language.

An eloquent summary of the speech perception capacity of infants was proffered by Ingram (1989):

> *The young infant is born with much greater ability than was ever thought just a few years ago. This fact makes the child's rapid linguistic development a year later less difficult to understand (though no less impressive!). It appears that this innate ability combined with a year's listening experience is sufficient for the young child to begin to recognize language-specific words around the end of the first year. Further, it appears that these perceptions are categorical in that the discriminations are more abrupt at specific acoustic parameters than at others. These two*

findings make the young infant's speech perception much more adult-like than was ever anticipated. (p. 96)

Suprasegmental Aspect: Production and Perception

Intonation patterns have been observed to emerge during Stage 2 (i.e., Kaplan and Kaplan) of the babbling phase. By Stage 3, these patterns begin to resemble those of adults. In his investigations, Halliday (1975) reported that a contrast between rising and falling intonation is produced by the 10th or 11th month. He stated, however, that this contrast is not present in adult speech; rather, it is an idiosyncratic system unique to the child. Based on their analysis, Bloom and Lahey (1978; also see the discussion in Ingram, 1989) concluded that the rise-fall contour of infant vocalizations may be an important precursor of sentence types, for example, statements, questions, and explanations. Other researchers suggested that early intonation patterns are precursors of the later process of determining old information from new information (i.e., pragmatic function) and of interpreting direct and indirect speech acts (Lucas, 1980; Ninio & Snow, 1996). In sum, a number of researchers have suggested that infants are sensitive to the suprasegmental aspects prior to the segmental aspects of speech (Eimas, 1985; Morse, 1974; see review in Crystal, 1987, 1997; Goodluck, 1991; Ingram, 1989; Menyuk, 1977). Additional discussion of the expression of communicative intents prior to the emergence of the first words is provided in the ensuing paragraphs.

Table 4-1 presents a summary of major points on segmental and suprasegmental development.

TABLE 4-1 A Few Major Points on Segmentals and Suprasegmentals

---

Segmentals

- One major characteristic of the beginning of the babbling stage is the emergence of pulmonic-lingual sounds. Pulmonic-lingual sounds are produced as air is interrupted when passing through the tongue along with vowel-like, or vocalic, sounds.

- The babbled consonants and vowels exhibit a phonetic resemblance to those that actually occur in the infant's home language.

(continues)

(*Table 4-1 continued*)

- During the babbling stage, the production of consonants moves from the back of the mouth to the front. Vocalic sounds occur initially followed by consonant-vowel (C-V) combinations. Next to occur are the vowel-consonant-vowel (V-C-V) combinations, then the vowel-consonant (V-C) combinations, and finally the reduplication of C-V combinations.

- Babbling blends into early speech and continues even after the appearance of words that are recognizable and understandable. Thus, the relationship between babbling and speech might best be viewed within a continuity framework.

- Infants can discriminate between speech sounds during the first few months of life.

- By the age of 3 months, infants respond differently to their mother's voice compared to those of other adult females.

- The infant's ability to discriminate between speech contrasts is superior to his or her ability to discriminate between nonspeech contrasts. This implies that sensitivity to speech or speech-like sounds may be unique to human infants during this period.

- Infants have an innate capacity to discriminate phonetic contrasts in any language of the world. However, with exposure to the specific language of their culture, they become adept with those contrasts that are found in their language.

Suprasegmentals

- Infants are sensitive to the suprasegmental aspect prior to the segmental aspect of speech.

- The rise-fall contour of infant vocalization is an important precursor of sentence types such as statements, questions, and explanations.

- Early intonation patterns are also precursors for the later process of determining old information from new information and for interpreting speech acts.

Prelinguistic Semantics and Pragmatics

Semantic development is often considered to be isomorphic with cognitive development; however, they are not exactly the same. A semantic category, such as a word, may be indicative of a nonlinguistic conceptual category, but it is not the same as this category (e.g., schema, frame, etc.). Nevertheless, it is safe to conclude that semantic development parallels observed patterns of behavior that correspond to different levels of cognitive development. Thus, prior to the emergence of the first words, semantic and cognitive precursors may be essentially the same.

The development of referents as well as communicative competence is dependent on cognitive processes, which emerge during the first 2 years or during one of Piaget's stages called *sensorimotor* (Piaget, 1952, 1977; also see Chapter 3). Prior to learning about object concepts and relational concepts, a child must develop the ability to organize information. This process is inoperable without certain concepts such as object permanency, that is, a stable world replete with persons, objects, and events. Object permanence refers to the understanding that things exists even when they are out of sight or when one is not experiencing them.

Prior to the emergence of intentional and meaningful communication, a child explores the environment for about 1 year. With this exploration comes the realization that persons, objects, and events are separate from the self. By acting on these persons, objects, and events, the child discovers object and relational concepts and realizes that she or he can have an effect on them. Piaget argued that the representations of objects are stored in the child's mind in the same manner in which they are experienced. That is, the stored information is reflective of the direct representations of sensory experiences and motor activities of the child. It has also been shown that the child's representations can be more abstract and may even exist prior to the direct interactive experiences with objects and other phenomena. It has even been argued that the precursors of object permanency exist in infants who are $3\frac{1}{2}$ months old. Thus, by the end of the first year with the existence of object permanence and the ability to form first words, the child embarks on a period in which most of the utterances are single words.

With respect to pragmatic development, the precursors of speech acts (Dore, 1974, 1975; Searle, 1969), the functions of speech acts (Halliday, 1975), and the overall communicative aspects of language (Bates, 1976; Ninio & Snow, 1996) also emerge during the prelinguistic period. Bruner (1975) stated that a child learns about functions, rules, and referential concepts of language while engaging in joint activities with a parental caregiver. These concepts and rules are also part of the semantic development of the child. Rules of interactions, for example, are learned as the child and parent/caregiver vocalize and respond to each other. The parent/caregiver considers the child's vocalizations a response; this in turn prompts a return response from the parent/caregiver. This interaction establishes the roles of speaker and listener, which are important to the communicative process.

These intentional and purposive behaviors have been observed as early as 4 months in the motor patterns of the child (Bates, 1976). The child's endeavors to reach for objects while vocalizing simultaneously has been interpreted as a form of communication. In essence, these vocalizations apparently can perform certain functions without conforming to the linguistic structures of the native-speaking adult. Halliday (1975) delineated several functions in the early linguistic development of his son: (a) instrumental (I want), (b) regulatory (Do as I tell you), (c) interactional (me and you), and (d) personal (Here I come). The interactional function was observed to emerge at 9 months; however, it has been observed as early as 4 months (Bates, 1976). Also, at 9 months, the personal function emerged. It should be remembered that the primary forms of communication during this prelinguistic period are cries, smiles, eye-gazing, and vocalization. All of this implies that the infant uses these behaviors to express his or her needs.

Prior to the age of 9 months, it is difficult to determine if a child's behavior is deliberate or intentional in attempting to obtain the attention of an adult. To ascertain this, some researchers have suggested a set of criteria that can be applied for evaluation purposes (Sachs, 1993):

1. *The child makes eye contact with the partner while gesturing or vocalizing, often alternating his gaze between an object and the partner.*
2. *The child's gestures and vocalizations become more consistent and ritualized. For example, a child named Annie used a gesture of opening and closing her hand rather than attempting to reach the object herself. The vocalization she used, "Eh, eh," was one that she consistently used in situations in which she wanted something. Another child would probably have used a different sound in the same situation, because this sound is not copied from adult speech but rather is a communicative signal invented by the child.*
3. *The child may gesture or vocalize and wait for a response from the partner.*
4. *The child persists in attempting to communicate if he is not understood and sometimes even modifies his behavior to communicate more clearly. (pp. 43–44)*

For a more detailed discussion of the development and assessment of these early intentional behaviors, the work of O'Kane and Goldbart (1998) is recommended.

There seems to be little question that the interactions between mothers/caregivers and infants are important for developing pragmatic functions, particularly those that involved turn-taking. Some activities that may facilitate the development of true turn-taking seem to take the form of ritualized games that occur between mothers and infants. Consider the following example:

> *When Sue was almost five months old, we first observed her mother, with Sue supine on the changing table and ready to be freshly diapered, throw a diaper over Sue's head and croon, "Where's the baby? Where's the baby?" She then removed the diaper and very brightly and enthusiastically called, "There's the baby!" Two weeks later, after her mother had carried out the routine through the two "where's the baby" utterances, Sue removed the diaper from her own face, and then her mother said, "There's the baby!" By the time Sue was six months old, Sue both covered her face with the diaper and removed it. . . . The moment Sue's mother noticed Sue was pulling the diaper over her face, she quickly sang out, "Where's the baby, where's the baby?" Sue pulled the diaper away from her face, and her mother said, "There's the baby!" During our next observation the mother was somewhat preoccupied as she diapered Sue. Sue pulled the diaper on and off her face with no response from her mother, who was jabbering about "baa, baa, black sheep." Again, Sue pulled the diaper on and off her face with still no response from her mother, so this time Sue provided an elongated vocalization herself after pulling the diaper off her face. Even though Sue "knows" that "where's the baby" has a sequence (face covered, vocalization with rising pitch, face uncovered, vocalizations with level or falling pitch), she doesn't know what the actions or the vocalizations mean or signify. It's a little routine she has learned to do with her mother. (Holzman, 1983, pp. 31–32)*

The debate on the emergence of intentional communication in infants is, of course, influenced by both cognitive-interactionists (e.g., followers and interpreters of Piaget's work; Piaget, 1952) and social-interactionists (e.g., followers and interpreters of Vygotsky's work; Vygotsky, 1978). The tensions and aspects of this debate on overall language development were discussed briefly in Chapter 3 of this text, particularly in the section on the relationship between language and cognition. There seems to be an emerging consensus that any explanation of the emergence of intentional communication and the effects this has on subsequent cognitive and linguistic development needs to consider three broad areas: (a) the biological basis for language development related to the maturation of physiological structures such as the central nervous system and language areas of the brain, (b) the nonlinguistic cognitive development of the child, and (c) the culture and experiences of the child with respect to significant caregivers in particular and meaningful interactive situations.

Table 4-2 provides a snapshot of some of the major issues of the prelinguistic period regarding the perception and production of infants as well as semantic and pragmatic precursors.

TABLE 4-2 Some Major Points of the Prelinguistic Period

Speech Production and Perception

- A lengthy period of very sensitive listening precedes the production of speech in infancy; infants appear to be tuned to human voices from just after birth.

- The very first sounds, cries, and babbles exercise and develop the capacities of the speech organs and the child's control over them.

- In the first months of life, infants begin to use their voices to control others and to get them to do things.

- In their first months, infants practice and perfect the habitual and significant sounds of the particular languages to which they are exposed.

- Many infants appear to use a set of personally evolved sounds to express their needs and meanings systematically.

Semantics and Pragmatics Precursors

- The development of referents and communicative competence are dependent on cognitive processes that emerge during the first 2 years.

- Prior to the emergence of intentional and meaningful communication, a child explores the environment for about 1 year. With this exploration comes the realization that persons, objects, and events are separate from the self.

- Mutual eye-gazing and patterns of inviting and ending eye contact are soon established by infants and caregivers. These sequences may have significance for the later turn-taking patterns of conversations when eye signals still remain important.

- The precursors of speech acts, the functions of speech acts, and the overall communicative aspects of language emerge during the prelinguistic period.

- In essence, during the first year, the infant develops the precursors for the language components—phonology, syntax, semantics, and pragmatics. By the end of the first year, with the onset of object permanence and control over sounds for the first words, the child proceeds into the one-word stage.

Note: Adapted from Cairns (1996) and Whitehead (1990).

LINGUISTIC DEVELOPMENT: FIRST WORD AND BEYOND

Prelinguistic development does not simply culminate with the emergence of the first words. In fact, the development of the later stages of this period may parallel the beginning stages of linguistic development (Gleason, 1993; Goodluck, 1991; Ingram, 1989). Occasionally, the child may engage in behaviors that emerged earlier in both the prelinguistic and the linguistic periods. This should not be taken to mean that the child is regressing; rather, the child may be increasing his or her understanding of the form, content, and use of language.

One way to view linguistic development, particularly grammatical development, is to use the stages of Brown (1973) based on mean length of utterance (MLU). Although this method is not adopted here, it is briefly discussed later to account for the development of inflectional morphemes. As with prelinguistic development, the development of the linguistic stages is continuous; the labels are used for the purpose of studying various parts of the stages (Cairns, 1996; Crystal, 1987, 1997). The reader should keep in mind that in discussing one component (say, syntax), it is often necessary to repeat some information about another component (semantics or pragmatics). This overlap is kept to a minimum; however, it does emphasize the difficulty in discussing one component of a language in isolation, especially in the early linguistic development—that is, the one-word and two-word stages.

The child's first words generally mark the beginning of linguistic development. Depending on the nature of the linguistic criteria established, different ages have been reported for the emergence of the first words. Dale (1976) stated three general requirements that have been cited repeatedly in the literature: (a) The child must demonstrate an understanding of the word; (b) the child must use the word consistently and spontaneously with reference to an object or event; and (c) the word must be recognized as one from a native-speaking adult's lexicon. It has been remarked:

> *Learning a word—its form and meaning—is no small task. It requires that one be able to identify the form of the word, its beginning and end, so that it can be picked out from the stream of speech and produced, eventually, in a form recognizable to others. And it requires that one learn what it means. This includes learning what parts of words mean, since knowing this offers children a way of expanding their current vocabulary much as adults do. (Clark, 1991, p. 31)*

Analyses of the first words and meanings and subsequent development are presented within the conceptual framework of the linguistic components in the ensuing paragraphs. In general, this discussion evolves around the use of one word, two words, three words, and beyond or, roughly, development during the first year, second year, third year, and beyond. It seems to be clear that syntactic analyses are not useful for determining the content of the first words; however, semantic analyses are relevant for this purpose (see discussion in Bloom & Lahey, 1978; also see Bloom, 1973; Brown, 1958). More specifically, it has been demonstrated that syntactic precursors do not appear until the end of the one-word stage (Bloom, 1973; Dore, Franklin, Miller, & Ramer, 1976). Syntax, as a linguistic component, does not emerge until sometime during the two-word stage; however, children may have a basic understanding of some two words-or-more phrases or sentences prior to the period labeled the two-word stage (Crystal, 1987, 1997; Goodluck, 1991; Ingram, 1989).

Table 4-3 presents a few general remarks on the use of the first words and beyond, some of which are elaborated on and discussed throughout the ensuing sections of this chapter.

TABLE 4-3 General Remarks on the Emergence of the First Words and Beyond

---

- First words can only be fully understood within the contexts in which they are uttered. Some of them are not just labels but stand for sentence-like commentaries or instructions.

- Two-word combinations are examples of early grammatical language; the words are put together to express the child's perception of actions and relationships.

- In the years from 2 to 4, children evolve grammatical rules that produce some errors of overgeneralization in plurals and tenses. They also invent verbs and nouns by analogy with conventional forms.

- Words refer to actual experiences and things in the world, but they also stand for concepts or classifications in the minds of speakers.

- Concepts are generalized categories; they classify similarities, differences, and hierarchies (or families) of connected ideas, objects, and happenings.

- Concepts are usually thought to have core meanings, perceptual information, and linguistic signs. Personal associations also play a part in the complex development of concepts.

- Thinking with concepts develops with language use.

Note: Adapted from Whitehead (1990).

Phonologic Development

Until the 1970s, there were two general groups of theories on the acquisition of phonology: behaviorism and nativism. As discussed in Chapter 3, the behaviorist theories are not in vogue, so only some attention to them is provided here. Olmsted's (1971) work was characteristic of this line of thinking. He attempted to demonstrate that children's phonological acquisition commences with the acquisition of the most frequent sounds (i.e., phones) and proceeds to the least frequent sounds of their language. The use of frequency as a major criterion is a salient principle of many behaviorist perspectives. In addition, the development of phones was considered to occur in tandem with the use of external rewards (i.e., praise and reinforcement) for improvement. Reward, or more precisely, reinforcement, is another important behaviorist principle.

The exemplar for the nativist position was the work of Jakobson (1968). Jakobson (1968) attempted to chart the order of phonemic acquisition by using his notion of distinctive feature analysis. He proposed several principles to delineate the order of acquisition. Only two are presented here: (a) The description of phonologic development should parallel the mastery of distinctive features, and (b) the system of phonemic contrasts of the child may not always be similar to that of adults in distinguishing between words. In essence, Jakobson argued—and to some extent this was also true of several behaviorists' theories—that the pattern of phonologic development in all children is systematic and universal. The universal sequence proposed by Jakobson was as follows: (a) Children initially differentiate vowels from consonants; (b) then, they make a distinction between oral stops and nasal consonants; (c) next, they distinguish between labial (lip) and apical (tip of tongue) stops; and (d) finally, they differentiate the high vowels from the low vowels. (A brief discussion of the mechanism and sounds of speech is presented in Chapter 5.)

There has been some evidence for aspects of Jakobson's theory; that is, the reality of distinctive features has been observed after the age of 2 years (Menyuk, 1968). It seems that after children have mastered a particular phonemic contrast, they generalize this knowledge to other phonemes with similar distinctive features. Nevertheless, there has been much criticism of both behaviorist and nativist theories, especially with their common assumption that development proceeds along a smooth systematic path with no regressions or individual differences. For example, there is ample evidence showing that some children regress in their pronunciation of words (i.e., words become less intelligible or mispronounced or loss of ability to pronounce words), and some children avoid certain words altogether due to the difficulty of pronouncing them. In essence, there appears to be a wide variation in the early phonologic development of children not accounted for by these early theories.

It seems that the cognitive theories (both cognitive and social) have been most productive in addressing the early development of phonology because of the emphasis on problem solving. That is, the child is attempting to solve problems with his or her pronunciation efforts (as well as other types of efforts). Within this framework, phonologic research has moved away from the phoneme as a unit of speech analysis to either syllables or whole words (Ferguson & Farwell, 1975). The findings indicate that a child's phonologic development does not proceed one sound at a time or by mastery of successive distinctive features. Instead, development occurs according to certain strategies or rules (see discussions in Crystal, 1987, 1997; Goodluck, 1991; Ingram, 1989).

To obtain a sense of the syllable as the minimal unit of perception, consider the following example: *dog*. The speaker/listener does not hear three distinct phonemes, for example, /d/ /o/ /g/, because of the influence of the vowel on the consonants. This phenomenon is labeled *coarticulation*. Thus, speech perception (for mature listeners) seems to be at the syllable level; that is, *dog* is perceived as one syllable or acoustic unit.

This shift in research approach to the syllable or word seems also to have shed more light on the speech perception-speech production issue. In general, the following three points, offered by Menyuk (1977), are still acceptable:

1. For the most part, perception precedes production.
2. Sometimes, both perception and production appear to be simultaneous, and occasionally, production precedes perception.
3. The sequence of phonemic development in perception may not be congruent with that of production.

Phonological development continues well beyond the first year and probably continues to be refined even in the early school years (Fowler, 1991; Gerken, Jusczyk, & Mandel, 1994). Most of the phonologic rules are acquired by around 6 to 8 years of age (Crystal, 1987, 1997; Goodluck, 1991; Ingram, 1989). From age 3 onward, the child attempts to acquire the rules associated with various inflectional endings of nouns and verbs (Brown, 1973). The more general rules of phonology are acquired prior to the acquisition of the specific or less general rules. As mentioned previously, the early stages of phonologic development cannot be described relative to phonemic contrasts or distinctive features. This development can be charted only after the acquisition of a certain number of words in the child's lexicon. The strategies that a child develops may relate these words to each other or to an adult model. In essence, these strategies may be dependent on the particular first words acquired by the child.

With respect to children's perception of speech, there is a shift from holistic (based on overall prosodic or acoustic shapes of syllables and words) to segmental (based on small phonemic units) during the late preschool period (Gerken et al., 1994; Jusczyk, Friederici, Wessels, Svenkerud, & Jusczyk, 1993). As discussed in Chapter 8, this is important for a phase termed *alphabetic reading* in which the letters correspond roughly to phonemes. This shift from holistic to segment-based strategies does not occur until there are a number of words in the child's lexicon. This also provides evidence for the well-documented relationship between vocabulary size and early reading ability. In other words, the child's development of fine within-word discrimination ability (phonemic representation) may be contingent on overall vocabulary size rather than on a specific age or general developmental level. If children's phonological encoding/representation systems are not well developed at the inception of formal reading instruction, it is argued that this impedes their progress in achieving a level of phonemic awareness for spoken words that is strongly related to fluent decoding of written words. This issue is discussed further in Chapter 8 of this text.

Before leaving phonologic development, a few comments should be made about the role of parents. It is clear that parental remarks, via the use of imitation and reinforcement as delineated by behaviorism, do not account for the development of their children's speech productions. However, parents do play a role in assisting children in improving the accuracy of their articulations in learning to speak. This is a subconscious effort on the parents' part and occurs during the first few years. In other words, this effort is not necessarily to correct speech as it is to improve understanding of the message. It is important to emphasize that parent-child interactions are indeed critical for language development, particularly with the use of language games and ritualized activities.

Table 4-4 presents a few highlights in this section on phonological development.

TABLE 4-4 Highlights of Phonologic Development

- Until the 1970s, there were two general group of theories on the acquisition of phonology: behaviorism and nativism. A predominant theme was that the pattern of phonologic development in all children is systematic and universal. Nevertheless, both groups of theories were criticized, especially with their

(continues)

(Table 4-4 continued)

common assumption that phonologic development proceeds along a smooth systematic path with no regressions or individual differences.

- There appears to be a wide variation in the early phonologic development of children.

- Cognitive theories (both cognitive and social) have been most productive in addressing this early phonologic development because of the emphasis on problem solving. That is, the child is attempting to solve problems in his or her pronunciation efforts.

- Children's phonologic development does not proceed one sound at a time or by mastery of successive distinctive features. Instead, development occurs according to certain strategies or rules. These strategies seem to be dependent on the particular first words that are acquired.

- Phonologic development continues well beyond the first year and probably continues to be refined even in the early school years. Most of the phonologic rules are acquired by around 6 to 8 years of age.

- With respect to children's perception of speech, there is a shift from holistic (prosodic or acoustic shapes of syllables and words) to segmental (e.g., phonemic units) during the late preschool period.

- If children's phonology is not well developed at the beginning of formal reading instruction, this can impede their progress in achieving a level of phonemic awareness for spoken words that is strongly related to the fluent decoding of written words.

Semantic Development: First Words, Meanings, and Vocabulary Growth

In all cultures that have been studied, most children are saying their first words by the time they are 1 year old (Cairns, 1996; Crystal, 1987, 1997). There is variability in the exact words used within a specific culture; however, these words do tend to refer to objects and events that are present (i.e., here and now). For example, the words tend to refer to objects that can move or be acted on by others, including the child. It is not uncommon to find words such as *dog, shoes,* and *car* in young children's vocabulary as opposed to words such as *sofa, ceiling,* and *lamp*—that are not easily acted on or manipulated by the child. Most of the early words are nominals; next in frequency is the action words (i.e., words that elicit or accompany action). Nominals and action words comprise the overwhelming majority of words in children's early vocabularies (Nelson, 1973).

An important aspect in the language growth of a child is the development of semantic or meaningful referents (Ingram, 1989; Lindfors, 1980; Lucas, 1980; Schlesinger, 1982). These referents reflect the organization of the child's knowledge concerning persons, objects, events, and relations (Bloom, 1973; Brown, 1973; Crystal, 1987, 1997; Ingram, 1989). Essentially, it is argued that these early relations must be analyzed relative to surrounding contexts. de Villiers and de Villiers (1978) provided a good overview of the ways in which the meanings of the first words have been described in the literature: (a) categorization of objects and events; (b) categorization of relations between self and other persons, objects, and/or events; and (c) categorization of relations between others and objects and/or events.

It should be kept in mind that a word might signify a referent, but the referent itself is not the meaning of the word. For example, if one tells a child—"Hey, look at the bird!," the referent is the actual bird, perhaps a cardinal, but this is not the meaning of the *bird*. This relationship between the word (or sign) *bird* and the referent (*bird*) is symbolic and arbitrary. How words are represented in the mind has been the subject of numerous debates, and of course, there are several theories—some of which focus on relations, features, or attributes of words (see Aitchison, 1994). Not all children's words are only referential, and the same words can have different meanings. For example, a child might say *juice* while pointing. If she is pointing to a glass, this usually means "I want some juice." If she is pointing to juice on the table, this could mean "I spilt some juice."

There was a substantial amount of early research on the nature of children's vocabularies. Researchers attempted to understand the semantic aspects that contribute to the development of words and meanings. A number of concepts were proposed, for example, functional (Nelson, 1973), perceptual (Clark, 1973, 1991), relational-categorical (Bloom, 1973), and relational (Greenfield & Smith, 1976).

Nelson (1973) investigated the nature of the first 50 words acquired and remarked that two-word combinations emerge after the acquisition of at least 50 words. Nelson reported her findings in six categories. The common category was general nominals, for example, *milk* and *dog*, which consisted of 51% of the data. Next with 14% of the data each were specific nominals (e.g., *mommy*) and action words (e.g., *give*). Nelson concluded that the words that are learned initially are those words the child can manipulate; that is, these words are functional.

Clark (1973) reported on the phenomenon of overextensions, that is, the use of a word to reflect a broader category than is appropriate. An example is the use of the word *daddy* to refer to all men encountered. Clark argued that overextensions might be based on perceptual attributes, which she classified into six categories: shape, sound, size, movement, taste, and texture. Her data revealed that the most common overextensions are concrete nouns occurring between the ages of 12 and 30 months. A more recent—albeit similar—rendition of Clark's view of the development of word meanings can be found elsewhere (Clark, 1991).

Underextensions as well as overextensions were reported by Bowerman (1973, 1988). *Underextension* refers to a word representing a narrower category than is appropriate. This phenomenon is difficult to determine because the child is using the label in a correct, albeit restricted manner. Bowerman asserted that underextensions, similar to overextensions, are related to perceptual attributes of objects. It is suggested that underextensions occur prior to overextensions.

Related to this issue is Clark's principle of contrast (see Clark, 1987, 1991). Clark argued that when children hear a new word, they assume that the word has a unique meaning. This implies that when children recognize a difference in the structure or form, they assume that there must be a difference in meaning. Debates on the concept of synonyms notwithstanding (also see the discussion in Chapter 2), children find it difficult to accept (at least in the early learning stages) that several words may share similar attributes (e.g., meanings) but have different forms. In addition, as noted by Johnson and Pearson (1984), children may also develop meaning rigidity—that is, they refuse to accept the fact that a word may have more than one meaning, including a variety of different meanings as in multimeaning words (e.g., *bank, check,* and *run*).

Semantic relations expressed during the two-word stage have been described extensively in the literature (Bloom, 1973; Bowerman, 1973, 1988; Cairns, 1996; Cruttenden, 1979). Only the most common relations are discussed here. It is possible to group these relations into eight categories: nomination, attribution, recurrence, possession, notice or exclamation, negation, location, and action. Examples of the first five are: nomination—*that car;* attribution—*big car;* recurrence—*more car;* possession—*mommy car;* and notice or exclamation—*hi car.* The categories of negation, location, and action may be subdivided into further categories. For example, negation may reflect nonexistence (*no cookie*) or disappearance (*all gone cookie*). Location may reflect a noun plus noun category (*mommy car*), verb plus verb (*walk car*), or noun plus prolocative (*car up there*). Action may reflect an agent-action category

(*Daddy read*), agent-object—noun plus noun—(*mommy sock*), or agent-object—verb plus noun—(*make cookie*). During this stage, the relations that initially occur in large quantities are possession, recurrence, negation, and location (for further details, see Bloom & Lahey, 1978).

In general, comprehension of words emerges before the ability to produce words, and this occurs at around the child's first birthday (Huttenlocher & Smiley, 1987; Nelson, 1973). There is a tremendous increase in the size of children's working vocabularies between ages 1 and 2 (Bates et al., 1988). It has been argued that vocabulary growth is rapid throughout the preschool and school years and highly variable among individual children. It has been difficult to estimate the size of children's vocabularies due to many problems, posed as questions, such as what is a word, what is a meaning, and what does it mean to know a word (Beck & McKeown, 1991; Nagy & Anderson, 1984; see also, the review in Paul, 1996, 1998a). As is expected, there are individual differences in vocabulary growth; for example, first graders from higher income backgrounds had about twice the vocabulary size of those from lower income ones. Higher vocabulary growth is almost always associated with children whose homes are considered literacy rich (e.g., numerous books) and exhibit strong parental involvement (e.g., parents read to and discuss books with their children).

As discussed in Chapter 8, the enormous explosion of vocabulary knowledge occurs with the advent of mature reading. That is, children—particularly good readers—learn the bulk of their vocabulary from reading extensively and widely. All readers learn words and meanings from context in a slow incremental fashion. However, readers must read widely because context cues are not revealing, especially the use of a single context that surrounds a particular word (see discussions in Paul, 1996, 1998a).

It is important to emphasize that new words (and meanings) are not simply added in a serial fashion to an already existing static and established vocabulary. The exposure to new words alters and refines the semantic representations of words and meanings and the relationships between words that are present in the child's vocabulary (Landauer & Dumais, 1997). One of the most important metalinguistic milestones is achieved when children understand what a word is as well as what a sentence is and so on. This metalinguistic awareness of words and sentences as well as others associated with the concept of print has important implications for developing literacy skills, as discussed in Chapter 8.

Table 4-5 presents some highlights of this section on semantic development.

TABLE 4-5 Highlights of Semantic Development

- Most children are saying their first words by the time they are 1 year old.

- There is variability in the exact words used within a specific culture; however, these words do tend to refer to objects and events that are present.

- Nominals and action words comprise the overwhelming majority of words in children's early vocabularies.

- The child develops semantic or meaningful referents that reflect the organization of the child's knowledge concerning persons, objects, events, and relations.

- There are several semantic models regarding the development of the first words—among them are functional (Nelson, 1973), perceptual (Clark, 1973, 1991), relational-categorical (Bloom, 1973), and relational (Greenfield & Smith, 1976).

- In general, comprehension of words emerges before the ability to produce words, and this occurs around the child's first birthday.

- Vocabulary growth is rapid throughout the preschool and school years and highly variable among individual children.

- Higher vocabulary growth is almost always associated with children whose homes are considered literacy rich and exhibit strong parental involvement.

- New words and meanings are not simply added in a serial fashion. Exposure to new words alters and refines the semantic representations of words and meanings and the relationships between words that are present in the child's vocabulary.

- An important metalinguistic milestone is reached when a child understand what a word, phrase, or sentence is.

Syntactic Development

Prior to the emergence of the two-word stage, there are syntactic precursors (Bloom, 1973; Dore et al., 1976; also see the discussion in Crystal, 1987, 1997; Goodluck, 1991; Ingram, 1989). The notion of syntax, or that word order is meaningful, is marked by the production of successive utterances that do not at this time function as connected or cohesive linguistic units. Bloom (1973), for example, reported that a 16-month-old child consistently used one word (e.g., *wide*) with a certain phrase. Bloom maintained that this lexical unit was not interpretable because it referred to anything and everything. Other notions of syntactic precursors include (a) the use of a nonsense syllable with a certain lexical unit (e.g., a word), (b) the reduplicated production of a single lexical unit (word) successively, (c) the production of a single phonetically unstable unit prior to a lexical unit, and (d) the production of two words in combinations consistently and restrictively (i.e., not with other word combinations).

The beginning of grammar, particularly syntax, commences with the combination of two or more words in sentences (Dale, 1976; de Villiers & de Villiers, 1978; Goodluck, 1991; Ingram, 1989). The syntactic activity during this period prepares the child for the later acquisition of the major transformations of the language (e.g., relative clauses and passivization). An important question during the two-word stage is whether children possess knowledge of subject and predicate and whether this knowledge is similar to that of adults. Several researchers suggested that knowledge of the basic grammatical relation between subject and predicate is possessed by children. Bloom and Lahey (1978), however, argued that such knowledge is not syntactic only but rather semantic-syntactic in nature. They described two kinds of relationships: linear syntactic relationship and hierarchical syntactic relationship (see the discussion in Crystal, 1987, 1997; also see Chapter 2 of this text). In the former, relational words (e.g., *more* and *away*) are combined with other words, and the meaning of the relational word determines the meaning relation of the two-word combinations. In hierarchical syntactic relations, these combinations involve the form classes of nouns and pronouns in relation to verbs. The meaning of these combinations (i.e., subject-predicate concepts), however, are not the same as the meaning of the individual words. In the latter combinations, children must know both the category of word-order relation between words and semantic relation between words. This position was also supported by Bowerman (1973, 1988). In addition, both syntactic and semantic complexity have been used as adequate indices in accounting for the acquisition of the inflectional morphemes by Brown (1973). Essentially, Brown maintained that both components overlap, making it difficult to distinguish their relative contribution.

Other researchers agree that knowledge of the subject-predicate relation is present at this stage, but it is better explained by pragmatic terminology (Bates, 1976; Greenfield & Smith, 1976). These investigators asserted that the use of word order by children is in accordance with a *given-new* concept. In the adult use of this concept, given or known information is presented first, followed by new or unknown information. It has been reported that in children the order is reversed. Thus, the first word in the two-word stage is the comment (unknown) about the topic (known), which occurs as the second word.

Additional in-depth reviews and discussions of two-word utterances can be found in Bloom and Lahey (1978) and Brown (1973). At the two-word level, children's utterances represent what can be considered a limited corpus of semantic relations. Examples of declarative sentences include *Mommy push* (agent and action), *Pull car* (action and object), *Mommy sock* (possessor and possession), and *That doggie* (demonstrative and entity). The three types of negation include *All gone cookie* (nonexistence), *No dirty soap* (rejection), and *No truck* (denial—because it refers to a toy car). There are two types of questions—yes/no (*Doggie there?*)—with rising intonation and *wh-* (use of words such as *what, where,* and *who*). From these examples, it can be seen that children are making comments about objects, events, and actions in their immediate environment. Similar results can be found in cross-linguistic studies (see discussions in Crystal, 1995; Slobin, 1979). Many scholars have argued that these results support the modularity hypothesis (Fodor, 1983) in which there is a language modality that is separate from cognition (see brief discussion in Chapter 3 of this text).

Cairns (1996) provided an eloquent description of the two-word stage that highlights information presented in this section on syntax (also see the section on semantics):

> *The two-word stage is as interesting when we consider what children do not say as when we consider what they do say. There are two classes of words,* content words *(also known as* open class*) and* function words *(also known as* closed class*). Content words are verbs, nouns, adjectives, and* adverbs, *which have independent meaning. Function words, on the other hand, are words that, while not without meaning, serve primarily grammatical functions. These are words such as conjunctions, articles, prepositions, and the like. During the two-word stage, the overwhelming majority of a child's words are content words, with very few function words. Neither do we find the copula or any system of modals (e.g.,* would, could, might*) or auxiliaries. Although an occasional pronoun such as* you *or* me *might be used, there is no system of pronouns, reflexives, and reciprocals (e.g.,* each other*). A system of quantifiers (e.g.,* each, every*) is also missing although individual quantifiers such as* some *may appear. In terms of content, these children do refer to events and objects displaced in space and time, but they do not use counterfactuals, hypothetical statements, or subjunctives. In terms of language use, they demand, but they do not persuade or drop hints. The subtleties of language come later. (pp. 43–44)*

Table 4-6 provides a few highlights of this section on syntactic development.

TABLE 4-6 Highlights of Syntactic Development

- The notion of syntax is marked by the production of successive utterances that do not at this time function as connected or cohesive linguistic units. An example is the use of one word with a certain phrase that can refer to anything and everything. This is one of several examples of syntactic precursors.

- The beginning of grammar, particularly syntax, commences with the combination of two or more words in sentences. During this period, the child is preparing for the later acquisition of the major transformations of the language (e.g., relative clause and passive voice).

- During the two-word stage, the child is beginning to acquire an understanding of subject and predicate. Some scholars argue that this knowledge of the basic grammatical relationship between subject and predicate is a type of semantic-syntactic knowledge rather than only a type of syntactic knowledge. Others argue that it is an example of pragmatic knowledge.

- At the two-word level, children's utterances represent what can be considered a limited corpus of semantic relations. This finding has been confirmed in cross-linguistic studies. Some scholars argue these findings lend support to Fodor's modularity hypothesis, which suggests a language modality that is separate from cognition and other areas.

- At the two-word stage, there are two classes of words, content words (e.g., nouns, verbs, adjectives, and adverbs) and function words (e.g., articles, conjunctions, and prepositions). The overwhelming majority of words are content words; very few function words are used.

Pragmatic Development

Of course, there is more to language use than just the demand aspect (see previous passage)—even up to and including the two-word stage. Pragmatic development entails the acquisition of semantic rules, which are necessary for engaging in purposive and intentional behaviors (Bates, 1976; Crystal, 1987, 1997; Lucas, 1980). The basic unit of analysis of pragmatics is the speech act (Searle, 1969). Speech acts have been investigated in very young children. For example, Dore (1974, 1975) attempted to describe the development stage of language acquisition by employing Searle's (1969) theory of speech acts. Several primitive speech acts were identified: labeling, repeating, answering, requesting an answer, requesting (action), calling, greeting, protesting, and practicing. Dore suggested that the one- and two-word semantic relations of children contain both a function and form and represent the content of the child's social interactions. Others disagree, however, that these early utterances have a form (Bloom & Lahey, 1978; Halliday, 1975). An interesting finding reported is that some of the primitive speech acts of the child are different from the adult's speech acts. These differences contribute to the difficulty of interpreting the intentions and purposes of the child. Dore maintained, however, that the development of clearer intentions and purposes parallels the acquisition of more advanced linguistic competency. Thus, the child eventually uses speech acts that are in accordance with those of the native-speaking adult.

The basic context for speech acts, or rather, communicative competence, is social interactions (see Chapter 3 of this text). As mentioned previously, during the prelinguistic period, the child expresses the beginnings of purposive and intentional behaviors in his or her motor patterns. Typical behaviors include crying, vocalizing, eye-gazing, smiling, and various attempts to reach for objects in conjunction with some of these behaviors. By the second year, due to an increase in mobility and cognitive structures, the communicative gestures consist of showing, giving, and pointing (Bates, 1976). This phase commences with the child showing an object to an adult. Then, the child engages in such behaviors as giving objects and pointing out objects (i.e., deixis). The major function of these acts is to direct the adults' attention to the object. The attention and acceptance of the adult/caregiver is important for the child. The emergence of the first words coincides with these early communicative behaviors of showing, giving, and pointing. A more detailed description of the substance and function of interaction/deixis can be found elsewhere (Lindfors, 1980; Lucas, 1980).

The functions of speech acts have also been reported by Halliday (1975). Halliday's Phase I, described earlier, contained four functions. Halliday maintained that during Phase II the child continues to master the functions of language by using utterances that resemble those used by adults. In addition, Halliday reported that a fifth function, *heuristic*, emerges during this phase, around the 13th or 14th month. This function entails the use of vocalization in exploring and learning about the environment. In the early heuristic period, a child demands the name of objects (see earlier passage by Cairns, 1996), and later on, this behavior evolves into questioning behaviors.

Halliday (1975) asserted that it is possible to make a distinction between the *mathetic* and pragmatic functions of language. The mathetic function is the use of language to learn about persons, objects, and events in the environment. The precursors of this function are the personal and heuristic functions. The pragmatic function refers to the regulation of others' behaviors and attempts to satisfy personal needs. The precursors of this function are the instrumental and regulatory functions. The interaction function contributes to the development of both the mathetic and pragmatic functions. In sum, Halliday argued that the functions of language are expressed in isolation prior to the age of 2 years. During the second year, however, a child's utterance contains both mathetic and pragmatic functions.

Table 4-7 provides a few highlights for this section on pragmatic development.

COMPREHENSION-PRODUCTION ISSUE

Central to the analyses of the first words (up to and including the three-word stage) is the long-standing comprehension-production issue. This issue—mentioned briefly previously—is similar to that discussed relative to the sounds

---

TABLE 4-7 Highlights of Pragmatic Development

- Pragmatic development entails the acquisition of semantic rules that are necessary for engaging in purposive and intentional behaviors.

- Speech acts have been investigated in very young children. Primitive speech acts include labeling, repeating, answering, requesting an answer, requesting (action), calling, greeting, protesting, and practicing. However, because the nature of some of these primitive speech acts are different from those of adults, it is often difficult to interpret the intentions and purposes of the child.

- The basic context for speech acts, or rather, communicative competence, is social interactions.

- The emergence of the first words coincides with early communicative behaviors of showing, giving, and pointing. The major function of these acts is to direct the adults' attention to the object.

- During the second year, the child uses language to learn about persons, objects, and events in the environment. The child also uses language to regulate others' behaviors and to satisfy personal needs.

- A prominent model for understanding the development of the functions of speech acts is that of Halliday (1975).

---

of speech, that is, the perception-production issue. The focus here is on the nature of the first words. Traditionally, the productions of children have received—and continue to receive—more attention than the corresponding comprehension of words. This situation is not due to a lack of interest but rather to the difficulty of measuring the comprehension of children (see discussions in Bloom & Lahey, 1978; Cairns, 1996; Crystal, 1987, 1997; Goodluck, 1991; Ingram, 1989).

In some cases, the one-word utterances of children seem to be analogous to the sentences of adults (Cairns, 1996; Ingram, 1989). This phenomenon is termed holophrastic speech, implying that children understand more than what they say. Although the word-as-sentence hypothesis has been discussed extensively, most of the past and ongoing evidence seems to support Bloom's (1973) argument that the extent of children's early knowledge is restricted to the lexical meanings, not the grammatical meanings, that is, syntax or relations between words.

The question of whether comprehension precedes production or vice versa has been investigated although perhaps it needs a different focus. In one exemplar study, for example, Huttenlocher (see review and discussion in Huttenlocher & Smiley, 1987) studied the performance of four 1-year-old children. The researcher devised procedures to assess comprehension by minimizing the influence of contextual cuing. A list of words with precise meanings, that is, those understood by the children, was obtained. This is contrary to Clark's (1973) and Bowerman's (1973, 1988) contentions that obtaining precise meanings is extremely difficult at this stage. Nevertheless, the results of this study also supported Bloom's (1973) arguments. Huttenlocher concluded that at the one-word stage: (a) The comprehension of children is dependent on contextual cues rather than on verbal comprehension, and (b) there are no instances of overextensions, thus, comprehension of lexical items precedes production.

In another classic study, Shipley, Smith, and Gleitman (1969) investigated the comprehension-production issues in two groups of children: one group used single-word utterances, and the other used telegraphic two- and three-word sentences. Commands were presented to these children in single words, telegraphic speech, or well-formed sentences. Conflicting results were reported. The single-word group responded best to commands of first words, thus substantiating the claim that comprehension precedes production at this stage. The telegraphic group, however, responded best to well-formed commands. This latter result cannot be interpreted in the same way as the former.

In sum, a number of scholars (Bloom & Lahey, 1978; Cairns, 1996; Crystal, 1987, 1997; Ingram, 1989) have suggested that different kinds of questions should be asked concerning comprehension and production. Instead of investigating which one precedes the other or the relationship between the two, there is a need to study the processes that underlie each and the relationship of the two processes to linguistic and cognitive development. This latter focus has been a topic in the ongoing language-cognition debates (see Chapter 3). It is still true that "the developmental gap between comprehension and speaking probably varies among different children and at different times, and that the gap may be more apparent than real" (Bloom & Lahey, 1978, p. 238).

LINGUISTIC MATURITY: THREE-WORD STAGE AND BEYOND

In essence, growing up with adults/caregivers within a language community, most children acquire the language (spoken or signed) of that community in an effortless manner. Throughout the preschool years (up to age 5 or so), there is a tremendous growth in all domains of language, phonology, morphology, syntax, semantics, and pragmatics. Initially, children's utterances beyond the two-word stage do not indicate any real increase in syntactic or semantic complexity.

After a while, as utterances move beyond the two-word stage, children utilize the same grammatical relations as observed for the two-word utterances, save for the encoding of additional grammatical relations. The progression of these utterances can be described by the processes of modulation and refinement. The basis of these processes is the acquisition of morphemes that alters meaning and form (Brown, 1973). The early syntactic-semantic utterances are modulated and subsequently expanded (or refined) into structures similar to those used by adults. Examples of this process include conjoining, expansion, elaborating, and embedding. An example of conjoining is: *Mommy make* and *Make cookie* becomes *Mommy make cookie*. In conjoining, two grammatical relations sharing a common term are conjoined with the redundant term deleted. An example of expansion is *My cookie all gone*. In essence, a noun phrase is often used to replace a simple grammatical relation. In this example, the subject is represented by a possessive noun phrase. An example of elaboration (from Brown, 1973) is *Adam ride horsie*. In analyses of declarative sentences, Brown and his colleagues found this pattern to be consistent and in the prescribed English order: agent-action-object-location. Beyond the two-word level, three or more elements of this pattern are included. In *Adam ride horsie*, there is an agent-action-object. An example of embedding is: *No cookie* and *Make cookie* becomes *Make no cookie*. *No cookie*, which expresses a functional relation, is inserted or embedded into *Make cookie* to form a grammatical relation. Thus, an increase in semantic information parallels the increase in structure complexity, and this phenomenon is reflected in the production of complex utterances (Lucas, 1980).

One of the most influential discoveries from the research of Brown (1973) was the delineation of the acquisitional order of morphemes, particularly the first 14 morphemes. This finding has influenced the development of several of the signed systems for deaf and hard-of-hearing students, particularly signed English and seeing essential English (see Chapter 6 of this text). It has also influenced research on the morphological development of deaf children. Cairns (1996) provided an excellent synopsis of this line of research, discussed in Table 4-8.

TABLE 4-8 Synopsis of Brown's (1973) Research on the Early Acquisition of Morphemes

---

Early Acquisition of Morphemes

1. *Present progressive.* This is the bound morpheme *ing* in a sentence such as "The kitty is sleeping." Children do not use the auxiliary *is* until much later. A typical sentence would be "Kitty sleeping."

2. & 3. *The prepositions in* and *on.* These, of course, are free rather than bound morphemes.

4. *Plural.* This refers to the orthographic *s* that is bound to nouns, as in *dogs.* Brown does not include in his list the acquisition of the irregular plural, such as *children* or *mice.*

5. *Past irregular.* Irregular past tense forms, such as *broke,* appear before regular past tense forms.

6. *Possessive.* This is also an orthographic *s,* as in "Grover's."

7. *Uncontractible copula.* The copula is the verb *to be.* It can be contracted in sentences such as "He is there," becoming "He's there," but not in environments such as "Here I am." "Here I'm" is not grammatical. It is in the latter environments that children first use the copula.

8. *Articles.* These are the free morphemes, *a, an,* and *the.*

9. *Past regular.* Regular past tenses are orthographically *ed,* as in *worked.*

10. *Third person singular (regular).* This again is an orthographic *s,* as in "He works." Note that the plural third person, "They work" is the

uninflected form of the verb, as used in infinitives such as "They like to work," without a bound morpheme.

11. *Third person singular (irregular).* This affects words such as *does* and *has.* Again, the plural is the infinitival form (*have* and *do*), with the exception of the verb *to be,* which becomes, "They are."

12. *Uncontractible auxiliary.* The auxiliary can be contracted in some cases; for example, "They are cheering" can become "They're cheering." But in "They were cheering" the auxiliary *were* cannot be contracted. Like the copula, the uncontractible form appears first in children's speech.

13. *Contractible copula.* See the example in number 7.

14. *Contractible auxiliary.* See the example in number 12.

Note: Taken from Cairns (1996, pp. 46–47).

Beyond the three-word stage, children begin to produce and comprehend linguistic forms and functions of a more complex nature. Now they are learning the general adult rules that govern the application of rules for the various linguistic components. Children play an active role by discovering regularities and formulating hypotheses regarding the application of the rules (Cairns, 1996; Ingram, 1989). Through the joint social interaction or deixis, children acquire semantic referents and functions for persons, objects, and events in their environment. The forms of the referents entail the combinations of the arbitrarily defined symbols from phonology, morphology, and syntax. The applications of linguistic form, content, and function correspond to a rule system (Bloom & Lahey, 1978; Crystal, 1987, 1997; Goodluck, 1991).

Beyond the three-word stage, the syntactic development of children consists of using the major transformations of the language (Cairns, 1996; Crystal, 1987, 1997; Goodluck, 1991). Initially, children adhere to a noun-verb-noun or subject-verb-object word order, which presents problems in some transformations, notably passivization. Nevertheless, the major transformations, for example, question formation (e.g., *wh-* and *yes/no* questions) and relativization (i.e., use of relative pronouns such as *who, whom,* and *that*) are acquired in a systematic manner. Within the question formation category, *yes/no* questions are acquired before *wh-* questions, and this in turn is acquired before tag questions (e.g., *You ate the cookie, didn't you?* or *You didn't eat the cookie, did you?*). There are also smaller acquisition steps within each group of questions. Further discussions of the acquisition process can be found elsewhere

(Cairns, 1996; Crystal, 1987, 1995, 1997). In general, most children have internalized much of the grammar of the language by the age of 4 or 5 years and have mastered nearly all of the grammar by age 9 or 10.

It is often forgotten just how rapid children develop their understanding of the grammar of the language. Even before the three-word stage, children have an understanding of the syntax of English that permits them to recognize the difference between the following two sentences: *Elmo is tickling Zoe* and *Zoe is tickling Elmo* (Golinkoff & Hirsch-Pasek, 1995).

This rapid growth in language form, content, and use enables children to use their language as a means of engaging in more complex information exchanges with adults and older children. One of the most important activities in which this becomes apparent is during book sharing, especially with significant others or adults. With an increasing sophistication of language, children can progress from naming people and objects in the pictures to asking and answering questions about the story. With the ability to produce and understand complex sentences, children can not only use *wh-* questions with words such as *what, when,* and *who* but can also handle questions that focus on abstract ideas—for example, *why* and *what if.* More important, children are able to handle discussions that entail people, objects, and events that are not present or in the immediate environment. As discussed in Chapter 8, this ability to address decontextualized information is extremely critical for the development of literate thought, particularly via the use of script literacy skills—reading and writing.

Returning to the area of pragmatics, children continue to learn and refine these language skills throughout the preschool period and well into adulthood (see review in Ninio & Snow, 1996). During the preschool years, children continue to work on conventional speech acts such as requesting, attention getting, describing, and the use of conversational skills, which entail turn-taking, topic contingency, topic development, and psychological presupposition (ensuring that speakers understand what you are saying by providing additional information).

Much of the work in the field of pragmatics describes how children learn the rules for using language in specific situations such as book reading, sharing time, and dinner-table talk (see review in Ninio & Snow, 1996). Through various literacy activities (e.g., book or story sharing), children understand differences in the use, tone, and style of language by characters in the story. In addition, they became familiar with and understand literary genres such as fiction, mythology, and nonfiction.

METACOGNITIVE DEVELOPMENT

With the increase in language knowledge, children began to develop what is called *metacognitive* skills. During the preschool years, metalinguistic insights about the language domains (e.g., phonology, syntax, semantics, and pragmatics) emerge and continue to develop throughout childhood and adolescence. This is a very critical area; its absence is noticeable in children who have language difficulties or who have not developed a high level of skill in the use of their language. Metalinguistically, children can use language for thought and for communication. This involves the ability to play with it, talk about it, analyze it componentially, and make judgments about acceptable versus incorrect forms. For example, children may play with and think about the sounds, word usage, different sentences, and some application of ideas. Traditionally, due to the heavy influence of Piaget's work, it was reasoned that metalinguistic development did not begin to emerge until about school age, especially during the late preoperation or early concrete operation stages of Piaget. However, it has been demonstrated that some children exhibit basic metalinguistic skills by the age of 3 years or even younger. In addition, a number of children possess a significant amount of metalinguistic insight about sentences, words, and speech sounds by the time they are 4 to 5 years old. Of course, metalinguistic skills continue to improve throughout the school years and reaches a very complex, mature level during what Piaget labeled the *formal operation stage.*

Chapter 8 further discusses a very important metalinguistic milestone: the appreciation or understanding of what a word is. When children comprehend the idea that things have names, they quickly proceed to the notions of phrases and sentences and other literacy labels that are critical for successful reading and writing activities. In the beginning, young children are not able to distinguish between the word itself and the object or action it represents. They cannot separate a sentence into its component words. Children have difficulty making metalinguistic judgments about the length of words. Subsequently, when children reach the stage of understanding the notion of a word and that this word is separate from its referent, they can develop their segmentation skills. Words such as nouns, verbs, and adjectives eventually are recognized as linguistic units, and this is a crucial developmental milestone. Finally, it has been argued that one of the most important skills for beginning reading is the child's ability to attend to and analyze the internal phonological structure of spoken words. This progression is from phonological awareness to phonemic awareness, and the use of phonics is deemed inappropriate if the progression has not been accomplished.

Table 4-9 provides a summary of salient points presented in the sections on linguistic maturity and the development of metacognition.

TABLE 4-9 Highlights of Linguistic Maturity—Three-Word Stage and Beyond—and Metacognitive Development

---

Linguistic Maturity: Three-Word Stage and Beyond

- Initially, children's utterances beyond the two-word stage do not indicate any real increase in syntactic or semantic complexity.

- During the early part of this stage, children engage in two general processes—modulation and refinement—that are driven and shaped by the acquisition of morphemes, which alter meaning and form. Examples of these processes acting on utterances are conjoining, expansion, elaborating, and embedding.

- The increase in semantic information parallels the increase in structure complexity (i.e., syntax), and this is reflected in the production of complex utterances.

- Children discover regularities and formulate hypotheses regarding the application of the rules. This process is now considered similar to that of adult language users.

- Children acquire semantic referents and functions for persons, objects, and events in their environment.

- Beyond the three-word stage, children's syntactic development consists of using the major transformations of the language (question formation, relativization, and passive voice; also see Chapter 2).

- Initially, children use a linear strategy for understanding sentences such as noun-verb-noun or subject-verb-object. Later, they develop more sophisticated strategies for dealing with hierarchical syntactic structures (also see Chapter 2).

- In general, most children internalize much of the grammar of the language by the age of 4 or 5 years and master nearly all of the grammar by age 9 or 10.

- With respect to pragmatic development during the preschool years, children continue to work on conventional speech acts such as requesting, attention getting, describing, and the use of conversational skills, which entail turn-taking, topic contingency, topic development, and psychological presuppositions.

- During the preschool years, there is an emergence of metalinguistic insights about the language domains—that is, the domains of phonology, syntax, semantics, and pragmatics.

- During this period, the emergence and development of metacognitive skills are critical for the subsequent development of high-level language use, including the development and enhancement of literate thought.

- Examples of early metalinguistic development include playing with and talking about language, analyzing language into components and parts, and making judgments about acceptable versus unacceptable forms.

- Some children exhibit basic metalinguistic skills by the age of 3 years or younger.

- By age 4 or 5 years, many children have a significant amount of metalinguistic knowledge about concepts such as word, sentence, and speech sounds. This type of knowledge seems to be critical for early literacy development. It is during this period that children begin to develop segmentation skills (i.e., syllables and phonemes), or rather, segmentation awareness begins to emerge. For this development to proceed, children need to understand that a word is separate from its referent.

LANGUAGE DEVELOPMENT AND DEAFNESS: A FEW REMARKS

Through observations of a young hearing child, say a 5 year old, in the home and school environments, it is possible to describe the nature of the language she or he is using. That is, one can label it as *Spanish, French,* or *English,* or even bilingual combinations such as *Spanish and English* and so on. It is much more difficult, of course, to determine the communicative and grammatical competence of this hypothetical hearing child.

On the other hand, describing the primary language development of a deaf child (and sometimes a hard-of-hearing child) is much more complicated. As discussed in Chapter 1, it is true that most deaf and hard-of-hearing children in the United States are exposed to English in infancy and early childhood. Quigley and Kretschmer (1982) averred that the description of this exposure needs to consider two issues: (a) the nature of the language input (i.e., American Sign Language or English) and (b) the nature of the communication mode used, that is, manual or oral.

Relative to these issues, it can be stated that some deaf and hard-of-hearing children are exposed to English (language input) via the use of speech (communication mode—oral). Other deaf and hard-of-hearing children may be exposed to English (language input) via the use of signs (communication mode—manual) or signs and speech (communication modes—manual and oral). Still others may be exposed only to American Sign Language (language input), which only involves the use of signs (communication mode—manual) as well as nonmanual cues (see Chapter 7 of this text). It can be argued that exposure to English in a signed form also involves some exposure to ASL because of a few overlapping aspects (mostly the lexicon) between the various English signed systems and ASL (see Chapters 6 and 7 of this text). Nevertheless, exposure to some aspects of ASL is not commensurate with exposure to ASL as a language input in the same way that exposure to or use of a few French words is not commensurate with knowledge of the French language. Of course, the nature of the exposure for deaf and hard-of-hearing children is also problematic and controversial (see Chapter 1 for a brief discussion of this concept; also see Chapters 5 and 6).

In light of this discussion, it might be surprising for the reader to discover in the ensuing chapters that there have been very few research studies that attempted to determine the communicative and grammatical assessment of deaf and hard-of-hearing children, especially with respect to exposure to oral English and/or the English signed systems. Some of the research involved retrospective studies employing script literacy assessments, that is, reading and writing, in evaluating the efficiency of language/communication approaches in developing the primary or performance form of English. This is not a direct way to understand the issue of primary language development, that is, the development of the conversational or performance aspect of a language manifested, for example, by speaking and/or signing. There are a few studies, however, that are developmental; these studies attempt to chart some aspect of primary or performance language development.

The dearth of research studies seems to reflect the difficulty of the task of evaluating the primary language development of deaf and hard-of-hearing students. Furthermore, the research approaches have been criticized as being too narrow or shortsighted. In some cases, the research approaches seem to be atheoretical or seem to lack a defining explanatory focus. That there needs to be more concerted research efforts has become a trite, simplified, overused generalization, and unfortunately, it needs to be said repeatedly.

FINAL REMARKS

With the information in this chapter and that discussed in the previous two chapters (Chapters 2 and 3), it is hoped that the reader has obtained a basic understanding and appreciation of the complexity and magic of language, particularly the acquisition of language. This development is truly remarkable, especially when one considers the major accomplishments during the first 3 years within the various language components. The advancement of researchers' knowledge has revealed the critical role of the prelinguistic period—a period in which the precursors for subsequent linguistic features can be observed. It is not difficult to imagine the deleterious effects of a disruption or disturbance during the prelinguistic period on later linguistic and cognitive development of individuals. In addition, it is also understandable (or will be in the ensuing chapters) why the development of a bona fide language as early as possible is one of the major issues facing educators of deaf and hard-of-hearing students.

There are a number of concluding—albeit tentatively concluding—remarks that can be made about language acquisition. Some scholars believe that the acquisition of language after childhood is still a poorly understood phenomenon. This acquisition, of course, is quite different from the native acquisition of one or more languages in childhood. In fact, this acquisition essentially epitomizes the problem for most deaf and some hard-of-hearing students who have not acquired a first language during the early childhood period.

With respect to the development of a first language for children with typical hearing, summaries of major points were presented throughout the chapter. Here, only a few highlights are provided of those summaries within two broad categories: prelinguistic development and linguistic development.

Prelinguistic Development

- During the first few months of life, infants can discriminate between speech sounds. By the age of 3 months, infants respond differently to their mother's voice compared to those of other adult females.

- Infants are sensitive to the suprasegmental aspect prior to the segmental aspect of speech. The rise-fall contour of infant vocalization is an important precursor of sentence types such as statements, questions, and explanations.

- In the first months of life, infants begin to use their voices to control others and to get them to do things. Infants practice and perfect the habitual and significant sounds of the particular languages to which they are exposed.

- Prior to the emergence of intentional and meaningful communication, a child explores the environment for about 1 year. With this exploration comes the realization that persons, objects, and events are separate from the self.

- In essence, during the first year, the infant develops the precursors for the language components—phonology, syntax, semantics, and pragmatics. By the end of the first year, with the onset of object permanence and control over sounds for the first words, the child proceeds into the one-word stage.

Linguistic Development

- First words can only be fully understood within the contexts in which they are uttered. Some of them are not just labels but stand for sentence-like commentaries or instructions.

- Two-word combinations are examples of early grammatical language; the words are put together to express the child's perception of actions and relationships.

- There appears to be a wide variation in the early phonologic development of children. This development continues well beyond the first year and probably continues to be refined even in the early school years. Most of the phonologic rules are acquired by around 6 to 8 years of age.

- Vocabulary growth is rapid throughout the preschool and school years and highly variable among individual children. New words and meanings are not simply added in a serial fashion. Exposure to new words alters and refines the semantic representations of words and meanings and the relationships between words that are present in the child's vocabulary.

- Beyond the three-word stage, children's syntactic development consists of using the major transformations of the language (question formation, relativization, and passive voice).

- By age 4 or 5 years, many children have a significant amount of metalinguistic knowledge about concepts such as word, sentence, and speech sounds. This type of knowledge seems to be critical for early literacy development. It is during this period that children begin to develop segmentation skills (i.e., syllables and phonemes), or rather, segmentation awareness begins to emerge. For this development to proceed, children need to understand that a word is separate from its referent.

- In general, most children internalize much of the grammar of the language by the age of 4 or 5 years and master nearly all of the grammar by age 9 or 10.

The next two chapters examine the acquisition of language by deaf and hard-of-hearing individuals with respect to a specific mode of communication, that is, oralism and total communication via signing and the signed systems. The development of American Sign Language is discussed in Chapter 7. In essence, these chapters address the primary language development of most deaf and hard-of-hearing students with respect to the development of English or American Sign Language.

In sum, the study of language continues to be an important task for scholars with the obvious need for further development of theory (i.e., understanding) and further improvement of instruction of—for the purposes here—English as a first or second language. It is often forgotten that the study of language is also critical for humans to understand themselves and others; indeed, this entity is a critical, defining element of our humanity. Some scholars believe that language is what separates us humans from other animals, including the primates (see discussion in Crystal, 1997). It seems that a proficient command of the benefits of language is only possible when it is acquired during early childhood. This raises some rather thorny, uncomfortable questions: What happens when language is not acquired during early childhood or at least by puberty? Does this mean that individuals have not or will not ever develop an important part of their humanity? and Without a full-blown language, is an individual less than human? There might not be complete or satisfying answers to these questions. Nevertheless, the next two chapters present some information that is relevant to these questions and others for deaf and hard-of-hearing children.

PRIMARY LANGUAGE DEVELOPMENT: PERSPECTIVES AND ISSUES COMPREHENSION QUESTIONS

1. In the beginning of the chapter, it was remarked that there is still much controversy surrounding theory and research on the language acquisition of children. What are some of the persistent disagreements?

2. Briefly describe what is considered to be the prelinguistic or preverbal period of language development. Why is there a renewed interest in research in this area?

3. Describe the following terms:

   a. segmental aspects

   b. suprasegmental aspects

   Discuss some of the major research highlights involving the development of the infant's perceptual and production skills with respect to both segmental and suprasegmental aspects (i.e., discuss the infant's perception [discrimination] and production of sounds during the first year).

4. What are some semantic (i.e., cognitive) and pragmatic precursors during the prelinguistic stage?

5. What milestone marks the beginning of linguistic development? Does this milestone indicate the end of the prelinguistic period? Why or why not?

6. There is no question that the development of language is quite remarkable from the emergence of the first words to the beginning of the three-word stage (i.e., from about 1 to 3 years of age). Discuss a few of the major developmental milestones/research findings with respect to:

   a. phonology

   b. syntax

   c. semantics

   d. pragmatics

7. With respect to the analyses of the first words, there has been much discussion on what is called the comprehension-production issue. What is this issue? What are some tentative conclusions?

8. It has been stated that linguistic maturity occurs beyond the three-word stage and throughout the preschool years. Briefly describe the language development of children during this period (e.g., syntax, semantics, and pragmatics). What is the nature of children's metacognitive development? Why is metacognition important?

9. According to the author, describing the primary language development of a deaf child is much more complicated than that of a hearing child. Why?

CHALLENGE QUESTIONS

(Note: Complete answers are not in the text. Additional research is required.)

1. Either obtain or make a videotape that contains about 15 minutes of the following three children (between 2 and 3 years old, same sex, same race, same socioeconomic status, etc.) at play with toys or engaged in an interaction with the mother:

   a. hard-of-hearing child (i.e., up to but not including the severe hearing-impaired level)

   b. deaf child who speaks (i.e., with severe to profound hearing impairment)

   c. child with typical hearing

   Listen to and analyze (with assistance from parents and/or professionals) the three language samples. Do you notice any quantitative (i.e., amount) differences or similarities? Describe them. Do you notice any qualitative differences or similarities? Describe them. [Try to describe the children's use of language with respect to types of words, phrases, etc. Be sure to include the contexts or situations in which the language is used. If possible, compare your findings with what was described in this chapter for children in the two-word stage—i.e., from about 2 to 3 years of age).

2. Using the same three children, observe the mother (or other professional) reading a story to each child, respectively. Are there differences in the rate of speech? In the style of reading (i.e., holding the book, pointing to the pictures, etc.)? In the type of questions asked? Are there differences in the child's responses to questions? In the child's remarks about the story (initiating remarks, not in response to questions)?

3. Show three pictures to children with typical hearing who are 3, 4, and 5 years old. Ask each child to tell you about the picture. (Ask parents or relevant professionals to suggest three fairly detailed interesting

pictures.) After a child responds, ask him or her if he or she can tell you more about the picture. Compare the responses of the three children for the pictures. With assistance, discuss the contents with respect to vocabulary (number of words, types of words, meanings of words, etc.), use of syntax, and Brown's research on morphology, discussed in this chapter, if relevant.

FURTHER READINGS

Atkinson, M. (1992). *Children's syntax*. Cambridge, MA: Blackwell.

Bruner, J. (1983). *Child's talk: Learning to use language*. New York: Norton.

Denes, P., & Pinson, E. (1973). *The speech chain: The physics and biology of spoken language*. Garden City, NY: Anchor Press/Doubleday.

Lorenz, K. (1954). *Man meets dog*. London: Methuen.

Tinbergen, N. (1951). *The study of instinct*. Oxford, UK: Oxford University Press.

Orality: Speech, Audition, and Speechreading

There is a great deal of confusion as to what is meant by oral method. I think it means generally the "speech-reading method." I believe that all children should be taught articulation, and taught to use articulation, but I do not think that all children should be taught by articulation, that is to say, speech-reading. All who can be successfully and readily taught by speech-reading should be so taught, and those who cannot should be taught manually—by which I mean that written language should be used by the teacher. In all cases, however, the mouth should be used by the pupil as his means of communication. In this sense I would use an oral system for all. "Speech," for all; "speech-reading" for as many as can readily profit by it. This is my opinion. (Alexander Graham Bell as cited in Cornett, 1990, pp. 149–150)

As indicated in this passage, Alexander Graham Bell's focus seemed to be predominantly on the development of speech, and this remains a fixture or major belief of members of the Alexander Graham Bell Association for the Deaf in which *The Volta Review* is its major scholarly publication (i.e., research journal). This passage (part of Bell's 1888 testimony before The Royal Commission of the United Kingdom on the Condition of the Blind, the Deaf and Dumb, Etc.) should be considered with respect to the prevailing technological knowledge in Bell's times. As noted by Cornett (1990), Bell and his contemporaries could not "foresee the tremendous potential value of tiny amounts of residual hearing" (p. 146). This might have also led to Bell's thinking about the use of speechreading to teach spoken language to individuals who have limited hearing and no strong prior development of the language. In addition, Bell could not foresee the integral relationships among speech, speechreading, and audition (residual hearing) that are now a staple in many oral education programs today. Without a doubt, these relationships have become apparent or are becoming apparent with the advances in technology in speech and hearing science (e.g., cochlear implants and tactile aids).

Nevertheless, according to Connor (1986), it is shortsighted to describe the oral method as one that simply entails "the use of speech and speechreading exclusively" (p. 118). It is possible to remark, at least, that speech, speechreading, and audition are major components that characterize this method—although there are other components or aspects (e.g., environment, instruction, curriculum, and parental involvement) that are necessary to ensure the development of English in both the spoken and written modes. The same can be said for descriptions of Total Communication methods (see Chapter 6). There are a number of sensory devices that are often used to develop or enhance speech and/or speechreading skills. The most obvious ones (at least relative to function) are amplification devices such as hearing aids and cochlear implants. Tactile aids are also used, sometimes alone, sometimes in conjunction with either hearing aids or cochlear implants (see discussion in Geers & Moog, 1994; McGarr, 1989). The major purpose of tactile (i.e., touch via vibrations) aids is often to enhance or assist the development of speech skills and, in some cases, speechreading skills.

Although all of these are elements of the oral method, it is not uncommon to find specific proponents who have either placed emphasis on one element or one kind of sensory input to be used in isolation or predominantly (see Levitt, 1989; Ling, 1976; Pollack, 1984). Nearly all proponents of oral education would agree with Ling (1984) that:

> *The philosophy of oral education is that hearing-impaired children should be given the opportunity to learn to speak and to understand speech, learn through spoken language in school, and later function as independent adults in a world in which people's primary mode of communication is speech. (p. 9)*

Because of the strong emphasis on speech development, much attention is devoted here to salient aspects of the physical process of articulation. The development of speech has had a tremendous appeal to parents, especially hearing parents of young children with hearing impairment. The following passage, published more than 30 years ago, still encapsulates the spirit of oralism for many hearing parents today:

The oral philosophy has a powerful appeal to parents of young deaf children. More than anything else, they want their deaf child to talk and to understand others through lip reading. This is particularly true of parents who have guilt feelings regarding their deaf child. If the child can be taught to speak and read lips well, somehow some or all of the guilt is relieved. (Hester, 1969, p. 154)

This chapter briefly discusses the oral English language development of students whose major mode of receptive and expressive communication is via the use of speech, speechreading, and audition. Although the focus is on students in oral programs, the findings of selective studies involving students in mainstreamed or inclusion programs are reported, including students who are classified as hard of hearing (see Chapter 1 of this text for a description). Also discussed in this chapter are students who have been exposed to and use cued speech (or cued language). Prior to synthesizing the results of these studies, some basic information is provided on the classification of speech sounds and a brief general description of the oral approaches, including the components of aural rehabilitation—speechreading and auditory training/learning. This information is necessary for understanding the general findings on speech perception, production, and intelligibility as well as understanding the research on oralism and deaf and hard-of-hearing students. The reader is referred elsewhere for additional information on speech and hearing, particularly anatomy, physiology, and the development of speech and hearing abilities (Boothroyd, 1984; Brownell, 1999; Erber, 1982; Levitt, 1989; Ling, 1976, 1989).

Given the breadth (i.e., wide range) of topics for this chapter, the selection of empirical and secondary (i.e., reviews and discussions) is limited but, hopefully, reflective of the major findings on and salient areas in oral education. Some discussion is devoted to issues of pediatric audiology, for example, early identification, early amplification, and the use of cochlear implants. There is no description of the various types of amplification systems (i.e., types of hearing aids, FM systems, etc.) or of the various types of hearing losses (for a readable account of these domains, including the importance of developing audition, see Epstein, 1999; Flexer, 1997; Lewis, 1995). As is the case for all chapters in this text, the coverage of selective issues is meant to be representative and balanced; however, more likely, the treatment is a reflection of the author's interests and interpretations.

CLASSIFICATION OF SPEECH SOUNDS

In Chapter 2, there was a brief discussion of the sound system of English, that is, phonology. The reader was introduced to concepts such as phonemes, segmentals, and suprasegmentals. Hopefully, a better understanding emerges as these concepts are discussed with respect to general findings on speech perception and production by deaf and hard-of-hearing students.

To understand speech sounds, the reader needs some basic understanding of speech mechanisms and production. Many of the structures of the body for producing speech are the same ones used for breathing and eating. These include structures such as the lungs, larynx (i.e., voice box, which contains the vocal folds or cords), tongue, and lips (Boothroyd, 1986; Ling, 1976; Stevens, 1992; Zemlin, 1968). The quality (i.e., resonance) of the speech sounds are affected also by three chambers or cavities known as oral (mouth), pharyngeal (throat), and nasal (nose). The air flow from the lungs becomes sound (i.e., on exhalation) when it is obstructed or constricted by the various speech mechanisms. For example, the vocal folds (two muscular flaps) can interrupt the flow of air by coming together and separating. (For a detailed illustration of these speech structures, see Boothroyd, 1986, and Zemlin, 1968).

In general, there are three categories of sound source—voicing, frication, and stop-plosives—that are responsible for producing two groups of speech sounds, or phonemes—consonants and vowels (for further discussion, see Boothroyd, 1984, 1986; Levitt, 1989; Ling, 1976; Stevens, 1992). *Voicing* refers to the vibrating movements of the vocal folds, resulting in voiced sounds. The frequency of the vibration is perceived as *pitch*, and the variations of frequency during speech production are perceived as *intonation*. When the air flow is constricted—that is, forced through a narrow opening—the result is a turbulence known as *frication*. The location of the narrow opening is called the *place of articulation*. For example, some sounds may involve both lips (bilabial as in /p/ and /b/) or the lower lip and upper teeth (labiodental as /f/ and /v/) and so on. The *stop-plosive* sound source results when the air flow is obstructed completely and then released quickly by the build-up of air pressure

It is difficult to determine the number of phonemes in English, mainly because of differences among the speakers of the language. Obviously, this applies to consonants and vowels (see discussions in Creaghead & Newman, 1985; Shelton & Wood, 1978). Table 5-1 displays a list of the most commonly heard consonants in English, and Table 5-2 provides a list of vowels.

Inspection of Table 5-1 reveals that consonants are typically categorized with respect to the manner of articulation indicated by the use of terms such as *stop-plosive, affricate, fricative, nasal,* and *vowel-like* (i.e., glides). Given the previous description of stop-plosion, the notion of stop-plosive consonants should be clear. In English, there are six common stop-plosive sounds, half of which are voiced and the other half voiceless. Affricates are generally similar to stop-plosives except that the air pulses are sustained for longer peri-

TABLE 5-1 A List of Consonants in American English

Place of Articulation

Type/Manner	Bilabial	Labio-dental	Inter-dental	Apico-alveolar	Fronto-palatal	Dorso-velar	Glottal
Stop-plosive	p (*p*at)			t (*t*ip)		k (*c*at)	
	b (*b*it)			d (*d*og)		g (*g*um)	
				d (*d*og)		g (*g*um)	
Affricate				tʃ (*ch*at)			
				dʒ (*j*et)			
Fricative	wh (*wh*at)	f (*f*it)	θ (*th*in)	s (*s*ip)	ʃ (*sh*ip)		h (*h*it)
		v (*v*et)	ð (*th*at)	z (*z*ip)	ʒ (a*z*ure)		
Nasal	m (*m*y)			n (*n*ap)			ŋ (so*ng*)
Lateral				l (*l*et)			
Semivowel	w (*w*ine)			r (ba*r*)	j (*y*et)		

Notes: *Stop-plosive: voiceless = /p/, /t/, and /k/; voice = /b/, /d/, and /g/.*
Affricate: voiceless = /t/; voice = /d/.
Fricative: voiceless = /wh/, /f/, /θ/, /s/, and /ʃ/; voice = /v/, /ð/, /z/, /ʒ/, and /h/
Lateral and semivowel are glides.
Nasal, lateral, and semivowel are voiced.
Note: *Based on Creaghead and Newman (1985) and Shelton and Wood (1978).*

ods of time. Fricatives, of course, involve the sound source of frication. Voiced fricatives involve both voicing (vocal folds) and frication. Vowel-like consonants are similar to vowels; there seems to be four common vowel-like consonants in English.

All vowels involve voicing (vibrations of the vocal folds), and the resulting sound is typically given its quality by the oral cavity. As indicated in Table 5-2, the differences among vowels are determined primarily by the placement of the tongue. The configurations of the lips and the pharyngeal cavity also play important roles in vowel production. Additional terms for classifying vowels are *tense* and *lax* (Creaghead & Newman, 1985; Shelton & Wood, 1978). Tense vowels require more muscular tension and adjustments than do lax vowels and are longer in duration. Long durations refer to long vowel sounds (as in *see* and *cope*), whereas short durations refer to short vowel sounds (as in *hit*

TABLE 5-2 A List of Vowels in American English

Tongue Positions

	Front	Center	Back
High	i (beat)		u (food)
	I (hit)		U (book)
Middle	e (rate)	ɝ (bird)	o (coat)
	ɛ (forever)	ʌ (up)	ɔ (caw)
		ɚ (letter)	
		ə (about)	
Low	ae (at)		ɒ (lot)
	a (lass)		ɑ (father)

Note: Based on Creaghead and Newman (1985) and Shelton and Wood (1978).

and *sit*). Diphthongs are often called *double vowels* (Boothroyd, 1986). The tongue may assume one position in the beginning of the sound and end up in another position on the completion of the sound. Both the tongue and the vocal tract (i.e., the oral cavity) modify the resonance and quality of the sound, which is actually a blending of sounds. Examples of diphthongs include /eI/, as in vacation, /aI/, as in hide, and /oU/, as in blow (Creaghead & Newman, 1985).

The rendition of consonants and vowels shows them as isolated sounds, not in connected speech. Some of the important concepts of connected speech are intonation, rhythm, and coarticulation (Boothroyd, 1986; Levitt, 1989; McGarr & Whitehead, 1992). As mentioned previously, intonation refers to the patterns of frequency and is perceived as pitch. Rhythm refers to the timing patterns of speech, involving the duration of specific sounds and syllables. Rhythm also concerns the periods of time between stressed (emphasized) sounds and syllables. These pauses contribute to speech rhythm. In coarticulation, the production of a speech sound in a word is affected by the production of the preceding and following sounds. For example, in a word such as *beam*, the speech mechanisms used for producing the /i/ (ea) sound is affected by the mechanisms for producing the /m/ sound, which involves the nasal cavity only. Thus, coarticulation means that sounds are combined. In this example, the /i/ sound and the /m/ sound are coarticulated or combined, resulting in a sound that is quite different when either one is produced in isolation. The principle of coarticulation applies to all words spoken in connected speech, and both consonants and vowels are affected.

GENERAL DESCRIPTIONS OF THE ORAL APPROACHES

This section provides a brief description of the oral approaches, including some of the major components such as speechreading (i.e., lipreading) and auditory training/learning. The framework for discussing the approaches adopted here is as follows: unisensory and multisensory. Cued speech (language) is included in the multisensory category. Although synonyms or examples for these approaches are provided, there is still some disagreement with and confusion caused by this classification framework. Perhaps they are not approaches but rather components of or emphases within the overall oral approach, as seems to be indicated by the synthesis of Connor (1986), presented previously.

Unisensory Approaches

In unisensory approaches, the major emphasis is placed on one primary distance sense, typically audition, with vision (another distance sense) (see Silverman & Kricos, 1990) or taction (nondistance sense) stressed or developed subsequently (see the research of Ling, Leckie, Pollack, Simser, & Smith, 1981). Approaches dealing with the development of residual hearing, or audition, have been known as primarily auditory, aural-oral, aural, auditory-verbal (Beebe, Pearson, & Koch, 1984), acoupedic (Pollack, 1984), acoustic (Erber, 1982), and auditory global (Calvert & Silverman, 1983). There is also an approach called the unisensory approach. In these approaches, children with hearing impairment engage in activities designed to encourage them to use their residual hearing only. Early amplification and proper auditory management (e.g., use of hearing aids and cochlear implants) are also essential features. Although the use of speechreading (or vision) is minimized initially, it will be developed or motivated as a result of the intense earlier focus on audition.

The use of the approaches focusing mainly on audition has been considered the traditional oral approaches, often labeled simply the *auditory-verbal practice* (Goldberg, 1993). There is a strong emphasis on developing skills in deaf and hard-of-hearing children to enable them to enter the mainstream of society. As is typical of these approaches, the focus is on the development of residual hearing to "promote optimal conditions for the acquisition of spoken language" (Ling, 1993, p. 187). Some of the major principles of the auditory-verbal approach are as follows (Goldberg, 1993, citing information from an organization called Auditory-Verbal International):

1. *Supporting and promoting programs for the early detection and iden- tification of hearing impairment and the auditory management of infants, toddlers, and children so identified;*

2. *providing the earliest and most appropriate use of medical and ampli- fication technology to achieve the maximal benefits available;*

3. *instructing primary caregivers in ways to provide maximal acoustic stimulation within meaningful contexts, and supporting the development of the most favorable auditory learning environments for the acquisition of spoken language;*

4. *seeking to integrate listening into the child's total personality in response to the environment;*

5. *supporting the view that communication is a social act, and seek- ing to improve spoken communicative interaction within the typi- cal social dyad of infant/child with hearing impairment and primary caregiver(s), including the use of the parents as primary models for spoken language development and implementing one-to-one teaching;*

6. *seeking to establish the child's integrated auditory system for the self- monitoring of emerging speech;*

7. *using natural sequential patterns of auditory, perceptual, linguis- tic, and cognitive stimulation to encourage the emergence of listening, speech, and language abilities;*

8. *making ongoing evaluation and prognosis of the development of lis- tening skills an integral part of the (re)habilitative process; and*

9. *supporting the concepts of mainstreaming and integration of chil- dren with hearing impairment into regular education classes with appropriate support services and to the fullest extent possible. (p. 182)*

The use of touch primarily, or the tactile-kinesthetic approach, is impor- tant for students who do not benefit much from the traditional oral approaches that focus on audition and/or vision (Calvert, 1986; Calvert & Silverman, 1983). The tactile-kinesthetic approach is based on a motor theory of speech pro- duction. It incorporates oral communication features such as speechreading, auditory training/learning, and intensive speech training. As in all other approaches, reading and writing activities (i.e., literacy skills) are also included.

Multisensory Approaches

Moores (1987) called the multisensory approach a "balanced" approach, and this is still an accurate, apt description. The balance refers to the equal stress on and development of the two primary distance senses, audition and vision. Similar to the unisensory approaches, early amplification and adequate auditory management are important features. For some students with hearing impairment, the combination of audition and speechreading has been shown to be more effective for understanding speech than the use of audition alone (Novelli-Olmstead & Ling, 1984). The multisensory approach may also include the use of a tactile component. This variation has been known as the *auditory-visual-tactile technique* (e.g., Messerly & Aram, 1980; Moores, 1987).

Cued Speech (Cued Language)

Cornett (1967, 1984), the creator of cued speech, classified this approach as a multisensory oral approach. Cornett was concerned with the difficulties of many deaf children in using traditional oral approaches. Despite best efforts in utilizing speechreading and residual hearing, many deaf and some hard-of-hearing students still do not receive a completely adequate spoken message. What seems to be lacking is an approach that permits a rapid, automatic, natural development of the spoken language of most home environments. Cornett's response to this issue is cued speech (also known as cued language) (Fleetwood & Metzger, 1998).

In general, cued speech is a method of communication in which one hand is used to supplement the information on the lips to ensure that the spoken message is clearly understood by the receiver. Cued speech provides an interesting perspective on a critical question that should be asked about any manual system for representing English: "Can a language that has traditionally been spoken and heard remain intact when conveyed with different articulators and in a different medium?" (Fleetwood & Metzger, 1998, p. 10). An affirmative answer to this question requires the acquisition of the phonology of a language because phonology represents the building blocks. In essence, phonology refers to both segmentals (vowels and consonants) and suprasegmentals (e.g., intonation, stress, and rhythm). As discussed in Chapter 6, this is a major problem with the use of the signed systems, especially if students can only access the manual movements of the systems and receive little or no information from the accompanying speech of the speaker/signer.

It is important to emphasize that cued speech entails the use of articulators and a medium that are different (theoretically) from those associated with speech. Fleetwood and Metzger (1998) coined the term *cuem*, which is roughly analogous to but not the same as speech. They stated that:

> *Cuem refers to an articulatory system that employs non-manual signals (NMS) found on the mouth and the hand shapes and hand placements of Cued Speech to produce visibly discrete symbols that represent phonemic (and tonemic) values. Neither the production or the reception of acoustic information nor of speech is entailed in the meaning of the term cuem. (p. 29)*

An understanding of a cuem requires an understanding of what is meant by hand cues (hand shapes and hand placements) and nonmanual signals. In cued speech, eight hand shapes are used in four positions either on or near the face (see Figure 5-1). These hand cues supplement the spoken signal. Each hand shape represents a group of consonants (i.e., consonantal phonemes) such as /h/, /s/, and /r/. Cornett (1967) attempted to address a major speechreading issue; many sounds look similar on the lips, for example, /m/, /p/, and /b/. Thus, each of these phonemes is associated with a different hand shape. That is, /m/ is associated with one hand shape, /p/ with another, and /b/ with a third hand shape. Likewise, different hand shapes are selected for /f/ and /v/ and for /t/ and /d/. To distinguish a consonant among the three in a group, the viewer needs to observe the lips of the speaker in conjunction with the consonant hand cues. Unlike the use of signs in the signed systems, the use of hand cues without the accompanying lip or mouth movements associated with speech is meaningless.

The hand positions near or on the face represents the vowels, that is, the vocalic phonemes. The composite movements of the hand shapes and vowel positions produce consonant-vowel pairs, resulting in words. Within this framework, it is possible to represent the consonantal and vocalic sounds of a word in a number of spoken languages. It is even possible, for example, to represent the different pronunciations of English words due to dialects (e.g., words such as *coffee, route, roof*, etc.). Vowel diphthongs (e.g., *oi* as in *boy*) are executed by a sequence of two different vowel locations. In short, the cued-speech user speaks and represents his or her speech phonemically.

Fleetwood and Metzger (1998) emphasized the importance of the nonmanual signals in the production of a cuem. NMS is rendered by mouth movements that are used to produce consonants and vowels (actually consonant and vowel phonemes). In American English, they have identified seven NMS for the consonants and three NMS for the vowels. For example, NMS A involves bilabial compression associated with the consonant phonemes /p/, /b/, and /m/. In other words, NMS A refers to the mouth movements that accompany the production of these sounds. NMS B involves upper teeth and lower lip for the consonant phonemes /v/ and /f/. Examples of NMS are provided in Figure 5-2.

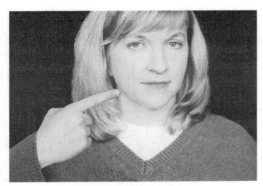

A

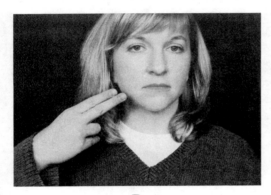

B

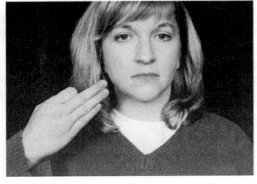

C

Note: Handshapes and Locations
Handshapes: Consonants
A: d, p, zh
B: k, v, tH, z
C: h, s, r

Figure 5-1 Hand Shapes and Positions of Cued
Speech/Language. *(continues)*

Note: Handshapes and Locations
Handshapes: Consonants
D: b, n, wh
E: t, m, f
F: l, sh, w

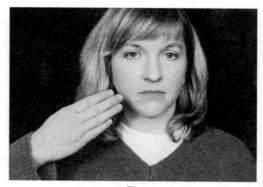

D

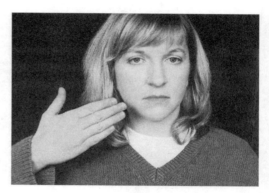

E

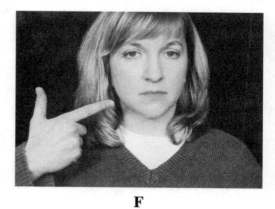

F

Figure 5-1 *(continues)*

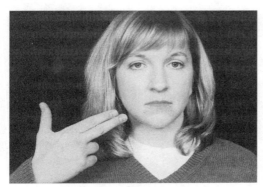

G

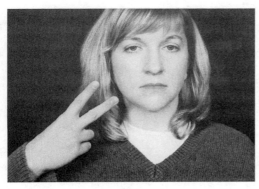

H

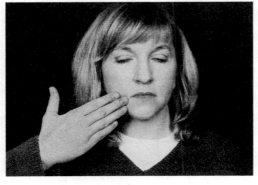

1

Note: Handshapes and Locations
Handshapes: Consonants
G: g, j, th
H: ng, y, ch
Locations for 'vowels'
   (point of contact)
1: corner of mouth

Figure 5-1 *(continues)*

Note: Handshapes and Locations
Locations for 'vowels'
(point of contact)
2: tip of chin
3: center of neck
4: non-contact movement:
begins 4 inches to side
of chin

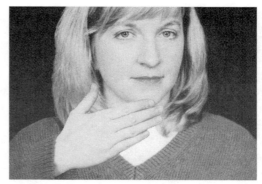

2

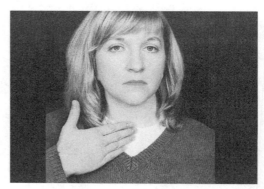

3

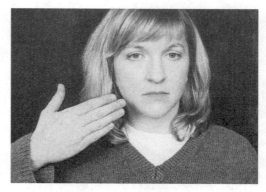

4

Figure 5-1
Source: Fleetwood & Metzger (1998).
See this source for further details.

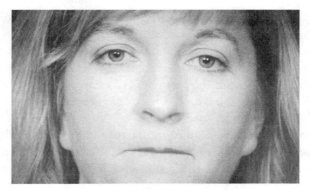

NMS A

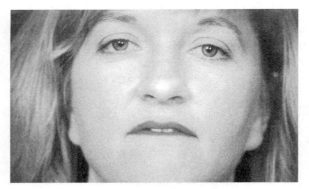

NMS B

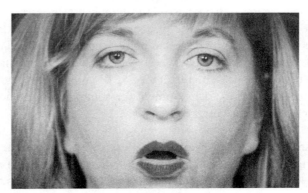

NMS C

Figure 5-2 Examples of Nonmanual Signals of Cued Speech/Language.
Source: Fleetwood & Metzger (1998).

When a specific hand shape is paired with a NMS, the NMS serves to assist the viewer in distinguishing among the group of phonemes associated with the same hand shape. For example, the hand shape 5 represents /m/, /f/, and /t/. However, there is a distinct NMS associated with each of these phonemes, and the particular NMS assists the viewer with the recognition process. Likewise, a particular hand shape or hand placement may serve to assist viewers in distinguishing phonemes (e.g., /m/, /p/, and /b/) that share the same NMS.

Although cueing entails a set of articulators and a medium different from those of speech, Fleetwood and Metzger (1998) argued that there is no real need for an acoustic signal or to represent phonemes via speech articulators only (also see Dodd & Campbell, 1987; Dodd & Hermelin, 1977). Furthermore, they maintained that "the act of cueing includes not only the rendering of phonemic information via cuem, but also the rendering of visibly distinct features (e.g., head thrust) which convey prosodic . . . and grammatical attributes" (p. 30). The assumption is that the cued articulators can represent the same range of abstract phonemic values as do the speech articulators, including the suprasegmental aspects such as intonation, stress, and rhythm.

If phonology is the building block of any language, then a litmus test for all invented communication systems for deaf and hard-of-hearing students is the extent to which they can convey the range of abstract phonemic values of that language. If this conveyance is adequate, then recipients should be able to develop phonological and phonemic awareness, which seem to be important for the development of English literacy skills. Theoretically, cued speech/language seems to have passed this litmus test. From a research standpoint, it needs to be shown that the phonemic awareness of children exposed to cued speech/language can be used to predict their subsequent literacy development, as is the case for children who have developed phonemic awareness through the use of speech articulators. As is discussed later, there seems to be some success in literacy development for some children who have been exposed to cued speech/language.

Despite the criticisms and shortcomings of the system and the need for further research, Cornett (1967) and his colleagues recognized the importance of developing a fluent and intelligible communication system between parents and their children. In essence, any contrived system needs to be accessible and capable of being learned by the average parent/caretaker. This system also needs to be clear and represent all of spoken language. Information that is added to the lips should be in sync with the rhythm and pace of speech. Finally, any typical young child must be able to learn this system without formal training and as part of the typical communicative environment of the home.

Table 5-3 provides a summary of the major aspects of the two groups of oral approaches—unisensory and multisensory.

TABLE 5-3 Highlights of the Oral Approach

- The major components of oral approaches are speech, speechreading, and auditory training/learning.

- It is possible to delineate two major groups of approaches: *unisensory* and *multisensory.*

- In unisensory approaches, the major emphasis is placed on developing one primary sense—typically, audition. Early identification and early amplification are essential endeavors. Vision and taction are often developed subsequently.

- There are a number of terms used to describe unisensory approaches, which focus primarily on audition, for example, primarily auditory, aural-oral, aural, auditory-verbal, acoupedic, acoustic, and auditory global. There is also an approach called unisensory.

- The approaches in the unisensory group should be considered traditional oral approaches, and the most recent general label used is auditory-verbal.

- In general, the use of touch primarily, or the tactile-kinesthetic approach, is reserved for students who do not benefit much from the traditional oral approaches.

- The multisensory approaches involve the use of both audition and vision in a roughly equal manner. It is considered to be a balanced approach. Early intervention and early amplification are considered important features—similar to the unisensory approaches.

- The multisensory approach may include a tactile component; this is labeled as the auditory-visual-tactile technique.

- In this text, cued speech/language is classified as a multisensory approach. It was meant for students who experience difficulty with the traditional oral approaches.

- In cued speech/language, eight different hand shapes are used to represent eight groups of consonants, and the hand positions near or on the face

(continues)

(*Table 5-3 continued*)

represent vowels. There are also identified nonmanual signals (NMS), which are mouth movements associated with the production of the sounds.

- Theoretically, it has been argued that cued speech/language is sufficient for representing the range of abstract phonemic values of a language. In other words, cued speech/language is sufficient for representing phonology, which is considered the building block of any language.

- If cued speech/language is adequate for reflecting phonology, then young users should develop phonological and, consequently, phonemic awareness, which seem to be critical for developing script literacy skills in that language.

THE AURAL REHABILITATION COMPONENTS: SPEECHREADING AND AUDITORY TRAINING/LEARNING

To develop spoken language, children need to be able to perceive and produce it (see Ling, 1989). Within the area of perception, it is possible to discuss the use of vision via speechreading and audition via auditory training/learning. Of course, perception is also enhanced by the use of assistive devices to aid vision and hearing such as tactile aids, hearing aids, cochlear implants, and even by the use of an approach called cued speech (cued language), discussed previously. At the very least, speech perception seems to involve the skills of detection (presence/absence), discrimination (same or different), identification (recognition), and comprehension (understanding). Much of the following information concerns speechreading due to the author's major interest in this area (the topic of his master's thesis); however, some pertinent information on auditory training/learning is also provided.

Speechreading

Speechreading (also known as lipreading) refers to the process of understanding a spoken message through observation of the speaker's face (Berger, 1972; De Filippo & Sims, 1988; Dodd & Campbell, 1987; Jeffers & Barley, 1971; O'Neill & Oyer, 1981; Silverman & Kricos, 1990). There has been much discussion on the description of speechreading. The debate focuses on whether speechreading should be considered as involving vision only (i.e., without speech or auditory cues) or as supporting the use of residual hearing via visual cues such as lip movements and facial expressions. This debate has a long illustrious history, and speechreading has been considered to be and used as a unisensory method, most likely because of the limitations of advances in amplification in the early part of the 20th century (see discussion in Silverman & Kricos, 1990). Due to the strong relations (actually correlations) between degree of hearing impairment and speech development, it is deemed necessary to study the effects of speechreading with and without the use of audition via amplification (see discussions in Conrad, 1979; Paul, 1988).

A number of frameworks have been proposed for studying speechreading ability, which is still considered somewhat of a subtle art (Silverman & Kricos, 1990). Perhaps the most feasible one is that of O'Neill and Oyer (1981), who delineated four broad areas: *speaker-sender, environment, lipreader-receiver*, and *code-stimulus*. The speaker-sender variable refers to factors associated with speakers, for example, articulation and rate of speech, speech features such as coarticulation and nasality, and dialects and other voice characteristics such as accents and styles. Not to be overlooked are the suprasegmental aspects such as intonation and rhythm (e.g., pauses and stresses). Finally, another interesting domain is the characteristics of the speaker's face such as size and movement of the lips and the effects of various aspects and visibility of the face (e.g., eyes, lips, areas around the eyes and lips, etc.).

Traditionally, the environment category has entailed a study of the effects of various types of lighting, visual and auditory distractions, and the distance between the speaker and the speechreader. Auditory distractions refer to the noise level of the room in which the speechreader is located. This is an important factor for speechreaders who are also dependent on the use of residual hearing. A room full of reverberation (e.g., echoes and other extraneous noises due to lack of carpeting) can cause considerable difficulty for the speechreader. One of the most important environmental issues is the angle of vision, which involves both horizontal and vertical perspectives. For example, if the speechreader is seated and the speaker is standing directly in front of the speechreader, the angle can be described as 35 degrees vertical, 0 degrees horizontal. If both the speechreader and speaker are seated and facing each other, this can be described as 0 degrees vertical and horizontal. With respect to classroom teaching situations, angle of vision can become a critical issue for deaf and hard-of-hearing children.

The most complex category is the lipreader-receiver one. In fact, it could be argued that this is the source of the major difficulty in understanding the development of speechreading and tends to give the impression that speechreading is still pretty much of a subtle art (Silverman & Kricos, 1990). Some speechreader-receiver factors include personality characteristics, prior or world knowledge, motivation or interest, linguistic competence, memory, and visual perceptual abilities. That there are interactions among these speechreader-receiver factors is an understatement. Consider the ensuing passage by Silverman and Kricos (1990), who are commenting on psychological effects associated with speechreading:

> *Pertinent are orientation to the specific situation in which oral exchange is taking place; concentration which may be vulnerable to fatigue after long periods of looking; alertness to changes in subject of conversation; interest in subject of conversation; background of the speechreader's information, the wider the better; emotional set and sociability that freely encourage association with others and provide opportunity for practice in speechreading, obsessive fear of making mistakes, or conversely, to be undaunted by them; motivation and perseverance; approval or avoidance; and the speechreader's language competency, whether hearing-impaired child or adult. (p. 24)*

Code-stimulus refers to the spoken message itself, including visibility of sounds, rate of transmission, vocabulary levels, and length and types of sentences. All of these variables have been problematic with respect to the development of speechreading measures. That is, there has been much debate on what types of words and longer discourses (e.g., sentences) should be included. If speechreading is viewed negatively by those who doubt its utility and feasibility, most likely this is due to the visibility of sounds. In other words, the ability to speechread is impacted by the similar looking characteristics of sounds—sounds that look similar on the lips of the speaker-sender. Consider, for examples, the sounds (or more precisely, the articulatory movements of) /b/, /p/, and /m/. It is extremely difficult—and probably impossible most of the time—to discriminate the following words in isolation and sometimes in running speech, depending on the syntax used: *ball, mall*; *bail, pail*; *mane* (or *main*), *pane* (or *pain*); *bat, pat, mat*; *bill, pill, mill*; and so on. There are numerous other clusters such as /f/ and /v/, /t/ and /d/, and so on that are associated with the anatomy and physiology of speech mechanisms. This was a major guiding principle for the development of cued speech/language with the association of consonants with selective hand shapes.

Most of the research on speechreading has been conducted with respect to the framework of O'Neill and Oyer (1981), discussed earlier. Investigators have looked at the effects of training on improving speechreading skills (Black, O'Reilly, & Peck, 1963; Crawford, Dancer, & Pittenger, 1986; Squires & Dancer, 1986), the effects of speechreading and vibrotactile aid training, and the effects of variables such as age, gender, and education (Dancer, Krain, Thompson, Davis, & Glenn, 1994). Effects from other aids and approaches such as cochlear implants and cued speech/language have also been documented.

There are several general remarks that can be made here with respect to the overall findings (for additional perspectives, see Conrad, 1979; De Filippo & Sims, 1988; Dodd & Campbell, 1987; Paul, 1988; Silverman & Kricos, 1990). A number of investigations attempted to describe the relations (statistically, this mean correlations) between (and among) speechreading and variables such as academic achievement, age at onset of hearing impairment, degree of hearing impairment, intelligence, linguistic skills, perceptual skills, and personality traits (for a detailed summary of early studies, see Farwell, 1976; also see De Filippo & Sims, 1988; Paul, 1988). Although it is possible to state some general effects of these studies, it is not possible to state definite clear patterns that could inform classroom practice for improving these skills in children who are deaf and hard of hearing. This does not denigrate the availability of instructional strategies for improving speech production and perception in children, especially in conjunction with sensory aids such as cochlear implants and the tactaid devices (see the extensive discussion in Geers & Moog, 1994; McGarr, 1989). However, it is still true that convincing measures of speechreading skill and aptitude still elude researchers. Probably, given the reasonable face validity of the multiplicity of factors that may influence speechreading performance, more intensive and comprehensive multivariate analyses are necessary.

It is not clear that what is learned during speechreading should guide what needs to be taught. This is not unlike the current debate on the teaching of reading (and writing). Proceeding with exercises on distinctions between sounds to more complex language may work for some individuals but not for all. In fact, this approach seems to be analogous to bottom-up approaches to reading (see Chapter 8 of this text; also see Paul, 1988, 1998a). What might be needed are approaches that are multidisciplinary and multifocused, taking into account the interactive effects of the numerous variables within the O'Neill and Oyer framework that have been studied in speechreading studies.

What is clearly needed is more research on young children who are deaf and hard of hearing. Much of the focus still seems to be on adults, both with typical hearing and hearing impairment (Dancer et al., 1994; Samar & Sims, 1983; Shepherd, 1982; Spradlin, Dancer, & Monfils, 1989). Via these studies, researchers seem to be obtaining a better understanding of variables such as age, educational level, gender, and—the long-standing one—practice. For example, Dancer et al. (1994) reported the following summary of results from their study:

1. *There were not statistically-significant effects of education on the speechreading scores of this sample of 50 persons, which consisted*

of higher than average socioeconomic individuals ranging in age from 20–69 and having no hearing or vision complaints.

2. *There was a statistically-significant effect of gender on speechreading scores: females scored higher than males.*

3. *There was a statistically-significant interaction between gender and practice on speechreading performance: females increased their performance from a first to a second trial; males did not.*

4. *There was a statistically-significant effect of age group on speechreading scores in females: 30- and 40-year old females scored higher than the other age groups. (p. 35)*

Despite the importance of studying adults, it is now known that the results on adults cannot be generalized indiscriminately to younger populations such as adolescents and children. Of course, some of the variables discussed and even some of the assessment materials used in the adult studies are also inappropriate for children. Nevertheless, scientists are still a long way from employing multivariate analyses on a multiplicity of factors within a multidisciplinary framework to understand and develop speechreading performance in young children and adolescents who are deaf and hard of hearing.

There is no question that the difficulty in understanding the speechreading performance in young children and adolescents is due in part to the difficulty in measuring this skill. In fact, the difficulties can be categorized within the O'Neill and Oyer framework, for example, speaker-sender (e.g., gender and speech rate), environment (e.g., live or filmed and lighting), listener-receiver (e.g., type of response required on assessment, i.e., effects of multiple-choice tests), and code-stimulus (e.g., use of nonsense syllables, words, sentences, and connected discourse) (see Berger, 1972; Jeffers & Barley, 1971; O'Neill & Oyer, 1981). Most speechreading tests are designed for the observer to render general qualitative remarks about the listener-receiver (e.g., *good, average, fair,* and *poor*) rather than to prescribe or diagnose specific instructional lessons. However, there are some that focus on specific areas such as consonants (Binnie, Jackson, & Montgomery, 1976).

In another technique (called tracking), the speechreader is required to shadow (i.e., repeat) word for word what is being presented by the speaker-sender (De Filippo & Scott, 1978). When errors occur, the speaker-sender and the listener-receiver engage in strategies to correct the situation. This technique seems to reflect what actually occurs during a speechreading situation; however, there is difficulty in addressing the issue of topic shifts or the difficulty of materials—both of which are impacted by listener-receiver variables such as prior knowledge and inferencing (see discussion in Paul, 1988).

It is not likely that there will ever be one complete test of speechreading or, at least, a test that can be administered in one sitting. With respect to this issue, Silverman and Kricos (1990) offered an eloquent summary:

> *Since existing speechreading tests fail to provide completely reliable and valid information, it has been suggested that a battery might consist of a number of tests including a measure of consonant recognition, word discrimination, identification of everyday sentences, and comprehension of connected speech. One notes with irony, however, that this battery approach differs little from Conklin's 1917 proposal for speechreading measurement. (p. 31)*

Table 5-4 provides a summary of major points discussed in this section on speechreading.

TABLE 5-4 Summary of Major Points About Speechreading

- Speechreading, also known as lipreading, refers to the process of understanding a spoken message through observation of the speaker's face.

- There seems to be a consensus that it is important to study the effects of speechreading with and without the use of audition (i.e., with and without the use of amplification).

- One of most productive frameworks for researching the effects of speechreading involves a study of factors in four broad areas: speaker-sender, environment, lipreader-receiver, and code-stimulus. There are a number of aspects within each broad area that can be examined in isolation or in combination with others. The most complex area seems to be the lipreader-receiver due to the numerous interactions of the aspects.

- There have been a number of research studies on the effects of speechreading within and across the four broad areas. It is possible to state general findings, for example, between (and among) speechreading and variables such as academic achievement, age at onset of hearing impairment, degree of hearing impairment, intelligence, linguistic skills, perceptual skills, and personality traits. However, these general findings do not offer useful or clear implications for classroom practice for improving the speechreading skills of deaf and hard-of-hearing children and adolescents. Thus, it is true that convincing measures of speechreading skill and aptitude are still elusive.

(continues)

(Table 5-4 continued)

- Not only is there a need for multidisciplinary and multifocused approaches and sophisticated analysis procedures, there is a great need for more research on young children who are deaf and hard of hearing. Much of the focus still seems to be on adults, both with typical hearing and hearing impairment.

- One of the biggest reasons for the dearth of research on young children is the difficulty in developing a reliable and appropriate measurement or test. Most likely, a battery of tests should be utilized; however, the contents and methods of these tests need to be different from what are used with adults.

Auditory Training/Learning

In addition to speechreading, another major component of aural rehabilitation is auditory training, also known as auditory learning (see discussion in Cole & Gregory, 1986; Osberger, 1990). Only a few brief remarks are presented here on this concept. In general, auditory training/learning refers to the use of techniques to assist children in their development of audition or use of residual hearing. In other words, the major goal is to enable children with hearing impairment to develop and use sound perception abilities. There are a number of teaching manuals available (see discussions in Erber, 1982; Sanders, 1982) that can be used with children, adolescents, and adults. Some programs, for example, use an analytic distinctive feature approach (i.e., for voicing, nasality, and sibilancy) (Hutchinson, 1990) that might be best suited for adolescents and adults.

Most of these early auditory training manuals for children emphasize or promote activities or conditions such as

> *wearing a hearing aid; participating in auditory exercises; having attention drawn to meaningful sounds; using sound for warning and arousal; modifying your own behavior so that the student must understand all or part of what you say through hearing alone; advising parents of the use of hearing and hearing aids. (Clarke School for the Deaf, 1971, p. vii)*

The beginning activities require children to discriminate nonverbal sounds such as bells and drums. After much practice in this area, the next step was for children to discriminate among speech sounds, words, and sentences.

With the development of powerful amplification systems, which has led to, for example, the increase of children with cochlear implants in school settings (Nevins & Chute, 1996) and the use of several aids in combination (e.g., tactile aids and hearing aids), much of the current emphasis is on developing listening skills. In other words, this current trend is to teach the child to learn to listen and learn by listening rather than to learn to hear (see discussions in Ling, 1986; Osberger, 1990). This current trend has been labeled *auditory learning*, in which activities for developing spoken language are related to the child's real-life experiences. Auditory learning stresses the comprehension of meaningful sounds, which is considered to be the highest level of auditory skills (Erber, 1982; Sanders, 1982). The other three levels—detection, discrimination, and identification—are important but are not sufficient for the development of listening skills. The concept of auditory learning has been influenced pervasively by research on pragmatics and the accompanying approaches for developing language functions in children with hearing impairment.

In several of the widely used auditory training/learning programs, there are both training and assessment components (see Erber, 1982; Thies & Trammel, 1983; Van Ert Windle & Stout, 1984). There is often a curriculum to be used in the development of auditory skills. For example, in a program called *Developmental Approach to Successful Listening* (DASL) (Van Ert Windle & Stout, 1984), three types of hierarchical auditory skills are emphasized: sound awareness, phonetic listening, and auditory comprehension. In general, this hierarchy is based on what can be expected in the development of audition in young children. As expected, during the sound awareness stage (also analogous to a general phonological awareness stage), the child becomes aware or is tuned in to amplified sounds. There is also a section on the use and care of personal amplification devices. The activities for developing phonetic listening are based on the speech training program developed by Ling (1976). Ling (1976; also see 1989) emphasized the need for children to perceive both nonsegmental and segmental features of speech. Finally, to develop auditory comprehension skills, children engage in activities that entail the discrimination and identification of common phrases. There is a progression from simple phrases to the comprehension of connected discourse.

With auditory learning, there is obviously a strong focus on the development of residual hearing—a critical component of auditory-verbal approaches. Some auditory-verbal programs emphasize lessons that develop children's auditory skills for discriminating phonemes in syllables and words in phrases. There are also activities for the development of auditory memory skills. For example, with infants and toddlers, Simser (1993) suggested the following activities (only a sample of items of increasing difficulty are presented here):

- *begin with repeated sound-word associations, e.g., tic-toc, tic-toc vs. moo-oo-oo, moo-oo-oo.*
- *identify known single items at the end of a sentence, e.g., "Give me the car," and then in the middle of a sentence "Put the car in the water."*
- *identify objects by listening to descriptive phrases, e.g., "It flies up in the sky, it has wings and you ride in it"—in closed and then open set.*
- *follow conversation of known topic.*
- *listen to a story and answer pertinent questions.*
- *follow conversation of undisclosed but familiar topic. (pp. 228–229)*

In essence, there are many common features across the various auditory learning approaches, especially those that stress auditory-verbal activities. Samples of activities for specific goals can be found in a number of sources (Erber, 1982; Sanders, 1982; also see the discussions of activities and strategies in Moog, Biedenstein, Davidson, & Brenner, 1994; Robbins, 1994; Simser, 1993).

Although the current auditory learning approach seems to be new, it should be highlighted that this approach, which is similar to the use of natural methods for teaching speech and language, has been in use for many years (McAnally et al., 1994; Moores, 1987, 1996). A brief discussion of current methods to develop and evaluate auditory and speech perception skills in children and adolescent can be found in Osberger (1990). The use of a computerized program to measure the effectiveness of auditory training stimuli has also been discussed (Tye-Murray, Tyler, Lansing, & Bertschy, 1990). Table 5-5 provides a brief summary of the major points in this section on auditory training/learning.

TABLE 5-5 A Few Summary Points on Auditory Training/Learning

- In general, auditory training/learning refers to the use of techniques to assist children in the development of audition or the use of residual hearing. This refers to the development of sound perception abilities.

- Traditional programs began with activities requiring children to discriminate nonverbal sounds such as bells and drums. After practice in this area, children were required to discriminate among speech sounds, words, and sentences.

- With the development and advancement in amplification (e.g., powerful hearing aids and cochlear implants), the current trend of programs is on teaching children to listen. That is, children learn to listen and learn by listening rather than to learn to hear. This approach has received the label of *auditory learning.*

- In auditory learning, the spoken language activities are related to the child's real-life experiences. The emphasis is on comprehension—which is considered to be the highest level of auditory skills. The other three levels—detection, discrimination, and identification—often associated with traditional approaches are important but not sufficient for developing listening skills.

- Many of the available programs have training and assessment components that are based on a curriculum. In general, auditory learning programs are an integral part of the auditory-verbal oral approach with its emphasis on the development of residual hearing.

GENERAL DISCUSSION AND RESEARCH SYNTHESIS OF SPEECH PERCEPTION, SPEECH PRODUCTION, AND SPEECH INTELLIGIBILITY

Because of what is often perceived as limited intervention success and the relative lack of strong experimental intervention studies, it is suspected that speech perception, production, and intelligibility are not popular or, in some cases, not politically correct topics in the field of deaf education. There is no question that it is difficult to develop or to assist the development of speech skills in many children with hearing impairment, particularly those with severe to profound hearing impairment. Nevertheless, there has been some success, although it varies across students and does not always reveal a strong pattern or generalization. Nevertheless, in the future, this success range might involve a greater number of children who are using digital hearing aids, advanced tactile aids, and of course, cochlear implants (see discussions in Geers & Moog, 1994; McGarr, 1989; Nevins & Chute, 1996; Stoker & Ling, 1992). In essence, there is a great deal of knowledge about the perception, production, and intelligibility of children with severe to profound impairment; however, the intervention knowledge is not commensurate with basic process knowledge.

There seems to be little doubt that there is an interrelationship among perception, production, and intelligibility, even if this interrelationship is not completely understood. Of course, there is more to learn about these three domains as well. To provide a basic description of these domains as well as a brief synthesis of research, the following discussion borrows heavily from a selected number of publications and reviews (Boothroyd, 1984; Calvert & Silverman, 1983; Carney, 1994; Dunn & Newton, 1994; Erber, 1982; Levitt, 1989).

Dunn and Newton (1994) presented a nice accessible discussion of the relationship between perception and production within their model for speech development. The development of speech is dependent on the perception of it. *Perception* refers to skills such as detection, discrimination, identification, and comprehension. The reader needs to keep in mind the manner in which perception is discussed here as opposed to the way it has been described in the literature on auditory training/learning (see previous discussion) to avoid confusion regarding the same use of this term. The development of articulatory-auditory representations in a cognitive manner (i.e., stored in the mind) is presumed to be the result of repeated exposures to the sounds of the language. For children with hearing impairment, there is a reliance on kinesthetic (i.e., proprioceptive), tactile, and visual information. If the development of articulatory-auditory impressions in the mind is lacking, Dunn and Newton (1994) argued that the "production of meaningful speech is probably impaired" (p. 125). And, this might also contribute pervasively to the difficulty many deaf and hard-of-hearing children have with the development of phonological and phonemic awareness of the English language.

The most common rendition of speech production has been that discussed by Ling (1976) in his speech development program; this was elaborated on by Dunn and Newton (1994) in their speech development model. In general, scholars have focused on two types of skills: *phonetic* and *phonological*. Phonetic skills refer to the production of distinct speech sounds (i.e., consonant and vowel phonemes), whereas phonological skills entail an understanding of the systematic patterns and meanings associated with the sounds in words. At both skill levels (phonetic and phonological), children need to deal with segmentals (consonants and vowels) and suprasegmentals (e.g., intonation, rhythm, and stress).

As stated by Dunn and Newton (1994) and others (Ling, 1976; also see the various articles in Stoker & Ling, 1992):

> Phonetic *skill is the motoric ability to produce speech sounds in a variety of phonetic contexts, independent of any meaning that these sounds may convey. Children must learn to coordinate the movements of the lungs, larynx, and articulators before they can produce intelligible speech. The second skill is* phonological, *which reflects the knowledge that sounds distinguish meaning and occur in systematic patterns in words. . . . For the hearing-impaired child, each of these skills must be practiced systematically. (p. 125)*

Speech intelligibility refers to what is understood by the listener. It is not uncommon to associate speech intelligibility predominantly with the speaker; that is, attention is typically stressed on the orality or speech output of the speaker, especially the type and number of errors. However, some scholars have preferred a more balanced approach, namely, one that considers both the speech production performance of the speaker and the listening/comprehension performance of the listener (see discussion in Carney, 1994). From one perspective, this balanced view is often a part of many studies in pragmatics, particularly those that have focused on the clarification request paradigm in young children (Ninio & Snow, 1996). In this paradigm, it is not the case that the speaker has produced speech errors (although that is certainly possible). Rather, it is the responsibility of the listener to ask for clarification if he or she has not understood the intent of the speaker's message. The listener might need to employ a number of strategies to understand the speaker's message. Of course, it is also the responsibility of the speaker to make himself or herself understood, and this might require the use of paraphrasing or rewording techniques.

If access to the auditory signal is limited or dysfunctional, then it is easy to conclude that many children with severe to profound hearing impairment will have difficulty or have had difficulty with the development of speech perception and speech discrimination abilities (French-St. George, 1986). This is another way of saying that speech perception, discrimination, and so on are pervasively affected by the degree of hearing impairment. Because speech is a continuous auditory signal, a number of children with severe to profound hearing impairment might experience difficulty in recognizing differences (sometimes minimal) in patterns of speech with respect to features such as time (e.g., pauses or gaps), intensity, and pitch. This results in difficulties in discriminating between sounds, syllables, words, and phrases at various levels. There are many manifestations of these skills. For example, children need to be able to separate a speech signal from background noise, to distinguish between voice and voiceless sounds, and so on. Students with mild hearing losses experience difficulty in hearing consonantal sibliants such as /f/ and /s/ and stop-plosives such as /p/ without amplification. Students in the severe impairment range experience difficulty with differentiating voiced consonants from voiceless ones. Many students with profound hearing losses might be able to perceive a few low-frequency vowels and nasals, even with the use of adequate, powerful amplification systems (see reviews in Carney, 1994; Dunn & Newton, 1994; French-St.-George, 1986).

There are a number of factors that affect speech intelligibility. Some are associated with the listener (e.g., experience), test materials, and of course, degree of hearing impairment (a good review of these areas can be found in Carney, 1994). Nevertheless, because of the effects of hearing impairment, the focus here is on speech production issues with both segmentals and suprasegmentals. As noted by Dunn and Newton (1994) and others, it is difficult to discuss these areas separately due to the reciprocal effects:

> The same mechanisms (i.e., lungs, larynx, articulators) are used to produce suprasegmental patterns, vowels, and consonants; therefore, a deficiency in one mechanism will often influence more than one aspect of speech. For example, poor laryngeal control can influence both voice quality and the voiced/voiceless distinctions between consonants. Just as it is artificial to describe these characteristics separately, it is also difficult to assess and treat them separately. While for the sake of clarity, they may be discussed separately, these complex relationships among suprasegmental patterns, vowels, and consonants must be kept in mind. (p. 123)

Despite the wide range of variability across students, even within the categories associated with degree of impairment (e.g., moderate, severe, and profound), it is possible to describe a few patterns of speech production errors. The patterns within suprasegmental and segmental categories should be viewed as part of a phonological system rather than unrelated errors (Dunn & Newton, 1994; Levitt, 1989). That is, many of the errors are similar to those made by younger children with typical hearing (also see the discussion of syntax in the research by Quigley and others in Chapter 8). In essence, the errors are reflective of quantitative difference (i.e., frequency) rather than qualitative differences (i.e., type). Differences between the two groups (hearing and hearing impaired) are most noticeable with the production of vowels and the development of suprasegmental features. In addition, Levitt (1989) remarked that for children with very poor speech intelligibility (i.e., close to zero), there is a large number of errors that appear to be idiosyncratic—that is, difficult to define in conventional speech terms.

Suprasegmental Aspects

Suprasegmental features refer to speech characteristics that accompany the production of vowels and consonants. A number of researchers have documented problems with several features, for example, respiration, rate, rhythm, stress patterns, and duration (see reviews and discussions in Dunn & Newton, 1994; Erber, 1982; Levitt, 1989; Ling, 1976). The speech rate of children with hearing impairment is often slower due to the excessive prolongation of vowels and consonants as well as prolonged and improperly inserted pauses in running speech. Children have difficulty producing syllables due to factors such as inappropriate rates of utterances and inability to differentiate stressed from unstressed sounds. Variables that affect the pitch and quality of children's speech include excessive breathiness, inappropriate quantity of nasality, and inappropriate variations and pauses in pitch. It is not uncommon for the voice quality of many students with severe to profound hearing impairment to be described as breathy or tense (Dunn & Newton, 1994; Erber, 1982; Levitt, 1989; Ling, 1976).

As noted by many scholars, these suprasegmental errors have an adverse effect on speech intelligibility. There seems to be a general consensus that many students with severe to profound hearing impairment have poor or inadequate control of their speech mechanisms, particularly the speech articulators and the breath-voice system. It seems that speech development programs or techniques need to assist these children to breathe and articulate at proper rates. However, it is possible that these problems will persist unless these children can take advantage of their residual hearing via the use of amplification, vibrotaction, or combinations of sensory devices.

Segmental Errors

As mentioned previously, the most noticeable segmental errors of children with severe to profound hearing impairment concern the production of vowels. In the production of vowels, these children do not utilize a sufficient amount of intensity, and this is often accompanied by excessive aspiration and nasality. Categories of common vowel errors include substitutions, dipthongization, and nasalization (see discussions and reviews in Dunn & Newton, 1994; Erber, 1982; Levitt, 1989; Ling, 1976). For example, children tend to substitute lax vowels for tense vowels such as the /I/ for /i/, producing a word such as *hit* for *heat*. Substitutions have also been noted for central vowels (e.g., *bet* to *but*).

Due to the nature of vowel production, it seems that children's difficulties are related to their poor coordination of the movement of the tongue. This limited or restricted range of tongue movement also affects the production of adjacent consonants. In fact, vowel errors almost always result in consonant errors.

With respect to consonants, two of the most discussed types of errors are omissions and substitutions. Students are likely to omit consonants that are produced near the center or back of the mouth (e.g., /t/, /l/, /k/, and /g/) rather than those produced near the front of the mouth (e.g., /p/, /b/, /f/, /v/, and /m/). From another perspective, consonants produced near the front of the mouth are easier to speechread than those in the center or back. Consonants that appear in the middle or final positions of words are more likely to be omitted than consonants in the beginning positions of words. There are omission errors involving unstressed syllables or verb endings (e.g., -s, and -ing). Again, many of these errors such as those involving unstressed affixes, plurals, and prepositions are made because the sounds are difficult to hear or speechread. Some of the errors, of course, might be due to an inadequate command of English language principles.

In the substitution category, consonants might be substituted for vowels. Consonant substitutions are often noticed for consonants that involved the same place of articulation. Thus, students might experience difficulty in distinguishing between nasals (/m/, /n/, and /ng/) and their counterparts, voiced stops (e.g., /b/, /d/, and /g/). Substitutions of voiced stops for nasal occur sometimes. Students might also substitute a voiced consonant (e.g., /b/) for a voiceless one (e.g., /p/). Stop consonants are often substituted for fricatives; however, fricatives for stop consonants are not as common. Affricates are typically substituted for other affricatives. Finally, there are a number of consonant errors that are due to difficulties in the manner of production; these involve consonants that have a high frequency range such as sibilants as well as blends (e.g., bl, sl, and cl) and clusters (e.g., str and scr).

Similar to the discussion of suprasegmental errors, the reasons for segmental errors have been considered to be due to poor control of the speech mechanisms. Levitt (1989), however, proffered another interesting perspective:

> By far the most common source of error, however, is that of lack of effort. The most obvious manifestation of this problem is the omission of consonants, particularly at the end of a word or phrase. Other related errors involve partial omissions in the production of diphthongs, affricates, and blends. The neutralization of vowels is also a manifestation of lack of effort and should not be regarded simply as improper placement of the articulators. (p. 30)

Table 5-6 presents a summary of major points discussed in this section on perception, production, and intelligibility.

TABLE 5-6 Major Points on Speech Perception, Production, and Intelligibility

---

- It has been and still is difficult to develop speech skills in children with severe to profound hearing impairment. Success varies across students and does not reveal a strong consistent pattern or generalization. There might be greater success in the future with the continued advances in amplification systems and cochlear implants.

- Based on repeated exposures to the sounds of a language, children develop and store articulatory-auditory representations in their minds. Some scholars argue that if these representations are lacking, it is extremely difficult—perhaps impossible—to develop meaningful speech. These representations are also necessary for developing phonological and phonemic awareness.

- In most speech programs for deaf and hard-of-hearing students, the focus is on developing two types of skills: phonetic and phonological. Phonetic skills refer to the production of distinct speech sounds such as consonants and vowels. Phonological skills require an understanding of the systematic patterns and meanings associated with the sounds in words.

- Traditionally, speech intelligibility has referred to what is understood by the listener; thus, the focus has been on the speech productions of the speaker whenever there are problems with intelligibility. Due to the influences of pragmatics, the focus has shifted to speaker-listener interactions. Although the speaker may make errors, the listener has a role to play as well in asking for clarification if the message has not been understood.

- Despite the wide range of variability across students, even within the categories associated with degree of impairment, it is possible to describe a few patterns of speech production errors with respect to suprasegmentals and segmentals. It should be kept in mind that many errors are similar to those made by younger hearing children. However, for children with very poor speech intelligibility (i.e., close to zero), there is a large number of errors that appear to be idiosyncratic—that is, difficult to define in conventional speech terms.

- Suprasegmentals features refer to speech characteristics that accompany the production of vowels and consonants. Researchers have documented problems with features such as respiration, rate, rhythm, stress patterns, and duration. In essence, many students with severe to profound hearing impairment have poor or inadequate control of their speech mechanisms, particularly the speech articulators and the breath-voice system.

- The most noticeable segmental errors of children with severe to profound hearing impairment concern the production of vowels. It seems that children's difficulties are related to their poor coordination of the movement of the tongue. This limited or restricted range of tongue movements also affects the production of adjacent consonants. In fact, vowel errors almost always results in consonant errors.

(continues)

(*Table 5-6 continued*)

- Similar to the research on suprasegmental errors, the reasons for segmental errors have been considered to be due to poor control of the speech mechanisms. At least one prominent researcher argued that a major reason for the errors is lack of effort.

RESEARCH ON ORALISM AND STUDENTS

There is no best method for synthesizing the research on the effects of the components of oralism on the development of speech, language, and literacy in English. The approach adopted here is to discuss some general findings on two broad groups of students—namely, those who have been labeled traditionally hard of hearing (i.e., up to and including the moderate level of impairment) and those who are considered deaf (i.e., severe to profound levels of impairment). The discussion of deaf students is placed (most of the time) in the context of research on these students in oral programs (mostly auditory-verbal but also multisensory ones) as well as those students exposed to cued speech/language and those in mainstream or inclusive programs. A few remarks are also made regarding the benefits of early amplification, the strong focus on audition (in auditory-verbal programs), and the controversy surrounding cochlear implants. Regardless of how the research is interpreted and despite the pesky generalization issues, there are some successful oral students with hearing impairment. Success can be interpreted in many ways; the focus here is on the development of English language skills including literacy skills and the ability to engage in literate thought in any mode. As will be seen in the ensuing sections, it is still difficult to explain why some students are successful and why some are not and to explicate the nature of the factors that contributed to their success or lack of success in the development of English. Of course, some scholars have proffered a few strong reasons for the success or lack of it; nevertheless, as indicated here and in the subsequent chapters on English signed systems and ASL, the development of functional and high-level English competency remains difficult for many deaf and some hard-of-hearing students despite the communication mode or approach used.

Research on Hard-of-Hearing Students

Similar to any definition of deafness, an adequate description of hard-of-hearing students for research purposes should include characteristics such as degree of impairment, age at onset, etiology, presence of additional disabilities, level of intelligence, and certain parental attributes such as involvement in the child's education, acceptance, socioeconomic status, and hearing status. As indicated in Chapter 1, students in the slight to moderate categories of hearing impairment (from about 27 dB up to 70 dB) (Acoustical Society of America, 1982) have been labeled *hard of hearing*. With improvements in amplification systems, it is not uncommon to find a number of students in the severe category (71 to 90 dB) with characteristics that are similar to those of the traditional hard-of-hearing students. With early amplification and early intervention, it is argued that the overwhelming majority of students with hearing losses up to and including the severe category can function in a primarily auditory mode (Ross, 1986, 1990). That is, these students can learn to speak, read, and write in English (or any other spoken language) in the same manner as their peers with typical hearing ability.

It is extremely difficult to determine the prevalence and demographic characteristics of hard-of-hearing students, specifically students who are integrated fully in general education programs (Commission on Education of the Deaf, 1988; Ries, 1986). Although some information is available on these integrated students, much of what is known concerns students who are receiving special education services in self-contained classrooms in public schools or the very few students who attend residential schools for deaf students. Many hard-of-hearing students, especially those with slight to mild losses, often are not identified until 2 or 3 years of age (Commission on Education of the Deaf, 1988; Northern, 1994). This has led to debates on early identification procedures in hospitals and the push for universal screening procedures (Barin, 1999) in conjunction with the obvious needs to reduce the gap between identification and intervention and to assess the effects of both early identification and early intervention.

The incidence of hard-of-hearing students still remains at about 15 to 16 for every 1,000 students in compulsory education. A large number of these students have unilateral hearing losses and may not wear hearing aids (Blair, Peterson, & Viehweg, 1985; Davis, Shepard, Stelmachowicz, & Gorga, 1981; Shepard, Davis, Gorga, & Stelmachowicz, 1981). In a number of reviews from the time of Pintner and Lev (1939) to the present, it has been well documented that the educational achievement of hard-of-hearing students is not commensurate to that of their hearing peers. In fact, the gap between the two overall groups seems to increase with age. In addition, it was not uncommon to report that older hard-of-hearing students were most likely to drop out of school on reaching the legal age. Traditionally, the achievement lag of hard-of-hearing students has been related to their degree of hearing impairment and also to the quality of support services.

Despite the quantitative delays, it has been documented that the language and achievement development of hard-of-hearing students is qualitatively similar to that of typically hearing students. Taking into account individual differences, there seem to be overall patterns such that hard-of-hearing students proceed through learning stages of speech and language, produce errors, and use strategies that are similar to those of peers who are typically hearing.

Table 5-7 provides a summary of the highlights of selected major studies focusing on the achievement of hard-of-hearing students.

TABLE 5-7 Summary of Selected Major Studies on Hard-of-Hearing Students and General Remarks

Research on Hard-of-Hearing Students

Study	Highlights
Kodman (1963)	Analyzed the academic performance of hard-of-hearing students whose hearing impairment ranged from 20 to 65 dB in the better ear (i.e., from slight to moderate). Average achievement level of these sixth-grade mainstreamed students was 3.8 years, which was more than two grades lower than that of hearing peers. Documented that only a third of these students wore hearing aids, and only one-fourth received speech and language services.
Quigley & Thomure (1968)	Found an inverse relationship between degree of hearing impairment and academic achievement; students with slight hearing impairment demonstrated a 1-year lag; students with moderate hearing impairment exhibited a 3-year lag when compared with grade-level hearing peers. First researchers to document the negative effects of even a slight impairment on academic achievement. Students who

exhibited losses up to 14 dB demonstrated a delay of about 1 year on a vocabulary subtest (i.e., word meaning). Despite this finding, it was not uncommon to find that students do not qualify for special education services unless their hearing impairment is at the mild or moderate level.

Balow, Fulton, & Peploe (1971)

Reported that the mean reading scores of the students with mild hearing losses were about one grade higher than students with severe and profound hearing losses in residential and/or special day-school programs.

Jensema (1975)

Reported an inverse relationship between degree of hearing impairment and academic achievement in a national sample of students in special education programs. Findings similar to those reported by Balow et al. (1971).

Davis & Blasdell (1975)

Syntactic development of students with hearing impairment was quantitatively different (i.e., reduced) but qualitatively similar to that of hearing students who were younger. For example, the hard-of-hearing students produced more errors than their hearing peers at all age levels compared, and the gap between the two groups increased with age. Nevertheless, the errors of hard-of-hearing students were similar to those made by hearing counterparts.

Davis, Shepard, Stelmachowicz, & Gorga (1981)

Students with mild to moderate impairment performed on a par with peers who were hearing in reading,

(continues)

(Table 5-7 continued)

	mathematics, and spelling. Gap between the two groups becomes significant for students with hearing losses greater than 50 dB.
Blair, Peterson, & Viehweg (1985)	Academic achievement lag of students with hearing impairment not as great as that documented by Quigley and Thomure (1968). Results are said to be due to the implementation of early adequate auditory management. That is, the academic performances of these hard-of-hearing students were also correlated positively to the length of time they had worn their hearing aids. Most impressively, the mean grade scores of the hard-of-hearing students were very similar to the norms associated with hearing students.

General Remarks

- In general, the achievement of hard-of-hearing students is not commensurate with that of hearing peers. Despite the quantitative delays, the language and achievement development of hard-of-hearing students is qualitatively similar to that of typically hearing students. In other words, hard-of-hearing students proceed through learning stages of speech and language that are similar to hearing peers.

- Most studies have documented a strong inverse relationship between degree of hearing impairment and achievement. That is, the greater the impairment, the larger the gap in achievement when compared to hearing counterparts. Even a slight hearing impairment can have negative effects.

- For hard-of-hearing students, the gap in achievement can be minimized and even eliminated in some cases if there is a strong educational management process including early identification, early amplification, and early intervention.

In essence, there are still a number of educators who agree with Ross (1986, 1990) and others that a well-planned program of educational management focusing on the development of oral skills should result in improvement in academic achievement for most hard-of-hearing students—perhaps for many deaf students. Despite the voluminous amount of research documenting the relationship between hearing loss and achievement, caution should be taken to assume that hearing loss alone can predict achievement. As discussed previously, a number of studies have reported that students with less severe hearing impairment (i.e., hard-of-hearing students) score significantly higher on achievement tests than those with severe to profound hearing impairment (see discussion in Allen, 1986). However, surprisingly, other studies have shown that students with severe to profound hearing impairment performed better than those with less severe hearing losses (for college students, see Saur, Popp-Stone, & Hurley-Lawrence, 1987). Thus, it seems that hearing impairment alone should not be considered the all-encompassing factor for academic achievement. There are numerous other factors that should be assessed, for example, motivation of students and parents, self-efficacy of students, quality of educational placement, quality of instruction, communication ease between students and significant others such as parents and teachers, and a priori academic ability and success (J. Davis, Elfenbein, Schum, & Bentler, 1986; Long, Stinson, & Braeges, 1991). As with so many other issues in education and deafness, these studies and others seem to argue against the quest for a single all-encompassing factor for academic achievement or, indeed, for any kind of achievement. Nevertheless, with respect to hard-of-hearing students—and as discussed next for deaf students—it is important to make improvements in all aspects of the educational management process including early identification, early amplification, and early intervention.

Research on Oral Deaf Students

This section synthesizes a sample of research on oral deaf students. The areas of research include studies that focus on general language development, literacy development, cochlear implants, cued speech (cued language), and survey studies. Similar to the research on hard-of-hearing students, the language and literacy development of most oral deaf students can best be described as qualitatively similar, albeit quantitatively different (i.e., delayed or slower). Some scholars argued that the success of some oral deaf students can be generalized to students with similar characteristics and educated in similar educational conditions (see the special monograph of Geers & Moog, 1994). In essence, there seems to be good results for some students who use sensory or amplification aids such as tactile aids or cochlear implants (Spencer, Tomblin, & Gantz, 1997; also see the discussion and review in Geers & Moog, 1994; McGarr, 1989; Nevins & Chute, 1996) and for students who are exposed to cued speech/language (see review in LaSasso & Metzger, 1998).

Studies Focusing on Aspects of General Language Development

Several studies have focused on specific aspects of language development, for example, phonology, syntax, semantics, and pragmatics. Some of the findings of earlier studies have been reiterated in later investigations. For example, Mavilya and Mignone (1977) examined the oral development of three deaf children from birth to 5 years of age. These investigators provided information on development during the prelinguistic stage (e.g., babbling) up through the first words of the linguistic stage and indicated that at least some deaf children can master aspects of speech and language at rates comparable to those of hearing children. This finding of quantitative similarity (i.e., comparable rates) was confirmed in a later study using the syllable as a unit of analysis (Ling et al., 1981).

It has been shown that the language systems of deaf children is rule governed; however, the rules are not applied systematically or consistently due to the impoverished or incomplete input of the auditory system (i.e., speechreading and residual hearing) (Dodd, 1976; Pressnell, 1973). This often resulted in uneven progress or a plateau in development despite an early period of rapid language development, reported previously. For example, at least with respect to syntax (Geers & Moog, 1978; Pressnell, 1973), the rate of development was slower than that of hearing children. Although older deaf children outperformed the younger ones, there were no significant improvements associated with age. In addition, children with hearing impairment acquired some syntactic constructions in a different order than that reported for hearing children. It was hypothesized that this difference was due to the unnatural order of teaching by the instructors. This has been the conclusion of other more recent studies on the unnatural order of instruction (see discussions in Wilbur, 1977, 1987; for second language students, see McLaughlin, 1984, 1985). The notion that the English language development of deaf children is rule governed, although the application of rules may be inefficient or not always systematic, has been a robust finding in the area of syntactic development (see the work of Quigley and collaborators; Russell, Quigley, & Power, 1976) as well as other domains of language.

A few studies explored specifically the development of semantics and pragmatics in children, especially young children, who are orally deaf. Similar to studies on the other components, it has been concluded that the development of children with hearing impairment is similar to—albeit slower than—that of comparable children with typical hearing (Skarakis & Prutting, 1977). In addition, many of these documented semantic and communicative functions are similar to those observed in children with typical hearing at 9 to 18 months of age (Halliday, 1975; Lucas, 1980; Ninio & Snow, 1996). It was also suggested that both types of functions, semantic and pragmatic, may not be differentiated in the early linguistic stages of children with profound hearing impairment.

This similar—but slower—rate of development was reported also in a study that focused on the development of temporal semantic functions (Jarvella & Lubinsky, 1975). It should be remembered that these semantic functions are difficult even for hearing children, most of whom achieve mastery around 8, 9, or 10 years of age (Lucas, 1980). In general, children with hearing impairment performed similarly to children with typical hearing when the temporal order in the sentences was preserved; that is, the use of the after clause first or the before clause second. The performance of children with hearing impairment, however, was inferior to children with typical hearing and only at chance level when the temporal order was reversed. A good review of research and practice involving pragmatics or communicative interactions can be found in the work of Kretschmer and Kretschmer (1988). Some data on the communicative interactions/efforts of very young children with hearing impairment can be found in the work of Yoshinaga-Itano and Stredler-Brown (1992).

The specific benefits of unisensory methods, especially the acoupedics approach, have been reported in several case studies (see discussion in Pollack, 1984). Long, Fitzgerald, Sutton, and Rollins (1983), for example, documented the achievement of a $4\frac{1}{2}$ year-old-girl. The language development of the girl was proceeding at a rate similar to her hearing counterparts. Much has been said about the benefits of traditional aural-oral (i.e., auditory-verbal) approaches, including research studies that support the importance and utilization of residual hearing (e.g., see discussion in Goldberg, 1993). It should be kept in mind that a number of students may receive greater benefits in approaches that utilize vision in conjunction with audition (and sensory aids, etc.) (see discussion in Ling, 1984), especially with the development of speech via the use of visual-based speech training.

It has also been argued further that most educational programs do not have adequate provisions for developing speech communication skills (Ling, 1976; Ross, 1990). Thus, adequate oral language development is not as commonly achieved with deaf children as it ought to be is an often repeated dictum throughout the years by strong proponents of oralism.

Table 5-8 provides a summary of the findings of selected salient studies in this section.

TABLE 5-8 A Few Highlights on Achievement of Oral Deaf Students and General Remarks

Study	Oral Deaf Students Highlights
Pressnell (1973)	Reported that the rate of syntactic development in children with hearing impairment was slower than that of comparable hearing children. Analyses of the spontaneous language samples revealed no significant improvement associated with age. Also reported that children with hearing impairment acquired some verb constructions in a different order than that reported for hearing children. Hypothesized that this difference was due to the unnatural order of teaching verbs by the instructors.
Dodd (1976)	Concluded that the phonologic systems of deaf children are in part rule governed and used by children with typical hearing at an earlier stage. Hypothesized that the systems are only partially rule governed due to the incomplete information provided by residual hearing and speechreading abilities.
Mavilya & Mignone (1977)	Reported that children began the babbling stage at 6 months, almost 2 to 3 months later than that observed for hearing children. Similar to hearing children, however, these deaf children were producing one and two words at 24 months. By the age of 30 months, these children began to use their voices with other deaf children. In addition, the three- to four-word stage emerged around

age 3. Finally, the children's speech began to approximate that of an adult around age 5.

Skarakis & Prutting (1977)   Concluded that the semantic and pragmatic development of young children with hearing impairment is similar to—albeit slower than—that of comparable children with typical hearing. That is, many of the semantic and pragmatic behaviors are similar to those observed in younger hearing children.

General Remarks

- Similar to the research on hard-of-hearing students, the language development of oral deaf students is qualitatively similar and quantitatively delayed when compared to peers with typical hearing ability. This has been observed for all language components, phonological, syntax, semantics, and pragmatics.

- In general, the language system of deaf students seems to be rule governed; however, the system might be only partially rule governed due to incomplete or inaccurate information provided by the oral skills of the students—namely, speechreading and residual hearing.

- The most impressive results are associated with the few students who are able to benefit greatly from an intensive traditional oral program or unisensory program involving early amplification and intervention.

Selected Studies on Literacy Development of Students in Oral Programs

Some of the most impressive results of traditional oral methods can be found in studies on students enrolled in indisputably comprehensive oral programs. In an earlier study, Lane and Baker (1974) compared the reading grade-level scores of former students at Central Institute for the Deaf (CID) to students with hearing impairment in other investigations. The reading achievement growth of the former CID students was 2.5 grades for a 4-year education period. This growth rate is much greater than that observed in national surveys (Allen, 1986; Center for Assessment and Demographic Studies [CADS], 1991; Trybus & Karchmer, 1977; also see the discussion and review in Paul, 1998a).

The success of orally trained students has been documented in recent studies and reviews (Geers & Moog, 1989, 1994; Luetke-Stahlman, 1988a). Students in intensive comprehensive oral education programs are more likely to develop better language, reading, and academic skills than are students in other educational programs and those exposed to approaches that do not completely represent the grammar of English (see Chapter 6 for a discussion of the signed approaches).

The study of Luetke-Stahlman serves as a representative example. Luetke-Stahlman (1988a) examined the performances of students with hearing impairment who were between the ages of 5 and 12. The students were exposed to two groups of approaches. One group of approaches consisted of oral English (OE) and other forms representing either a language (e.g., American Sign Language) or—what Luetke-Stahlman considered—a fairly complete representation of a language, seeing essential English [SEE I], signing exact English [SEE II], or cued speech [CS]). The other group consisted of approaches that are not considered to be a complete representation of a language (e.g., signed English [SE], manual English, and pidgin sign English—English-based signing or contact signing). The researcher controlled several variables statistically, for example, age and aided and unaided hearing acuity.

The results indicated that the students exposed to OE and other systems in this group of approaches performed significantly better than students in the other group on six of the seven measures used. Luetke-Stahlman (1988a) concluded that it was important to be exposed to instructional approaches that are either a bona fide language or a complete representation of a language.

It can be inferred from the Luetke-Stahlman study that students who are deaf and who have a working knowledge of the performance form of English may acquire adequate English literacy skills. This issue has been investigated extensively and supported by more recent studies (Geers & Moog, 1989; Spencer et al., 1997). In addition, as discussed previously in this chapter, these studies have shown that some important factors associated with the development of literacy include the exploitation of residual hearing, early amplification, and educational management as well as the development of oral English language ability.

It is interesting to note that many of these factors have been documented as important for students with severe to profound hearing impairment in Total Communication programs, as discussed in Chapter 6 of this text (Delaney, Stuckless, & Walter, 1984; Moores & Sweet, 1990). It might not be obvious that most of the factors support the very strong relationship between the performance (especially, oral) and script literacy (i.e., print) forms of a language such as English.

The development of oral English and subsequent literacy skills is becoming evident in children with cochlear implants (Spencer et al., 1997). Spencer et al. (1997) examined 40 children from kindergarten through 12th grade. Results of the study were compared with those on deaf and hard-of-hearing students in the national survey by Furth (1966) and the study by Krose, Lotz, Puffer, and Osberger (1986).

In general, Spencer et al. (1997) observed that their subjects with cochlear implants attained higher reading levels than children with similar levels of hearing impairment in other studies. They reported that their children continued to improve their reading skills, and the famous age performance gap, often observed in comparison with hearing counterparts, was not as pronounced. Spencer et al. also reported better results than those by Lane and Baker (1974), discussed previously in this section.

As impressive as these data are, the reader should exercise caution in interpreting the findings as evidence for the all-encompassing factor of using cochlear implants. As indicated previously, there are several factors that need to be considered with respect to reading achievement. In essence, there is no intent here to denigrate the findings of this study; however, reading involves much more than the ability to hear the speech signal.

Table 5-9 provides a summary of the major highlights of the studies on literacy and oralism.

TABLE 5-9 A Few Highlights on Literacy and Oral Deaf Students and General Remarks

Oral Deaf Students

Study	Highlights
Lane & Baker (1974)	Reported that the reading achievement growth of the former Central Institute for the Deaf (CID) students was much greater than that observed in national surveys.
Doehring, Bonnycastle, & Ling (1978)	Examined the language comprehension abilities of CID students, some of whom were integrated in regular education programs. Found that the students

(continues)

(Table 5-9 continued)

performed at or above grade level on reading tasks. Concluded that the performances of the CID students were influenced by their intensive auditory-oral training.

Luetke-Stahlman (1988a)

Examined the performances of students with hearing impairment who were exposed to two groups of approaches. One group of approaches consisted of forms representing either a language (ASL) or a fairly complete representation of a language (via a signed system). The other group consisted of approaches that are not considered to be a complete representation of a language (via a signed system). Results indicated that the students exposed to forms that are representative of a language performed significantly better than students in the other group on six of the seven measures used.

Geers & Moog (1989)

Argued that the primary oral form of English is indispensable. The researchers proffered several statements to explain the well-developed language and cognitive skills of many of the students in their study. For example, they concluded that: "The primary factors associated with the development of literacy in this orally educated sample are good use of residual hearing, early amplification, and educational management, and—

	above all—oral English language ability, including vocabulary, syntax, and discourse skills" (p. 84).
Spencer, Tomblin, & Gantz (1997)	Concluded that about 25% of the children in their study were reading at or above grade level, and about 20% were within 8 months of their respective grade level. Observed that their subjects with cochlear implants attained higher reading levels than children with similar levels of hearing impairment in other studies. Reported that their children continued to improve their reading skills and the infamous age-performance gap, often observed in comparison with hearing counterparts, was not as pronounced.

General Remarks

- Some of the most impressive literacy results can be found in studies on students enrolled in indisputably comprehensive oral programs using traditional oral approaches—specifically, auditory-verbal approaches. Readings scores are almost always higher than those of oral students in other types of programs.

- Oral deaf children who have a combination of favorable factors such as at least average intellectual ability, early educational management, and strong family support have the potential for developing higher literacy scores than is reported for children with hearing impairment in general.

- It is possible that the summary statement of the Geers and Moog (1989) study can be generalized to orally educated students with similar experiences: "The primary factors associated with the development of literacy in this orally educated sample are good use of residual hearing, early amplification, and educational management, and—above all—oral English language ability, including vocabulary, syntax, and discourse skills" (p. 84).

A Few Remarks on Studies of Individuals with Cochlear Implants

This section presents a few critical remarks about the research on cochlear implants, which perhaps has generated the bulk of the current controversy in the field of deaf education. Cochlear implants should not be considered to be a panacea or an all-encompassing factor. This view has been echoed by others (see discussions in Geers & Moog, 1994; Nevins & Chute, 1996), who have implied that sometimes it is not always clear whether the benefits are due solely to the use of cochlear implants. However, in conjunction with effective educational practices, it can be argued that cochlear implants do play a critical role in the improvement of English speech, language, and literacy.

That cochlear implant technology is an anathema for many members of Deaf culture should not be a surprise, given the current understanding of the cultural perspective. It seems that many members of Deaf culture believe that cochlear implant technology represents a threat to Deaf culture, and there might be a tendency to reject prospective members who have had implants. This view has been expressed by one of Deaf culture's most vocal proponents, Harlan Lane (1992): "Among the biological means aimed at regulating and ultimately eliminating deaf culture, language, and community, cochlear implants have historical antecedents, then, in medical experimentation on deaf children and reproductive regulation on deaf adults (p. 216)."

In considering an implant for their children, parents need to be aware of the social and political issues; however, ultimately they need to make a decision that they feel is best for them and their children. This decision, however, should be based on their understanding of the benefits and disadvantages, informed by empirical research. A well-balanced accessible discussion of the major issues and findings on cochlear implants can be found in Nevins and Chute (1996). These authors also discussed the important issues of management.

The effects of cochlear implant have been documented. For example, in general, children with multichannel cochlear implant experience perform better than children who wear hearing aids on tests of speech perception (Tyler, Fryauf-Bertschy, Gantz, Kelsay, & Woodworth, 1997), speech production (Tye-Murray, Spencer, & Woodworth, 1995), and measures of language acquisition (Miyamoto, Svirsky, & Robbins, 1997) and literacy (Spencer et al., 1997). One of the most comprehensive discussions of the effects of cochlear implants (as well as the use of tactile aids) was documented in a monograph (Geers & Moog, 1994). With respect to the positive results that were observed, Geers and Moog (1994) cautioned that:

The results reported in this monograph must be interpreted in light of the sample studied and the educational setting in which they participated. There were children who were judged to have at least a fair prognosis for developing spoken language as a primary means of communicating. Their parents and teachers were highly supportive of this overall goal. The children were taught individually or in small groups of two to eight children by trained and experienced teachers of the hearing impaired for the entire school day. They had daily access to audiologists and technicians who assured that the sensory aids (cochlear and tactile) *[emphasis added] functioned appropriately. It is possible that the results reported here may be generalizable only to children who share these characteristics. (pp. v–vi)*

There is no doubt that there have been failures or poor results—many of which are not often published in scholarly journals—neither are there doubts of false promises and horror stories, as related by Lane (1992). Perhaps it is difficult to trust the results of researchers who might have a vested interest in the benefits of cochlear implants; however, the same can be said for researchers who have a vested interest in the failures of this technology.

Whether cochlear implants can facilitate and be responsible in part for assisting children with hearing impairment to perform on a par with children with typical hearing in the areas of English speech, language, and literacy is, of course, an open question. Nevertheless, if there is such an entity as unbiased documentation, perhaps the 1995 National Institutes of Health (NIH) *Consensus Statement on Cochlear Implants in Adults and Children* fits this criterion (NIH Consensus Program Information Service). This report documented improvements in speech perception (via speechreading and implants) in postlingually deaf adults. Similar levels of improvement were not documented for prelingually deaf adults; however, many of these individuals seem to derive satisfaction from the use of the implants and continue to wear them (e.g., for hearing environmental sounds). There is variability across children with cochlear implants; nevertheless, improvements in speech perception and production have been documented.

This variability has also been reported for children who wear hearing aids (see discussion in Nevins & Chute, 1996) and is typically attributed to factors such as age at onset of the hearing impairment, age of implementation of the implant, the quality of the management program, and mode of communication of the children. The NIH (1995) document reported that the performance of children with implants might be commensurate over time with those who are successful hearing aids users. There seem to be clear benefits for children who were implanted at a young age; that is, their speech production (e.g., of segmentals and suprasegmentals) were more accurate than children with comparable hearing impairments who were using tactile aids or hearing aids. This report also remarked that the oral language development of deaf children with implants is a slow, labor-intensive process, and most of the time, the performance is not commensurate to that of their peers with typical hearing.

The NIH (1995) document also reported on other issues related to cochlear implants. In any case, it is this type of consensus report that is needed for a highly controversial issue such as cochlear implants. Cochlear implant technology represents an opportunity and a choice for parents and their deaf and hard-of-hearing children. The author agrees with Nevins and Chute (1996), who remarked:

> *The impact of the cochlear implant on the field of deaf education is only beginning. Early trends seem to indicate the potential for earlier mainstream placement which has a concomitant impact on the field of regular education and society at large. True mainstreaming, in the sense of full participation in the mainstream of school and society, can only be accomplished if proper assessment and follow-up are components of the process. (p. 201)*

Also, if researchers continue to produce relatively unbiased research documentation of the effects of cochlear implants, they should have a better understanding of why and for whom this technology produces the greatest benefits.

Research on Cued Speech

Research on cued speech has been conducted on students in the United States and other countries. The use of cued speech in the United States seems to be increasing (Quenin & Blood, 1989; also see the discussion in Fleetwood & Metzger, 1998; LaSasso & Metzger, 1998). Examples of early research are the works of Ling and Clarke (1975) and Clarke and Ling (1976), who analyzed the receptive abilities of students who had been exposed to CS for 2 years. The test stimuli consisted of cued and noncued words, phrases, and sentences. Results indicated that students understood cued stimuli significantly better than noncued stimuli. Cued words were easier than cued phrases, which were easier than cued sentences. The investigators also reported that the students' phonetic (i.e., pronunciation) errors can be grouped into patterns that can be addressed in a systematic remedial speech and language program.

Nicholls and Ling (1982) analyzed the speech reception abilities of Australian students with hearing impairment exposed to cued speech for 4 years. Test stimuli were presented under seven conditions that resulted from all possible permutations of three variables: audition, cues, and speechreading. The scores of the students for two conditions, speechreading plus cues and audition, speechreading, and cues, were significantly higher than those for all other conditions. In addition, the use of cues did not negatively affect the students' abilities to speechread or to use their residual hearing. The researchers concluded that CS might be a viable option for students with severe to profound hearing impairment who cannot progress adequately in conventional oral education programs.

Mohay (1983) studied the effects of cued speech on the English language development of three children—two had a profound hearing impairment and one child had a severe hearing impairment. The children started their education in a traditional oral program and then transferred to a CS program. The researcher observed that the children's use of word combinations (i.e., two or three words) increased after exposure to cued speech. It was suggested, however, that certain factors such as growth in cognitive ability might have been responsible for the increase in production rather than the use of CS.

More recent studies on hearing adults (Abraham & Stoker, 1984; Chilson, 1985) and adults with hearing impairment (Gregory, 1987) have provided additional support for the positive effects of cued speech on speechreading skills. In general, the adults obtained significantly higher speechreading scores on speech stimuli presented with cues. Thus, many of these studies seem to confirm the results of a survey by Quenin and Blood (1989): "Cued Speech is viewed as a vehicle for conveying spoken language and as a tool in speech development" (p. 288).

The assumption that the use of cued speech has a positive effect on the development of a language, particularly reading skills, has been discussed. Liedel and Paul (1991) argued that cued speech may play a critical role in the development of rapid word identification skills (i.e., bottom-up skills) for reading. The development of rapid word identification skills in English is dependent in part on the cognitive representation of the phonological and morphological properties of English. Liedel and Paul proposed a model in which cued speech is part of an interactive-interaction bilingual-bicultural program for ASL-using deaf students. This model is based on a social-cognitive interactive view of reading. In addition, this model is another example of a recent survey finding: "Cued Speech may be a component of both oral and total communication approaches to teaching hearing-impaired students" (Quenin & Blood, 1989,

p. 288). Another similar perspective on the use of cued speech in a bilingual-bicultural program was offered by LaSasso and Metzger (1998).

Cornett (1991) also recognized the role of cued speech in the development of reading via the development of phonological awareness. This recognition is based on some research evidence and on the fact that Cornett designed the CS system to reflect the phonological aspect of any spoken language. In emphasizing the importance of cued speech for reading, Cornett quoted the concluding paragraph of a study by Alegria, DeJean, Capouillez, and Leybaert:

> *To come back to our initial point, the present work strongly suggests that the lexicon developed by the deaf with Cued Speech has properties that are equivalent to the phonology of the hearing subjects. In both cases the internal representations of the words are compatible with their orthographic representation. This allows the use of phonological coding to identify unfamiliar words and, as said before, can prime the whole process of reading acquisition. (Cornett, 1991, p. 36)*

This passage in the study by Alegria, DeJean, Capouillez, and Leybaert (as cited in Cornett, 1991) provides the major reason, in the author's view, for the success of cued speech in the development of literacy for some deaf and hard-of-hearing children and adolescents. As discussed previously, access to phonology is a critical feature for learning a language, including learning to read and write in that language. This access in part is responsible for the success of some children and adults in improving their visual speech reception and speechreading skills and the success of cued speech for some children with cochlear implantation (for a good review on phonology and cued speech/language, see LaSasso & Metzger, 1998).

With respect to literacy, access to phonology is necessary for the development of phonological and phonemic awareness, which seem to be critical (or at least facilitative) for the development of rapid automatic word identification skills in reading, although this assertion is in need of further research. A number of researchers have argued that the acquisition of phonology is not dependent on the rendering of acoustic information (Dodd & Campbell, 1987; Dodd & Hermelin, 1977; Fleetwood & Metzger, 1998; also see the review in LaSasso & Metzger, 1998). In fact, cued speech/language, which involves a different set of articulators and a different medium, seems to be sufficient for some deaf individuals to develop the use of a phonological code in short-term memory and representations of phonological information cognitively. This is because information rendered in cued speech represents the same range of abstract phonemic values as does speech in the spoken languages in which cued speech has been researched (see previous discussion of the work of Fleetwood & Metzger, 1998). As remarked by Leybaert and Charlier (1996), deaf children who are exposed to cued speech early in life seem to rely on internal phonological representations to perform tasks involving rhyming, remembering, and spelling, and this reliance is similar to that noted for children with typical hearing. The crux of the matter is that children need "complete, well-specified perception of the phonetic contrasts of spoken language" (Leybaert & Charlier, 1996, p. 246), and cued speech seems to fulfill that requirement.

Table 5-10 provides a few major highlights of salient studies and reviews of cued speech (cued language).

TABLE 5-10 Highlights of Research on Cued Speech/Language

- In early studies, it was documented that students understood cued stimuli significantly better than noncued stimuli. Cued words were easier than cued phrases, which were easier than cued sentences.

- The use of cues has not been found to affect negatively the students' abilities to speechread or to use their residual hearing.

- In studies on adults, it was observed that individuals obtained significantly higher speechreading scores on speech stimuli that were presented with cues.

- Cued speech/language might have a major role in the development of reading skills, particularly via the development of phonological and phonemic awareness. More research is needed in this area.

- In one study, it was stated that deaf children who are exposed to cued speech/language early in life seem to rely on internal phonological representations to perform tasks involving rhyming, remembering, and spelling. This reliance was reported to be similar to that noted for children with typical hearing.

SELECTED SURVEY STUDIES

Additional insights into the success of orally educated individuals have been reported in several survey studies (Goldberg & Flexer, 1991; McCartney, 1986; Ogden, 1979; Roberts & Rickards, 1994a, 1994b). In one study, it was remarked that oral adults in "this group is atypical in comparison to the national population and the national hearing-impaired population"; that is, they "have better than average education, careers, and annual salaries" (McCartney, 1986, p. 135).

With respect to these studies, there are several limitations that should be discussed briefly. Utilizing self-reports produces subjective data, although self-views should be considered as one source of information. With children in the surveys, parents are often requested to assist in completing the question-naire; thus, this is not a direct assessment of the self-perceptions of the par-ticipants. The greatest limitation—and one that needs to be kept in mind with all empirical studies—is the generalization of the results to other groups of individuals with hearing impairment. To proffer generalizations, it is impor-tant to be cognizant of the characteristics of the sample in the study. For exam-ple, in a study involving Australian children from age 7 to 17 years with hearing impairment ranging from mild to profound (mean = 79 dBHL), Roberts and Rickards (1994a, 1994b) cautioned readers in generalizing their findings because of several issues:

> *All children had been involved in the same early intervention program operating within an integrated setting with an auditory/oral emphasis and were primarily from middle class families. . . . The cross-sectional design adopted in this study limits the ability to distinguish between stu-dent characteristics and advantages associated with early intervention in accounting for the students' amplification usage, communication practices, and speech intelligibility. Examination of only bivariate rela-tionships in the present study, and the interdependence between the edu-cational setting and degree of hearing loss, further restricts interpretation of the data. (1994a, p. 199)*

With these caveats in mind, it is possible to present some findings of the surveys, which are generally similar and consistent across the selected ones examined here. In the studies by Ogden (1979) and McCartney (1986), the adult individuals attributed their success to several factors mentioned previ-ously, namely, early education, early amplification, parental involvement, and oral communication skills. They also felt that it was important to have the desire to be integrated into general education programs and the mainstream of soci-ety. Similar findings were reported in a later study by Goldberg and Flexer (1991), who used a consumer survey to investigate the status of graduates of auditory-verbal programs.

Roberts and Rickards (1994a, 1994b) analyzed questionnaires that were completed by Australian children (with assistance from parents, if necessary) between the age of 7 and 17 years. These children were graduates of an integrated auditory-oral preschool program in Australia. The major focus of the study (reported in two articles) was on the children's perceptions of factors such as amplification usage, communication practices, speech intelligibility, academic achievement, use of support services, and friendship patterns. The researchers also studied the relationships between the perceptions and students' characteristics (e.g., degree of hearing impairment, etc.). The researchers remarked that "overall, the findings of this survey appear to reflect the auditory/oral integrated preschool educational experience these children received" (p. 222, 1994b). Notably, most of the children wore hearing aids, had hearing friends, used speech as their major mode of communication, and perceived their academic achievement as average or above average.

In sum, there is a need for additional survey and follow-up studies involving current students and graduates of oral education programs, particularly programs that are intensive and comprehensive. As mentioned previously, the results of survey studies should be interpreted with caution; however, they can offer some insights into the values and attitudes of the participants. It seems to be clear that students, parents, and educators need to be committed to and value the development of adequate oral communication skills and literacy, although this is not an easy process. Perhaps it is true that oral students "must have innate qualities to be oral" (McCartney, 1986, p. 140).

FINAL REMARKS

The major intent of this chapter is to describe the effects of oralism on the development of English speech, language, and literacy skills in deaf and hard-of-hearing children and adolescents. To provide a context for some of these effects, it was necessary to present some basic information in four broad areas: (a) classification of speech sounds, (b) descriptions of prominent oral English approaches, (c) discussion of critical components such as speechreading and auditory training/learning, and (d) research synthesis of speech perception, production, and intelligibility.

Throughout the chapter, highlights and summaries of major points are provided. Here, a few of those summary remarks are selected to be representative of the information in following areas: speech, speechreading, and auditory training/learning; hard-of-hearing students; and oral deaf students.

Speech, Speechreading, and Auditory Training/Learning

- It is difficult to develop speech skills in children with severe to profound hearing impairment. Success varies across students and does not reveal a strong, consistent pattern or generalization. Greater success in the future is expected with the continued advances in amplification systems and cochlear implants.

- There have been numerous research studies on the effects of speechreading. General findings have been documented, for example, between (and among) speechreading and variables such as academic achievement, age at onset of hearing impairment, degree of hearing impairment, intelligence, linguistic skills, perceptual skills, and personality traits. However, these general findings do not offer useful or clear implications for classroom practice for improving the speechreading skills of deaf and hard-of-hearing children and adolescents. Thus, convincing measures of speechreading skill and aptitude are still elusive.

- The current trend of auditory-verbal programs is on teaching children to listen. That is, children learn to listen and learn by listening rather than to learn to hear. This approach has received the label of *auditory learning*. Spoken language activities are related to the child's real-life experiences. The emphasis is on comprehension—which is considered to be the highest level of auditory skills. The other three levels—detection, discrimination, and identification—often associated with traditional approaches in auditory training, are important but not sufficient for developing listening skills.

Hard-of-Hearing Students

- In general, the achievement of hard-of-hearing students is not commensurate with that of hearing peers. Despite the quantitative delays, the language and achievement development of hard-of-hearing students is qualitatively similar to that of typically hearing students.

- Most studies have documented a strong inverse relationship between degree of hearing impairment and achievement. The greater the impairment, the larger the gap in achievement when compared to hearing counterparts. Even a slight hearing impairment can have negative effects.

- For hard-of-hearing students, the gap in achievement can be minimized and even eliminated in some cases, especially if there is a strong educational management program including early identification, early amplification, and early intervention.

Oral Deaf Students

- Similar to the research on hard-of-hearing students, the language development of oral deaf students is qualitatively similar and quantitatively delayed when compared to peers with typical hearing ability. This has been observed for all language components, phonological, syntax, semantics, and pragmatics.

- In general, the language system of deaf students seems to be rule governed; however, the system might be only partially rule governed due to incomplete or inaccurate information provided by the oral skills of the students—namely, speechreading and residual hearing.

- Deaf children who have a combination of favorable factors such as at least average intellectual ability, early educational management, and strong family support have the potential for developing higher literacy scores than is reported for children with hearing impairment in general.

In essence, at least two general patterns seem to emerge in the literature on deaf and hard-of-hearing students. One, there is (or can be!) an inverse relationship between degree of hearing impairment and academic achievement. That is, the more severe the hearing impairment, the more apparent the performance gap between these students and those with typical hearing. In fact, this performance gap seems to become wider as the students with hearing impairment become older. However, it was argued that this inverse relationship should be stated with caution. Hearing impairment should not be considered an all-encompassing factor for academic achievement. In addition to social-emotional, instructional, and parental factors, consideration should be given to all aspects of the educational management process, including early identification, amplification, and intervention. The time lag between identification and the implementation of adequate amplification and intervention components also needs to be reduced.

The second major pattern that has been documented repeatedly is: The language and literacy development of both hard-of-hearing and deaf students is qualitatively similar to that of children with typical hearing. The notion of qualitative similarity means that taking into account individual differences, deaf and hard-of-hearing students proceed through stages, produce errors, and use strategies that are generally similar to those of children with typical hearing. Of course, a number of deaf and hard-of-hearing children produce more errors and use ineffective strategies—due in part to the perception of an incomplete or inadequate auditory signal. Nevertheless, this qualitatively similarity hypothesis supports the use of materials and practices similar to those used for children with typical hearing, with adjustments made more often for rate of presentation rather than type or manner of presentation. Another perspective on this pattern: The understanding of the learning process of hearing children can be applied to advance the understanding of the process for deaf and hard-of-hearing children. And, the converse is also true.

There is no question that some deaf and many hard-of-hearing students are or have been successful as a result of the oral approaches, particularly the auditory-verbal approach and cued speech/language. However, it is also possible to find successful deaf and hard-of-hearing students who have been exposed to nontraditional oral approaches (e.g., multisensory). Because of the variability across students, care should be taken in making generalizations about the effectiveness of the various approaches. As noted in this chapter, there is a need for more complex research designs and, more specifically, a need for additional, rigorous, unbiased research syntheses. The latter point is critical for obtaining a better understanding of some of the effects of the new technology—namely, the use of cochlear implants.

Even if there is some consensus on factors that contribute to the oral success of deaf and hard-of-hearing students, this does not mean that these approaches will work for the vast majority of students with severe to profound hearing impairment. Nevertheless, the oral approach does work for some students, and oral education is preferred by many parents. The focus should be on determining why and for whom oral education approaches are most effective. With the advances in technology, there might be opportunities for more students to achieve success in the development of English speech, language, and literacy. It is suspected that, despite best efforts, scholars might not progress too far beyond the mystique or magic of oralism that causes some scholars to call speechreading a subtle art (Silverman & Kricos, 1990) and others to remark that oral students "must have innate qualities to be oral" (McCartney, 1986, p. 140).

ORALITY: SPEECH, AUDITION, AND SPEECHREADING

COMPREHENSION QUESTIONS

1. List and briefly describe the three categories of sound source that are responsible for producing consonants and vowels.

2. Provide one example (using a word) for the following categories of consonants and vowels. The first example has been done for you.

   Consonant: stop-plosive: /b/ as in *ball*.
   a. nasal
   b. affricate
   c. fricative

Vowel: high front: /i/ as in *beat*
   a. low front
   b. high back
   c. midfront

3. Describe the following concepts of connected speech:
   a. intonation
   b. rhythm
   c. coarticulation

4. Describe the major tenets of the following oral approaches for deaf and hard-of-hearing children:
   a. unisensory approaches
   b. multisensory approaches
   c. cued speech/language (e.g., consonants, vowels, and NMS)

5. If phonology is the building block of any language, then what is the litmus test for all invented language/communication systems for deaf and hard-of-hearing students? According to the chapter, does cued speech/language pass this litmus test? Why or why not? Do any of the English sign systems pass this litmus test (as discussed briefly in this chapter)? Why or why not?

6. Describe the following terms:
   a. speechreading
   b. auditory training/learning
   c. balanced approach to speech intelligibility

7. For studying speechreading ability, O'Neill and Oyer (1981) proposed a useful framework that focuses on four broad areas. Discuss and provide one example for each of the four areas.

8. The chapter provided several general remarks with respect to the overall findings of research on speechreading. Discuss some of these remarks. What type of research is still needed? Is it difficult to measure or assess speechreading skill? Why?

9. Although there is a wide range of variability across students with hearing impairment, it is possible to describe a few patterns of speech production errors. What are some of these patterns for suprasegmental and segmental aspects?

10. In the research on oralism, what are some general findings for hard-of-hearing students with respect to quantitative and qualitative development of language and literacy?

11. With respect to the research on oral deaf students, discuss some general findings of studies presented within each of the following categories:
    a. general language development
    b. literacy development
    c. cochlear implants
    d. cued speech/language
    e. survey studies

Are any of the general findings for deaf students similar to those presented for hard-of-hearing students?

CHALLENGE QUESTIONS

(Note: Complete answers are not in the text. Additional research is required.)

1. There is the assumption that cued articulators can represent the same range of abstract phonemic values as do the speech articulators, including suprasegmental aspects such as intonation, stress, and rhythm. What specific lines of research (or research questions) should be generated to test this assumption? (Think of areas such as phonological and phonemic awareness, the relationship between phonemic awareness and early reading development, the development of speech production and perception, and so on).

2. Given the existence of unisensory and multisensory oral approaches, including the use of cued speech/language, is it possible to determine (scientifically or logically) which approach should be used initially with a particular deaf or hard-of-hearing child? Does this chapter offer a sufficient amount of information for rendering such a decision? What do you think should be the guidelines? What is the theoretical or research support for your guidelines? Should a particular oral approach be assessed periodically? What guidelines would you recommend for this periodic assessment?

3. What are your views on cochlear implants? Can you support your views with theoretical and/or research data? Is there a positive linear relationship between cochlear implants and reading achievement? Why or why not? Is there a problem with constructing questions on linear

relationships—for example, a linear relationship between digital hearings aids and achievement, between Ling's speech method and English language development, and so on? Why or why not?

4. Do you think that advances in technology such as digital hearing aids or cochlear implants will eradicate the Deaf culture? Why or why not? Should deaf children (younger than 18 years old) of hearing parents have the opportunity to benefit from such technology? Why or why not? Who should make this decision?

FURTHER READINGS

Beebe, H. (1953). *A guide to help the severely hard of hearing child*. Basel, NY: Karger.

Cole, E. (1992). *Listening and talking: A guide to promoting spoken language in young hearing-impaired children*. Washington, DC: Alexander Graham Bell Association for the Deaf.

Goldstein, M. (1939). *The acoustic method*. St. Louis, MO: Laryngoscope Press.

Hodson, B., & Paden, E. (1983). *Targeting intelligible speech: A phonological approach to remediation*. San Diego, CA: College-Hill Press.

Pollack, D. (1970). *Educational audiology for the limited-hearing infant*. Springfield, IL: Charles C. Thomas.

CHAPTER

6

Signed Systems

*T*here are several other communication systems for deaf children that have been around for some time. These language alternatives fall into two categories: modifications to sign communication, typically intended to make it more English-like, and modifications to spoken communication. . . . Each alternative has its proponents, and anecdotal evidence concerning the successes of particular children with particular systems is not hard to find. This is not to say that one of these alternatives, or another yet to be invented, might not prove effective in facilitating the education and interpersonal communication of deaf children as a group or for particular deaf children. . . . However, we will not be in a position to decide which way of expressing language is best for which children until appropriate, scientific evaluations have been made. (Marschark, 1997, p. 62)

One of the most controversial debates in the education of children with severe to profound hearing impairment is the type of signed system that should be used by teachers and significant others. Despite the importance of this issue and despite the 25-plus years of use of some of the signed systems, there is no clear picture on the most effective system to adopt. This lack of clarity seems to be somewhat reflective of the manner in which the signed systems are used; that is, none of the signed systems is used widely, although practitioners do extract signs from a few systems, notably signing exact English and signed English. In essence, aside from the use of seeing essential English in

235

a school system in Texas, it seems that signed English and signing exact English are "the only MCE [manually coded English] systems now used in total communication programs in the United States" (Stewart & Luetke-Stahlman, 1998, p. 36; also see Marschark, 1997). Because all systems are based somewhat on English, it is assumed that the indiscriminate borrowing of signs from several systems is appropriate and desirable. However, this undermines the issue of representation as discussed in Chapter 1. There are several questions of interest here, at least. What exactly do these systems represent? How much of English is represented by a particular system? How much of English needs to be represented by a particular system? Can spoken English really be represented by a signed system? Does simultaneous communication entail the ability to perceive information on the lips (i.e., via speech) and on the hands (i.e., via signs) simultaneously? If so, what is the nature and extent of the perception process? Another issue that needs to be addressed in detail is whether it is possible to speak and sign simultaneously in a consistent systematic manner and not violate the system rules for executing signs. Finally, one of the most interesting areas of research has been the manner in which the systems are perceived by deaf and some hard-of-hearing students. This is a rather complicated issue to investigate because there is no linear relationship between sign input (i.e., reception/perception) and sign output (i.e., execution/performance). This is similar to the problematic relation between perception and production in the spoken language literature. Nevertheless, this should cause many educators to rethink and reflect on the goals of using any particular signed system or even to speak and sign simultaneously as in phrases such as simultaneous communication or Total Communication.

It needs to be reemphasized that using a mode of communication does not mean that one is using a specific language-teaching method. Each signed system is purported to represent the structure of English; however, when viewing the signs only, this representation seems to be only at the morphological and syntactical levels, albeit imperfectly. Phonology (see Chapter 2) can only be received via the students' use of their oral skills—that is, speechreading and use of residual hearing (see discussions in Akamatsu & Stewart, 1998; Drasgow & Paul, 1995; Fleetwood & Metzger, 1998; LaSasso & Metzger, 1998; Wilbur, 1987). The rules for representing certain aspects of English such as past tense and plurality vary across the systems. Deaf and hard-of-hearing students are not taught English but rather exposed to a particular system or some form of signing as a medium of instruction. The assumption is that the students either know English or will internalize the rules of a specific system and the language that it represents, namely, English.

In this chapter, the focus is on selected English-based signed systems, including the Rochester method, that have been developed for educational purposes. First, the basic tenets of a few systems are described, especially how each system attempts to represent the structure of English. This is only a brief introduction to the principles of the major signed and manual systems, and the reader is directed to the original sources for more details. Next, the chapter provides a synthesis of the major (albeit meager) research findings regarding the effects of the systems on the development of English. Admittedly, this is actually a global perspective that reflects much of the available research. This global perspective has been criticized for its shortcomings (Drasgow & Paul, 1995; Paul & Drasgow, 1998); however, it is reflective of much of the research that has been conducted on this issue. The last section of the chapter presents some tentative conclusions that are based on the available data, with implications for further research efforts.

TOTAL COMMUNICATION

Total Communication (TC) is another one of those terms that seems to cause clarity and confusion at the same time. On the one hand, TC is defined by whatever works for a particular child, for example, speech, speechreading, audition, signs, print, and so on, as well as combinations of these items. Apparently, TC is better known as the use of simultaneous communication, that is, the use of speech and signs in a simultaneous manner. On the other hand, for some reason, the use of American Sign Language (i.e., solely) does not seem to be a part of TC programs although it could fit into the TC philosophy. Many of the signs in the various signed systems used in TC are taken from the lexicon of ASL; however, this is a misleading and incomplete statement. Using ASL vocabulary in an English word order actually strips the grammatical functions of the ASL signs, especially because a number of ASL signs are also accompanied by important nonmanual (e.g., facial clues, shoulder shrugs, and puff cheeks) aspects that are not typically present in English signing (see Chapter 7 of this text). The inclusion or discussion of ASL within the TC philosophy is the cause of several misconceptions on the nature and use of ASL (Woodward & Allen, 1988).

Roy Holcomb, a deaf graduate from the Texas School for the Deaf and from Gallaudet University, is considered the father of Total Communication (Gannon, 1981). By the 1980s, most (about two-thirds) of the educational programs for deaf and hard-of-hearing students adhered to the philosophy of Total Communication (again, to mean speaking and signing simultaneously) (Stewart & Luetke-Stahlman, 1998). However, the use of simultaneous communication or manual communication methods is not new. Historical records reveal that signing and finger spelling were used to teach students to read and write as early as the 15th century (McClure, 1969; Moores, 1996).

The notion of signed systems, that is, using signs from a sign language to represent the structure of a spoken language, is not new either. During the 18th century, Abbe de l'Epee (1712–1789) and his successor, the Abbe Sicard (1742–1822) attempted to adapt the sign language of their students to conform to the structure of the French language. This novel approach to create a French-based signed system was the precursor to the English signed systems developed in England and the United States during the 1960s and 1970s. A more detailed account of these events can be found elsewhere (McAnally, Rose, & Quigley, 1994; McClure, 1969; Moores, 1987, 1996).

MANUALLY CODED ENGLISH

There are a number of reasons why manually coded English systems were developed. The two major ones are the attempt to represent the structure of English, particularly English words and word parts, and to provide an avenue for parents to learn and use signing without learning a new language (for a readable discussion of these reasons, see Stewart & Luetke-Stahlman, 1998).

For most individuals involved with deaf and hard-of-hearing students, the selection and use of sign has become a very complicated and confusing matter. Part of the confusion stems from the sheer number of communication systems that are available with names such as the Rochester method, seeing essential English, signing exact English, manual English, linguistics of visual English, conceptually accurate sign English (CASE), signed English, pidgin sign English, and contact signing. Most of these manual English codes were designed specifically to reflect the morpho-syntactic structure of written standard English in a visual, manual (use of hands) manner. Because the signed systems are morphologically based, the signs represent the English morphemes of written words (Akamatsu & Stewart, 1998; Raffin, 1976; Wilbur, 1987). It should be stressed that representing morphemes via signs or finger spelling is not the equivalent of representing morphemes via print. In fact, finger spelling is eally a representation of English letters that are combined to produce morphological-based words. This does not denigrate the contributions of the signed systems, including finger spelling, to assisting deaf and hard-of-hearing children in their attempts to understand morphology and syntax despite the imperfection of this representation (see Chapter 2 for a discussion of morphology and syntax).

The signed systems, with their focus on English morphology, are quite different from cued speech/language, with its focus on English phonology, which is considered the building blocks of the language, at least from the standpoint of linguistic principles (Fleetwood & Metzger, 1998).

There are several assumptions about the signed systems, all of which purport to represent English. Only one is highlighted here: It is permissible to borrow or combine signs from different systems to communicate concepts because all systems are variations of one language, English. This assumption is neither supported or refuted by the available research (Marschark, 1997); nevertheless, it is problematic. The rules for creating and using signs in one system are different from those for signs in another system. Borrowing signs (including inflectional and derivational markers; see Chapter 2) might make it difficult for deaf and hard-of-hearing children to receive consistent input so that they can form reliable hypotheses about the language they are attempting to learn. With limited and for the most part unambiguous input, learners intuitively discover underlying, unspoken regularities or rules. Although it is possible for practitioners to learn and use a specific system, for example, signing exact English, consistently and systematically (see discussion in Stewart & Luetke-Stahlman, 1998), most signing in education programs for deaf and hard-of-hearing students seems to be unrelated to a specific system. In other words, most practitioners are simply speaking and signing simultaneously, using signs from probably signed English and signing exact English without adhering to a specific set of rules from any signed system, save for following an English word order. Thus, deaf and hard-of-hearing children might be exposed to different rules in a haphazard or ambiguous manner and might not internalize the grammatical aspects of English. In addition, unlike cued speech/language, the signed systems, although they contain related overlapping features, are not representations of the various dialects of English. This is another reason why borrowing or combining signs, particularly in a haphazard or unsystematic fashion, does not seem to be theoretically sound.

Perhaps this can become clearer with an analogy. Suppose a deck of cards represents signs from the various English signed systems. Now in the world of cards, it is possible to play a number of games, each with its own set of rules. Suppose that card games such as Go Fish, Gin Rummy, and Skip-Bo represent different signed systems with different sets of rules. It might be possible to see similar patterns (i.e., overlapping use of similar signs) across these card games, not to mention the numerous variations within each game. Imagine playing cards in a haphazard fashion within each particular game (i.e., similar to the idiosyncratic use and borrowing of signs). In this case, the rules of one game might be followed along with the rules for the other card games.

Is it possible to learn Go Fish, Gin Rummy, and Skip-Bo at the same time, especially when not all of the rules are applied systematically or consistently? Can one say that a person knows how to play cards (i.e., sign English) in general although a particular game (i.e., signed system) is not strictly speaking a version (i.e., dialect) of the Overall Card Game of English? Perhaps this analogy is crude and is not the same as learning a code or language. Perhaps also the analogy does not capture the overlapping features or rules among the various signed systems or even represents the reality of the actual use of the systems. Nevertheless, it is argued here that although it is possible that one is learning to play cards (i.e., signing something like English), it is not certain what game (i.e., signed system) it is one is playing, except that one might not be playing any of them well. It could be said that one is playing cards haphazardly, which might be sufficient for a limited recreational purpose (i.e., similar to communicating basic needs in some form of English signing). Analogically, the author is just not convinced that one could learn English via signing in this manner. Of course, it is assumed for the sake of the analogy that it is possible to learn English via the use of or exposure to any particular signed system in a systematic or consistent manner.

This situation could become even more complicated if educators who are learning ASL incorporate ASL-like features into their English signing, with the use of ASL-like signs constrained by semantic and pragmatic aspects (see discussion in Akamatsu & Stewart, 1998). On the one hand, this approach might be one way to resolve the visual processing issues associated with the signed systems (discussed later). In addition, it might provide a bona fide avenue for improving English literacy skills, especially with respect to second-language principles (see Chapter 9 of this text). Nevertheless, unless there are natural grammatical rules for such incorporation (such as that exist between contact languages or pidgins), the haphazard incorporation of ASL-like features might become as problematic as the haphazard use of English signing, discussed previously.

The ensuing sections discuss a few of the signed systems, including the Rochester method and a form of signing that does not have a brand name but refers to the use of speaking and signing simultaneously. As stated previously, only a few major points are provided, and the presentation is based on the theoretical representation of the systems to the grammar of English— proceeding from most representative to least representative. The placement of the systems on a continuum from most to least is based on the nature and extent of their representation of a written English word. That is, the more a word is represented, the more the system is considered representative of English. Table 6-1 demonstrates how one word, *indescribable,* is represented by the

---

TABLE 6-1 Representation of *Indescribable* by Four Manual Systems

---

English sentence: *That is indescribable.*

Rochester method (finger spelling): Each letter is represented by a finger spelled hand shape.

Example: i-n-d-e-s-c-r-i-b-a-b-l-e

Signing exact English (SEE II): Two sign markers (*in-* and *-able*) and an initialized American Sign Language (ASL) sign meaning *explain, describe* are used to convey the message.

Example: IN- DESCRIBE -ABLE

Signed English (SE): The ASL sign for negation (*not*) is used along with the initialized sign for *describe* (same as SEE II).

Example: NOT DESCRIBE

English sign: There are probably several different ways to express this word. One common way is to use two ASL signs together. In the context of the sentence, the words, *can't explain,* is what the signer means.

Example: CAN'T EXPLAIN

Note: Adapted from Paul and Quigley (1990, p. 162). Underlined letters in SEE II and SE indicate that the finger-spelled hand shape is used for that sign.

manual aspects of four systems—Rochester method (i.e., finger spelling), signing exact English, signed English, and English signing. With this in mind, Figure 6-1 illustrates the placement of the various manual systems on a continuum from least to most representative of English (see Figure 6-1).

Within this contentious framework, the Rochester method is considered be most representative of written standard English. The least representative of the manual English codes has several labels that have caused considerable confusion in the research and scholarly literature. The term used in this text is *English signing* or *English sign* (in the second edition of this text, *English-based* or *English-like signing* was used). The other systems in between these two extremes that are discussed are seeing essential English, signing exact English, and signed English. Keep in mind that the descriptions of these systems

Signed Communication Approaches				
Least Representative of English		Most Representative of English		
•			•	
English signing	Signed English	SEE II	SEE I	RM

Note: English signing is also known as contact signing, conceptually accurate sign
English (C. A. S. E.), sign English, signed English, and pidgin sign English (archaic).
SEE I = seeing essential English
SEE II = signing exact English
RM = Rochester method

Figure 6-1 Relationships of Signed Communication Approaches to the Written Structure of Standard English.

are prototypic with respect to their stated rules for creating and using signs. The changes to the systems and the perception of them by deaf and hard-of-hearing students have become prominent research issues, which have led to major criticisms of the prototypes. A few studies are discussed in-depth because of the author's interest in them; in addition, they illustrate the typical manner in which research has been conducted to assess the effects of the system on the learning of English.

Finger Spelling and the Rochester Method

This section discusses research on the Rochester method and research on the finger spelling component only. In recent years, finger spelling has received increased interest because of its purported benefits for assisting deaf and hard-of-hearing children in learning English, particularly orthography and morphology (Grushkin, 1998a, 1998b; Padden, 1998a). It is considered the natural route for deaf students, particularly those who know ASL, for progressing through the stages of spelling and the alphabetic system, the system on which written English is based.

Finger spelling (dactylology) is a means of representing the alphabet and number system. Obviously, it is an integral part of the Rochester method; however, it is used for various purposes in all signed systems, including American Sign Language. In the United States, there are 23 distinct hand shapes that are used to represent the letters of the English alphabet (see Figure 6-2).

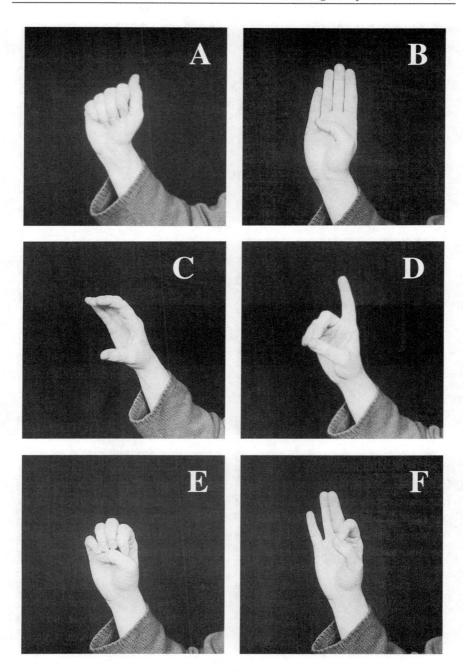

Figure 6-2 The Finger-Spelling Alphabet. *(continues)*

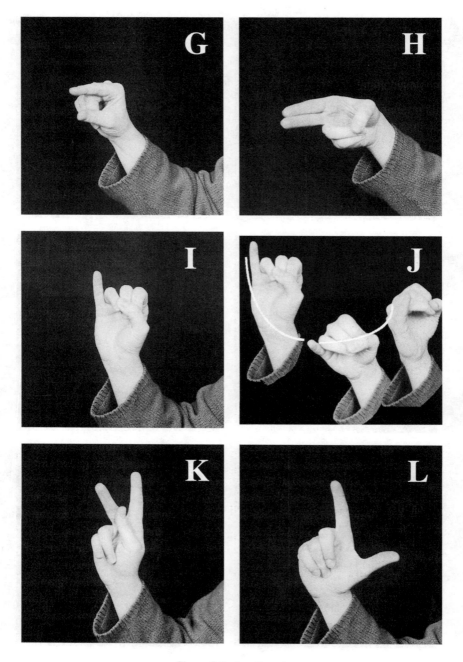

Figure 6-2 *(continues)*

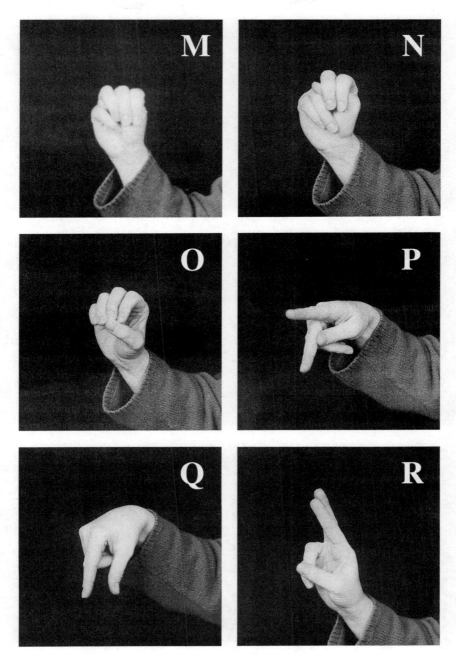

Figure 6-2 *(continues)*

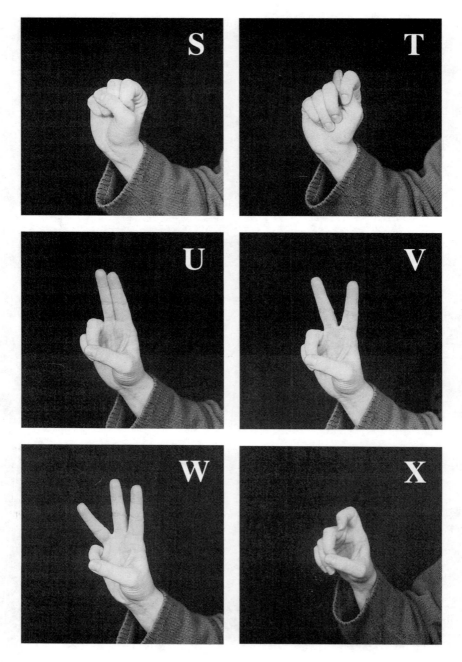

Figure 6-2 *(continues)*

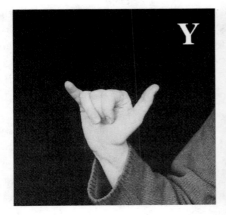
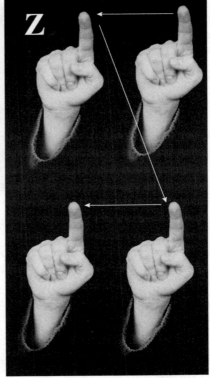

Figure 6-2

Three hand shapes in two different positions are used to represent a total of six letters (i and j; k and p; and g and q). Some countries (e.g., United States and France) use a one-hand alphabet that represent their respective writing system, whereas others (e.g., England and Australia) use a two-hand alphabet.

It should be emphasized that finger spelling is a code that represents the letters of the English writing system. There are obvious differences between finger spelling and writing, particularly in the areas of representation, presentation, and processing. Writing is permanent (i.e., captured and decontextualized) and reflects the alphabetic system in an agreed-on arbitrary manner. In English, writing is a reflection of the relations between phonemes and graphemes (e.g., orthography) (see Chapter 8). Readers can proceed at their own pace and reread whenever necessary. Finger spelling is typically transitory (it can, of course, be executed repeatedly) and represents conversations in contextualized situations (i.e., live and face-to-face). In one sense, finger spelling is similar to the Morse Code in that it is a representation of English letters with no direct relations to English phonology. Thus, when used in contextualized situations, the receiver is not cognizant of the various sounds that can be associated with the same letter in different words (e.g., b*a*t, b*a*ll, and g*a*ve) or the fact that some letters are affected by preceding or following letter/sounds (i.e., coarticulation).

Chapter 7 presents some evidence on the processing of finger spelling by deaf children of deaf parents. Only a few remarks are made here on the use of finger spelling by some young deaf children. In essence, the processing of finger spelling seems to be or might be different for deaf children of deaf parents as compared to that of deaf children of hearing parents. In any case, by age 3, young children are able to finger spell letters in a sequential manner, and subsequently, they begin to observe the relationship between finger spelling and the letters in print (see Padden, 1991). Wilbur (1987) stated that skilled finger spellers execute words as units, called movement envelopes, not as sequence of letters (also see Padden, 1998a; Padden & LeMaster, 1985). Thus, it is not uncommon to find that many finger spellers omit letters (i.e., finger-spelled hand shapes) during rapid delivery. The experienced finger speller can still comprehend the message due to the redundancy and contextualization of the conversations. In some cases, knowledge of the grammar of English is beneficial. Stuckless and Pollard (1977) argued that individuals must have a high-level proficiency in English to comprehend and produce advanced finger spelling of words, particularly if finger spelling alone is used predominantly or often. Learning finger spelling by itself, however, is not a normal learning situation because this requires a great deal of effort and training. As indicated previously, language learning is not dependent on formal training.

Research on the Rochester Method

Historically, the Rochester method originated at the Rochester School for the Deaf in New York during the late 1870s (Quigley, 1969; Scouten, 1967). In the Rochester method (RM), finger spelling and speech are used simultaneously. In Russia (previously the Soviet Union), this method has been called *Neooralism,* indicating that initially, finger spelling was used to supplement oral approaches in teaching deaf and hard-of-hearing children and adolescents (see discussion in Moores, 1987, 1996).

During the 1950s and 1960s, the Rochester method was widely used in special education programs for deaf and hard-of-hearing students (Quigley, 1969). By the late 1970s, however, it was present in only a few programs, particularly at the secondary educational level (Jordan, Gustason, & Rosen, 1979; Jordan & Karchmer, 1986). Finger spelling by itself is now used mostly as a supplement in the various signed systems (see readable discussions in Marschark, 1997; Moores, 1996; Stewart & Luetke-Stahlman, 1998).

Quigley (1969) conducted a major study of the effectiveness of the Rochester method. He examined the performance of deaf students (i.e., with profound hearing impairment) from nine residential schools in the United States. In this longitudinal research project, Quigley reported that students exposed to the Rochester method performed better than those exposed to simultaneous communication on selected language-related subtests (e.g., vocabulary and reading) of the Stanford Achievement Test (SAT). Nevertheless, this researcher also documented that the reading level of average 18-year-old students with hearing impairment was approximately seven grades below that of their hearing peers. With respect to young preschool children, students taught with the RM performed better in reading (on the SAT) and on measures of written language (writing ability) than students taught with oral methods in these schools. This latter finding was confirmed in a later study by Moores, Weiss, and Goodwin (1978). Moores et al. found that students exposed to RM performed better than those in either oral or TC (i.e., simultaneous communication) programs.

Research on Finger Spelling: Selected Studies

Stuckless and Pollard (1977) examined the ability of college-age deaf students to process both print and finger spelling. They reported that the processing ability of students was strongly related to their level of English competence. In addition, it was noted that print was easier to process than finger spelling. This might be due to the permanent nature of print; in fact, this finding has been confirmed in other studies that compared print with the language/communication approaches such as English signing and other signed systems (see reviews in Moores, 1987; Quigley & Kretschmer, 1982).

Looney and Rose (1979) demonstrated that finger spelling can be used as an effective aid in teaching certain English morphemes such as *-ed* and *-er*. Twenty-four prelingually deaf students, age 8 to 15 years, participated as subjects. After demonstrating the ability to express through writing and finger spelling a few basic English kernel patterns (e.g., *The boy is happy* and *The girl walked down the hall*), the subjects were randomly assigned to three groups. One group was exposed to the Rochester method, another to print, and the third group was the control group. The two treatment groups were exposed to a systematic, 4-week instruction of selected morphological rules, that is, those involving past tense inflectional suffixes (e.g., *-ed*) (see Chapter 2). The researchers administered pre- and posttests to assess the students' ability to recognize, select, determine grammaticality, and produce the appropriate past tense morphemes.

The results indicated that both treatment groups made significant gains, whereas the control group failed to demonstrate such a trend. In addition, no significant differences were reported between the two treatment groups. This led the researchers to conclude that finger spelling as well as print are useful in representing inflectional suffixes when taught in a systematic manner. It was also noted that maximum benefits resulted when students have some understanding of basic English sentence patterns. Finally, the researchers emphasized that it is important to provide systematic and consistent instruction over a period of time.

The manner in which finger spelling is used in the classroom has been the subject of a few studies. An early classic study documented the fact that practitioners are not using finger spelling in a systematic consistent manner (Reich & Bick, 1977). In an interesting update on this early study, Akamatsu and Stewart (1989) investigated the use of finger spelling by five trained teachers of deaf students. They found that these teachers did not frequently employ finger spelling in several situations. For example, when finger spelling was used, it was primarily for the purpose of conveying a specific English word. The clarity of finger spelling use varied with the intent of finger spelling, that is, to use or teach a specific English word. Nevertheless, the findings on the clarity issue motivated the answer to one of the researchers' important questions:

What are deaf children expected to do with the finger spelled words of their teachers? They are expected to learn English words and their spellings, to recognize the words in print, and to write them correctly. How they can learn all this in the relative absence of clear and accurate finger spelling models is still an open question. (Akamatsu & Stewart, 1989, p. 369)

The role and importance of finger spelling for the development of rapid word identification skills needs further study. For example, it has been reported that some good deaf readers use both finger spelling and a phonological code for the temporary retention of linguistic stimuli in short-term memory (Hanson, Liberman, & Shankweiler, 1984; also see the reviews in Hanson, 1989; Paul &

Jackson, 1993). There seems to be little evidence that poor readers predominantly used either finger spelling (i.e., beyond the mere copying of words letter by letter) and/or a phonological code.

It has been argued that development in finger spelling correlates with the developmental progression in written language, that is, proceeding from holistic (logographic) to analytic (orthographic) processing (see Grushkin, 1998a, 1998b; Padden, 1991, 1998a). The interplay of ASL and finger spelling in deaf children's writing development (Padden, 1998a) is covered in Chapter 7.

As discussed previously, the connection between finger spelling and print is not made until the child is about 3 years old, and many deaf children (up to 11 years old) are often surprised to discover this connection (Hirsh-Pasek & Freyd, 1983a, 1983b). It has been suggested that finger spelling might be a useful mechanism for assisting deaf children in recognizing or learning about words in print (Hirsh-Pasek, 1987). This requires a conscious effort on part of teachers, and it might be possible to increase deaf students' recognition of printed words to match their finger-spelled vocabulary. This is assuming, of course, that finger-spelled words reflect or are analogous to word identification skills, not merely a copying of the letters of the word in a letter-by-letter fashion. There are a number of studies and reviews that have documented the fact that deaf students are aware of the orthographic and morphological systems of English, particularly with the assistance of finger spelling (Hirsh-Pasek, 1986, 1987; Hirsh-Pasek & Freyd, 1983a, 1983b, 1984). Whether it is possible to learn about English orthography or at least to advance to a higher, mature level is debatable in light of the strong interrelations among phonology, morphology, and orthography. Some scholars, notably Adams (1990, 1994), do not believe that orthography can be taught but must be experienced and learned via the ongoing act of reading. It might be possible for deaf and hard-of-hearing children and adolescents to perform this feat via the use of finger spelling and engaged reading activities. Some scholars have argued that finger spelling, due to its visual properties and connection to print, is one of the best routes to take to assist in the growth of literacy skills, especially in the context of ASL/English bilingual-bicultural programs (Grushkin, 1998a, 1998b; Padden, 1991, 1998a).

Table 6-2 presents a summary of the major research findings and a few remarks about finger spelling.

TABLE 6-2 Summary of Findings of Selected Studies for Finger Spelling and General Remarks

Research Findings on Rochester Method (RM)/Finger Spelling

Study	Findings
Quigley (1969)	The average 18-year-old student exposed to RM was reading at about the fifth-grade level. Quigley remarked that finger spelling (or rather, the Rochester method) is not a panacea.
Stuckless & Pollard (1977)	The processing ability of deaf students was strongly related to their level of English competence. They noted that print was easier to process than finger spelling. This might be due to the permanence of print.
Looney & Rose (1979)	Finger spelling can be used as an effective aid in teaching certain English morphemes such as -ed and -er. To observe the benefits, there is a need for strong systematic instruction over a period of time.
Akamatsu & Stewart (1989)	The clarity of finger-spelling use varied with the intent of finger spelling, that is, how it is used to teach an English word. Researchers argued that there needs to be additional research on how deaf children learn to finger spell in the absence of clear, complete teacher models.

General Remarks

- The Rochester method is the use of finger spelling and speech simultaneously.

- Finger spelling is a code that represents the letters of the English alphabet; however, there are differences between finger spelling and English writing.

- The processing of finger spelling of deaf children of deaf parents might be different than that of deaf children of hearing parents.

- Skilled finger spellers perceive and execute words as units called *movement envelopes.*

- It is not uncommon to discover that many skilled finger spellers omit letters during rapid delivery. This does not seem to affect the comprehension of the message by the receiver due to the redundancy and contextualization of the conversations.

The SEE Systems: Seeing Essential English and Signing Exact English

The SEE systems refer to two signed systems: seeing essential English (SEE1) (Anthony, 1966) and signing exact English (SEE2) (Gustason et al., 1980; Gustason & Zawolkow, 1993). Because of the overlap in sign-formation principles and historical background, it is feasible to discuss the two systems together. SEE II is covered in greater detail because of the widespread use of its signs (Gallaudet Research Institute, 1985; Jordan & Karchmer, 1986) or, perhaps, the system as a whole (Stewart & Luetke-Stahlman, 1998).

A group of professionals, parents, teachers, and administrators met in California in 1969 to discuss the problem of representing English manually, as described next:

> *The main concern of the original group was the consistent, logical, rational, and practical development of signs to represent as specifically as possible the basic essentials of the English language. This concern sprang from the experience of all present with the poor English skills of many deaf students, and the desire for an easier, more successful way of developing mastery of English in a far greater number of such students. (Gustason et al., 1980, p. ix)*

This meeting resulted in three signed systems, which were originally similar but now are different: SEE I, SEE II, and linguistics of visual English (Wampler, 1972). Two of the 10 tenets agreed on by these members were:

- "Any specific sign should mean one thing, and one thing only, and

- English should be signed as it is spoken. This is especially true of idioms." (Gustason, 1983, p. 41; cf., Gustason, 1990)

Both SEE systems categorize English words into three broad groups: basic (e.g., *girl*), compound (e.g., *butterfly*), and complex (e.g., *runs*). Basic words may be whole or complete words (e.g., *girl* and *the*) or bound roots, as in *hospice* in *hospital*. Compound words are two or more basic words put together, as in *butterfly* and *understand*. Complex words are basic words with inflections (e.g., -*ing*) and affixes (e.g., *un*- and -*ness*), as in *walked, girls, unhappy,* and *sadness*. The selection or use of a sign to represent a word and its parts is based on a two-out-of-three rule involving sound, spelling, and meaning. Consider the word *run* in the following sentences.

1. The girl hit a home *run.*
2. There is a *run* in my stocking.
3. I like to walk not *run.*

The same sign is used for run in all three sentences because two of the three criteria are met: sound and spelling. This situation is similar for many English words with multiple meanings. Additional signs function as sign markers and correspond to the morphological aspects of the words, that is, inflections and affixes. For example, in the word *slowly,* the root, or base word, is *slow,* and the suffix marker is -*ly.* Some examples of SEE II sign markers are illustrated in Figure 6-3. There are 74 invented sign markers in SEE II (Stewart & Luetke-Stahlman, 1998).

One of the major differences between the two SEE systems is their treatment of a basic word. This difference results in the use of more invented sign markers for SEE I as well as more signs to represent a word. In addition, in SEE II, not all the affixes need to be executed by a sign marker. For example, it is permissible to drop a middle affix (i.e., use no sign) in a multiple-affix word if this does not result in ambiguity, a loss of meaning or understanding. As remarked by Stewart and Luetke-Stahlman (1998):

> *The word* examination *is signed EXAM + -tion without the sign marker* -ine *(as in EXAM + -ine) because there is no such word as* examtion. *It is expected that the person watching the signing will be able to fill in the missing part of the word. This, of course, assumes that the person is already familiar with the correct English word. For very young deaf children or for those who are just learning English, the forms of words that are signed without all their affixes have to be taught.*
>
> *Where dropping an affix would create ambiguity in meaning, the affix is retained.* Developments, *for example, is signed DEVELOP + -ment + -s to distinguish it from the sign for* develops *(DEVELOP + -s). (p. 88)*

Another major difference between the SEE systems is in the use of ASL-like signs. As much as possible, SEE II incorporates an ASL sign if it translates into only one English word. This principle applies to words in any of the three groups, that is, basic, compound, or complex. Thus, ASL signs are used to represent words such as *baseball, can't,* and *careless.* (Some ASL signs, such as the one used for *careless,* may have multiple English meanings or interpretations, e.g., not careful, not diligent, etc.)

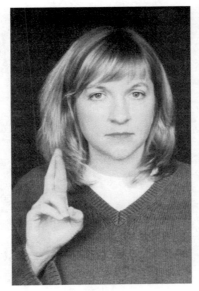

–er, –ar, –or

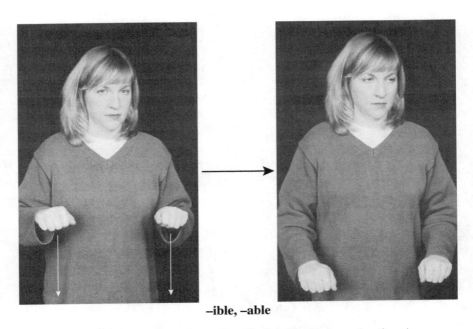

–ible, –able

Figure 6-3 Examples of Signing Exact English Sign Markers. *(continues)*

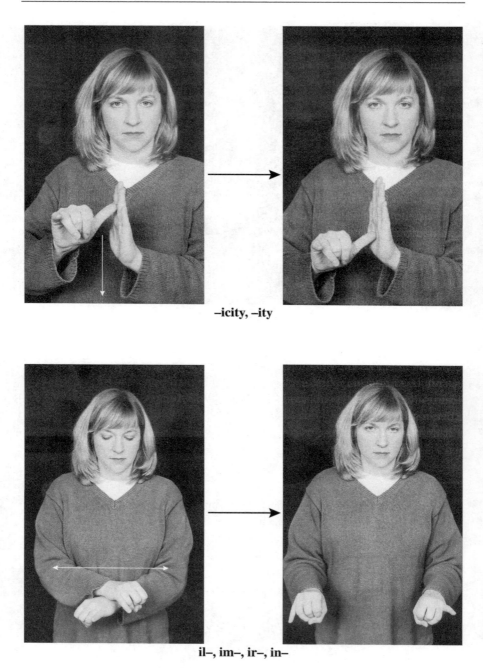

–icity, –ity

il–, im–, ir–, in–

Figure 6-3 *(continues)*

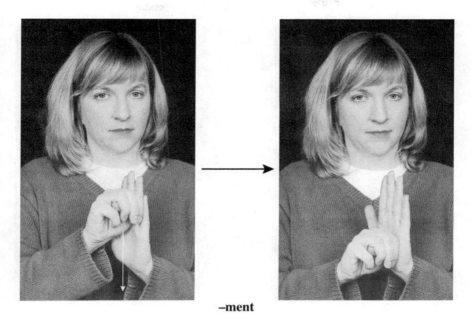

−ment

Figure 6-3

In sum, some of the major principles for SEE II are as follows (Gustason et al., 1980, pp. xiii–xiv; cf. Gustason & Zawolkow, 1993; Stewart & Luetke-Stahlman, 1998).

1. *English should be signed in a manner that is as consistent as possible with how it is spoken or written in order to constitute a language input for the deaf child that will result in his mastery of English.*
2. *A sign should be translatable to only one English equivalent.*
3. *When the first letter is added to a basic sign to create synonyms, the basic sign is retained wherever possible as the most commonly used word (e.g., basic sign for MAKE is retained whereas the sign is made with C-hands for CREATE and P-hands for PRODUCE [see Figure 6-4].*
4. *When more than one marker is added to a word, middle markers may be dropped if there is no sacrifice of clarity (e.g., the past tense sign is added to BREAK to produce BROKE, but BROKEN may be signed as BREAK plus the past participle or -EN).*
5. *While following [these] principles, respect needs to be shown for characteristics of visual-gestural communication.*

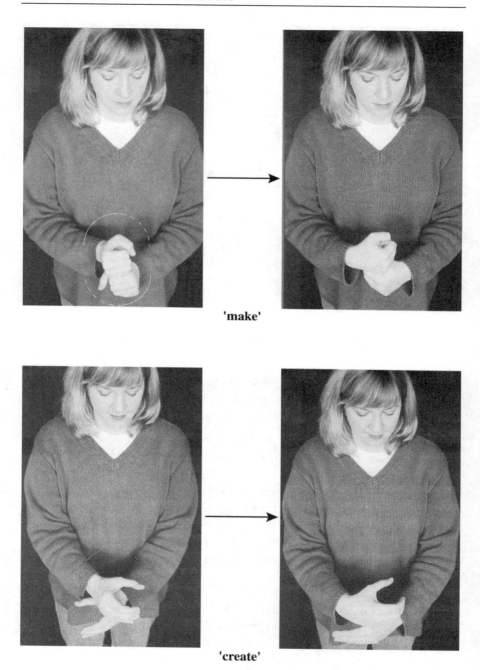

'make'

'create'

Figure 6-4 Signing Exact English Signs: MAKE, CREATE, and PRODUCE. *(continues)*

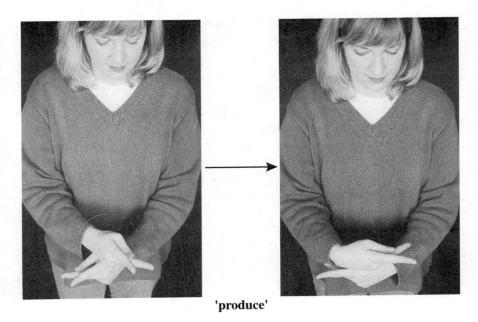

'produce'

Figure 6-4

Finally, Gustason et al. (1980; cf. Gustason & Zawolkow, 1993; Stewart & Luetke-Stahlman, 1998) also listed suggestions for the development of new signs, that is, signs for English words that are not contained in the SEE II dictionary:

1. *Seek an existing sign. Check other sign language texts. Ask skilled signers in your community, especially deaf native signers.*
2. *Modify an existing sign with a similar or related meaning. Generally, this means adding the first letter of the word to a basic sign.*
3. *Consider finger spelling. This depends, of course, on the age and perceptual abilities of the child, and the length and frequency of use of the word in question.*
4. *If all else fails, and you must invent, try to stay as close as possible to ASL principles. (p. xv)*

An in-depth treatment of the manner in which SEE II (Gustason et al., 1980) handles the pronouns and verbs of English as well as the formation of new words can be found in Wilbur (1987).

Research on Seeing Essential English

H. Schlesinger and Meadow (1972) described the primary language acquisition of four deaf children. Three of their subjects were exposed to at least some SEE I signs. The beginning of these subjects' exposure to SEE I ranged from 15 months to 3 years of age. Fairly substantial development was observed in both syntax and vocabulary, and some support was found for Bloom's (1970) two-word syntactic-semantic relations. The data on one subject were analyzed with respect to the pivot-grammar proposed by Braine (1963a, 1963b), the counterfindings on pivot-grammar argued by Brown (1973), and the semantic relations proposed by Bloom (1970). It was reported that the bulk of the data supported Brown's arguments against pivot-grammar. In addition, the use of two-word/sign utterances by this subject seemed to support Bloom's contention that such utterances tend to expose a variety of structural meanings in relation to the surrounding content cues. For example, this subject signed/spoke: *Daddy shoe.* This is an example of the agent-object relation in which the subject is attempting to tell her father to remove his shoes and get into the sandbox with her.

The data on another subject focus on the acquisition of some English morphological rules. It was found that this subject, exposed to SEE I markers at age 3, began to use the markers by age 4. In sum, on the basis of spontaneous language samples and tests of grammatical competence (Menyuk, 1963), it was concluded that these deaf children were acquiring grammatical competence in the same sequence as hearing children; however, the rate of development was slower.

Raffin and his associates (Gilman, Davis, & Raffin, 1980; Raffin, 1976; Raffin, Davis, & Gilman, 1978) focused on the use of SEE I markers by students, especially sign markers representing some of the most common English morphemes such as -s (plurality and third-person singular), -ly (adverb), -er (comparison), and -ed (past tense). The findings indicated that the order of acquisition of the markers of students with hearing impairment was qualitatively similar to the acquisition order of hearing students (Brown, 1973). In other words, students with hearing impairment proceeded through developmental stages at a slower rate than and produce errors similar to those of younger hearing students. It was also observed that the acquisition and use of the SEE I markers were influenced pervasively by teachers' use of the markers. That is, the more systematic and consistent teachers were in using the sign markers, the more likely students were to acquire and use them.

In a more recent investigation, Washburn (1983) discussed the educational achievement results of students in three public school districts who had been exposed to seeing essential English. Based on an analysis of scores from 1977 to 1981, the researcher stated that the average reading grade levels of SEE I students were from one to two grades higher than those of other students with hearing impairment in other programs. In addition, the SEE I students in grades 11 and 12 of one program scored in the top 20% of all hearing high school students taking the reading comprehension subset of the Stanford Achievement Test. The mean reading level of the top group was slightly above the seventh grade. Experimental research, however, is needed to determine if the use of SEE I actually leads to or causes a higher difference in scores for students exposed to this method.

In the research by Luetke-Stahlman (1988a), students exposed to SEE I were considered to be in a group that had been exposed to a system that was a fairly complete representation of the structure of English. This type of exposure was deemed to be responsible for their performance on the battery of tests in this study (this study is discussed in detail in "Research on Signing Exact English").

The results confirmed the findings of an earlier study by Deal and Thornton (1985); however Deal and Thornton argued that much more research is needed on the assumptions of the so-called more complete signed systems. These researchers investigated the comprehension level of deaf students who were exposed to stories via the use of SEE I and sign English (a synonym for English signing or the archaic, contentious pidgin sign English). Although the results indicated that the SEE I trained students outperformed the sign-English-trained students, "the overall comprehension scores for both groups was less than or equal to 50%" (p. 275). Washburn (1983) also remarked that "the use of SEE [I] is not a panacea, not the 'answer' to the vexing problem of providing English for the deaf youngster" (p. 29).

Research on Signing Exact English

As mentioned previously, the signs from the lexicon of signing exact English are widely used, perhaps the most widely used of all signed systems. Numerous educational materials are also available on the use of SEE II (Gustason, 1983; Stewart & Luetke-Stahlman, 1998). The two classic studies to be discussed are Babb (1979) and Luetke-Stahlman (1988a).

Babb (1979) examined the performance of students with profound hearing impairment who had been exposed to SEE II. Half of the students were taught by SEE II in the school only. The other half were exposed to this system in the home and also at school. Babb compared the performance of the two groups on subtests of an achievement test, on a test of receptive knowledge of certain syntactic structures, and measures of written language (i.e., assessing their ability to write sentences, etc.). In addition, the results of these groups were compared to those of the groups in the Brasel and Quigley (1977) study and to the scores from a national survey of academic achievement of hearing-impaired students (DiFrancesca, 1972).

Deaf students exposed to signing exact English in the home and school environment performed significantly better than did those students exposed to SEE II only in school. This seems to provide further support for the importance of the home environment for educational achievement. In addition, the achievement scores of the home-plus-school group were higher than those of a national sample of students with hearing impairment.

It is interesting to note that the home-plus-school group performed as well as the best group in the Brasel and Quigley (1977) study in which students were probably exposed to signed English (i.e., simultaneous communication or the archaic pidgin sign English [PSE]). Signing exact English appears to be more representative of the structure of English than is English signing (archaic PSE). It follows, then, that students exposed to SEE II should perform better than those students exposed to English signing on English-based achievement and diagnostic tests. Why this was not the case in the study by Babb (1979) is not clear. It is possible that the parents and teachers using SEE II had problems adhering to the principles of the system in forming and producing signs. Practitioners sometimes omit signs or sign markers because of the cumbersome nature of some signed systems or the difficulty in signing and speaking simultaneously (Marmor & Pettito, 1979; Strong & Charlson, 1987). It might also be possible that there are visual constraints on the perception of these systems by deaf children, some of whom seem to alter the signs when producing them. This issue is discussed in-depth later in the chapter.

With respect to use, Luetke-Stahlman (1988b) reported that some teachers can use SEE II consistently and systematically. Furthermore, students exposed to this system perform well on literacy measures. For example, Luetke-Stahlman (1988a) examined the performance of students, age 5 to 12 years, who were enrolled in public, private, and residential schools. Several variables were statistically controlled, for example, age and aided and unaided hearing acuity. Students with hearing impairment in one group had been exposed to oral English, cued speech, SEE I, SEE II, and American Sign Language. The other group had been exposed to signed/manual English and PSE. The literacy battery consisted of tests involving passage comprehension (using a cloze procedure in which every nth [third, fourth, fifth, etc.] word is deleted, as in *The boy hit ____ ball*), vocabulary, and syntax. In general, the results indicated that students exposed to SEE II (as well as oral English and cued speech/language, SEE I, and ASL) performed significantly better than the other group (i.e., signed/manual English and PSE) on six of the seven measures used. Luetke-Stahlman (1988a) argued that the:

> *Results of the study indicate that students exposed to instructional inputs that are either languages (English or ASL) or systems that attempt to completely encode spoken English tend to score higher on selected tests of achievement than do students exposed to input that does not correspond as highly to English. (p. 359)*

The findings that some deaf and hard-of-hearing students exposed to SEE II (or other complete manual codes) can acquire a few complex grammatical aspects of the English language (e.g., morphology and syntax) and may become good readers have been supported by some recent scholarly works (Gaustad, 1986; Luetke-Stahlman & Milburn, 1996; Schick & Moeller, 1992). Some possible reasons for this success and whether it can really be attributed to the use of a particular signed system, such as SEE II, are discussed in the last section of the chapter.

Table 6-3 presents a summary of some major research findings as well as a few remarks on the SEE systems, particularly SEE II.

TABLE 6-3 Synopsis of Major Research Findings on the Seeing Essential English (SEE I) and Signing Exact English (SEE II) Systems and General Remarks

---

Research Findings on Seeing Essential English (SEE I)

Study	Findings
Schlesinger & Meadow (1972)	It was concluded that deaf children were acquiring English grammatical competence in the same sequence as hearing children; however, the rate of development was slower.
Gilman, Davis, & Raffin (1980); Raffin (1976); Raffin, Davis, & Gilman (1978)	The acquisition and use of the SEE I markers were influenced pervasively by teachers' use of the markers. The more systematic and consistent teachers were in using the sign markers, the

(continues)

(Table 6-3 continued)

	more likely students were to acquire and use them.
Washburn (1983)	SEE I students in grades 11 and 12 of one program scored in the top 20% of all hearing high school students taking a reading comprehension subtest of the Stanford Achievement Test.
Deal & Thornton (1985)	The results indicated that the SEE I-trained students outperformed the sign-English-trained students; however, the overall comprehension scores of both groups were less than or equal to 50%.

Research Findings on Signing Exact English (SEE II)

Babb (1979)	Results indicated that the group exposed to SEE II in the home and at school performed significantly better than the group exposed to SEE II at school only.
Luetke-Stahlman (1988a)	Results indicated that students exposed to SEE II performed significantly better than students exposed to signed/manual English or pidgin signed English on six of the seven measures used. It was concluded that good results are often associated with systems that adequately represent English (see Chapter 5 for another view on this research study).

General Remarks

- The SEE systems refer to two signed systems: seeing essential English and signing exact English.
- Both SEE systems categorize English words into three broad groups: basic, compound, and complex.

- One major difference between the two SEE systems is the treatment of a basic word. This difference results in the use of more invented sign markers for SEE I as well as more signs to represent a word.

- Another major difference between the two systems is the use of American Sign Language (ASL) signs. It seems that SEE II incorporates more ASL signs (i.e., ASL-like signs) than does SEE I.

- SEE II seems to be the more widely used of the two SEE systems and one of the most widely used signed system in educational programs. However, it is suspected that the signs of SEE II are widely used, not the system per se.

Signed English: Description

The rationale for signed English (SE) is somewhat similar to the other systems discussed previously. According to Bornstein and his colleagues:

> *Signed English is a reasonable manual parallel to English. It is an educational tool meant to be used while you speak and thereby help you communicate with deaf children.*
>
> *Here is the basic reason for developing a manual system parallel to speech: Deaf children must depend on what they see to understand what others say to them. (Bornstein et al., 1983, p. 2)*

Similar to the other systems, there are two groups of signs in SE: sign words and sign markers. The SE dictionary contains 3,100 sign words (also see Stewart & Luetke-Stahlman, 1998). The words were compiled from lists of typical children's spoken language and from vocabulary lists used by young deaf children in homes and classrooms. A number of signs are ASL-like signs; however, there are signs that are invented and signs that are borrowed from other signed systems (Stewart & Luetke-Stahlman, 1998; Wilbur, 1987).

In general, the use of a sign is based on its entry (i.e., bold-face type) in a dictionary of standard English (no specific dictionary is mentioned). Bornstein et al. (1983) remarked that there are exceptions due to (a) numerous English multimeaning words with several lexical entries and (b) disagreements among lexicographers on what constitutes a lexical entry and what meanings should be included in a specific lexical entry.

The 14 sign markers represent the most common inflectional and derivational morphemes in the language of typical young children. Figure 6-5 illustrates the SE markers.

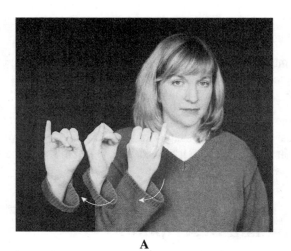

A

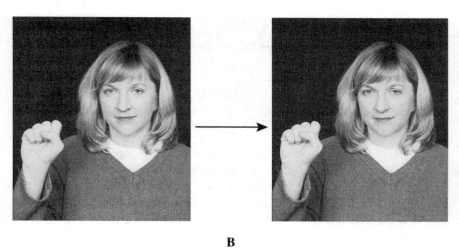

B

Figure 6-5 Signed English Sign Markers. *(continues)*
    Note: A: verb form: -ing as in
                playing.
          B: possessive: 's as in dog's.

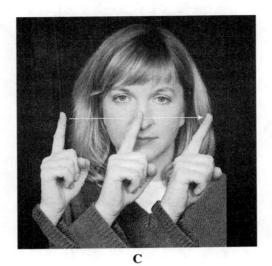

Figure 6-5 *(continues)*

Note: C: irregular plural nouns
(sign the word twice)—
example: mice.
D: adverb: -ly as in happily.

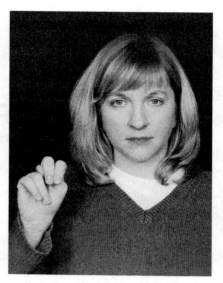

E

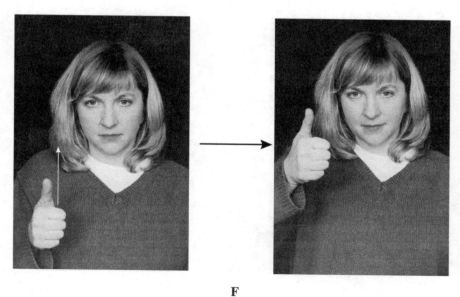

F

Figure 6-5 *(continues)*
Note: E: participle as in gone.
F: comparative: -er as in smarter.

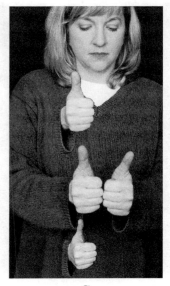

G

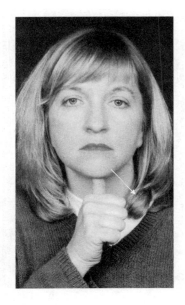 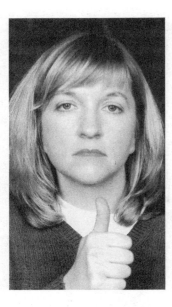

H

Figure 6-5 *(continues)*

Note: G: superlative: -est as in tallest.
H: opposite of: un-, im-, in-, etc.
as in unhappy, impatient, etc.

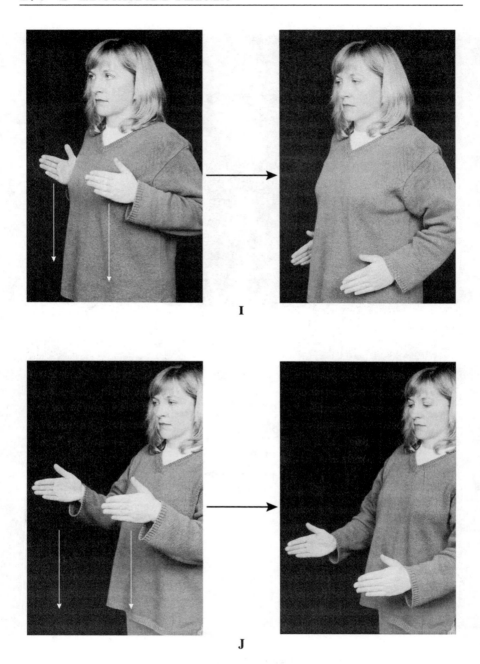

Figure 6-5 *(continues)*
Note: I: agent sign for person as in teacher.
J: agent sign for thing as in washer.

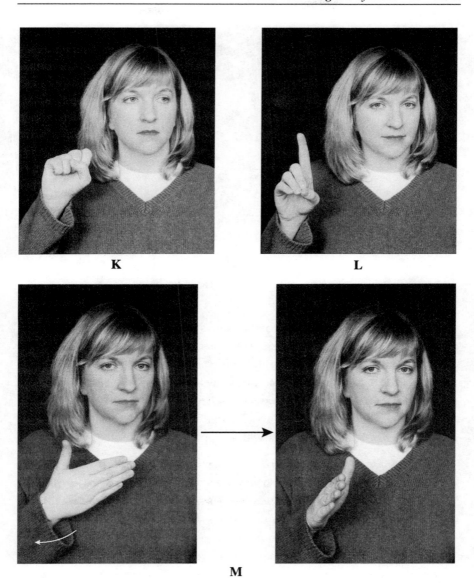

Figure 6-5 *(continues)*

Note: K: regular plural nouns: -s as in cats;
3rd person singular: -s as in writes.
L: regular past verbs: -ed as in learned.
M: irregular pat verbs as in saw.

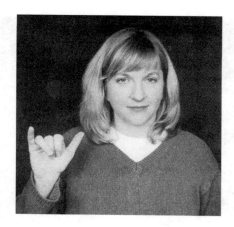

N

Figure 6-5
Note: N: adjective: -y as in cloudy.
Source: Bornstein et al. (1983).

The inclusion of only a few markers was to ensure that parents, teachers, and students learn to use the system and use it well. The creators felt that the other systems were too cumbersome and were not likely to be learned effectively (Bornstein, 1990). SE is used mostly with young deaf children; however, it is also used with older children as well (see Stewart & Luetke-Stahlman, 1998).

SE is executed in an English word order, that is, paralleling the exact spoken utterances. Some basic rules with exceptions include:

One sign for each English word: There are a number of phrases, proper nouns, and compounds, of two or more words, in this dictionary which are represented by a single sign word. These exceptions are, for the most part, ideographic, unambiguous ASL signs. Some examples are: after a while, of course, Santa Claus . . . *and* yo-yo.

One sign word for a separate English dictionary entry: There are two or more signs for a number of single English dictionary entries such as back, blind, brush, fall, glass, right, watch. *The various signs represent different meanings of the same English word. For example, the noun* fall *and the verb* fall *are etymologically related; however, the common and well-established signs for these words are too ideographic to be used interchangeably. Thus the two words will be represented by two different sign entries.*

> *One sign word plus one sign marker: Because the use of the agent marker does not preclude a noun form further assuming a plural or possessive form, we permit the use of two sign markers in this one instance; for example, work + agent + plural, or speak + agent + possessive. (Bornstein et al., 1983, p. 8)*

Research on Signed English

Several studies have been conducted on the effects of signed English on the development of English language skills. Bornstein, the creator of SE, and his associates explored the effects of signed English on primary language development in English (Bornstein, Saulnier, & Hamilton, 1980; Bornstein & Saulnier, 1981). They conducted a longitudinal study of 18 students with severe to profound hearing impairment enrolled in residential and day schools.

After 4 years, the researchers reported the growth in receptive and expressive skills of vocabulary and syntax. Similar to the findings of previous studies, the results show that students proceed through developmental stages similar to those of younger hearing children. As expected, the rate of development of the deaf and hard-of-hearing students was markedly slower. For example, it was reported that the vocabulary growth was half of that observed in the average hearing student. Specifically, the English language expressive abilities of the 9-year-old deaf and hard-of-hearing students were found to be equivalent to those of 3- to 4-year-old children with typical hearing.

In a follow-up investigation 1 year later, Bornstein and Saulnier (1981) focused on the students' use of the 14 signed English markers. Compared to SEE I and SEE II, signed English has very few morphological markers. The results, however, showed that most students do not use the markers consistently or systematically. In fact, even after 5 years of exposure, the students were using only half of the 14 SE sign markers.

The findings of Bornstein and his collaborators seem to question whether English morphological structures can be represented manually with contrived signs. It may also be that the students understand the concepts of past tense (as in *walked*) or present progressive (as in *I am running*) but are expressing these concepts in other ways. For example, the students may prefer to express their understanding of a sentence, question, or story by using ASL, ASL-like signs, or signs that reflect the visual and motor properties of typical signed languages (Maxwell, 1983; Stewart, 1985; Supalla, 1986, 1991). It appears that many students have not learned or internalized the rules of English morphology. Thus, they are not able to express these rules by using symbols that represent them. On the other hand, the argument has been advanced that the signed systems are incompatible with the visual and manual mechanisms of individuals who are predominantly dependent on sign for communication purposes.

In a more recent study, Gardner and Zorfass (1983) examined the oral language development of a 3-year-old child with a severe hearing impairment. The child was exposed to SE from the age of 13 months. As the oral development (i.e., speech) of the child increased, the use of signs or sign markers decreased. The child benefitted enormously from the use of amplification. This indicated that audition was the primary mode of receiving communication, rather than vision, which is not the case for most students with severe to profound hearing impairment. The results of this case study provide further support for the importance and relevance of audition in the development of spoken language skills such as speech and speechreading.

There is some evidence that the placement of SE signs above words impacts positively the reading comprehension scores of deaf students (Robbins, 1983; also see the discussion in King & Quigley, 1985). Other research has shown that this technique can be used to improve students' word identification skills (Stoefen-Fisher & Lee, 1989). These positive results should be interpreted with caution because SE does not deal with complex English words, that is, words that involve markers not included in the system. The limitations of the system relative to advanced literacy skills has been demonstrated by the work of Luetke-Stahlman (1988a). Finally, there are problems in using signs in the printed form, especially for the purpose of reading. It was remarked:

> *One problem the authors have struggled with is that they can follow the left-to-right convention for writing words in sequence but cannot use that convention for sequencing of sign actions within words; e.g., a right-handed sign that moves from the mouth to the ear moves backward and slightly to the right; the reverse image illustrated (as one would see the signer) shows the sign moving to the signer's right, which means it moves to the reader's left. This right-to-left movement disrupts the left-to-right sequence of standard print. Such backtracking could lead to omissions of the final parts of signs or to the reversal of two parts. (Maxwell, 1987, pp. 345–346)*

In essence, it should be noted that the overall results of the use of the SE system have not met the expectations of its creator (see Bornstein, 1982). This has led to a modification of the theory of using SE (Bornstein, 1982); that is, Bornstein felt that the structure of English does not need to be completely represented all or even most of the time. In addition, the completeness of this representation becomes less critical as the individual becomes older. These statements seem to be relevant but only for those deaf and hard-of-hearing students who have a fairly good command of English and can infer the missing elements. In addition, as argued by Stewart and Luetke-Stahlman (1998), it is most critical to teach/expose deaf and hard-of-hearing children to those English structures not represented by signed English or any signed system because these structures cannot be derived or inferred without a reasonable proficiency in English. Theoretical debates aside, there is no compelling evidence that many individuals who are deaf or hard of hearing have acquired a high level of competency in either the performance or script-literacy mode of English via the use of signed English.

Table 6-4 provides a summary of major research findings as well as a few general remarks on signed English.

TABLE 6-4 Summary of Research Findings on Signed English (SE) and General Remarks

---

Research Findings on Signed English

Study	Findings
Bornstein, Saulnier, & Hamilton: (1980); Bornstein & Saulnier (1981)	Analyzing the students' use of the SE markers over a 5-year period, it was found that very few students were using the markers consistently. In fact, even after 5 years of exposure, the students were using only half of the 14 SE sign markers.
Bornstein (1982)	The completeness of representing English structure becomes less critical as the deaf individual becomes older. That is, it is argued that it is not necessary for English to be represented completely for older students (i.e., adolescents).
Gardner & Zorfass (1983)	Results of this case study provide further support for the importance of audition in the development of spoken language skills such as speech and speechreading.
Robbins (1983)	Placement of SE signs above words positively impacted reading comprehension of deaf students.

(continues)

(Table 6-4 continued)

General Remarks

- Similar to the other signed systems, there are two groups of signs in SE— sign words and sign markers.

- With respect to the sign words, there are 3,100 signs. The 14 sign markers represent the most common inflectional and derivational morphemes in the language of typical young children.

- In addition to signing exact English, signed English is used widely in educational programs, especially with young children.

- Signed English should not be confused with sign English or signed English, both of which are often associated with English sign or signing. These two terms do not have a set of rules for producing signs and do not utilize 14 sign markers consistently and systematically, as mandated by Bornstein's system—signed English.

- Despite the appeal of placing SE signs above words in children's books, there are several problems with this approach due to the left-to-right conventions associated with reading English (e.g., image of signs is reversed—as one would see the signer).

English Signing: Description

It is extremely difficult to describe systematically and completely much of the signing that occurs in Total Communication classrooms. Traditionally, this type of simultaneous communication has been labeled *pidgin sign English,* a phrase still used in the research literature (see Marschark, 1997) although it is not technically accurate (see Cokely, 1983; Paul & Jackson, 1993; Stewart & Luetke-Stahlman, 1998). This type of signing, labeled *English signing* in this text, may entail the use of a few contrived sign markers (e.g., *-ing* and *-ed*) or perhaps no markers at all. This description is even applicable to individuals who are deaf and who attempt to sign to persons who are hearing and who do not know ASL. As with the signing of individuals who are hearing, there are variations in the signing of individuals who are deaf. However, it is likely that the signing of individuals who are deaf, especially those with a limited knowledge of English, contains a number of ASL-like grammatical aspects. It is possible that the sign order (syntax) may also vary depending on whether a person knows ASL and/or English; however, English word order is typically followed.

A more recent term that has been used to describe this type of signing is contact signing, also labeled *sign English* or *conceptually accurate sign English* (CASE) (however, cf. Stewart & Luetke-Stahlman, 1998). Stewart and Luetke-Stahlman (1998) provided a description of contact signing:

> *When used by a person whose first language is English, contact sign-*
> *ing means putting ASL signs in English word order with elements of*
> *English grammar left out and ASL features added. This is the perspec-*
> *tive of hearing parents and deaf people who acquire proficiency in*
> *English before learning to sign. But contact signing is also used by Deaf*
> *people whose first language is ASL. For them it means omitting some of*
> *ASL's grammatical features and adding some English ones to organize*
> *the ASL signs. Contact signing takes various forms along a spectrum,*
> *depending on the users' knowledge of ASL and English. The point is that*
> *people blend features of the two languages to make communication*
> *easier. (p. 119)*

Because contact signing entails a blend of ASL and English, this still might not describe the majority of signing that occurs in public school classrooms for deaf and hard-of-hearing students, especially by hearing teachers who were not trained in ASL and/or one of the specific signed systems. It should be emphasized that contact signing (similar to the archaic PSE) is not a signed system; thus, there are no specific rules for forming or executing signs save for the notion of producing effective communication. This contributes to the wide variation among users. In addition, the use of ASL-like signs in the signed systems is or may be quite different from the use of ASL-like or ASL signs in contact signing. In light of these factors and others, it is difficult to describe the signing of any individual. A better understanding of signing requires not only a study of the signing in various situations but also the education and training of that person relative to sign.

Consider a few other factors. Some teachers may find it difficult to adhere to the principles of some of the signed systems or may not like certain signs for given English words. Consequently, they may search for or borrow signs from other systems or other people (including those who may use contact signing). Other teachers may use a signed system but modify it (drop some markers) to fit their interests and needs. These reduced, inconsistent, unpre-dictable variations of signing may combine some grammatical aspects of ASL with those of the various signed systems within an English word order. In addi-tion, as mentioned previously, research shows that some practitioners, teach-ers, and parents are not systematic or consistent with their use of some signed systems (Marmor & Pettito, 1979; Strong & Charlson, 1987; Swisher, 1984). The results of the combination of this type of signing with contact signing or with other types of signing are not known.

With this in mind, the nature of contact signing is still far from clear. The signing of both hearing and deaf individuals in bona fide English/ASL contact situations needs to be researched further. Finally, the signing interactions between teachers/parents (mostly hearing) and children and among children also need to be studied further. It is not clear whether these interactions can really be described as examples of contact signing, especially when a number of these children come from homes in which parents do not sign English well.

The foregoing discussion should clarify why it is often difficult to synthesize the findings of studies that examine the effects of English signing (or PSE or contact, sign English). This type of signing is so idiosyncratic that there are variations across individuals in the same school, indeed, even in the same classroom. Whether these variations are critical for understanding the effects of this type of signing on English language and literacy remains to be seen. Ironically, English signing may be widely used (see discussions in Stewart & Luetke-Stahlman, 1998); however, the acquisition of this mode of communication or its effects will remain elusive until researchers attempt a systematic clear description. Until then, it is difficult to understand research documenting the benefits of this type of signing. Likewise, it is difficult to understand the criticisms of this type of signing for the same reasons.

With these caveats in mind, the achievement of students exposed to this form of communication in early childhood, including in school settings, is described, based on a few selected investigations. Because of the dearth of experimental research, it is difficult to conclude that the use of this particular form of signing causes the achievement of these students or to specify what it is that contributes to the development of English. Furthermore, as discussed later, studies that continue to assume a direct unitary relation between type of signing and English achievement are oversimplifying the processes and influences involved in the acquisition of a complex phenomenon such as the English language. Finally, the studies discussed in this section used several other terms for what is labeled here as *English signing;* examples include *manual English, pidgin sign English, sign English, signed English, simultaneous communication,* and *Total Communication.* Until further research clarifies this situation, it is permissible to classify these terms and others, for example, *contact signing* and CASE, within the general descriptive phrase used in this text—*English signing* or *English sign* (however, cf. Stewart & Luetke-Stahlman, 1998). In fact, these terms may all be for all practical purposes roughly similar (e.g., as *sofa* is roughly similar to *couch*).

Research on English Signing

The first study examined is one that described the communication approach used in school and at home as Total Communication. Griswold and Cummings (1974) investigated the expressive vocabulary of 19 preschool deaf children, age 2 to about 5 years old. Results indicated that a composite vocabulary list of 493 words and expressions were used by 2 or more students. However, the size of the vocabulary was smaller than that reported for hearing children of comparable ages. In spite of this, the composition of the vocabulary of the deaf children was similar to that of hearing children regarding (a) the proportion of nouns and verbs, (b) the number and usage of specific prepositions, (c) the usage of numbers (words), and (d) the usage of specific question words. The deaf children, however, differed from the hearing children in that they rarely used connectives, articles, and auxiliary/modal verbs. These investigators concluded that a correlation existed between the size of the vocabulary and two other variables: the length of time spent in a preschool program and the amount of exposure to Total Communication in the home environment.

In another study, Crandall (1978) studied the developmental order of manual English morphemes. The subjects used a communication approach labeled as *manual English*. Manual English entailed the use of signs from an ASL lexicon and sign markers representing morphemes (e.g., *-ed* and *-ly*), demonstratives (e.g., *this* and *that*), and articles (e.g., *a, an,* and *the*) from SEE II and from a basic text on manual communication (O'Rourke, 1973). Twenty pairs of hearing mothers and their young deaf children served as subjects. In particular, Crandall was interested in ascertaining whether the development order of the morphemes used by the deaf children was (a) related to age, (b) similar to that of hearing children of comparable age, and (c) related to their mother's use.

In general, all three hypotheses were supported. Mixed results, however, were obtained for the first hypothesis. It was reported that the deaf children's production of the inflectional morphemes did not increase significantly with age. The mean number of morphemes per utterance, however, did show an increase with age. Relative to developmental order, it was found that the first six morphemes used by the deaf children were similar to those documented for hearing children (Brown, 1973). This finding is consistent with those obtained in other studies (Raffin, 1976; Raffin et al., 1978; Schlesinger & Meadow, 1972). Finally, Crandall (1978) remarked that the mother's use of the morphemes influenced the child's use of these same morphemes. This last finding is typical of others in that it reveals the importance of the language stimuli in the home environment. However, the findings should be interpreted with caution given the current understanding of language acquisition.

Exposure—albeit important and influential—does not describe the complete picture of language acquisition and use.

Layton, Holmes, and Bradley (1979) examined the emergence of semantic relations in deaf children in a PSE-using environment. Three children, ages $5\frac{1}{2}$, $6\frac{1}{2}$, and 7 years, 7 months, served as subjects. They had been exposed to signing 9 to 15 months prior to the inception of the study. Signing is taken to mean a Total Communication system in which speech is simultaneously combined with manual signs, predominantly selected from an ASL lexicon. The signs needed for inflections and articles were selected from SEE II (Gustason, Pfetzing, & Zawolkow, 1975). The subjects were exposed to signed/spoken utterances that were one-word/one-sign in advance of their productions. For example, a subject at the one-word/one-sign stage was exposed to two-word/two-sign sequences.

The findings indicated that the semantic-syntactic categories of the deaf subjects were proportionately different from those reported for younger hearing children at less developed and equivalent linguistic levels (Bloom, Lightbown, & Hood, 1975). For example, hearing children produced more recurrence utterances (e.g., *more*), whereas deaf subjects produced more state, negation, and attribution utterances (for examples and detailed explanations, see Bloom & Lahey, 1978). It was noted that these latter types of utterances did not emerge until a later stage of hearing children's development. The investigators attempted to account for these differences by suggesting that (a) deaf children were exposed to advanced categories prior to their understanding of the basic concepts and (b) that the differences may be due to a difference in age, that is, the older deaf subjects processed at a more sophisticated cognitive level than that of the younger hearing subjects in the study by Bloom et al. (1975). Finally, the researchers argued that instructors of children with hearing impairment should be aware of the normal developmental patterns of children who are hearing.

The studies presented thus far seem to indicate that the use of English signing may be effective for primary language development if it is used in the home and if its practitioners use structures that follow the developmental patterns of hearing children. The work of Brasel and Quigley (1977) is representative of what is known about the effects of English signing (in this case, manual English) on the development of English literacy skills. The research design permitted the investigation of the effects of type of communication (oral and manual), type of language (ASL and English), and intensity of early language input. Eighteen deaf students between 10 and 19 years of age were located in each of four language groups: manual English (termed PSE), average manual (considered ASL), intensive oral, and average oral. The intensive oral group represented those students who received intensive oral training involving both the school and the parents. The parents of the average oral group left the education of their children to the schools. The parents of the manual English and average manual groups were deaf parents, whereas those of the two oral groups had normal hearing.

The results indicated that the manual English group significantly outperformed both oral groups on five of the six major syntactic structures as measured by the Test of Syntactic Abilities (Quigley, Power, Steinkamp, & Jones, 1978). In addition, the manual English group significantly outperformed all other groups on all subtests of the Stanford Achievement Test. On the Paragraph Meaning subtest, the manual English group's mean score was about 7 years, which was nearly 2 years better than the nearest group, intensive oral. The overall mean score of the manual English group on the SAT was about 5 years.

The findings of the Brasel and Quigley (1977) study were interpreted as indicating that both form of communication and type of language input are essential variables in the language development of deaf children and that manual English might be a superior system for teaching some deaf students. It is still not clear how or how much of English should be represented manually. For example, the manual English group in the Brasel and Quigley study read as well as both the SEE II (home-plus-school) group in the Babb (1979) study and the high school SEE I group in the Washburn (1983) investigation.

Delaney et al. (1984) suggested that exposure to manual communication is not sufficient by itself for developing English literacy skills. The achievement levels of three groups of students with profound hearing impairment were compared in a school that changed from oral education to Total Communication education. The results showed that the TC students had higher achievement levels than both the transitional students (i.e., exposed to oral and TC methods) and the oral students (i.e., exposed to oral methods prior to the change). The achievement level of the TC students was similar to that of the best group in the Brasel and Quigley (1977), Babb (1979), and Washburn (1983) studies. Delaney et al. stated that several other factors were probably responsible for the students' achievement level, for example, involvement of parents and school personnel, well-established curricula, and the presence of some oral communication skills.

Table 6-5 presents some of the major highlights of the various studies on English signing and a few general remarks about the nature of English signing.

As discussed previously, the results of Luetke-Stahlman (1988a) do not support the findings of Brasel and Quigley (1977) or Delaney et al. (1984). In conjunction with the findings of the study by Deal and Thornton (1985), it seems to be clear that no specific signed system (or even English signing) is superior for all or even most students with hearing impairment. This does not

TABLE 6-5 Summary of Research Findings on English Signing and General Remarks

Research Findings on English Signing

Study	Findings
Griswold & Cummings (1974)	It was concluded that a positive correlation existed between the size of vocabulary and two other variables: the length of time spent in a preschool program and the amount of exposure to Total Communication in the home environment. Researchers stated also that the composition of the vocabulary of deaf children was similar to that of hearing children in several areas. There were differences also between the two groups.
Brasel & Quigley (1977)	Findings were interpreted as indicating that both type of communication and type of language input are essential variables in the language development of deaf children and that manual English might be a superior system for teaching deaf students.
Crandall (1978)	In general, the developmental order of the morphemes used by deaf children was similar to that of hearing children of comparable age and related to their mother's use of the morphemes.
Layton, Holmes, & Bradley (1979)	Findings indicated that the semantic-syntactic categories of deaf subjects were proportionately different from those reported for younger hearing children at less developed and

equivalent linguistic levels. It is possible that these differences are due to the fact that the deaf subjects were older than the hearing children and/or were exposed to advanced categories prior to their understanding of the more basic concepts.

Delaney, Stuckless, & Walter (1984)

Findings indicated that exposure to manual communication is not sufficient by itself for developing English literacy skills. Several other factors were probably responsible, for example, involvement of parents and school personnel, well-established curricula, and the presence of some oral communication skills.

General Remarks

- It is extremely difficult to describe systematically and completely much of the signing that occurs in Total Communication classrooms. This signing, called English sign or English signing, varies from individual to individual due to the absence of established rules often associated with a signed system. Strictly speaking, English signing is not a signed system similar to the other systems with rules such as signed English, signing exact English, and seeing essential English. English sign may entail the use of a few contrived sign markers or no markers at all depending on the proclivity and ability of the individual user.

- There have been many terms or labels associated with English sign, for example, *Total Communication, simultaneous communication* (i.e., SimCom), *sign English, signed English* (not Bornstein's system), *manual English, conceptually accurate sign English,* and *contact signing.* Whether these terms are similar—that is, similar to dialectical variations (e.g., *sofa* for *couch*)—needs to be clarified by further research.

- A better understanding of English signing requires not only a study of this type of signing in various situations but also a discussion of the education and training of the person who is using English sign.

(continues)

(Table 6-5 continued)

- Because of the difficulty of describing English sign, it is extremely difficult to synthesize and interpret the findings of research studies in which subjects are purported to use English sign or some other label in this category (e.g., contact signing, etc.).

necessarily mean that any type of signing is effective or that future research will not reveal the beneficial effects of specific types of signing.

In lieu of conclusive, convergent research findings, it is difficult for parents and teachers to decide on the use of a particular system. In addition, the purposes of the selection may vary from communicating basic needs to developing English language and literacy. Although it might be possible for many students, particularly older deaf and hard-of-hearing students, to develop a sufficient level of skills for interpersonal, everyday, contextualized communicative interactions, their ability to engage in higher literate thought functions (e.g., making inferences and drawing conclusions) may be limited (see Musselman & Akamatsu, 1999). The lack or underdevelopment of a bona fide language, for example, ASL or English, is certainly one reason; however, there are others, some of which are discussed in the last chapter of this text (Chapter 12). Furthermore, it is debatable whether the use of any signed system by itself (i.e., without accompanying accessible perception of speech) can contribute effectively to the development of English language and literacy skills, as discussed in the next section.

SIGNING AND THE DEVELOPMENT OF ENGLISH: BRIEF SYNTHESIS AND RECOMMENDATIONS FOR FURTHER RESEARCH

This section summarizes briefly some of the major points on the relationship between signing and the development of English that have been discussed in this chapter. In addition, some areas for further research are provided. That the choice of signing, whether a particular signed system or American Sign Language, continues to be problematic and controversial on both a theoretical and practical level can be gleaned from the vitriolic debates in the literature. Part of the impetus for this debate has been the working paper by Johnson, Liddell, and Erting (1989) and the subsequent responses in the form of open letters and journal articles (a sample includes Dragsow & Paul, 1995; Paul, 1994; Paul & Dragsow, 1998; Ritter-Brinton, 1996). As usual, it is not uncommon to hear accusations of misrepresentation of research, narrow or biased interpretations, or interpretations based on poor research. Despite the headaches and confusion these debates might cause parents and educators, this type of exchange is actually healthy as long as it does not result in mere name-calling and inaction with respect with the need for further scientific research. Although the information in the ensuing paragraphs represents the author's perspective, it is not offered as *the* perspective. Hopefully, it and other views will engender ongoing research efforts. Three broad points (in the form of bullets) are listed and a few remarks are made on each one separately.

- There is no convergence of research to indicate the superiority of any of the signed systems for the development of English, including English literacy, for all or even most deaf and hard-of-hearing students or to determine adequately which system should be selected for a particular student.

This is a critical problem in the field of education for deaf and hard-of-hearing students. Convergence requires a sufficient number of scientific studies that can be subjected to a research synthesis or a metaanalysis. There are specific guidelines (albeit contentious) for conducting these syntheses. Ironically, this situation has been noted by some researchers involved with hearing children who attempted to synthesize the available scientific research on literacy and deafness in a national report (Snow et al., 1998).

Although the author is open to a variety of research paradigms, for example, quantitative, qualitative, or critical, only the quantitative and qualitative paradigms seem to be reflective of the scientific approach. To establish policy, which affects large groups of students, it is necessary to conduct a number of quantitative and qualitative studies and to synthesize the findings. Qualitative studies allow one to focus on individuals, that is, a teacher, a parent, or a student, but this focus by itself is not sufficient for making generalizations and establishing policy for groups unless attempts are undertaken to conduct quantitative analyses of a number of similar qualitative studies. Whatever the purpose, the fact remains that there is a dire need for more scientific research on the signed systems, including their use by parents and their deaf children.

It is possible to find successful students who have been exposed to any one of the signed systems. However, the reasons why a particular system is successful for a particular student are still not clear. A better understanding of this issue is not forthcoming if researchers continue to view the development of the English language or English literacy as unitary skills or if they continue to view the acquisition of a particular signed system itself as a unitary phenomenon. This leads to the next two broad points.

- There is a need to understand specific contributions of the various aspects of each sign system or communication mode to the development of specific components of the performance mode of English.

There are several remarks to be made on this complex point. The performance mode refers to the use of English in face-to-face or live interactions between individuals and groups. It is often forgotten that the acquisition of English essentially means that individuals have a tacit or intuitive understanding of rules associated with components such as phonology, morphology, syntax, semantics, and pragmatics (see Chapter 2 for discussion of pragmatics and semantics). In other words, individuals have a good working knowledge of the form, content, and function of a language. Research on the representation, production, and reception of signs should be considered with respect to these language components rather than on a global level only.

One line of research has focused on the use of specific signed systems by practitioners. The few studies that exist indicate that it is difficult for many practitioners to adhere to principles for forming and producing the signs and for executing these principles faithfully in a consistent manner. This often leads to signs or sign markers that are omitted periodically during communicative interactions. In essence, this means that practitioners are leaving out information relative to English structure. On the other hand, there is evidence that it is possible to become adept at speaking and signing simultaneously with a specific signed system. One major concern here is that researchers cannot accept at face value that a particular system is in fact being used consistently and systematically in a particular school or classroom. Describing in detail the signing of the teachers (e.g., via analyses of videotapes) needs to be a critical part of every study that attempts to discuss the effects of a specific type of signing on a particular area of students' achievement or performance. Admittedly, this is time-consuming and difficult, and it becomes extremely problematic when subjects are drawn from several classrooms either within the same school or across schools or school districts. This is not an issue of dialect or signing dialect (although that may be important); the issue is one of how and how much of standard English is represented. In addition, due to wide variations in the use and understanding of English signing or contact signing, the author cannot see any systematic cumulative progress in the understanding of the effects of this communicative mode without attempts to describe these signing situations adequately so that others can effectively evaluate the merits.

Related also to this line of thinking is what needs to be represented to convey English as a language. The argument in this chapter is that most of the signed systems only convey, albeit imperfectly, information on the morphological and syntactic structures of English. This is the case when the focus is on only the signed (signs and sign markers) portion of the systems. Although the signs of the systems are executed with speech in a simultaneous manner, there has been no systematic research on the relative and combined contributions of each component (i.e., speech and/or sign). There seems to some relationship between the use of the signed mode and children's acquisition of some aspects of English morphology, at least in younger children. However, unless children are perceiving adequately all aspects of the spoken message, they are not being exposed to the phonological component of English, including segmentals (i.e., vowels and consonants) and suprasegmentals (e.g., intonation and rhythm). The phonological component represents the building blocks of any language, and in one sense, it facilitates the acquisition of other components such as morphology, syntax, and semantics. With respect to English, this means that the full range of phonemes (i.e., the abstract values) must be represented, typically via the use of articulators, which might not need to be those associated with speech.

The most recent research seems to reveal benefits associated with the more representative systems such as SEE I and SEE II; however, it is possible that benefits depend on the students' access to as much of the English language as possible. Thus, if students cannot access the sound system or cannot speechread and are solely dependent on the signs, then all things being equal, there should be more favorable results associated with the systems most representative of English via the use of signs, assuming that these students do not have difficulty processing the system (see ensuing paragraphs). However, if students do equally as well with the systems that are least representative of the structure of English, it might be that such representation is adequate for these students because they are accessing information from the simultaneous presentation of speech and signing. Of course, there are other possibilities that may be as idiosyncratic as the number of students exposed to signing. It is possible for students, up to a point, to abstract morphological and orthographic information from print, and this contributes further to their understanding of English. Nevertheless, unless more specific research paradigms are utilized, specifically, experimental designs, the list of possibilities may be endless, and it will be difficult to reach a consensus on the merits of the various signed systems.

The last issue to be discussed with respect to this complex point is the learnability of the signed systems. The learnability issue has been investigated by several researchers (Gee & Goodhart, 1985; Maxwell, 1983, 1987; Supalla, 1991). Even if practitioners become proficient in the simultaneous use of speech and signing within a particular system, it still might be difficult for deaf students to learn the system and, thus, the language that it purportedly represents.

The rate of delivery or the manner of representation by the users of the signed systems may be incompatible with the perception or production capabilities of deaf and hard-of-hearing receivers. The evidence for this assertion can be seen in children's alterations of grammatical elements (morphology and syntax), which result in either an odd pattern of use (e.g., Maxwell's work) or an increase in the rate of signed production by the receivers (e.g., the work of Gee and Goodhart). Supalla (1991) and others suggested that these alterations reflect the processing capabilities of the eye. This might explain why a sign language such as ASL is or should be easier to process than a signed system based on a spoken language such as English. Nevertheless, the major point here is that if deaf and hard-of-hearing children have difficulty processing the signed portions of the various signed systems, they will not be able to internalize the grammatical rules of English, which the systems are intended to represent. Finally, it is possible that this incompatibility issue is only evident for those students who are predominantly dependent on the signed portion. Whether this is also the case for students who actually utilized information from both the spoken and signed modes simultaneously remains to be researched.

Perhaps one approach to addressing these processing difficulties is the attempts to incorporate more ASL-like features in the English signing of teachers (Akamatsu & Stewart, 1998). The manner in which this approach will affect the development of English, including English script literacy skills, needs to be researched.

- Research on the effects of signed systems on the development of English literacy skills needs to shift from global, all-encompassing correlational approaches to more specific, experimental explorations on the acquisition of specific literacy skills.

Only a few remarks are presented here because the complexity of literacy is discussed in detail in Chapter 8 of this text. It has become clear that English literacy is not a unitary skill; that is, an individual needs to develop a number of lower and higher skills and orchestrate them in a manner that permits the construction of meaning at several levels—word, phrase, sentence, paragraph, and entire passage. For many deaf and hard-of-hearing students, improvement in literacy might require intervention and enrichment activities on many levels simultaneously and independently.

The major problem with most of the existing research on the signed systems, including ASL, is the narrow focus on establishing a correlational link between the use and/or exposure of a specific system and the subsequent development of English literacy. Establishing this correlation is a necessary first step perhaps; however, it does not provide insights into the why and the how that often results from the use of painstaking, systematic, creative experimental research designs. Furthermore, conducting these simple correlational studies undermines the complexity of the literacy process. English literacy (i.e., reading and writing) requires more than just a knowledge of the performance (e.g., speech and/or sign) form of the English language. Granted, it is critical for deaf and hard-of-hearing students to have a bona fide working knowledge of English, including an intuitive, tacit understanding of the rules associated with the structure such as phonology, morphology, syntax, semantics, and pragmatics. However, the relationship between the performance and literacy modes is complex, interactive, and reciprocal. For many deaf and hard-of-hearing students, including many students who are considered at risk for reading and writing, these relationships are extremely difficult to learn without an enormous investment of time, energy, and resources via interventions. And, it should be clear that simply knowing a signed system (and hopefully English) or American Sign Language is not sufficient for developing a high level of achievement in reading and writing.

There are many lines of research that need to be undertaken. One of the major issues is the development of rapid word identification skills, which seems to be dependent on a working knowledge of phonology (e.g., phonological awareness) and morphology (e.g., word parts) and the ability to use this knowledge to comprehend the words in print, which is based on an alphabetic system (i.e., phonemic awareness, phoneme-grapheme link via orthography, etc.). A working knowledge of English is indeed important and facilitative for literacy development; however, there are numerous other skills that are also critical. Researchers' understanding of the English literacy process and deafness cannot grow substantially if they are confined to the findings from simple research designs that have been utilized in much of the research on the signed systems and English literacy.

FINAL REMARKS

This chapter attempts to present some major highlights on the development of the performance mode of English via the use of selected signed systems, including the use of the Rochester method and its finger-spelling component. Relative to the TC approaches, operationalized as MCE systems and the use of English signing or contact signing, a sample of findings from research studies on students with severe to profound hearing impairment was synthesized. Summary remarks are presented in the last section; here a few points are highlighted.

There is evidence that some deaf students can acquire a high level of competence in English as a first language via the use of several of the signed systems. The recent evidence seems to favor those systems that are considered to be most representative of the grammatical structure of English, notably seeing essential English and signing exact English. However, most deaf and hard-of-hearing students do not attain this lofty level, suggesting that there is no superiority of any of the signed systems, including English signing, Rochester method, or finger spelling, for all or even most children and adolescents. These results do not undermine the contributions of some signed systems to assist children, especially young children, in acquiring an understanding of a few of the basic morphemes—that is, some morphological knowledge of English. Nevertheless, if the litmus test is functional literacy or on-grade level literacy in English, then it must be concluded that all systems have not contributed substantially to this goal for most deaf and hard-of-hearing adolescents.

There seems to be several reasons for this relative lack of success. Some hypotheses that have been proffered in this chapter are

- the inconsistent and unsystematic use of the signed systems by many practitioners, resulting in an impoverished or inadequate exposure to the structure of English, as well as difficulties in assessing the merits or contributions of specific systems;

- a relative lack of understanding of how much of the English structure can be represented by the systems and the fact that the phonological component of English may be lacking if the focus is only on the signed portion;

- the nature of the representation of English by the signed systems being incompatible with the visual processing capabilities of many deaf students, especially if the students are predominantly dependent on the signs and sign markers; and finally,

- the limitations of current research designs that seem to underestimate the complexity of the development of English language and English literacy skills.

Whether the acquisition of English is or should be easier for ASL-using deaf students is one of the topics of Chapter 9. There seems to be the assumption, supported by some evidence, that under comparable conditions, ASL might be essentially easier and faster for many deaf students to acquire at a proficient level than are the manually coded English systems. The nature and acquisition of American Sign Language is discussed briefly in the next chapter.

SIGNED SYSTEMS
COMPREHENSION QUESTIONS

1. Describe the concept of Total Communication. Is the use of American Sign Language part of the TC philosophy? If so, in what way?

2. The author stated that there seems to be several problematic assumptions about the signed systems; however, only one was discussed in this chapter. Describe that problematic assumption.

3. Discuss the major tenets of the following systems:
   a. Rochester method (including finger spelling)
   b. The SEE systems: seeing essential English and signing exact English. What are some differences between the two SEE systems?
   c. Signed English
   d. English signing (including all synonyms or related terms)

4. Which system is considered to be most representative of the structure of English? Least representative? What determines the placement on the continuum from least representative to most representative? Does representation consider the issue of phonology?

5. Discuss the salient research findings of the following manual systems (refer to specific studies):
   a. Rochester method (including finger spelling)
   b. Seeing essential English
   c. Signing exact English
   d. Signed English
   e. English signing

   With respect to representation (see Question 5), is there sufficient research to argue that the most representative systems provide the greatest benefits? Why or why not?

6. Why is it so difficult to describe and do research on English signing, especially as this is presumed to be the most widely used type of signing in educational programs?

7. Discuss briefly some of the major points on the relationship between signing and the development of English that were presented in the chapter (See "Signing and the Development of English").

8. In general, it was concluded that the signed systems have not been successful in developing English language and literacy skills. What are some reasons (hypotheses) for this relative lack of success?

CHALLENGE QUESTIONS

(Note: Complete answers are not in the text. Additional research is required.)

1. At the beginning of the chapter, the author posed several important questions: What exactly do these systems represent? How much of English is represented by a particular system? How much of English needs to be represented by a particular system? Can spoken English really be represented by a signed system? Does simultaneous communication entail the ability to perceive information on the lips (i.e., via speech) and on the hands (i.e., via signs) simultaneously? If so, what is the nature and extent of the perception process? What did the chapter offer with respect to these questions? Did the chapter provide complete explicit answers? If not, do you think that there are adequate answers available? Why or why not?

2. The author stated that there is no linear relationship between sign input (i.e., reception/perception) and sign output (i.e., execution/performance). What does this statement mean?

3. Is there a sufficient amount of information (e.g., scientific or logical) to select a particular English signed system for initial use with children? If not, do you think there will ever be adequate information to make a decision? Why or why not? Is it possible to state guidelines for selecting a particular system? If so, what do you recommend? Can you find research or theoretical support for your guidelines?

4. If phonology is the building block of a language, how do deaf students become exposed to the phonology of English (both segmental and suprasegmental aspects) via the use of a signed system? Is it possible to understand or internalize the morphology and syntax of a phonetic language such as English without access to phonology? Why or why not?

FURTHER READINGS

Blasdell, R., & Caccamise, F. (1976). *Factors influencing the reception of finger spelling.* Houston, TX: American Speech and Hearing Association.

Evans, L. (1982). *Total communication: Structure and strategy.* Washington, DC: Gallaudet University Press.

Garretson, M. (Ed.). (1990). *Communication issues among deaf people: A deaf American monograph.* Silver Spring, MD: National Association of the Deaf.

Schein, J., & Stewart, D. (1995). *Language in motion: Exploring the nature of sign.* Washington, DC: Gallaudet University Press.

Walworth, M., Moores, D., & O'Rourke, T. J. (1992). *A free hand.* Silver Spring, MD: T.J. Publishers.

American Sign Language

7

L anguage is the most important attribute of many minority groups, and it has been so for deaf Americans. American Sign Language is not poor English; it is unique. It not only differs from English in its syntax and vocabulary, its visual form is so strange to hearing people that for decades it was not recognized as a language. The significance of sign language to deaf people is obvious from their history. With very few exceptions, the associations, conventions, clubs, and marriages of deaf Americans uniformly reflected the importance of sharing this communication method. They found it rapid, facile, and precise, unlike speech or speechreading. (Van Cleve & Crouch, 1989, p. 106)

Prior to the 1960s, much of the knowledge about the acquisition and development of language has been based on the systematic investigations and study of spoken languages such as English, French, and German (Blumenthal, 1970; Bonvillian, 1999). Much has been written about the search for the origins of language and the evolution of language, which purportedly proceeded from nonverbal hand signals to articulations as in speech (see an eloquent, brief discussion in Crystal, 1987, 1997). Communication via speech was considered to be a natural evolutionary process that freed the hands for other important activities. In fact, sound is considered to be the most universal and natural medium for the transmission and reception of language. There are clearly more spoken languages than written counterparts (or representations). This strong bias or focus on spoken languages has led some scholars to postulate strong interrelations among speech, language, and thought.

One of the best, and unfortunate, examples of this strong focus can be seen in the seminal work of Myklebust (1964), who exerted a considerable influence on the thinking of a generation of researchers and teachers of deaf and hard-of-hearing students. In his attempts to understand the effects of lack of hearing on individuals, Myklebust reasoned that the signing behaviors of deaf individuals did not constitute a bona fide language. Because deaf individuals did not possess a language, he argued that they had extreme difficulty in engaging in abstract thinking or problem-solving activities (see discussions in Moores, 1987, 1996; Paul & Jackson, 1993). Interpretations of Myklebust's work have led to many implications regarding the development of language and cognitive abilities of deaf individuals, including:

- Speech is equal to language

- Speech is important for the development of abstract thought

- The use of signs interferes with the development of speech

As discussed in Chapter 3, Moores (1987) characterized this period of scholarly thought on deafness as Deaf as concrete. That is, it was generally assumed that deaf students were concrete thinkers, exhibiting enormous difficulty in performing abstract, logical, problem-solving tasks. For the most part, this was due to their inability to internalize a language, namely, a spoken language such as English.

This connection of speech to language was so ingrained that it was not uncommon to hear many educators of deaf and hard-of-hearing students describe the Sign Language of Deaf individuals (later known as American Sign Language) as a substandard or low form of English or as a street language. In fact, many Deaf people themselves also felt that the manner in which they sign in their homes and clubs was not the proper way to sign in formal or educated places, especially in the presence of hearing or educated people. Despite more than 30 years of research on American Sign Language, there are still ongoing debates on its linguistic status (see *Deaf American*, 1990) and on whether Deaf people actually constitute a true cultural group (Padden, 1998b).

In any case, Myklebust was certainly not alone in his skepticism about the language of signs. Thus, he should not receive all or even most of the blame for the misconceptions that were engendered, some of which still exist. The interesting question now is: Why has there been a flurry of research on sign languages, particularly American Sign Language? The juxtaposition of Deaf people and the use of signing has been observed throughout recorded history (Schein & Stewart, 1995). What is the reason for the burgeoning interest in this area at the present time?

Perhaps the major reason for the preponderance of research efforts has been the realization that sign languages are indeed bona fide languages on a par with spoken languages. Spoken languages are not superior to sign languages; in fact, there is no linguistic evidence for the assumption that some languages are intrinsically superior to others. Accepting these assertions should have a domino effect on some issues mentioned previously: Speech does not equal language; speech is not the only avenue to abstract thought; and so on. Clearly, there is an intimate relation (or relations) between language and thought; however, the medium for conveying and receiving language does not have to be based on sound. This is not only true for sign languages, but it might also be the case for the use of cued speech/language.

Bonvillian (1999) offered an eloquent discussion of another critical reason for the growth of research on sign language development:

Investigators realised that the systematic study of sign language acquisition provided a way to answer important questions about human language abilities. One question of interest was whether there were effects of language modality on language acquisition. This question sparked a series of investigations to determine how much children's sign language acquisition resembled children's spoken language acquisition. A second question that intrigued investigators was whether the human brain processed sign languages in much the same way as spoken languages. When researchers interested in this topic studied the development of young children, they often focused on the children's hand preference as they signed as an indicator of cerebral hemispheric involvement in sign production. A third question of interest was whether hearing individuals who failed to acquire a spoken language could make progress in acquiring a signed language. If so, then this finding would indicate that signed and spoken languages were not processed identically and might open up a lot of opportunities for speech-limited individuals. A final question of interest to investigators was whether the varying ages and settings in which deaf children learned to sign affected their level of sign language mastery. In answering this question, researchers might be able to gain insights into how much of language development was the product of environmental factors and how much the product of innate mechanisms. (p. 278)

As can be seen in this passage, the study of American Sign Language and signed languages in general has spawned many different lines of research with, of course, a common interest in the human capacity to learn a language. Despite such broad and deep lines of research, this text is intended to be modest in the discussion of the nature and acquisition of ASL. In the first section of this chapter, a brief overview and some historical background on the evolution of American Sign Language are presented. Next, the general nature of ASL is described, focusing on its roles as a sign language and as a minority language within the United States. Also mentioned briefly is how ASL differs from English and from the English signed systems. Then, a linguistic description of ASL is provided, with attention devoted to language components, for example, phonology, morphology, and syntax. The selection of features associated with the language components is motivated by the intent to highlight differences between ASL and English. Due to the growing call for ASL/English bilingual/bicultural programs, it is important to show how ASL differs from English and from the English signed systems that were described in Chapter 6. As a result, concepts such as nonmanual features, incorporation, modulation and inflection, classifiers, and the use of space are briefly discussed. This section of the chapter ends with a summary of differences between ASL and English.

The next section describes some of the general findings on the acquisition of American Sign Language based on selected psycholinguistic and sociolinguistic research studies. These findings are also presented with respect to the various language components. Finally, the role of finger spelling in ASL is discussed briefly, including its possible role in English literacy, and some insights are provided into the critical period hypothesis and sign language acquisition.

BRIEF OVERVIEW AND HISTORICAL BACKGROUND

To the casual observer, it might be easy to see how the term *compensatory* can be and has been applied to the signing behavior of deaf individuals (see discussion in Myklebust, 1964). In other words, to compensate for their insufficient or lack of auditory ability, deaf individuals have attempted to develop a communication system to meet basic needs. However, this compensatory issue is not only controversial but also does not capture the strong interrelations among language, thought, and the development of identities, for example, personal and social—as discussed in Chapter 2 of this text. It also neglects to consider the fact that American Sign Language, as an example, is a bona fide language and has been in existence for a long time.

The history of the evolution of ASL, as any other historical account, is dependent on a point of view, and obviously, some points of view are promoted more loudly and ostentatiously than others. Indeed, it is quite difficult to be neutral about history; thus, it is important to read a variety of voices to obtain a broad and hopefully accurate and complete picture (Bender, 1970; Lane, 1984, 1992; Moores, 1996). One simple way of viewing this situation is to argue rightfully and, perhaps, accurately that varieties of sign languages have existed in America for as long as there have been deaf people (Stokoe, 1960; Woodward, 1978). It is possible that a number of these signs or gestural behaviors were esoteric; that is, they are means of communication developed among a few deaf people to communicate with hearing people or to communicate among themselves. The lack of a rich deaf community with multiple users of sign probably accounts for the limited range and development of these linguistic items. This is only conjecture because there has been no systematic documentation on the structure of these early varieties of sign in America.

On the other hand, there is some documentation of signs used by isolated deaf communities, especially communities in frequent contact with hearing communities in the same location. Groce (1985) reported on deaf and hearing individuals who resided on Martha's Vineyard (an island). An hereditary form of deafness resulted in a high percentage of deaf individuals on this island. As a consequence, many hearing inhabitants knew sign language, and deaf individuals were integrated pervasively into the social, political, and economic milieus on the island. Woodward (1978) reported on a somewhat similar phenomenon on another island, Providence Island, located in the Caribbean. Woodward also hypothesized that there were a number of sign languages/signed systems or varieties of sign on both Martha's Vineyard and Providence Island and elsewhere in young America during the 17th and 18th centuries.

According to several historical accounts, Thomas Hopkins Gallaudet and Laurent Clerc are credited with bringing the *Abbe de l'Epee* sign language (French Sign Language) to America and with establishing the first school for the deaf in 1817. In essence, this story can be placed in a historical context of language approaches/methods that have been used with deaf and hard-of-hearing children and adolescents (see McAnally et al., 1994). In other words, the discussion of the evolution of ASL in the United States is intertwined with the debates on the best methods for teaching language to children and adolescents.

The dominant figure of the 18th century was the Abbe de l'Epee in France. The Abbe first used the signs of deaf people as the language of instruction. He later developed this language into a sign system to approximate the vocabulary and syntax of the French language. This involved creating signs for words and signs and other devices to function for inflections, tenses, articles, and other grammatical parts of French. This system was continued and elaborated on by the Abbe Sicard, de l'Epee's successor, who also compiled an extensive dictionary of signs. The great similarities between this approach and the modern-day approaches in the United States of conforming sign language to the structure of English via the English-based sign systems are obvious.

Laurent Clerc was one of Sicard's prized pupils, and he described Sicard's method (see McAnally et al., 1994). Sicard's method was the forerunner of the structured approaches to language development in the 19th century. Returning directly to the use of sign language in the United States, it should not be concluded that when Gallaudet and Clerc arrived, deaf people began to use French signs in 1817, mainly because they did not have a language until that time (Baker & Cokely, 1980; Lane, 1984). As noted previously, there may have been several sign languages already in existence. As remarked eloquently by Baker and Cokely (1980):

> *Common sense tells us that possibly several different signed languages were used by the 2000 or more deaf people living in this country in the early 1800's. Certainly they were not all just waiting around for someone to give them an effective way of communicating! (p. 50)*

In any case, it is probably true that the signed system of the Abbe de l'Epee was combined with many of the signs or sign languages that were already in use by deaf people. From this combination, one might assume that American Sign Language was born. It is also possible to argue that ASL and other sign languages have become more conventional and rule governed—that is, more arbitrarily defined in a linguistic sense since its inception—as is the case for the evolution of any other language.

The combination of existing deaf sign and the French method was not without controversy and is very similar to the ongoing debates today re the interrelationships among American Sign Language and the various English signed systems. Bebian, a former student of Sicard, who was, of course, a student of de l'Epee, strongly criticized the use of French method with the bulk of the focus on the teaching of the French grammar, particularly French writing. His remarks seem to have transcended time and are still applicable for the current situation:

> *The more profoundly these signs decompose the sentence—thus revealing the structure of French—the further they get away from the language of the deaf, from their intellectual capacities and thinking. That is why the deaf never make use of these signs among themselves; they use them in taking word-for-word dictation, but to explain the meaning of the text dictated, they go back to their familiar language. (Bebian as cited in Lane & Phillip, 1984, p. 23)*

GENERAL NATURE OF AMERICAN SIGN LANGUAGE

Let's begin by stating that American Sign Language is a visual-gestural and rule-governed language. The rules that governed ASL have been published since the 1960s in a number of books (Baker & Cokely, 1980; Klima & Bellugi,

1979; Liddell, 1980; Stokoe, 1960; Stokoe, Casterline, & Croneberg, 1976; Wilbur, 1987). These two major characteristics, visual-gestural and rule governed, are critical to consider together to demonstrate similarities and differences between ASL (and other sign languages) and spoken languages, particularly English and the English signed systems in America.

As a visual-gestural language, American Sign Language is particularly structured to accommodate the visual capacities of the eye and motor capabilities of the body. Indeed, this accommodation issue is a major criticism of the English signed systems. ASL entails both manual and nonmanual features. The manual features pertains to the shapes, positions, and movements of the hands, whereas the nonmanual features refer to the movement of the cheeks, lips, tongue, eyes, eyebrows, shoulders, and the body (e.g., for body shifts). Most of the information in ASL is presented and conveyed in front of the signer's body. In essence, native signers communicate by executing systematic manual and nonmanual body movements. As is discussed later, space and movement play important linguistic roles in all sign languages.

Because ASL (and other sign languages) uses gestures and nonmanual movements, this often engenders a number of misconceptions and, in many cases, a source of discomfort for individuals who attempt to learn this language. In the author's beginning classes at the university, there are a number of students who fixate strongly on his hands, failing to notice that the nonmanual aspects are also critical for conveying information. They become extremely uncomfortable with using their bodies and faces, mainly because they are simply not used to this type of expression. Some of them even laugh nervously at the author's facial "distortions" (e.g., pulling eyebrows together, raising eyebrows, puffed cheeks, etc.).

Related to these observed phenomenon, Stewart and Luetke-Stahlman (1998) remarked:

> *Many people who learned to sign when they were adults are reluctant to accompany their signing with appropriate facial expressions and body movements. Years of speaking and a social taboo on physical expressiveness in conversation may explain this. Their reluctance is at odds with the fact that many physical expressions are part of everyday speech. For example, consider the way we shrug our shoulders, turn the palms up, and make a face when we say "I don't know." ASL should feel just as natural once social inhibitions about signing and using your body to communicate are removed. (p. 63)*

To say that ASL is rule governed means that the formation, sequencing, and execution of signs are governed by a finite set of rules that needs to be learned or acquired. Similar to other languages (e.g., spoken languages) that are widely used within a specified geographical region, ASL has a number of dialects and other varieties of expressions. It is possible that these variations are regional in origin (i.e., dependent on where one resides); however, there are numerous other factors that contribute to the diversity of sign usage—for example, the age at which the language is learned, the influence of the home environment, race, gender, and the educational background of the signer. Not to be ignored also is the fact that a minority language such as ASL is influenced by the majority language of society, which is English in the United States. The influence of English on ASL has been manifested in several ways—the use of finger-spelled loan signs (e.g., the signs for NO GOOD, JOB) and the placement of adjectives before nouns (e.g., BLUE CAR as opposed to CAR BLUE; RED HOUSE as opposed to HOUSE RED). These examples are illustrated in Figure 7-1.

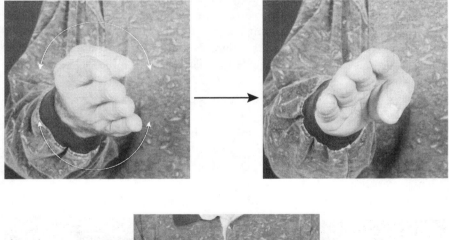

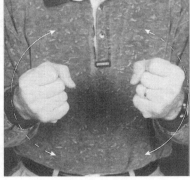

"blue car"

Figure 7-1 A Few Examples of the Influence of English on ASL. *(continues)*

This does not mean, however, that ASL does not have its own grammar; all minority languages within majority-language cultures exhibited these and other types of influences.

Before proceeding, a few additional brief comments about the nature of this influence should be made. Unless a minority language or culture attempts to create an extremely isolated existence, there is bound to be influences from the majority language and culture. It is also possible—and in the author's view desirable and necessary—that the influence is bidirectional (or multidirectional, depending on the complexity of the situation). The immediate and long-range implications of this discussion can be seen in the ongoing debates on majority/minority values, the concept of multiculturalism, and use of terms such as *empowerment* and *oppression* when discussing the economic and political conditions of members of minority and ethnic groups in this country. These and other more specific issues (e.g., educational goals and the use of the minority

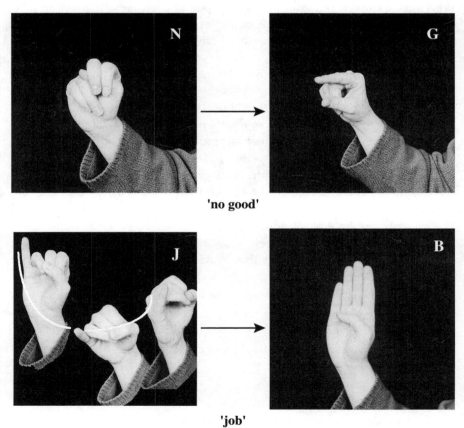

'no good'

'job'

Figure 7-1 *(continued)*

language as a first language) are contentious with respect to the establishment and implementation of bilingual and/or second language programs. The discussion of ASL/English bilingual programs is one of the major topics of Chapter 9 of this text.

Despite the nature and extent of reciprocal influences, it is important to highlight a few salient differences between ASL and English, including the English signed systems. The obvious difference of grammar has already been mentioned. However, the grammatical differences manifested themselves in unique ways, specifically with reference to the use of gestures and space. For example, it should be obvious (although many people still seem surprised) that ASL, similar to other sign languages, does not involve the use of speech sounds, which are part of what can be called the articulatory-auditory loop. In addition, native signers do not read or write their messages. In other words, ASL and other sign languages do not possess a literacy mode, which functions analogically as print does for some spoken languages. The lack of a literacy form has caused some educators to view ASL (and other languages without written forms) as a less prestigious language. This perception, of course, has no linguistic merit.

Not only is the grammar of ASL different from that of English, but it is also different from that of the various signed systems designed to represent the structure of English (Lou, 1988; Wilbur, 1987). Despite the overlap of signs between ASL and some signed systems, there are important differences in the various components such as phonology, morphology, syntax, and semantics. For example, the phonological system of ASL is rule governed, permitting a finite number of features such as the number of allowable hand shapes. Some hand shapes that correspond to the initialization of signs in, for example, the SEE systems are not allowable (i.e., grammatical) in ASL. That is, these hand shapes violate phonological principles.

To provide examples of a few other differences between ASL and the English signed systems, consider that in American Sign Language (Baker & Cokely, 1980; Wilbur, 1987):

1. Space may be used to designate and distinguish individuals (e.g., as in the use of pronouns). The area in front of the signer is reserved for second person pronouns; the areas to the sides for third person pronouns.

2. Questions are indicated by the use of eyebrow movements and head tilts.

3. Reduplication (repeated movements) is used to express notions such as plurality, degree, or emphasis.

4. Grammatical boundary is marked by the use of pause between signs or sign sequences.

5. The spatial area can be varied to correspond to louder or quieter signing.

Additional examples of this discussion are discussed and illustrated in the next section on the linguistic description of American Sign Language. Because ASL entails the use of signs and other gestures without accompanying speech, there have been doubts about its status as a language for a long time. In addition, individuals have thought that sign language is universal (only one sign language) due to the so-called iconic properties (discussed later). Crystal (1997) provided an eloquent description of these issues:

> *Popular opinions about the manner are quite plain: sign language is not a real language but little more than a system of sophisticated gesturing; signs are simply pictorial representations of external reality; and because of this, there is just one sign language, which can be understood all over the world. It is now clear, from the results of the first research studies of this subject, dating from the 1960s, that all of these opinions are wrong.*
>
> *A clear distinction must be drawn, first of all, between sign language and gesture. To sign is to use the hands in a conscious, "verbal" manner, to express the same range of meaning as would be achieved by speech (especially by grammar). By contrast, gesturing is far less systematic and comprehensive; there are in fact very few hand gestures, and these are used in an ad hoc way to express a small number of basic notions. Everyone can gesture; but few have learned to sign. (A similar point can be made about facial expressions and body movements.)*
>
> *Some of the hand movements of sign language can be plausibly interpreted by non-signers because they reflect properties of the external world (they are* iconic*); but the vast majority of signs are not. It is possible that many of the signs were iconic when they were first devised, but little information is available about this point in the past, which some have speculated may be as early as the origins of human language. In any case, whatever the original situation, the iconicity has been lost in most instances because of the influence of linguistic change, which affects sign as it does spoken language. (p. 222)*

LINGUISTIC DESCRIPTION OF ASL

It is always a challenge for linguists to describe a new language using a particular type of notational system. Eventually, the goal is to describe the rules that govern phonology, morphology, syntax, semantics, and pragmatics. With respect to the phonology of a spoken language, it is no easy feat to categorize the sounds of a foreign language, especially in running speech. After considerable experience, the linguist can detect the beginning and ending of words. In addition, the linguist might eventually recognize the existence of sounds that are different from his or her own. In general, much of the focus of these descriptive efforts is on phonology, which as discussed previously in this text, represents the building blocks of any language.

In describing ASL, the best place to begin is to discuss its phonology and proceed to the other components. The approach to this process is roughly similar to what was described earlier for a spoken language. More detailed descriptions of the grammar of ASL can be found elsewhere (Baker & Cokely, 1980; Liddell, 1980; Wilbur, 1987).

Phonology: A Brief Introduction

The phonology of a sign language such as ASL is not based on sound; rather, it involves hand movements, positions, and shapes. A breakthrough in establishing the legitimacy of ASL commenced with the seminal work of William Stokoe (1960). Stokoe proposed that signs contained a finite number of linguistic traits that can be combined to produce a number of concepts in the lexicon of a language, that is, the vocabulary of that language. Stokoe investigated the formation of signs, which he labeled *cherology* (from the Greek root *cheir* for *hand*). Cherology is analogous to phonology (i.e., study of speech sounds). Just as a spoken word can be analyzed with respect to phonemes as in English, a sign can be broken down into cheremes. Cherology has not been widely adopted; linguists prefer the term *phonology*, which can be applied to any language and refers to the building blocks such as phonemes and so on.

Stokoe (1960) identified three major formational aspects that distinguish one ASL sign from another. These correspond to the shape of the hand—hand shape or configuration—(*designator* or *dez*), the location (i.e., place of articulation) of the sign (*tabulation* or *tab*), and the movement of the hand (*signation* or *sig*). Stokoe and his collaborators developed a system for documenting the aspects of a sign (Stokoe et al., 1976). A sample of this system is shown in Figure 7-2.

With respect to these phonological features, research has documented that there are about 40 distinct hand shapes and 20 distinct locations (Liddell & Johnson, 1989; Stokoe et al., 1976). Of these three phonological features, the tab, or location aspect, is the one that is most often produced accurately by young children learning American Sign Language, and hand shape is produced least accurately (Siedlecki & Bonvillian, 1993). One possible explanation for this might be that the location features are relatively broad in nature and do

Sample of tab (location) symbols

0   zero, the neutral place where the hands move

U   chin, lower face

[ ]   trunk, body from shoulders to hips

α   wrist, arm in supinated position (on its back)

Sample of dez (hand shape) symbols (some also used as tab)

A   compact hand, fist; may be like "a", "s", or "t" of manual alphabet

5   spread hand; fingers and thumb spread like "5" of manual numeration

C   curved hand; may be like "c" or more open

3   "cock" hand; thumb and first two fingers spread, like "3" of manual numeration

X   hook hand; index finger bent in hook from fist, thumb tip may touch fingertip

Sample of sig (hand movement) symbols

>   rightward movement

<   leftward movement

T   movement toward signer

ℓ wiggling action of fingers

x   contactual action, touch

Note: Adapted from Stokoe, Casterline, and Croneberg, 1976.

Figure 7-2 Sample of Stokoe's Notational System.

not require the fine distinctions often associated with the other features such as hand shape and hand movement.

Since the work of Stokoe, a fourth formation aspect has been proposed—orientation (Lane & Grosjean, 1980; Wilbur, 1987). Originally, orientation referred to the direction or position of the palm of the hand, that is, up, down, or to the right or left. This feature is instrumental for making distinctions between, for instance, the sign for SHORT (as in brief period of time) and the sign for TRAIN (as in vehicle for travel). This is illustrated in Figure 7-3.

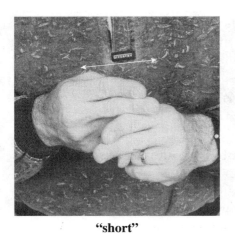 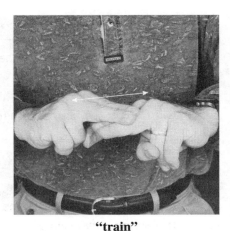

"short"   "train"

Figure 7-3 Signs for SHORT and TRAIN.

More recently, however, researchers referred to orientation of the articulators or hands with respect to the body. About 10 distinct orientations have been identified (Liddell & Johnson, 1989; Stokoe et al., 1976).

Many studies of sign phonological acquisition have relied predominantly on Stokoe's model for describing the formational structure of the signs in American Sign Language. To illustrate how the system works, consider the sign, KNOW. Typically, the sign KNOW is executed on the forehead (or in proximity to the forehead). The tab (location) symbol for the forehead or upper brow is selected. The hand shape for KNOW resembles a flat-hand salute with the palm facing down (or to the floor of a room). This combination requires a dez (hand shape) symbol and another tab (location) symbol. Finally, the sig (movement) symbol selected is one that indicates movement toward the signer (e.g., tapping of the fingers on the forehead).

Morphology, Syntax, and Semantics: Selected Features

There are a number of grammatical features of ASL that can be described. The focus here is on a few selected aspects that serve to highlight major differences between American Sign Language and the English signed systems, for example, the use of nonmanual cues, incorporation, modulation and inflection, and the use of classifiers. The ensuing paragraphs discuss how these features are reflective of grammatical elements of ASL associated with morphology, syntax, and semantics. An in-depth description of these and other features can be found elsewhere (Baker & Cokely, 1980; Klima & Bellugi, 1979; Liddell, 1980, 1995; Liddell & Johnson, 1989; Wilbur, 1987).

Nonmanual Features

In general, nonmanual features refer to those features that do not involve the hands (i.e., manual aspects). In this domain are aspects such as facial expressions (e.g., puffed cheeks and pursed lips), movements of the eyes and eyebrows (e.g., eye gaze, raising the eyebrows, and pulling the eyebrows together), and movements of other body parts (e.g., protruding tongue and moving the shoulders and/or head forward or backward). In essence, nonmanual features refer to facial grammar and body grammar of ASL.

Consider the ASL signs for the following declarative sentence: *You want coffee*. This simple sentence can be expressed by the use of three ASL signs for the three separate words, *YOU*, *WANT*, and *COFFEE*. By raising the eyebrows and tilting the head forward, this declarative sentence can be changed to a yes/no question: *DO YOU WANT COFFEE?* At the end of this signed sequence, the signer may also point an index finder at the addressee (i.e., person to whom the signer is talking).

The use of the eyebrows and shoulder movements is also critical for asking *wh*- questions such as *What do you want? Where are my shoes?* In this case, the eyebrows may be squint or raised and pulled together, and this is accompanied by a tilting of the head. Occasionally, the signer may shift his or her body forward, and sometimes, the shoulders are raised. Eye contact between the signer and the addressee is established at some point during the execution of the signed question. For sure, there is eye contact during the sign for the *wh*- words such as *what, when, where,* and *how*.

The expression of questions in ASL can be contrasted with how questions are executed in several of the English signed systems such as signed English, signing exact English, or seeing essential English. For example, none of the English signed systems employs the use of nonmanual signals as grammatical devices. The focus is typically on representing the words and the type of sentence (i.e., statement or question) visually via signs. For example, in the following sentence, *Do you want coffee?*, there might be a sign for every English word as well as for the question mark, amounting to a total of five separate signs. A good discussion of these differences can be found in Wilbur (1987).

Other facial movements in American Sign Language such as pursed lips and puffed cheeks add intensity to the meaning of the signs; that is, they serve to qualify the descriptions. For example, it is possible to change the meaning of *LARGE* to *ENORMOUS*, *SMALL* to *TINY*, *RECENT* to *JUST RECENT*, *DISTANT* to *REMOTE*, and so forth.

Incorporation

In American Sign Language (and other sign languages), it is possible to embed two or more concepts in the execution of a sign. This process is termed *incorporation* and can be seen in the use of negation (e.g., the signs for *DON'T KNOW* and *DON'T WANT*), numbers, and directional signs (e.g., signs such as *GIVE, INFORM*, and *TEACH*) (Baker & Cokely, 1980; Wilbur, 1987). This is another major difference between ASL and the English signed systems.

Consider the use of numbers in which the number sign (e.g., sign for *1, 2*, or *3*) is incorporated into the time sign (e.g., for *DAY, WEEK, MONTH*, or *YEAR*). For example, consider the sign for *MONTH*, which is made with the index finger of one hand (the dominant hand) sliding down the index finger of the other hand (the nondominant hand). If a two hand shape is used to make the month-like sign, then this is interpreted to mean *TWO MONTHS*. Similarly, the dominant hand shape can be changed to a different number, and this changes the month meaning—for example, three hand shape for *THREE MONTHS*, four hand shape for *FOUR MONTHS*, and five hand shape for *FIVE MONTHS*. Other examples can be shown for the following phrases: *ONE WEEK, TWO WEEKS FROM NOW, THREE YEARS AGO*, and so on.

Additional examples of number incorporation indicate the age of a person or the time of day, for example, *1 YEAR OLD, 5 YEARS OLD, FOUR O'CLOCK, THREE IN THE AFTERNOON*, and so on. According to Baker and Cokely (1980), some signers feel comfortable incorporating numbers up to nine, whereas others might stop at four or five.

Another form of incorporation involving the use of directional signs (GIVE, TEACH, etc.) indicates the subject and object of a sentence. Specifically, the subject-object distinction depends on the direction of the sign such as the one for *GIVE*. If the GIVE sign begins near the signer's body and moves outward to the person in front of him or her, this means *I GIVE YOU*. Moving the sign from the signer's body to the signer's right or left (i.e., to a person on the right or left) is interpreted as *I GIVE HIM OR HER*. Conversely, if the sign begins with the addressee and moves toward the signer, this means, *YOU GIVE ME*. Moving from the right or left (person on the right or left) toward the signer conveys the meaning, *HE OR SHE GIVES ME*. Figure 7-4 illustrates examples of incorporation involving numbers and directionality.

Modulation and Inflection

Another major difference between ASL and the English signed systems can be seen in the use of inflection (also called *modulation*) (for an extensive, clear treatment of this concept, see Baker & Cokely, 1980; Wilbur, 1987). In many English signed systems, contrived signs are used/invented to inflect words,

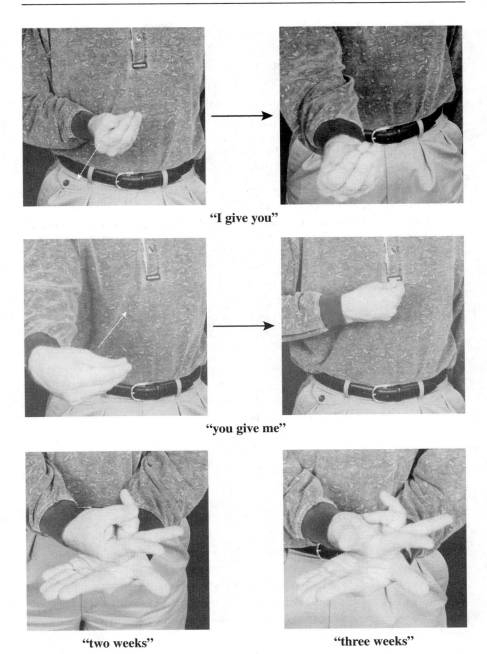

"I give you"

"you give me"

"two weeks"   "three weeks"

Figure 7-4 Examples of Incorporation in ASL.

for example, by adding inflectional suffixes and other types of inflections. Examples include pluralization such as changing *cat* to *cats* or *ox* to *oxen* and past tense of verbs such as changing *walk* to *walked* or *run* to *ran*. For example, in some English signed systems (notably, signed English and signing exact English), some of the signs that are used to indicate these inflections are the *s* hand shape (for *girls*), the *d* hand shape (for *walked*), and the FINISH sign made with one hand (for *ran*).

In American Sign Language, modulation/inflection is indicated by changes in the movement, place of articulation, or hand shape of a particular sign. It is possible to discuss this concept with respect to, at least, classifiers (next section), nouns, pronouns, verbs, adjectives, and time signs. Only a few examples are presented here because ASL has an extensive modulation/inflection system. In fact, it has been argued that "the functions of inflectional processes in ASL greatly exceed those in English" (Wilbur, 1987, p. 115).

With respect to some nouns, one way to indicate plurality is to repeat the noun sign itself; typically, the repetition is executed once. It seems that the use of the repetition movement is applicable to only a few noun signs; however, there is continuing research in this area. For example, the sign for *CAT* can be repeated to indicate the plural of CAT—*CATS*.

Verb signs may be repeated to agree with the plurality of some noun signs. In addition, verb signs can be modulated to indicate that a particular action (e.g., eating) occurred more than once (e.g., several times a day) or occurred over a period of time (e.g., eating continually). As is discussed later, the duration aspect is expressed by a slow repetition (i.e., reduplication) of the sign accompanied by wide circular movements. Finally, verb signs can be subjected to a number of modulations that can be translated in English as, for example, adverbs and verb aspects (e.g., progressive BE plus ING).

Reduplication (i.e., repetition), mentioned previously, can also be used with time signs. For examples, the signs for *WEEK, MONTH,* and *YEAR* can be repeated to indicate concepts such as *EVERY WEEK* or *WEEKLY, EVERY MONTH* or *MONTHLY,* and *EVERY YEAR* or *YEARLY.* This aspect of regularity can even be applied to the days of the week. For example, the sign for *WEDNESDAY* can be changed to express the meaning *EVERY WEDNESDAY.* In essence, this change (i.e., modulation) entails moving the specific hand shape downward in a vertical line in front of the signer. To indicate *EVERY OTHER WEDNESDAY*, the signer can add what is called a *hold* movement while moving the hand shape downward. Examples of modulation involving time signs are illustrated in Figure 7-5.

Time signs also can be modulated to express the concept of a repeated and long period of time. To express duration, the signer uses a slow repetition

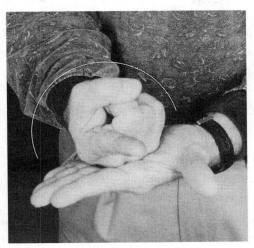

"every week"
or
"weekly"

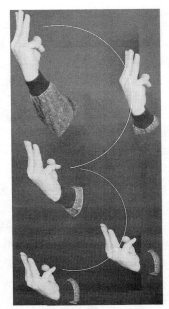

"every other Wednesday"

Figure 7-5 Examples of Modulation in ASL.

along with wide circular paths. In this manner, the sign for *ONE WEEK* can be modulated to express the meaning *FOR WEEKS AND WEEKS*. Similarly, the sign for *ONE MONTH* can be modulated to express the meaning *FOR MONTHS AND MONTHS*. As described by Baker and Cokely (1980; also see Wilbur, 1987):

> *This modulation seems to use both the slow intense movement that is used to show* duration *and the repeated movement that is used to show* repetition *or* regularity. . . . *This modulation involves a straight movement toward the place of contact (the passive hand), followed by a slow, intense movement . . . while the hand moves in an arc back to the place where the straight movement begins. This cycle is repeated (usually twice) and is often accompanied by a rocking movement of the head/body and an intense opening and closing of the mouth. (pp. 189–190)*

One other example involving two time signs are mentioned here. Consider the sign for *ONCE*. This sign can be reduplicated in a regular manner to express the concept of *SOMETIMES*. If the sign is repeated slowly and accompanied by circular movements (for duration), it expresses the concept of *ONCE IN A WHILE* or *OCCASIONALLY*. Similarly, the sign for the concept of *AGAIN* can be reduplicated regularly to express the concept of *OFTEN* and repeated slowly with circular movements to express the concept of *OVER AND OVER AGAIN*.

This is only a brief treatment of modulation/inflection. At the beginning, it was mentioned that the English signed systems tend to use additional signs to express modulation; often, these are contrived signs to address the changes/inflections of nouns (e.g., plurality), verbs (e.g., tense), adjectives (qualification), and other form classes. To highlight this treatment and contrast it with modulation in ASL, consider the following English phrases in which each word is expressed by a sign (or more, depending on the word) and the accompanying possible ASL descriptions. The reader should keep in mind that many of the ASL modulation examples are also accompanied by nonmanual movements involving the head and face.

English	*Possible ASL Descriptions*
very, very, big house	modulation of the HOUSE sign
eats continually all day long	modulation of the EAT sign
every other Monday	modulation of the MONDAY sign
really, really important	modulation of the IMPORTANT sign
extremely slow walk	modulation of the WALK sign
working quickly	modulation of the WORK sign
running very fast	modulation of the RUN sign
just recently	modulation of the RECENT sign

a long, long, long time ago   modulation of the PAST sign
extremely exhausted   modulation of the TIRED sign

Classifiers

One of the major and perhaps most interesting differences between ASL and English is the use of classifiers. There are a number of classifier languages; ASL is one, English is not. The presence of classifiers in ASL was initially reported by Frishberg (1975); since then, there have been numerous studies and descriptions of this grammatical feature (for a review, see Wilbur, 1987). In a simplified fashion, classifiers have been described as: "particular hand shapes that have general-purpose meanings" (Marschark, 1997, p. 57). Baker and Cokely (1980) remarked that:

> *Classifiers are basically hand shapes that are used in particular ways to represent the location and/or movement of a person or thing, or to describe certain characteristics of a person or thing, such as its shape, size, and texture. The palm orientation and movement of classifiers often vary to represent different things or to describe certain actions or characteristics of the referent. (p. 321)*

On the basis of this passage, classifiers can be categorized and refer to animate/inanimate, shape, size, and arrangement. For example, with respect to size, one can show large or small; with respect to shape, one can illustrate dimensions (one, two, and three), vertical/horizontal aspects, and descriptions of the surface of the objects.

There is, of course, more to this notion of classifiers than that which can be discussed here in this brief chapter (see the extensive discussion in Wilbur, 1987). In general, because classifier hand shapes have a certain meaning associated with them that is separate from their use in a particular sign, they can be utilized in creative ways to demonstrate a wide range of expressions in American Sign Language. Using a vehicle classifier (see Figure 7-6), the signer can describe the movement and results of a car in an event such as DEMOLITION DERBY in which cars bump into each other incessantly until there is only one remaining car that can move. That car is the WINNER.

A list of common classifiers used in ASL is presented in Figure 7-6 with descriptions. As can be seen in the figure, this list has classifiers for a person (whole and just legs), vehicle, airplane, and objects.

Use of Space

The last feature of ASL to be discussed here is the use of space, which is yet another aspect that can be contrasted with the manner in which it is used in

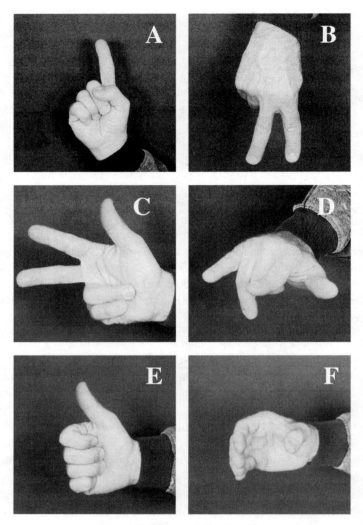

Figure 7-6 Sample of ASL Classifiers.

Note:
A: General person (animate): G-hand, usual orientation is fingertip up.

B: Person by legs: V-hand, usual orientation is fingertips down for 'stand,' 'walk,' 'kneel,' but may have other orientations.

C: Vehicle: 3-hand, orientation is fingertips sideways (as opposed to the numeral '3,' which has its citation orientation fingertips up), may be used for car, motorcycles, boats, trains, etc.

D: Plane handshape, may be used for airplanes.

E: Stationary object taller than it is wide (also may be used as dummy general object): A-hand, used in place of objects such as bottle, house, lamp.

F: Hollow, curved object with rim: C-hand, plam facing sideways, can be used for glasses, cups, jars, etc.

Source: Adapted from Wilbur (1987, p. 90).

the English signed systems. A few brief remarks have already been made about this feature previously; however, some elaboration is necessary. In essence, linguistic and paralinguistic information are conveyed by the spatial dimension in ASL. This is not the case in any of the signed systems. Space in the English signed systems is merely that rectangular area in front of the signer's body that is needed for the execution of signs.

In ASL, space is used as a grammatical device (i.e., to express syntactic and semantic relations) to communicate information related to time and location. It is probably best to view the signing space as a three-dimensional bubble (a metaphor from Crystal, 1997). Essentially, this entails the area directly in front of the signer from slightly below the waist to about one-half of an arm's length above the head (for some signs). The bubble includes the area in front of the signer as well as those areas to the right and left. This is considered a comfortable bubble; the signer might proceed outside the bubble for emphasis or exaggerated signing. Most of the signing, however, is executed within this bubble.

The use of a comfortable range of space notwithstanding, the real differences between ASL and English signing become evident in the linguistic principles associated with the use of space in ASL. This can become obvious, for example, with the use of classifiers, discussed previously. With respect to the notion of time and location, it has been remarked that (Crystal, 1997):

- *Time relationships can be expressed by dividing the space into neutral (present), further forward (future), and further back (past) areas; these areas can then be used both for tense forms and for time adverbs* (then, now, next, last, *etc.*).
- *Several persons (pronouns) can be distinguished using different spatial areas;* you *is front-centre; one third-person form is signed to the right; another to the left; and others divide up the intervening space. Moreover, once a space is established for a given person, it is normally "reserved" for that person for the remainder of the conversation.*
- *The whole spatial area can be enlarged or confined to express "louder" or "quieter" signing. (p. 224)*

ASL and English: Brief Summary of Differences

The previous section attempts to provide a few examples of differences between ASL and the English signed systems. These differences are due to those between the two languages, ASL and English. The focus earlier was on some major differences in morphology and syntax. A brief summary is presented here.

In English, and consequently in the signed systems, derivational and inflectional word parts are added to the base word or word stem in a linear or sequential pattern (*talk + ed*; *improve + ment*). From the brief rendition earlier, it should be clear that the morphological system of American Sign Language is simultaneously based. Signs are not simply affixed to the beginning or end of a sign stem or base sign. There are alterations in the movement of the sign itself (e.g., duration, repetition, and speed) that result in morphological changes. Another way of describing this phenomenon is: Signs are nested within movement contours. These movement contours are not affixed to the beginning or end, but rather, they occur simultaneously with the sign (see the discussion of modulation and incorporation).

The previous section contained a brief discussion of ASL syntax, or rather, ASL syntax was demonstrated via the use of classifiers, sign space, and some aspects of both pronouns and verb systems. It should be remarked that English adheres to a subject-verb-object word order, which is important to show grammatical relations. Of course, this word order can become quite complicated and confusing due to the use of hierarchical structures such as the use of relative clauses, passive voice, and other instances of embedded or conjoined structures. ASL also has a basic SVO word order; however, this pattern does not seem to dominate the syntactic structure of ASL (Isenhath, 1990; Liddell, 1980). There is quite a bit of variability in the sign order of ASL due to the existence of nonmanual features and the use of space (e.g., spatial syntax) (Baker & Cokely, 1980; Liddell, 1980; Wilbur, 1987). As discussed previously, one of the most interesting uses of spatial grammar can be seen in expression of vehicle or person classifiers. The variability of morphology and syntax in ASL is rule governed.

THE ACQUISITION OF ASL: PSYCHOLINGUISTIC AND SOCIOLINGUISTIC CONSIDERATIONS

Researchers' knowledge of the acquisition of American Sign Language and how ASL is used in a variety of social situations has been the result of psycholinguistic and sociolinguistic studies (see reviews in Bonvillian, 1999; Drasgow, 1998; Lane & Grosjean, 1980; Liddell, 1995; Newport & Meier, 1985; Wilbur, 1987). Researchers have focused on an array of issues such as the comprehension and production of the first signs, how signs are stored in memory, and the development of finger spelling by ASL-using deaf children of deaf parents (as opposed to English-signing deaf children of hearing parents). The manner in which deaf individuals process and use ASL is influenced by a number of linguistic and social factors, for example, the age at which ASL is required, the age at onset of deafness, the hearing status and socioeconomic status of the parents, the educational level of the deaf individual, and so on. One of the most interesting lines of debate has been whether ASL needs to be described in a sociolinguistic manner (i.e., how it is used in the community) rather than a pure linguistic one (i.e., independent of use via introspections). This has been influenced by various accounts on the nature of American Sign Language, especially in contact situations with individuals who possess knowledge of a range of English signing (see the discussions in *The Deaf American*, 1990).

Another intense, interesting line of research concerns whether there are parallels or similarities between the development in a sign language and that in a spoken language. Bonvillian (1999) offered a nice synopsis of the reasons for the importance of this question:

> First, if language acquisition processes were shown to be the same, this would indicate that language was a higher cognitive process that transcended the modality of expression. Second, if the processes were the same, then investigators could study linguistic processes in sign and then extrapolate their findings to languages in general. And, third, if the course of acquisition were found to be different across modalities, then many of the assumptions in linguistic theory about universal processes would need to be changed. Clearly, much was riding on the answer to this question. (p. 280)

This section highlights a few early exemplar studies on the acquisition of American Sign Language. It also provides a brief summary of findings on salient issues such as parallel/similarity between sign and spoken languages, early sign production, the notion of babbling, and a few studies on syntax, semantic, and pragmatics. The discussion of ASL acquisition is organized into two broad areas: (a) phonology and related aspects (e.g., babbling, first signs, and iconicity) and (b) grammar (i.e., morphology and syntax), meaning (i.e., semantics), and use (i.e., pragmatics). The reader is referred elsewhere for in-depth analyses of these areas (Bonvillian, 1999; Klima & Bellugi, 1979; Liddell, 1980, 1995; Wilbur, 1987).

Phonology: Babbling, The First Signs, and Iconicity

Much of the research on signing has focused on the acquisition of vocabulary and grammar; only recently has there been an interest, perhaps renewed interest, in sign phonology (see review in Bonvillian, 1999). In fact, this is also true in the studies on spoken language; that is, in recent years, there has been a proliferation of investigations on the development of phonological and related knowledge (e.g., the developmental sequence of sounds, the issue of phonological and phonemic awareness, and so on). With respect to sign languages, specifically American Sign Language, there has been some research on the nature of babbling, iconicity, and of course, the acquisition of the first signs. As is typical of these studies, there have been comparisons between the development of spoken language and that of a sign language.

As discussed previously, the acquisition of a spoken language begins during the prenatal period, that is, during the time the fetus is developing. In this respect, one can argue that the processing and development of a spoken language is advanced when compared to that of a sign language. Most 6- to 7-month-old fetuses can hear; thus, the human fetus has been responding to human voices from the beginning of life, most specifically, the fetus responds to the pregnant mother's voice (see discussion in Locke, 1993). Chapter 4 also describes the newborn's range of auditory processing skills, which are quite impressive. It should be remarked that hearing infants with no sign language experience also are able to discriminate between gestures with respect to the movement contrasts in the signs of ASL (Carroll & Gibson, 1986). In essence, visual language discrimination skills are also developing from the time infants are able to utilize visual abilities.

Babbling

There has been a preponderant amount of debate on the role of babbling to the subsequent language acquisition process. One line of research considers babbling to be a direct precursor to language development. Within this purview, infants are exercising and playing with the speech mechanisms; however, they are not attempting to engage in intentional behavior per se (i.e., to talk). A second line of research focuses on the effects of the infants' babbling on significant others, particularly the parents. Within a sociocultural paradigm, this reciprocal relation between infant's babbling and adults' response contributes to the development of language because language is considered to be a socialization process.

There has been an interesting debate also on the vocal babbling behavior of deaf infants and whether hearing infants actually engage in manual babbling (Bonvillian, 1999; for a readable account, see Marschark, 1997). Based on his understanding of the research, Bonvillian (1999) argued that vocal babbling in deaf children is delayed when compared to that of hearing children. Marschark (1997), however, provided a much more elaborate interpretation. Marschark argued that the early vocalizations of deaf infants have a range of sounds that are quite similar to those of hearing infants of hearing parents. Then, there seems to be a decrease in both variety and frequency, whereas the babbling of hearing infants continues to increase and becomes more complex up to the production of their first words and beyond. In essence, the relative lack of complex babbling development during this period seems to have pervasive effects on the development of a spoken language for social and communicative intents for deaf children of hearing parents. Or to put it another way, because the continuing development of babbling is essential for subsequent language development, deaf children of hearing parents already are at a disadvantage in the language acquisition process, specifically with respect to the development of a spoken language. Even with early amplification and intervention, the babbling and early vocalizations of deaf children of hearing parents still seem to be fewer in variety and frequency when compared to those of hearing infants of hearing parents.

The situation is quite different for deaf infants of deaf parents, at least with respect to manual babbling. Manual babbling refers to the repetitions of the components of a sign (i.e., shape or movement). The emergence of manual babbling has been reported to occur during the latter half of the first year (Meier & Willerman, 1995; Petitto & Marentette, 1991). This seems to indicate that deaf infants of deaf parents have a language advantage over deaf infants of hearing parents. In this case, the reference is to the development of a sign language for social and communicative intents for deaf children of deaf parents. This development is advanced when compared to the development of a spoken language for deaf children of hearing parents during the early language acquisition period. Because there is an increase in manual babbling for these deaf children, similar to that of vocal babbling for hearing children, there is also an increase in the reciprocal interactions between deaf infants and significant others, particularly parents.

Marschark (1997) provided an eloquent—albeit poignant—description of this difference between the early language development of deaf children of deaf parents and that of deaf children of hearing parents:

> *In general, deaf parents show greater awareness of the communication needs of deaf children than do hearing parents. This awareness results in part from their own experiences, but they also are likely to be more sensitive to visual signals from their children, and they clearly will have a better channel of communication with them via sign language. Some hearing parents also are very aware of cues from their young deaf children about the success or failure of communication. Most, however, lack competence and confidence in their signing abilities, and these attributes can make it more difficult for them to adapt to the needs of their children. For their part, hearing fathers tend to have even poorer sign skills than hearing mothers—presumably one reason (and perhaps a partial cause?) for mothers taking on a proportionally greater caregiving role than they do with hearing children. (p. 103)*

Bonvillian (1999) remarked that there seems to be some disagreement concerning the nature and extent of manual babbling among hearing infants who are not exposed to a sign language. The babbling response seems to be innate, and both vocal and manual aspects have been reported for both deaf and hearing children. For example, Petitto and Marentette (1991) reported a higher incidence of manual babbling in deaf infants learning to sign than in hearing infants who are learning to speak. They interpreted their findings to mean that (a) babbling emerges from a general single language capacity and that (b) the language capacity was functional without respect to the type of language input or modality. On the other hand, Meier and Willerman (1995) reported similar levels of manual babbling in both deaf and hearing infants (who were not exposed to sign). In essence, Meier and Willerman argued that manual babbling occurred without regard to language input or modality. In addition, Meier and Willerman suggested the importance of neuromotor aspects for both vocal and manual babbling. With respect to the differences between these two studies, Bonvillian (1999) argued that:

It is clear that additional research will be needed in the future to resolve the role of neuromotor development in both vocal and manual babbling. For the present, we can conclude that there is strong evidence for babbling in both language modes at about the same ages. (p. 281)

Selected Aspects of Phonology

One of the main phonological foci of other early studies on American Sign Language was the acquisition of hand shapes (see review in Hoffmeister & Wilbur, 1980). In general, similar to hearing children learning a spoken language, deaf children acquire easier (unmarked) linguistic elements prior to the more difficult (marked) linguistic elements. McIntire (1977) provided a good example of this finding. McIntire studied the acquisition of hand shapes in one deaf child at ages 13, 15, 18, and 21 months. This researcher reported that pointing and grasping hand shapes were acquired initially (e.g., A, S, L, 5, C, and BABY O). The acquisition of more complex hand shapes (e.g., H, W, 8, and X) occurred with the increasing maturity of cognitive and physical abilities. In addition, substitutions produced by the subject involved similar phonological elements, for example, using the 5 hand shape instead of the F hand shape to sign *CAT*. This phenomenon parallels substitution of phonemic elements in hearing children. Thus, the phonological development of deaf children appears to be similar to the phonologic development of hearing children. That is, both groups of children proceed from easier, less marked linguistic elements to more difficult, more marked elements, and both substitute easier, similar linguistic elements for more difficult ones.

There seems to be a general acquisitional sequence for hand shapes, and more recent studies have attempted to explain this process (Boyes-Braem, 1973/1990; Siedlecki & Bonvillian, 1997). One major hypothesis is that the development of hand shapes is constrained (or guided) by the anatomical and physiological development of the hands. That is, in the use of early signs, children tend to produce four basic hand shapes—5-open hand, G-index finger extended, B-flat hand, and A-fist—most often and accurately. With the further development of their hands, they learn to execute the other hand shapes that are more complex. Their production also becomes more accurate and consistent due to the increase in their vocabulary knowledge. There may also be other factors that impact the formation of a sign, particularly the developmental sequence of hand shapes. Most interesting, a couple of major factors are sign input and sign context (i.e., the richness of the environment). These findings have also been reported for children and adolescents learning a second language. That is, one of the major criticisms of second language programs is the lack of natural language models, which often resulted in the use of stilted language or inadequate development across all of the language components (e.g., phonology and syntax) of the second language. A good summary of some additional major findings on other phonological features can be found in Wilbur (1987) and Bonvillian (1999).

The First Signs and Beyond

Comparisons have been made between the ages at which children say their first words and those at which they execute their first signs. Research on hearing children has documented the production of the initial words between the ages of 10 and 14 months. A broader age range has been documented for the production of the first signs by deaf children, from about 7 months (Hoffmeister & Wilbur, 1980; Orlansky & Bonvillian, 1985) to about 13 months (Schlesinger & Meadow, 1972). Reporting on studies on both hearing and deaf children, Marschark (1997) remarked that the first signs have been reported to emerge around 9 months of age. In essence, it has been difficult to determine when either the first words or first signs emerge in both deaf and hearing children. The first utterances, whether signs or words, are actually approximations of the adult forms and may not be the actual intentions of the child. In other words, these are utterances without communicative intentions or purposes. Depending on parental survey or observations can be misleading because parents tend to read more into their actual observations or documentations of the utterances.

There have been attempts to compare the early language development in sign language with that of spoken language. For example, Bonvillian (1999) synthesized the data from two longitudinal studies (Bonvillian, Orlansky, &

Novack, 1983; Folven & Bonvillian, 1991) that he argued accounted for "much of the information about early sign production" (p. 281). In the earlier mentioned two studies, there were 22 children, deaf and hearing, whose language development was examined for selected periods (i.e., from 4 months to beyond 2 years). These data were compared with those on the spoken language development of 18 hearing children in the work of Nelson (1973). Considerable variations in the emergence of first signs, two signs, and other language milestones were documented and were consistent with findings of the variations in spoken language development. In general, there were many similarities between the development of sign language and that of spoken language with respect to the emergence of referential usage (i.e., intentional communication such as naming new objects, relations, and so on), and there was considerable overlap of vocabulary items in both modes of development. For example:

> Both the signing and speaking children named many of the same objects, actions, persons, and properties that were common to their environments. Indeed, the same vocabulary items that occurred most often among the sign-learning children (e.g., cookie, Mommy, Daddy, hot, car, no, shoes, milk, dog) also were the most frequent entries in the lexicons of the children learning to speak. (Bonvillian, 1999, p. 285)

There were, of course, a few differences with respect to the rate of growth of vocabulary and the use of function items (as opposed to content items). However, the evidence in the realm of phonology suggests a general similarity in development for both sign and spoken language.

Iconicity

The last issue to be discussed here in the phonological realm is that of iconicity, which seems to generate interest and causes problems for unsophisticated observers of sign language usage. Much of the debate has been on the role of iconicity in the memory and acquisition of ASL signs. Iconicity is the purported pictorial relationship that exists between a sign and its meaning. It is possible to trace the formation of a sign to a real-world attribute and assume that this contributes to the acquisition of that sign. That is, there is assumed to be an association between the sign and the real-world aspect that it resembles. For example, the sign for *CAT* involves the stroking of the upper side or sides of the lip, indicating the whiskers of a cat. Iconicity implies that signs are pictorial or ideographic in nature and are not part of a real language.

Research on adults and young children indicates that iconicity does not determine the relationship between a sign and its meaning (see discussions in Bonvillian, 1999; Markowicz, 1980; Wilbur, 1987). For example, when signs were presented to nonsigners, it was found that these individuals could not guess the meaning of the signs on the basis of the so-called picturability of the signs. There is also evidence that iconicity does not play a major role in the acquisition of initial signs or in the memory of signs for young children (Klima & Bellugi, 1979; Orlansky & Bonvillian, 1984; Wilbur, 1987). Thus, similar to the relation between a spoken word and its referent, the relation between a sign and its referent is also arbitrary and must be learned.

In sum, there seems to be general developmental similarities between sign language and spoken language in the area of phonology. In both modes, phonological development requires a few years for proficiency, and the development of features (i.e., phonemes) seems to be sequential. The easier sign and spoken phonemes are acquired before the more difficult and complex ones. There are, of course, individual differences in the acquisition process. Perhaps the most interesting parallel is that the development of phonology in both language modes is constrained or guided by the anatomical and physiological development of the body. For speech, this entails the speech mechanisms (e.g., the articulators of the mouth), whereas for sign, this entails the manual mechanisms (e.g., the hand and fingers).

Grammatical, Meaning, and Use Aspects

There have been studies that focused on the acquisition of syntax (i.e., grammar), semantics (meaning), and pragmatics (use) in ASL. Similar to the studies on phonological development, researchers have had an eye on not only charting developmental patterns but also comparing them with those of a spoken language, notably, English.

Describing the syntax of ASL has proven to be an interesting challenge. Siple's (1978) remarks still hold true: "It is easy to say that the grammar of ASL is uniquely its own; but it is more difficult to identify and describe the actual syntactic devices used" (p. 10). Nevertheless, the secrets of ASL are slowly being uncovered as investigators unravel syntactic devices such as reduplication, verb directionality, and the use of nonmanual cues, mentioned previously (also see the discussions in Liddell, 1980, 1995; Wilbur, 1987). The study of these devices is important for a description of word order in American Sign Language. In addition, nonmanual cues are critical for the production of structures such as negation, question formation, and relativization (Liddell, 1980).

Only a few early studies and subsequent reviews are presented. The ones selected here as examples focused on three structures: negation, pronominal reference system, and classifiers. Again, the major impetus for selecting and discussing these studies is to show the similarities across language modalities, that is, across both spoken and sign languages.

Negation

Hoffmeister and Wilbur (1980) reviewed a number of studies investigating the beginning stages of the acquisition of negation. In general, in the earlier stage, the use of the sign for *NO* is present as well as the more frequent negative head shake. The latter stage is characterized by the emergence of two signs *NOT* and *CAN'T.* Similar to hearing children learning a spoken language, the notion of *CAN'T* is acquired prior to that of *CAN.* In sum, it was concluded that these developmental stages appear to parallel those reported for hearing children learning English (Brown, 1973).

These findings have been supported by subsequent research studies (Anderson & Reilly, 1997). Anderson and Reilly (1997) reported that ASL-using deaf children begin to express the concept of negation at about 1 year of age. This expression, similar to that reported by Hoffmeister and Wilbur (1980), took the form of a negative head shake to signify a rejection of others' comments or suggestions. This is also about the same time (1 year of age) that hearing children began to express negation via the use of nonverbal gestures. Anderson and Reilly remarked that deaf children were able to express negation via the use of negative signs by the time they were 18 months old. Again, this is roughly the same age as when hearing children have the word *no* in their vocabulary.

Pronoun Reference System

Hoffmeister and Wilbur (1980) described a study on the acquisition of the pronominal reference system of ASL. A deaf child of deaf parents served as a subject. Results were presented in five stages. In Stage 1, for example, they reported that pointing behaviors refer to objects that are visible in the immediate environment; for example, the signer, objects in view. The subject indicated a possessor-possessed relationship by initially pointing to an object and then pointing to the self. Analogously, Nelson (1973) and Bates (1976) also found similar deictic (pointing) gestures that preceded the spoken language development in young hearing children. These pointing behaviors of the deaf child also were the precursors to other pronominal concepts, for example, plurality, the use of *THAT* and *ALL*, which are later executed by formal adult signs. By Stage 3, the previously learned operations began to refer to events and objects not in the immediate environment. By Stage 4 (age 4 years, 2 months), reflexivization (i.e., use of the SELF signs as in YOURSELF, MYSELF, and so on) emerged as a set. Finally, the researchers concluded that this deaf subject had mastered the ASL referential system by Stage 5 (4 years, 5 months of age).

These findings were supported in a more recent review (Petitto, 1987). In essence, at approximately 2 years of age, young children using ASL employ the use of pointing gestures to refer to pronouns in their signing utterances. Again, this is about the same age that hearing children incorporate the use of pronouns in their conversations.

Classifiers

Kantor (1980) studied the acquisition of ASL classifiers by deaf children. Similar to classifiers in some spoken languages, ASL classifiers appear as part of syntactic forms (e.g., the verb or the noun) and reflect certain semantic properties of their noun referents. Nine deaf children, age 3 to 11 years, of deaf parents served as subjects. Similar to other studies on acquisition of ASL, these findings indicated a developmental sequence similar to that identified for hearing children learning a spoken language (Menyuk, 1977). In particular, it was reported that classifiers emerged around age 3 and were mastered by 8 or 9 years of age. It was concluded that classifiers are not acquired as lexical items but rather as a complex syntactic process. As mentioned previously, the concept of classifiers represents a very complex system. A more recent and detailed discussion of classifiers can be found in Wilbur (1987). In sum, Kantor suggested that rule acquisition in both ASL and spoken languages is affected by similar phonological and syntactical environments.

Semantic Relations

Newport and Ashbrook (1977) conducted a study to compare the emergence of semantic relations in deaf children learning ASL as a first language to that of hearing children learning English as a first language. Five young deaf children served as subjects. In general, the findings indicated that the existence relation emerged prior to action relations, which preceded state relations. In addition nonlocatives emerged prior to locatives. A detailed description of these relations can be found in Bloom and Lahey (1978) and Lucas (1980) (also see a brief discussion of relations in Chapter 4). It was concluded that the sequence of the acquisition of semantic relations by deaf children was similar to that reported for hearing children despite the differences in modality and syntax.

Form, Meaning, and Use

Kantor (1982) also conducted phonologic, syntactic, semantic, and pragmatic analyses on data obtained from interactions of two deaf mothers with their deaf children. This researcher was interested in (a) describing the modifications of deaf mothers in communicating with their children and (b) describing the developmental sequence of deictic (pointing) behaviors and modulated verbs in deaf children exposed to ASL. In general, Kantor reported that the deaf mothers, similar to hearing-speaking mothers, modified their language to fit the child's, that is, they used more simple and direct sentence structures. The developmental sequences of the pointing behavior and verb modulations were essentially similar to those reported early in this section by Hoffmeister and Wilbur (1980). In addition, Kantor suggested that pointing in the early stage indicated a few semantic relations, for example, the use of demonstratives (e.g., *THIS* and *THAT*). Additional semantic and pragmatic functions emerged at a later stage with the occurrence of locatives, pronominals, and indexing referents present in the context.

Acquisition Studies: Brief Summary

Only a few studies were presented here to demonstrate similarities across language modalities. A number of studies have focused on American Sign Language and English (for a discussion of the verb system, see Anderson & Reilly, 1997; Meier, 1987). The bulk of the evidence strongly supports the existence of many developmental parallels between American Sign Language and English. Of course, there are some differences with many of them due to individual variations. The similarity hypothesis needs to be accepted with caution because the findings are based on few longitudinal studies. Clearly, there is a need for additional studies.

In sum, the evidence is clear for general developmental similarities. It is much more difficult to investigate whether there are identical similarities across language modalities. Bonvillian (1999) proffered a synthesis of the similarity issue, which can be used as a guideline for future research:

> *Aspects of language acquisition that depend more on cognitive development (e.g., onset of referential language) appear to be virtually identical. Aspects of language acquisition that depend more on the development of control of production components (e.g., onset of recognisable words and signs) appear to differ considerably in their emergence across modality. Thus, the timetable of early vocabulary development often favors children learning to sign. (p. 291)*

FINGER SPELLING IN AMERICAN SIGN LANGUAGE

Chapter 6 presented a discussion of finger spelling with respect to its use in the Rochester Method and also for representing the letters of the alphabet of

English. This section provides a few brief remarks on the use and development of finger spelling in American Sign Language. It has been argued that the development of finger spelling in deaf children who know ASL is different from this development in deaf children who are attempting to learn English as a first language (Padden, 1991, 1998a; Padden & LeMaster, 1985). Consequently, it has been suggested that a better understanding of these differences is necessary to clarify the manner in which finger spelling is used by deaf children in their attempts to acquire English writing skills. Additional discussion on the use of finger spelling can also be found in Chapter 9 of this text, which focuses on bilingualism and second language learning.

The Use of Finger Spelling in ASL

Not all signed languages have a manual system for representing the symbols used in the dominant spoken languages for the printed form (e.g., letters, characters, and syllables) (Padden, 1991, 1998a). In the United States, there are 23 hand shapes to represent 26 English letters. *Finger spelling* is the popular term used to refer to the manual system of ASL.

In general, whole sentences of English words are not finger spelled unless a particular English sentence is finger spelled for emphasis or unless there is an attempt to capture a specific figurative usage in English (e.g., *It's raining cats and dogs*). When words are finger spelled in ASL, they usually refer to proper names or titles of individuals and places. In addition, in education settings, finger spelling is often used to reflect specific mathematical and scientific terminology as well as the terminology used in other learned situations (e.g., medical, legal, and government). In these instances, finger spelling can represent all letters of any English word and can be utilized for all of that word's meanings in English.

In essence, it has been stated that "fingerspelling is a marked manual system (compared to natural signed languages), imported into ASL putatively for representing foreign words" (Padden, 1998a, p. 105). This raises an interesting question: Should the use of finger spelling be referred to as the use of English? There is no simple answer to this question; however, Padden (1998a) offered an interesting perspective:

> *From a structural point of view, however, it is one thing to call finger spelling borrowed vocabulary and another to call it "English." First, it represents English in alphabetic, not spoken form. Second, its vocabulary is extremely selective, consisting largely of nouns, with verbs very rarely represented. Furthermore, signers do not finger spell sentences except in situations where one is attempting to represent extended English*

text verbatim. For the most part, finger spelling occurs only as words interspersed in signing. With this kind of distribution, it would be stretching any definition of a human language to call finger spelling "English." More accurately, finger spelled words are largely foreign vocabulary used as a resource within the larger resource of ASL. (p. 106)

The Development of Finger Spelling and English Writing

One way to understand the relationship of finger spelling in ASL and English writing is to describe its use by young children (deaf or hearing) of Deaf parents (Akamatsu, 1982; Padden, 1991; Padden & LeMaster, 1985). Several general patterns have been observed in these few studies. Finger spelling is used by young children who have not yet acquired the skills to read or write English (although some children may be in the emerging writing stage with the use of scribbling). Nevertheless, the main point here is that knowledge of English is not a prerequisite for using finger spelling, and children learn about the connection to English much later.

Perhaps the most provocative assertion is that finger spelling is a unique system with its own formational rules. The organization of finger spelling is such that it has connections with the written language systems of spoken languages rather than being a specific representation of a particular system. Evidence for this assertion can be seen in the manner in which young children of Deaf parents finger spelled words. These children do not finger spell the letters of words in a letter-by-letter sequential fashion. Furthermore, the finger spelled words are not synchronized with the manner in which the words would typically be pronounced (i.e., by syllables). The expression of finger spelled words seems to be governed by movement units or contours that resemble the movement activity found in the use of sign. Padden (1998a) highlighted a few examples from her studies:

> *One father reported that his daughter used different movement contours for finger spelling "rice" and "ice." R-I-C-E was finger spelled with a distinctive semicircle, but I-C-E, with a short opening and closing of the fingers. Another child, recorded on videotape, attempts to spell D-E-L-L, but uses a single L hand shape throughout while using the distinctive bounce for doubled letters. (p. 107)*

Again, it is emphasized that the children in these studies did not know English and at the time were not aware of the connection of finger spelling to English letters. Thus, one interpretation of these findings is that deaf children need to learn the association between finger spelling and English letters. Knowledge of English letters may not be essential for the acquisition of finger spelling. However, on the other hand, it seems to be critical for children to understand some of the morphological properties of American Sign Language to acquire finger spelling. In fact, Padden and others argued that children need to understand the foundations of finger spelling within ASL before they can understand the connection of finger spelling to the letters of English (i.e., the alphabetic principle).

Padden and others argued that deaf children can learn adequately about English orthography and its alphabetic system primarily via the use (i.e., mediation) of finger spelling and ASL. Within this framework, there is no need to manipulate or acquire the performance form (i.e., speech and/or sign) of spoken English prior to or in conjunction with learning the written form. The complex discussions of the merits of this viewpoint can be found in both Chapter 8 and Chapter 9. Regardless of the debate, it is clear that much more research is needed on the interrelations among finger spelling, ASL, and the English writing system.

CRITICAL PERIOD AND AMERICAN SIGN LANGUAGE

Chapter 3 mentions briefly the concept of a critical period for language acquisition, known as the critical period hypothesis (also see Lenneberg, 1967). This is the view that a specific period for language acquisition exists during which it needs to be acquired to be learned in a proficient manner. The strong form of this hypothesis asserts that the critical period extends from early childhood (actually within the first 3 years) to about puberty. The earlier a language is acquired, the better. In any case, it is extremely difficult for an individual to learn a language as he or she ages, and this difficulty is compounded after puberty. In fact, the strong form asserts that a full-blown first language is almost impossible after puberty.

Throughout this text, it has been reiterated that language needs to be acquired as early as possible for an individual to develop a high level of literate thought that is conducive for success in society (see Chapters 1 and 12). Although it has been and is still difficult to ascertain the critical period hypothesis, there seems to be a consensus that the early development of language is essential for the subsequent development in the psychological, social, and emotional domains as well as for the acquisition of script-literacy skills.

It is possible to obtain a good perspective on the critical period hypothesis from the research that has been done on deaf adults, especially those who were children of hearing parents and/or who have learned a language (English or ASL) at various ages during their formative years. A few remarks are provided here, based predominantly on the work of Mayberry and her associates (Mayberry, 1994; Mayberry & Eichen, 1991; Mayberry & Fischer, 1989). The reader is reminded that it is not uncommon for many students with severe to profound hearing impairment to begin their formal schooling period with little or no proficiency in a social-conventional language. In many cases, these students of hearing parents struggle with the language acquisitional process for their entire school career. For example, they may graduate from high school with a literacy level on the third- or fourth-grade level.

Mayberry and her collaborators examined the relationships between the ages at which deaf individuals began learning to sign and these individuals' abilities to use their language skills as adults. Mayberry (Mayberry & Fischer, 1989) documented several general patterns in her investigations. For example, there was a strong positive correlation between length of sign experience and performance on the experimental tasks. That is, adults with a greater amount of years in signing performed significantly better than other adults with fewer years of signing experience. In addition, the researcher found that the number and type of errors were related to the age at which sign language was acquired. For example, adults who learned to sign at a younger age produced more semantic errors (e.g., confusing meaning such as *older/younger*) than phonological errors (e.g., confusing hand shapes, hand movements, and hand location). On the contrary, the older sign learners produced more phonological errors than semantic errors. The older learners also produced more errors and more different types of errors than the younger learners.

In another study, Mayberry (Mayberry & Eichen, 1991) examined the sign language skills of deaf adults whose experience in signing ranged from about 21 to about 60 years. Despite the lengthy amount of experience among the participants, there were differences in performances that were related to the age at which they learned to sign (e.g., early childhood or adolescence). For example, the younger sign learners (i.e., those who learned to sign early in life) tended to produce more grammatically acceptable utterances in ASL and to perform better on a test of ASL sentence recall. In essence, despite the lengthy sign experience of many participants, the age at which they learned to sign became a critical factor in their performance.

In a subsequent analysis, Mayberry (1994) demonstrated that learning a language in early childhood in any modality (speech and/or sign) positively influences the learning of subsequent languages. Mayberry compared two groups of deaf students. One group of students learned ASL after acquiring a certain level of proficiency in English; in this case, most were considered to be bilinguals. The second group had experienced much difficulty in learning

English and thus learned ASL during adolescence. In essence, both groups had learned ASL; however, the first group had a better understanding of English and had levels of proficiency in a first language (English) at an earlier age. Results indicated that the first group (bilinguals) performed significantly better than the second group (late learners of one language, ASL) on ASL tasks. That is, the first group made significantly fewer errors. Even more interesting, this first group produced more semantic errors than phonological errors, resembling the early ASL learners in Mayberry's other investigations. On the contrary, the late learners of one language (ASL) produced more phonological errors than semantic errors.

In sum, although Mayberry's findings will not end the debate on the critical period hypothesis, they do seem to provide strong support for the notion that linguistic and cognitive performance are affected by the age at which a first language is acquired. Even more important, the benefits associated with early language acquisition are independent of a specific language modality (speech and/or sign).

FINAL REMARKS

Traditionally, the study of spoken languages has contributed to much of the prevailing linguistic thinking. The study of sign languages, however, has only recently attracted the attention of linguists and psycholinguists. The major objective of this chapter is to provide a brief introduction to the nature and acquisition of American Sign Language and to demonstrate how it is different from English and the English signed systems.

There is general agreement that ASL is a bona fide language, although there seems to be some disagreement on how ASL is used or should be described—that is, linguistically or sociolinguistically. Recent research has shown general similarities between development in sign languages and that in spoken languages. Parallels in processing and in developmental stages have been observed between ASL signers and speakers of English. Additional research is necessary to determine the manner in which skills can be transferred from a sign language to a spoken language. Within this arena, one of the most interesting lines of research has been the nature of finger spelling in ASL and whether it can be used to mediate an understanding of the written language system of English. The last section of this chapter discusses how the study of ASL has contributed to the ongoing debate on the critical period hypothesis.

A few of the major highlights of this chapter are as follows:
- American Sign Language was born from a combination of the sign system of the Abbe de l'Epee, brought over by Gallaudet and Clerc, and the varieties of signs that were already in use by deaf people in America.

- As a visual-gestural language, American Sign Language is particularly structured to accommodate the visual capacities of the eye and motor capabilities of the body. Manual features pertain to the shapes, positions, and movements of the hands, whereas the nonmanual features refer to the movement of the cheeks, lips, tongue, eyes, eyebrows, shoulders, and the body.

- Similar to any other language, ASL is rule governed, which means that the formation, sequencing, and execution of signs are governed by a finite set of rules that needs to be learned or acquired.

- There are a number of major differences between ASL and English, including the signed systems that are based on English. Most of the differences discussed in the chapter concerned the components of morphology and syntax, including the issues of nonmanual grammar, incorporation, reduplication, directionality, and the use of spatial grammar.

- There is still some controversy regarding the issue of babbling. Nevertheless, both vocal and manual babbling have been observed in both deaf and hearing infants of deaf parents. It is possible to conclude that there is strong evidence for babbling in both language modes (sign/speech) at about the same ages.

- With respect to general developmental similarities, one interesting parallel is that the development of phonology in both speech and sign modes is constrained or guided by the anatomical and physiological development of the respective articulators.

- With respect to general developmental similarities in spoken and sign languages, Bonvillian (1999) argued that:

Aspects of language acquisition that depend more on cognitive development (e.g., onset of referential language) appear to be virtually identical. Aspects of language acquisition that depend more on the development of control of production components (e.g., onset of recognisable words and signs) appear to differ considerably in their emergence across modality. (p. 291)

- Finger spelling is a unique system with its own formational rules. The organization of finger spelling is such that it has connections with the written language systems of spoken languages rather than being a specific representation of a particular system. Development of finger spelling in ASL is dependent not on knowledge of the alphabetic system of English but on increasing understanding of the morphological properties of ASL.

- Research on the critical period hypothesis and ASL (a) seems to provide strong support for the importance of early language acquisition and (b) reveals that the benefits of early language acquisition are independent of a specific language modality.

At this point in the text, the reader has been exposed to major findings associated with the language/communication approaches—oral English (Chapter 5), Total Communication (Chapter 6), and American Sign Language (this chapter). Despite the importance of this issue, there is a great need for additional research, especially with respect to the development of English literacy skills. Nevertheless, it is not often remembered that literacy is much more than language development—although, theoretically, it is part of the overall language comprehension process. The nature and development of English literacy are discussed in the next chapter.

AMERICAN SIGN LANGUAGE COMPREHENSION QUESTIONS

1. American Sign Language as well as other sign languages have been in existence for a long time, possibly throughout recorded history. What are some reasons for the increase of research on sign languages, particularly American Sign Language? (Consider the work of Bonvillian (1999) as well as other comments in the beginning section of the chapter.)

2. Describe a few perspectives on the history of the evolution of American Sign Language. What are some important events or issues in this evolution? (For example, consider the situation of language teaching methods, the development of a signed system, etc.)

3. Discuss the following phrases about ASL:
   a. visual-gestural, rule-governed language
   b. manual features
   c. nonmanual features

4. List and describe the four basic phonological (cherological) parameters of a sign in ASL.

5. Discuss the major highlights of the following selected features of ASL:
   a. nonmanual features
   b. incorporation
   c. modulation and inflection

    d. classifiers

    e. use of space

6. Discuss some of the major differences between American Sign Language and English, including the English signed systems. (You should focus on form and grammar, especially morphology and syntax.)

7. With respect to the research on phonology, provide a summary of points related to

    a. babbling

    b. the acquisition of hand shapes

    c. the first signs

    d. iconicity

8. Discuss some of the major research findings on grammatical (i.e., syntax), meaning (i.e., semantics), and use (i.e., pragmatics) in the acquisition of ASL. (Consider the studies on negation, pronouns, classifiers, and semantic relations.)

9. Based on psycholinguistic studies, is it possible to argue that there are developmental parallels between American Sign Language and English? If so, provide some examples. If not, why not?

10. Describe the role and use of finger spelling in American Sign Language. Is finger spelling the use of English? Does finger spelling have a role with respect to the development of English writing skills? What does it mean to say that finger spelling is a unique system with its own formational rules?

11. What are some of the main points in the section entitled: "Critical Period and American Sign Language?" Can the information in this section of the chapter be related to that from Chapter 1 on literate thought? In what way? (Also see Chapter 12.)

CHALLENGE QUESTIONS

(Note: Complete answers are not in the text. Additional research is required.)

1. In general, most scholars agree that

    • speech is not equal to language

    • speech is not important for the development of abstract thought

- the use of signs does not interfere with the development of speech

Provide some reasons and research support for these assertions. Do you think that speech is important for the development of English literacy skills? Or, do you think that speech is simply a manifestation of underlying phonological skills that are needed for phonemic awareness? (A perspective on phonemic awareness can be gleaned from Chapter 8 of this text.)

2. Conduct a literature review on the concept of the critical period hypothesis. Do you think the work of Mayberry (in this chapter) provides conclusive evidence for the hypothesis? Why or why not? Having read Chapters 5, 6, and 7, you now know that many if not most children with profound (and possibly severe) hearing impairment who have hearing parents do not develop proficiency in a first language, notably English, by the time they start their formal education period (ages 3, 4, or 5). Given the later performances of many of these students on achievement tests, can this be offered as indirect evidence for the critical period hypothesis? Why or why not? Given what you now know, what do you propose to ameliorate this situation? Do you think ASL should be the first language for all or most children with severe to profound hearing impairment, even if this is not the desire of the hearing parents? Why or why not?

3. Consider the following scenario:

ASL is a visual-gestural language that does not involve the meaningful use of speech sound for receiving and expressing information. Given typical language developmental patterns, it is quite possible that a number of deaf children of deaf/Deaf parents (i.e., parents who are both audiologically deaf, profoundly hearing impaired, and culturally Deaf) would not be encouraged by the parents to develop their residual hearing because it is simply not needed for their language. In fact, it is possible that they would not use amplification at all.

Should this be acceptable to the larger community of professionals and educators? There is some research (see Chapter 5) that early amplification/identification is critical for the development of residual hearing and, consequently, for the development of English language and literacy (although for the latter, it is not hearing per se that is the issue). The later the amplification, the fewer the benefits (or more difficulty) from the use of the remaining hearing. Is this a moral issue? Should it be a legal issue? Should parents be legally required to engage in early amplification/identification if their child is diagnosed with a hearing impairment? Why or why not?

4. Do you think it is possible to learn to read and write a phonetic language such as English without ever hearing or speaking it? Do you know of any cases? If so, why are these students successful? Is it clearly the case of knowing only a sign language such as ASL? Is this question similar to the linear relationship ones that have been asked previously in this text? How is it possible to proceed from the primary conversational form of a visual-gestural language to reading and writing in a phonetic language? (Some perspectives on these issues can be gleaned from Chapters 8 and 9; however, additional outside reading of other literature is necessary.)

FURTHER READINGS

Baker, C., & Padden, C. (1978). *American Sign Language: A look at its history, structure, and community*. Silver Spring, MD: T. J. Publishers.

Bishop, D. (1990). *Handedness and developmental disorder*. London: MacKeith Press.

Kimura, D. (1993). *Neuromotor mechanisms in human communication*. New York: Oxford University Press.

Stokoe, W. (1972). *Semiotics and human sign languages*. The Hague, the Netherlands: Mouton.

van Uden, A. (1986). *Sign languages of deaf people and psycholinguistics: A critical evaluation*. Lisse, Netherlands: Swets & Zeitlinger.

CHAPTER

8

Script Literacy: Development of Reading and Writing

To completely analyze what we do when we read would almost be the acme of a psychologist's dream for it would be to describe very many of the most intricate workings of the human mind, as well as to unravel the tangled story of the most remarkable specific performance that civilization has learned in all its history. (Huey, 1908/1968, p. 8)

What drives reading and writing is this desire to make sense of what is happening—to make things cohere. A writer achieves that fit by deciding what information to include and what to withhold. The reader accomplishes that fit by filling in gaps . . . or making uncued connections. All readers, like all writers, ought to strive for this fit between the whole and the parts and among the parts. (Tierney & Pearson, 1983, p. 572)

These passages, used in the second edition of this text, are still relevant and thought provoking, and they continue to epitomize, in the author's view, the way a number of theorists and researchers feel about the processes of reading and writing (or reading and literacy). The importance of literacy skills for a society such as in the United States and the enormous difficulty that a substantial portion of the American population has in acquiring an adequate, highfunctional proficiency level have been the subject of numerous debates, research, and reports, most notably, the national reports by Anderson, Hiebert, Scott, and Wilkinson (1985) and Snow et al. (1998). Even more interesting, and problematic for many deaf and some hard-of-hearing students, is the growing consensus that phonemic awareness is essential for beginning reading progress and for the subsequent development of advanced literacy skills. To put it succinctly and briefly here, phonemic awareness is the awareness that language is composed of small units of sounds called phonemes (i.e., vowels and consonants) that correspond to the letters of an alphabetic writing system such as that of English (see Chapter 2 for a discussion of phonemes). In other words, understanding the basic alphabetic principle requires an awareness that spoken language can be analyzed into separable words and that words can be segmented into sequences of syllables and phonemes (i.e., representing sounds and letters).

Phonemic awareness, albeit efficient, is not the only avenue for understanding the alphabetic principle; orthographic knowledge, for example, is also helpful and indeed may be an important route for students needing intervention programs (see Snow et al., 1998, for a review). Of course, there is more to reading (and possibly writing) than just an awareness of words and phonemes; yet, this awareness is critical for the development of rapid automatic word identification skills in reading. And, as discussed in this chapter, it is not likely for students to develop adequate reading comprehension skills if they are struggling to identify the words on the page. In addition, with respect to the complex—albeit not adequately understood—relations between reading and writing, it can be argued that fluent, organized writing ability will also be difficult for many individuals to attain.

There seems to be little doubt that reading and writing skills are highly valued and important in a scientific technological society such as that which exists in the United States. It could be argued that high-level literacy skills are reflective of the ability to think at high levels; that is, the ability to think in a rational, logical, complex, reflective manner often associated with the Western world consciousness or in societies that have written languages (however, see Chapters 1 and 12 for another perspective). One needs to read and perhaps write to continue to learn and perhaps survive in literate societies. In other words, reading and writing skills contribute to and are examples of the literate mind as well as tools that might be necessary for participating in and reaping the benefits of the social, economic, and political realms of mainstream society in the United States.

The plan for the chapter is as follows. Initially, the processes of reading (and literacy) are briefly discussed, as gleaned from prominent theoretical models of both reading and writing developed by theorists who have studied literacy in children who have typical hearing ability. It should be clear that this information is also critical for and applies to literacy in deaf and hard-of-hearing children and adolescents. In fact, it is becoming clear that there are certain fundamentals for all children who are attempting to learn to read and write in English, including in English as a second language (see reviews in Adams, 1990; Snow et al., 1998). It is emphasized that our either-or debates (e.g., phonics vs. whole language, word identification vs. comprehension, etc.) are counterproductive and do not emanate from a synthesis of the research findings. For example, despite the tendency to emphasize either word identification or comprehension in reading, it is becoming clear that word identification facilitates comprehension and comprehension facilitates word identification. The research on writing is also discussed; however, the author's bias (and perhaps scholarly interest) influences him to frame this discussion around the reciprocal effects of reading and writing. Thus, much of what is said has been influenced by his understanding of reading. A portion of the chapter is devoted to synthesizing and presenting the results of numerous studies on literacy (i.e., reading and writing) and deafness. It is demonstrated that the strong interrelations among language, reading, and writing relative to the English language account for much of the difficulty of many deaf and some hard-of-hearing students in obtaining advanced literacy skills. Banking on the discussion in Chapter 6 on the signed systems, there seems to be little doubt that the sign-print connection is not commensurate with or not similar to the speech-print connection, especially in light of what is known about the importance of phonological and phonemic awareness. Thus, it seems that the cross-modal properties of speech and print are different from those of sign and print. The last section of the chapter proffers some guidelines for developing script literacy in deaf and hard-of-hearing students and provides suggestions for further research efforts.

The major emphasis in this chapter is on script literacy, that is, the development of skills often needed for accessing and interpreting information that has been captured either typographically or chirographically—or what Olson (1994) termed, *The World on Paper*. There is some discussion of critical literacy, which is the ability to use language for activities that involve problem solving, making inferences, and other reasoning endeavors (Calfee, 1994). However, much of the information about critical literacy is presented in the last chapter of this text (Chapter 12), which includes a detailed discussion of the related concept of literate thought, that is, the ability to think reflectively, rationally, logically, critically, and creatively.

Table 8-1 provides a brief description of literacy-related terms to assist the reader in understanding those concepts as presented in this chapter.

Table 8-1 Brief Description of Literacy and Related Terms

- *Alphabetic principle*—The system on which English writing is based. There is an association between the limited set of phonemes from spoken language and the limited set of letters of the English alphabet. Knowledge of the alphabetic principle refers to an awareness that words are composed of letters that are related to phonemes (or phonemic segments) from spoken language.

- *Comprehension*—There is no acceptable description of comprehension save that it refers to *understanding*. Formally, comprehension refers to the individual's ability to construct a model of meaning relating to either spoken language (i.e., listening comprehension) or written language (i.e., reading comprehension).

- *Context clues*—To figure out the meaning of word, words, or phrases, the reader might use the information—that is, context clues—that surrounds these items in the sentence. For example, the reader might reread a sentence that contains an unknown word. Although using context clues is a helpful strategy for comprehension breakdowns, a reader should not engage in this process frequently. That is, frequent conscious use of context clues to understand a word or words impedes overall comprehension efforts. In fact, this might be indicative of a difficult passage for the reader.

- *Context factors*—The emerging sociocultural models of literacy are strongly concerned with the effect of context on reading and writing development. In this sense, context refers to the environment, situation, and time frame in which literacy occurs. For example, sociocultural proponents argue that understanding a passage depends on the effects of the reader's home environment as well as social, historical, and cultural influences. In addition, classroom and school environmental factors play major roles. It is also important for the reader to understand the period or environment of the time the story was written (e.g., the influences, background, and times of the author).

- *Conventional spelling*—This refers to the rules that govern the manner in which letters are used to represent the sounds/words of speech. This also refers to a particular sequence of letters in a word.

- *Decoding*—Traditionally, this is the conversion of print symbols (i.e., letters) into sounds (i.e., mostly via syllables or words). For some deaf and hard-of-hearing students, this conversion process might result in alternative representations (see *Internal coding strategy*).

- *Dialect*—A regional or social variety of language use, typically indicated by a difference in pronunciation, grammar, or vocabulary usage. This output differs from the standard language or speech pattern, often called the standard dialect of the culture.

- *Emergent literacy*—In general, the period of literacy development that culminates into conventional literacy. This is different from the concept of readiness in which the focus is on getting children ready for literacy. With emergent literacy, there is a recognition that children engage in literacy-related behaviors and activities that are precursors to and important for the development of later skills. In addition, these early behaviors evolve into the more conventional ones. In one sense, a good analogy is the relationship between babbling and the first words, as discussed in Chapter 4.

- *Fluency*—The ability to identify words and comprehend text in an automatic rapid manner. This also refers to the reader's ability to coordinate word identification and comprehension in a smooth manner.

- *Inferential ability*—This is another concept that is difficult to define or describe satisfactorily. In reading instruction, it is often referred to as the ability to perform tasks such as drawing conclusions, getting the main idea, generalizing, and answering high-level questions such as text-implicit and script-implicit questions (as discussed later in this chapter as Question-Answer Relationships [QARs]). In essence, to make inferences, the reader needs to supply information (i.e., fill in the gaps) that is not explicit in the passage. Inferential ability also refers to the reader's attempts to paraphrase or to build a model of what the text means.

- *Internal coding strategy*—This is related to the concept of decoding, discussed previously. As discussed later, deaf and hard-of-hearing children might employ one or more coding strategies, for example, sign, dactyl (finger spelling), visual (mostly print), and speech (i.e., phonological or phonemic aspects). Internal coding strategy refers to the representation of information in short-term (working) memory (also see Chapter 3).

- *Invented spelling*—In one sense, this is an idiosyncratic spelling system invented by a child and based on letter names and/or sounds. It is considered a developmental milestone on the way to conventional spelling ability. Other names for this process are *creative spelling* and *estimated spelling*.

(continues)

(Table 8-1 continued)

- *Letter blends/clusters*—Letter blends and clusters are combinations or strings of letters (i.e., consonants) in words. Some common blends are *bl, cl, sl, br, sm, sn,* and *sw.* Clusters refer to a series of consonants at the beginning or the end of words such as *str* in *stray* and *strong* and *ks* in *looks* and *books.*

- *Letter/sound knowledge*—This refers to the knowledge of sounds that are associated with the various letters. Formally, this entails the phoneme-grapheme link or the relationships between phonemes and their representative graphemes. Another way of stating this is the knowledge of consonants and vowels, their combinations, and their representations in letters.

- *Literacy*—Traditionally, this includes reading and writing; specifically, activities that involve the production and comprehension of printed texts.

- *Literary genre*—A category of literary composition. Some possible examples include fiction, fables, nonfiction, plays, poems, or prose.

- *Literate thought*—Another concept that is difficult to describe or define. In this text, it is described as the ability to think reflectively, creatively, logically, and rationally. It is related to inferential ability.

- *Metacognition*—In general, this means thinking about thinking. With respect to literacy, it refers to the individual's ability to think about comprehension. That is, the individual engages in comprehension monitoring (understanding or evaluating what is read) and comprehension repairs (figuring out unknown words or confusing information). The answering of questions, application of prior knowledge, and all forms of inferential activities are forms of metacognitive behaviors.

- *Orthography*—The study of the representation of spoken language via the use of letters, diacritical marks, and spelling. Orthographic awareness refers to the understanding of these representations. For example, an individual knows what letters represent and is familiar with specific spelling patterns and strings of letters. (A *diacritic* is a mark added to a letter, as in résumé or in proper names, to indicate a specific phonetic value or to distinguish words that are graphically similar.)

- *Phonemic awareness*—Simply put, this is an awareness that words are composed of or can be segmented into phonemes (e.g., *cat* into /c/ /a/ /t/). Many scholars believe that this awareness is critical for proceeding to conventional spelling and reading development. It is also related to an understanding of the alphabetic system, the system on which English writing is based.

- *Phonics*—The use of instruction that assists children in understanding the systematic relations between sounds and letters—that is, letter-sound correspondences. Phonics instruction requires that children possess both phonological and phonemic awareness skills (see phonemic and phonological awareness). Good examples of phonics instructional techniques can be found in Durkin (1989) and Johnson and Pearson (1984).

- *Phonological awareness*—This is a general awareness of the sound system of a language. Individuals recognize that spoken language contains structures that are separate from meaning. By focusing on the internal structures of words, children can hear or recognize chunks of sounds such as syllables and rhymes. Children might be made somewhat aware of smaller units of sounds such as phonemes; however, phonemic awareness usually develops after the general phonological awareness and typically requires instruction. One of the manifestations of phonological awareness can be seen in the way children play with words by repeating them and by the rhymes that children either make up or remember.

- *Print awareness*—This type of awareness is necessary if children are to proceed with vocabulary and reading development. Children need to understand what is meant by reading—for example, there is information on the page. They need to understand the basic relationship between oral language and printed language. Some of the areas in which children may need assistance are as follows:

  1. Concepts of text features or print: letter, word, sentence, question, and dialogue.

  2. Vocabulary for discussing books: cover, page, story, character, title (name), author (writer), and illustrator (artist).

  3. How to handle books: hold right side up, turn pages, where to begin reading, attend to the spaces in text, and reading from left to right, top to bottom.

  4. Book structures: title page, chapters, and table of contents.

- *Prior knowledge*—This is a term that is also difficult to describe or define. In general, prior knowledge (also known as *background knowledge*) refers to the stock of information that individuals have on a particular topic, word, event, and so on. As discussed in this chapter, there is a strong relationship between prior knowledge and reading comprehension. In essence, when applied (as via metacognitive skills), prior knowledge can assist readers in tasks such as making inferences and in applying information to other stories

(continues)

(Table 8-1 continued)

or incidents. It is difficult to determine just how much prior knowledge is necessary to understand or comprehend a particular story because it is not always clear what is meant by understanding or comprehending. Two broad types of prior knowledge have been discussed: passage specific and topic specific. Passage-specific prior knowledge is often described as information that is needed to answer literal and inferential questions given the information in the story. That is, the answers to the questions can be inferred using the information in the text. Topic-specific prior knowledge refers to the general background that individuals have about a particular topic—which seems to proceed beyond what is offered in a particular story. That is, individuals know more about a topic than is presented in a story on that topic. It has been argued that topic-specific prior knowledge is essential for a better understanding of the topic and for an adequate understanding of many passage-specific questions that are often asked in classroom settings.

- *Reader factors*—This refers to factors associated with the reader. The most typical ones are intelligence, socioeconomic status, background or prior knowledge (of topics, language literacy, etc.), motivation/interest, and metacognitive ability. With respect to deaf and hard-of-hearing students, there are others that can be added, for example, factors associated with hearing impairment (see Chapter 1) and type of internal coding strategy (see *internal coding strategy;* also see Chapter 3).

- *Structural analysis*—An instructional technique that is designed to assist children in analyzing unfamiliar words in print by focusing attention on the meanings of known parts within the words. Structural analysis addresses word parts such as bound and free morphemes (see Chapter 2 of this text). Using structural analysis, children might be able to apply their understanding of known elements (i.e., morphemes) to figure out the whole unknown word. For example, a child may know the word *ice*, but may have difficulty with the word *reice*. By focusing on word parts, the child might be able to combine his or her understanding of *ice* and *re-* and make an educated guess about *reice*.

- *Syllable*—This is a unit of spoken language, typically a unit of rhythm, often expressed by a vowel sound alone or a combination of a vowel with one or more consonants that either precedes or follows the vowel. Analyzing a word (i.e., figuring it out) via the use of syllables is one strategy used for word identification; however, it should be used judiciously due to the complexity and problems it might cause for children. Examples: *Fire* has two syllables; *book* has one syllable; and *beautiful* has four syllables.

- *Task factors*—This entails a broad area with the most common foci in the research on deaf and hard-of-hearing students on assessment (i.e., the measurement of reading and writing) and purpose (i.e., the purpose or goal for reading or writing a particular selection). With respect to assessment, there has been some research on the effects of certain tasks or formats for assessing reading, for example, the use of multiple choice and cloze procedures. Other research has documented the effects of the wording of questions at the end of passages, which have influenced the answers selected by deaf and hard-of-hearing students (e.g., word association strategies). With respect to purpose, the emphasis has been on the various reasons for reading a passage, for example, to scan or skim for a quick review or essential information or highlights, to study or remember intently for recall or test purposes, or to argue for a position or case.

- *Text factors*—This refers to factors associated with the text such as letters, words, syntax, figurative expressions, genre (see *literary genre*), and print conventions such as punctuations, headings, capitalizations, indentations, and markings such as bold, italics, and underlines. Much of the early research on deaf and hard-of-hearing students focused on text factors with some attention to reader factors (see *reader factors*).

- *Word identification*—A number of phrases have been associated with word identification, for example, *word analysis, word recognition, word attack,* and *decoding* (see Johnson & Pearson, 1984). Despite the debates on the differences among these terms, at least two seem to be used commonly and interchangeably—*word recognition* and *word identification.* At a simple level, word identification refers to the identification of a word by the reader by either pronouncing it or, in the case of many deaf readers, by signing it (Finger spelling presents problems in this area; see discussion in this chapter; also see Chapter 7). Identifying a word does not necessarily mean that the reader knows the meaning of the word. To identify a word, a reader might use a number of strategies and information relating to phonology (e.g., phonics), morphology (e.g., structural analysis), syntax (e.g., contextual analysis—i.e., placement of the word in the sentence structure), semantics (e.g., word meaning, contextual analysis), or a combination of strategies and information. Rapid word identification skills are considered essential for reading comprehension development.

Note: For additional information on the literacy terms, readers should consult the following sources—Adams (1990), Durkin (1989), Johnson and Pearson (1984), and Snow, Burns, and Griffin (1998).

348 ■ LANGUAGE AND DEAFNESS

DESCRIPTION OF THE LITERACY PROCESS

It should be clear that the answer to the question What are reading and writing? depends on one's worldview, particularly one's paradigm (see discussions in Ritzer, 1991, 1992). From one perspective, it has been asserted that reading and writing are constructive, multicontextualized entities involving an array of processes such as linguistics, cognitive, social, and political (Pearson & Stephens, 1994). It is possible to categorize factors into a number of frameworks such as text (e.g., orthography, grammar, and genres), reader/writer (e.g., prior knowledge, metacognition, and affective behaviors), task (e.g., purpose of reading/writing and type of assessment used), context (e.g., cultural influences and school effects), and the interactions or combinations of these areas (see Table 8-2).

Table 8-2 A Few Factors Associated With Text, Reader, Task, and Context

---

Text (Print Knowledge)

Letter knowledge

Letter-sound correspondences

Orthography

Word meanings

Syntax

Other discourse structures

Literary genres

Reader

Prior knowledge

Metacognition (strategies)

Inferential ability

Motivation/interest

Task

Purposes of reading/writing

Setting or time issues

Evaluation issues

Context

Social and cultural areas

Classroom culture

Home environment

Note: Additional information on many of these factors and related terms is presented in Table 8-1. Also see Chapter 2.

A substantial number of researchers have used a single-perspective lens (e.g., positivism or constructivism) and have focused on effects within one of these areas, whereas others have emphasized interactions or combinations of two or more areas. To be considered complete or adequate, any model of literacy needs to incorporate aspects of all areas mentioned (text, reader, task, and context), delineate major components within the areas, discuss internal processes, and demonstrate relationships between and among the components.

There is no widely accepted description of the reading and literacy process, although several frameworks have been proposed (Paul, 1998a, 1998b). One useful framework was proposed by McCarthey and Raphael (1992). These scholars attempted to categorize models into three broad areas: cognitive information processing, naturalism, and social constructivism. In the second edition of this text, much of the attention was devoted to the cognitive information processing models, which were further subdivided into bottom-up, top-down, and interactive, based on the framework of Samuels and Kamil (1984). Eloquent critiques of these frameworks and models can be found in several sources (Antonacci & Hedley, 1994; McCarthey & Raphael, 1992; Mitchell, 1982; Samuels & Kamil, 1984). Table 8-3 depicts some of the basic principles of the three broad frameworks, and Table 8-4 provides a few tenets of broad cognitive models (i.e., within the cognitive information processing framework) known as bottom-up, top-down, and interactive.

Table 8-3 Selected Points and Critiques of Three Major Literacy Frameworks

Cognitive Information Processing
Principles

- Reading and writing consist of similar underlying processes, including a number of subprocesses.

- Lower level processes should become automatic and fluent so that readers/writers can concentrate on higher level processes associated with the construction of meaning.

Critique

- A better understanding of the problems of poor readers and writers has emerged; however, it is not clear how poor readers and writers become or can become good readers and writers.

- Implications for instructional practices seem to be limited or not clear.

Naturalism
Principles

- A heavy focus is placed on the individual; for example, it is the individual who must interpret the world and construct his or her own personal meaning via reading and writing activities.

- Strong emphasis on child-centered or child-directed literacy activities; formal or teacher-controlled instruction, especially of specific skills, is deemphasized or discouraged.

Critique

- The notion that literacy development is similar to physical or biological development is open to debate.

- The role of the teacher or the social environment in the development of literacy has been downplayed or minimized.

Social Constructivism
Principles

- The promotion of the view that all knowledge, particularly human knowledge, is socially constructed.

- It is argued that language, cognition, and literacy are not entities unto themselves; rather, they are manifestations of social and cultural processes.

Critique

- It is difficult to test empirically some of the major tenets.

- This view may lead to radical relativism with respect to knowledge, including literacy knowledge.

Note: Based on the discussion in McCarthey and Raphael (1992) and Paul (1998a).

Table 8-4 A Few Tenets and Criticisms of the Broad Cognitive Models

Bottom-Up or Text-based Models

- There is a great deal of emphasis on the recognition (identification) of letters and words.

- The process begins with the perception of letters and words on the page, proceeds through the analyses at several successive levels involving larger units such as phrases and sentences, and culminates with the construction of meaning at the top, that is, in the readers' minds.

- The models have demonstrated the importance of knowledge of the alphabet system.

- The use of context clues in a deliberate manner actually plays a minor role in lexical access in highly literate readers.

Criticism of the Bottom-Up Models

- Readers do not read words letter by letter in a left-to-right fashion. Nevertheless, they do process all the letters of words.

- Word identification is mediated by phonological recoding; however, readers can access some words through a visual route. Readers still need to use a phonological recoding process for many other words.

(continues)

(Table 8-4 continued)

- The ability to identify words automatically and effortlessly is critical but not sufficient for reading comprehension.

Top-Down or Reader-based Models

- The only purpose of reading is comprehension, and this should be emphasized from the beginning.
- Reading is said to begin with the information that is in the readers' heads, not with what is on the printed page.
- In one top-down model, reading acquisition is similar to language acquisition.
- Models have shown that reading is a predictive process and that an adequate knowledge of the culture and specifically the language in which one is trying to read are important.

Criticism of the Top-Down Models

- These models do not adequately explain how young children learn to read.
- There is no adequate explanation of what skilled readers do whenever there is a breakdown in comprehension.
- One of the major weaknesses is the dependency on context for comprehension. It has been demonstrated that context does not accelerate the identification of words or accelerate the derivation of word meanings.
- Models fail to notice that difficulties in the use of context cues during reading for word identification purposes is not strongly related to reading comprehension problems that exist in readers.

Interactive Models

- These models emphasize the reader as an active information processor whose goal is to construct a model of what the text means.
- Comprehension is driven by preexisting concepts in the readers' heads as well as by the information from the text.
- The construction of meaning requires the development and coordination of both bottom-up and top-down skills and occurs at many different levels of analysis such as lexical, syntactic, schematic, planning, and interpretative.

Criticism of the Interactive Models

- In schema-interactive models, it is not clear how schema is developed initially. There does not seem to be adequate descriptions of the relationships between and among schemata.

- The manner in which schemata contributes to the understanding of a text is not completely or adequately understood.

- These models do not seem to address a variety of word identification strategies or problems associated with comprehension beyond the sentence level.

Note: Adapted from Bernhardt (1991), Grabe (1988), and Samuels and Kamil (1984). Criticisms based on Paul (1998a).

Another, perhaps more comprehensive manner for categorizing perspectives can be found in the text by Ruddell et al. (1994). The five major categories expounded are cognitive processing, sociocognitive processing, transactional, transactional sociopsycholinguistic, and attitude influence. In a previous text on literacy and deafness (Paul, 1998a), particularly in the chapters on script literacy, it can be seen that the author has been heavily influenced by cognitive processing models, particularly the works of Adams (1990, 1994) and Rumelhart (1994). Rumelhart framed reading and literacy as an interactive process in an attempt to explain the relations among letters, letter clusters, words, syntax, and semantics. Adams (1990) discussed the interactions among four components, which she labeled *phonological, orthographic, meaning,* and *context.* These influences, as well as some others, are evident in the discussion of reading and literacy in the present edition of this text.

Tierney (1994) offered a good critique (i.e., similarities and differences) of the five frameworks mentioned earlier. Similar to the attempts in Chapter 3 of this text for language models, Tierney attempted to frame his discussion of the reading and literacy models with respect to the continuing debates and influences of epistemology, for example, the tensions between absolutism/relativism or among positivism/constructivism/postmodernism. In addition, Tierney noted, as have others, that it is not simple and easy to proceed from the models to implications for instruction and curriculum. This remark was also made in Chapter 3 of this text with respect to language theories. In comparing the various models, Tierney remarked that:

Drawing from literary criticism, anthropology, linguistics, schema the-
oretic notions of text processing, social psychology, and observation of
readers, writers, and teaching, the model builders describe in varying
degrees the nature and role of the following:

- *the influence of context;*
- *the role of background knowledge;*
- *readers' or writers' experiences with text, purposes, values, motiva-*
  tions, and stances prior to their encounters with a text;
- *the nature of the reader's or writer's meaning-making, especially in*
  terms of hypothesis-testing;
- *the role of predictions, selective attention, self-monitoring, and imag-*
  ing and affective dimensions of reading;
- *the role of text features such as the propositional content, cohesion,*
  and organization;
- *peer influences on meaning-making;*
- *the role of teachers and classroom practice in literacy learning; and*
- *some of the expected outcomes of literacy learning, including the func-*
  tions that literacy encounters might serve as well as what might be
  considered the norms that govern any judgment of the adequacy of
  response. (pp. 1169–1170)

Most of the current perspectives on reading (and writing) can be traced
to early views on reading, particularly during the 18th and 19th centuries
(Bartine, 1989, 1992). Then, as now, there were a number of acrimonious
debates on whether meaning resided in the text, the reader/writer, or somewhere in between or above. These positions depended on how thinkers view
the nature of the contact between reader/writer and text. In addition, there
were discussions of the relationships between spoken English and written (text
based or script) English, including whether these relationships needed to be
taught or caught. Similar to the present push for multidisciplinary or interdisciplinary approaches, these frameworks in the past were influenced by the
work of individuals in various disciplines or domains such as rhetoric, literary criticism, linguistics, psychology, and pedagogy as well as by long-standing
debates in philosophy on notions such as empiricism, rationalism, and
phenomenology.

Admittedly, this is a rather broad, abstract—perhaps sketchy—overview
of models of the reading and literacy process; however, it is hoped that it encap-

sulates the tensions and dissensions that exist in this field, which have polarized theorists, researchers, and educators, even those who work with deaf and hard-of-hearing students (see discussions in Paul, 1997, 1998a, 1998b). It is still important for educators to be aware of the current thinking on reading and literacy from the perspectives of theorists and metatheorists. To discuss reading and writing in a more relevant manner, that is, more relevant to educators and other practitioners, a brief synthesis is provided of some of the major findings in three sources, Adams (1990), Anderson et al. (1985), and Snow et al. (1998).

THE DEVELOPMENT OF LITERACY: A BRIEF, SELECTIVE OVERVIEW

Researchers' understanding of literacy is the result of research from a variety of disciplines (e.g., psychology, sociology, political science, philosophy, linguistics, literary criticism, etc.), settings (e.g., laboratory, home, school, learning centers, etc.), and perspectives (e.g., cognition, socialization, language, instruction, culture, and politics). All of these areas are important; however, it has been difficult to paint a coherent picture (see discussions in Ruddell et al., 1994; Snow et al., 1998). The focus of this section is to discuss the development of conventional reading; that is, the independent activity of accessing the form (i.e., written code) to construct (or obtain) meaning. The notion of meaning is complex; nevertheless, there is a message in the text that can be comprehended and, obviously, interpreted in many different ways depending on the cultures and experiences of the reader/writer. In addition, there is a purpose for engaging in this activity, which includes enjoyment, obtaining information for studying and taking a test, and enlightenment. It is not the intention here to provide a comprehensive picture of literacy; instead the remarks focus on a few major areas of script literacy and emphasize that the access to the form of printed materials requires many skills—one of the most important ones is an understanding of the alphabetic system. This understanding is facilitated by phonemic awareness, that is, the notion that words can be separated into phonemes, which are manifested by the letters on the page.

With respect to conventional reading, it is often forgotten that all readers oscillate between the form (i.e., structure of letters, words, etc.) and meaning (i.e., comprehension of the words, sentences, story, etc.). This oscillation depends on skills, experiences, and purposes of the readers/writers. Preschool children (and even many poor readers) who have heard a story a number of times might pretend to read the story or even make up portions of it due to the fact that they have not learned to decode words yet. Beginning readers with some knowledge of the alphabetic system may read (via saying words out loud) the story slowly or disfluently, implying a strong attention to form. Both groups of children are interested in the meaning or message. Even mature readers oscillate between form and meaning. These individuals proceed on automatic pilot until they come to unknown words or concepts that disrupt the meaning-making process and compels them to take action to resolve the conflict (Adams, 1990; Anderson et al., 1985).

As most educators know, the acquisition of literacy skills begins prior to the mandatory school period. Without delving too deeply into the debate on when children can or should actually read and write, suffice it to say that literacy development is related to other age-related developmental timetables. Children who are deaf or hard of hearing need to be considered at risk because of the difficulty in developing age-appropriate literacy skills, however unappealing this might sound to strong cultural proponents of deafness. Most of these children, but certainly not all, do not exhibit age-appropriate developmental skills (e.g., language, cognitive, social, and sensory) as they progress through the early childhood period. Even culturally Deaf children who know ASL as a first language are at risk, similar to other second-language learners. However, culturally Deaf children are also at risk because of a sensory condition or deficit or whatever word is acceptable to most educators in this contentious field. An intact auditory-articulatory loop—albeit facilitative—is not necessary for developing literacy skills; however, it does contribute to the understanding of the sound system of a language, such as English, on which the writing system is based. Ultimately, an individual needs to have cognitive awareness of this representation system, even if it is not developed peripherally via the auditory-articulatory loop (i.e., the hearing-speaking connection).

Given the controversies surrounding the development of oral skills in deaf and hard-of-hearing children, it is important to emphasize that phonological and phonemic awareness, mentioned previously, are not the same as speech perception. As discussed in Chapter 5 on oralism, speech perception is the ability to detect and discriminate the sounds associated with a particular language. Because of the overlap of processing between speech perception and hearing ability, it is no surprise that children with severe to profound hearing impairment also have poor speech discrimination skills. Even some children with otherwise typical intact hearing may have difficulty making discriminations among speech sounds. For a number of varied reasons, children who possess poor speech discrimination skills have difficulty acquiring phonological awareness. In addition, many young children with typical hearing who perform satisfactorily on tests of speech discrimination may exhibit weak phonological awareness. In essence, for young children, phonological awareness, not speech perception or discrimination, is a good predictor of subsequent success in reading during the first few grades of school.

What does phonological awareness and phonemic awareness mean? The term *phonological awareness* refers to a general overall appreciation of the sounds of speech as distinct from their meanings. *Phonemic awareness* entails an understanding that words can be divided into a sequence of phonemes. Children with typical hearing develop phonological awareness during the preschool years, and the demonstration of this type of awareness manifests itself in the correction of their speech errors and the playing with a variety of sounds. The beginning stages of phonemic awareness become evident with the appreciation of activities such as alliteration (*Peter Piper* and *rat-tat-tat*) and rhymes. However, it is difficult for many preschool children to proceed to a more advanced level of phonemic awareness involving a conscious understanding or recognition of phonemes (i.e., vowels and consonants). In fact, without instruction, few children are able to engage in activities such as recognizing differences of initial (*bat-pat*) or ending sounds (*lab-lap*) or advanced ones such as leaving off a letter, resulting in a different sounding word (or sequence of letters) (*slap* to *lap*) (Adams, 1990, 1994; Snow et al., 1998).

It is also important to clarify the difference between phonological and phonemic awareness and phonics. *Phonics* refers to instruction in the manner in which the sounds of speech are represented by letters and spellings. For example, children may learn that the letter *P* represents the phoneme /p/ and may be exposed to the various ways by which the long vowel sounds are manifested (see the discussion in Durkin, 1989). Thus, with the use of phonics, it is assumed that children have a working awareness of the phonemic composition of words. In fact, children who lack phonemic awareness are unable to participate adequately in phonics lessons. They will have great difficulty in sounding and blending new words, in remembering words for subsequent lessons, and in learning to spell. On the other hand, there is some research showing instruction that focuses on developing a working awareness of phonemes affects the reading and spelling growth of children in a positive manner. These results have been obtained with typical (i.e., nondisabled) as well as with various at-risk populations (see Adams, 1990; Snow et al., 1998).

Difficulty with the use of phonics notwithstanding, the research on phonological and phonemic awareness still has important implications for deaf and hard-of-hearing students. For example, Chaney (1992) reported that performance on phonological awareness tasks by hearing preschoolers was highly correlated with general language ability. More interesting, it was the measures of syntactic and semantics skills rather than those of speech discrimination and articulation that strongly predicted phonological awareness differences among the hearing children. These findings indicate that phonological awareness (and other metalinguistic skills) develop in tandem with that of general language skills during the preschool years. This presents enormous challenges for parents and educators who work with deaf and hard-of-hearing children, especially with those children who come to school with minimal competency in any language and who have difficulty acquiring English as a first or second language. In fact, there is some evidence of a similar strong relationship between a reasonable level of syntactic competence and the ability to use vocabulary knowledge in deaf individuals (see Kelly, 1996). Thus, difficulties in one aspect of the reading process seem to affect the development and use of other aspects.

There have been a number of studies that have shown a strong relationship between children's ability to read and their ability to segment words into phonemes (Liberman, Shankweiler, Fischer, & Carter, 1974; see review in Adams, 1990). Subsequent studies have confirmed this close relationship for children in the early grades (Ehri & Wilce, 1985; Perfetti, Beck, Bell, & Hughes, 1987) and even throughout the later school years (see discussion in Snow et al., 1998). There seems to be little doubt that phonemic awareness is important, and this should be considered in the design and implementation of any literacy program for all children.

It is important to mention that some children (certainly some deaf children) (see Andrews & Mason, 1986; Ewoldt & Hammermeister, 1986) can proceed from print to meaning, particularly with the use of a sight word/sign approach. In fact, Snow et al. (1998) seemed to indicate that this is a productive route for young deaf children who might be able to interact and progress with print (also see Williams, 1994). However, whether most deaf children and adolescents can reach a high literate level in English via the sight word/sign approach is debatable. The overwhelming, indirect correlational evidence regarding the relationships among phonological recoding, working memory, and reading level seem to suggest otherwise (see later discussion in this chapter).

What seems to be important (albeit not absolutely necessary) is for children to develop an understanding of the alphabetic principle, which entails the relations between letters and sounds. Because phonemes are units of sounds represented by the letters of the alphabet, an awareness of phonemes is critical for understanding the logic of and using the alphabetic principle. It should be remarked that literacy can be considered to be broader than reading; however, the point here is that children need to use the principles of the writing system to assist them in constructing a model of what written texts mean or even to compose written texts. Although there are many and varied influences on subsequent literacy and academic achievement, it can be argued that some of the more important early childhood skills include an understanding of letter names and shapes, phonemic awareness, and interest in literacy. In addition, it should be reemphasized that there is more to accessing and interpreting texts than phonemic awareness. Children need to develop comprehension and metacognitive skills, and this process can begin during the preschool years.

Table 8-5 provides highlights and a discussion of terms for this section on the development of literacy.

Table 8-5 Highlights of the Development of Literacy

- Literacy has been studied from a variety of academic disciplines; however, a complete coherent picture is still not available.

- With respect to conventional reading, all readers need to deal with both the form (e.g., structure of letters and words) and meaning (e.g., comprehension of words and sentences). The amount of time and effort that is needed for each area (form and meaning) depends on skills, experiences, and purposes.

- In general, the development of literacy is related to other age-related developmental timetables.

- Phonological and phonemic awareness are not the same as speech perception. For example, many young children with typical hearing who perform satisfactorily on tests of speech discrimination may not have adequate phonological awareness.

- Phonological awareness, not speech perception or discrimination, is a good predictor of subsequent success in reading during the first few grades in school.

- Phonemic awareness entails an understanding that words can be divided into a sequence of phonemes. (See Table 8-1 for some information on phonological awareness, phonemic awareness, and phonics.)

- Phonological awareness (and other metalinguistic skills) develops in tandem with that of general language skills during the preschool years.

- Both phonological and phonemic awareness are important for understanding the logic of the alphabetic system, the system on which English writing is based.

A Few Remarks on Early Literacy Development

Much has been written about the early literacy development of children, which is influenced by their interactions/attempts with print and by the reciprocity of what they understand (i.e., their models of written language) and how they are attempting to further and deepen their understanding (Sulzby & Teale, 1987). To move into the alphabetic system, particularly with respect to orthographic development, children need to understand that print (i.e., orthography) is drastically different from pictures (see review in Ehri, 1991). In essence, word identification requires an understanding that words are composed of letters that represent sounds. Even the ability to spell (particularly conventional spelling) requires some understanding of these relationships.

Regardless of the type of initial or home language, it cannot be overemphasized that it is important for all children to acquire an understanding of how the English language is represented in print, especially if English literacy is a desirable goal. As expected, this is a gradual, sometimes arduous, process. One important milestone is the understanding of the concept of a word. What is being referred to is beyond the concept of things have names. During the preschool years, children begin their understanding of the use of words in phrases and sentences and as entities whose sounds are arbitrarily related to their meanings (Chaney, 1989). Eventually, children make distinctions between words (with a few lingering mistakes after formal schooling) and determine the referents for the words. In short, children proceed from whole sentences to smaller units such as phrases and then to words; they learn that a sentence is composed of smaller parts. Children also understand (not didactically) that the various grammatical functions and forms such as nouns, verbs, and adjectives and function words such as articles, conjunctions, and prepositions really are individual units or words. With respect to English literacy, this metalinguistic process needs to continue until children can attend to and analyze the internal phonological structure of spoken words (or their representative equivalents).

In addition to accessing and using the principles of the alphabetic system, children need to recognize that comprehension of an author's message requires reflection. It is clear (see the work of Olson, 1994) that literacy development requires that individuals recognize that language is an object of thought, in and of itself. As mentioned previously and throughout this text, the acquisition of a language for communication and for thought is a major obstacle to literacy development for many deaf and some hard-of-hearing children. Some of the components of this mind-boggling acquisition process were discussed in Chapter 4. It is truly remarkable how children proceed through the various components (e.g., phonology, syntax, semantics, and pragmatics) prior to formal schooling. Research on the early period of literacy development has revealed some very interesting findings (see reviews in Adams, 1990; Snow et al., 1998). During this early or emergent literacy period, children understand that certain kinds of intonations and wording are used with books and other written materials. Children who are read to frequently and enjoy such reading begin to recite selected words, phrases, or longer discourses that are specific to particular books. Selections such as *horse, I am Sam, Sam I Am,* and others not only indicate a playing-with-words-to-learn scenario but also, might be the beginning of the development of their social and personal identities or at least an indication of their interests in selected topics or stories. With an increase in their linguistic development, children become able to engage in conversations with peers and adults, especially for sharing the contents of literate materials such as books and magazines. In essence, children progress from a focus on names of objects in pictures to asking questions about the stories. With the advent of their ability to produce complex sentences, children are able to discuss abstract ideas, including concepts that are not present (or concrete) and those that occurred in the past. This use of decontextualized language is heavily dependent on the development of a bona fide linguistic system and, as discussed previously (Chapter 1), critical for the development of literate thought.

It is also important to discuss the reciprocal relations of reading and writing, particularly the manner in which writing is developed during the early years (Sulzby, 1996). During this period, writing tends to become an active arena in which children practice their developing skills of reading texts, that is, familiar texts. Children identify letters and learn letter-sound correspondences and may engage in invented spelling. Via their early written language productions, they are beginning to understand their growing knowledge of letters, sounds, and words. In fact, these productions show that children are actually developing literate thinking skills with respect to script literacy texts.

Word Identification and Comprehension

This section provides a few selective remarks on the development of word identification and comprehension skills. These issues are addressed in detail elsewhere (Paul, 1998a). Additional details and more eloquent descriptions can be found in Adams (1990) and Snow et al. (1998). With respect to word identification, the section provides some insights into the nature and process of word identification with a few comments on the importance of morphology. The discussion on comprehension is brief and restricted to a broad overview of a few issues relative to word knowledge, prior knowledge, and metacognition.

Word Identification

Word identification has been known by several other labels, namely, *word recognition, word attack, word analysis,* and *decoding* (Johnson & Pearson, 1984). Typically, word identification means that readers can pronounce the word regardless of whether they know the meaning(s) of that word. For many deaf children, signing the word is a close analogy, although it is on a whole-word level, which may or may not involve letter-sound relations for many members of this population. This is necessary to mention because sight word reading is actually facilitated by the use of phonological recoding skills (i.e., decoding via the conversion of letters to sounds) for many skilled readers (see the discussion in Ehri, 1991). In light of the information in Chapter 5, it is possible to argue that cueing a word (i.e., via cued speech/language) is roughly similar to pronouncing it. At this point, it can be averred that finger spelling a word, letter by letter, is not the same as word identification. However, finger spelled loan signs could be considered similar to word identification in some sense. Keeping in mind the skills of speech along with the earlier remarks, it is easy to see why assessing word identification skills in many deaf and some hard-of-hearing children is a formidable challenging task. It has been hypothesized that cueing a word would be a stronger predictor of early reading skills than either signing or finger spelling it. This is based on the premise that cued speech/language is a more feasible route for developing phonological and phonemic awareness. Of course, this is in need of more empirical research using designs similar to what have been used for typical hearing children.

Word identification is not only critical for beginning readers, but it is also an ongoing task for skilled readers as well because it is necessary (albeit not sufficient) for comprehension of print materials (see Adams, 1990, 1994). The word identification process begins with the focusing of the eyes on the letters on the page (i.e., visual processing). The range of focus is limited (Rayner & Pollatsek, 1989); thus, readers need to fixate on many words during the reading process. The reason for this is that readers can only perceive accurately a range of 5 to 10 letters to the right of the fixation point.

Adams (1990; also see Snow et al., 1998) provided an eloquent analogy by remarking that visual processing initiates the spark of recognition and other associated processes. The associated processes involve phonological, orthographic, and meaning (i.e., semantic) information. Most important is the activation of a phonological decoding process, which as discussed previously, concerns the relations between phonemes and graphemes. The exact nature of this combination of processes involving, for example, phonological and visual-orthographic information, is the subject of much intensive research, often motivated by hypotheses generated within the modularity framework (Fodor, 1983) or the parallel distributed processing model (connective or interactive) (Rumelhart et al., 1986). The following remarks by Adams (1990) are still representative of the current consensus (also see the review in Snow et al., 1998): "The emerging view is that skillful word recognition involves both direct visual processing and phonological translation. However, these two routes stand, not as independent alternatives to one another, but as synergistic parts of the same process" (p. 105).

As suggested by Adams, the processes of phonological decoding and orthographic knowledge are related; however, each contributes differently to the reading process, especially for the identification of words. Phonological decoding is concerned with the phonological structure of words, whereas orthography is concerned with the representations of these structures. With numerous experiences with words, readers can bank on the complementary contributions of these two processes. However, the ability to read new words seems to require an increase of experience and understanding of orthography, which needs to include phonology (Adams, 1990; Snow et al., 1998). In essence, this requires a closer attention to the string of letters that make up a word. Children who have developed this sensitivity are adept at pronouncing nonwords and at creating made-up nonwords, which are reflective of the phonological/orthographic complementary process.

There is still considerable debate on the importance and extent of phonological mediation (conversion of letters to sounds) at the sublexical level (i.e., within the word) with respect to the retrieval of a word (including its meaning) from memory. There is evidence for substantial phonological mediation (Berent & Perfetti, 1995) to occasional mediation (Besner, 1990; Paap & Noel, 1991) to no phonological mediation. Despite these differences, it seems that for skilled hearing readers, phonological information along with other information about the word—meaning, syntactic elements, and orthographic identity—are retrieved due to the close associations of these processes.

The role of morphology in the word identification process is still open to question (Feldman, 1994; Nagy, Winsor, Osborn, & O'Flahavan, 1994). It is not clear whether words are separated into morphological components prior to or after identification. There seems to be evidence that an awareness of morphology contributes to the learning of words, especially their spellings and meanings within the structure (syntax) of sentences (Nunes, Bryant, & Bindman, 1997). Nunes et al. (1997) delineated acquisitional stages that reflect children's spelling of inflectional morphology such as -ed, which represents the regular past tense for English. In essence, children seem to progress from early phonetic spellings (e.g., *kist* for *kissed*), driven by phonological sensitivity, to conventional spellings based on morphology. In addition, once children have learned the conventional spellings of words, they may overgeneralize them to other words (e.g., *sofed* for *soft*, due to the similar sounding endings of *soft* and *kissed*). Nunes et al. (1997) argued that progress toward a complete mastery of the spelling system of English requires a deep sensitivity to morphology and syntax. In essence, the road to mature spelling skills, as well to mature reading, is paved by the synergistic contributions of phonology, morphology, and syntax.

Comprehension: Word Knowledge, Prior Knowledge, and Metacognition

Each of these broad areas can be and have been discussed in book-length treatises. There seems to be an emerging consensus that an understanding of and improvement in the comprehension ability of children requires that they have adequate proficiency in word knowledge, prior knowledge, and metacognition.

Although there are still debates on the relations between vocabulary knowledge and comprehension, there seems to be little doubt that word knowledge contributes to, indeed correlates with, reading comprehension (Anderson & Freebody, 1985; Becker, 1977; Stahl & Fairbanks, 1986). What skilled readers know about words is mind-boggling. Not only do they know a large number of words (breadth), but they also have an in-depth knowledge of words, including multiple meanings, nuances, and figurative uses. They even know features that are common to two or more words (e.g., as in synonyms) and features that different across two or more words (e.g., as in antonyms). Skilled readers can use words to express analogies (e.g., part to whole) or categories (e.g., types of print materials as in books, pamphlets, magazines, journals, etc.) (for examples of synonyms, antonyms, and analogies, see Chapter 2).

Ironically, much of this knowledge about words is not taught; rather, skilled readers develop their understanding via varied and extensive reading experiences and reflections on the words. This does not mean that skilled readers do not need the benefits of some explicit instruction. Although reading in context contributes to word knowledge, this happens in small increments because it is difficult to use context cues to infer word meanings (Shu, Anderson, &, Zhang, 1995; also see Paul, 1996, 1998a, for a review). Many readers, especially poor readers, do not learn much about the words that they encounter in context. That this is the case for poor readers needs to be emphasized strongly. Poor readers are not likely to possess a range of skills that enables them to use context effectively and are not likely to read widely to benefit from multiple exposures to the words.

Vocabulary learning is so complex that it is counterproductive to set this up as an either-or situation, that is, incidental reading versus vocabulary instruction (see discussion in Beck & McKeown, 1991). Many educators, particularly those who work with deaf and hard-of-hearing students, tend to underestimate the contributions of interpersonal interactions—student to student, parent to child, and teacher to student—to the growth of vocabulary knowledge. In other words, it is not only the use of effective instructional techniques such as semantic-elaboration techniques (e.g., semantic maps and semantic feature analyses) that are important, but also, the quality and quantity of interactions are critical to the development of independent word learning skills. Effective discourses on words, topics, and other literacy-related areas require that students have a bona fide language for communication and thought. Of course, it is helpful if this language matches the language of print; otherwise, English needs to be approached as a second language.

It is best to consider prior knowledge and metacognition together because prior knowledge is most effective when it is applied (either activated or enriched) during the reading process, and metacognition, in one sense, addresses the application of prior knowledge via the use of strategies. Skilled readers use their world knowledge to comprehend the literal aspects of text and to make inferences for the nonliteral aspects. In addition, skilled readers use their prior knowledge to comprehend words (Anderson, 1985; Anderson & Pearson, 1984; Pearson & Fielding, 1991). The application of prior knowledge is even critical for performing reading tasks such as drawing conclusions, finding the main idea, and relating the text information to other similar themes from other texts. Although there is much debate on how this information is organized and retrieved—or even if *organization* and *retrieved* are the appropriate terms for the processes (Spiro, Vispoel, Schmitz, Samarapungavan, & Boerger, 1987)—there is little question that comprehending, learning, and remembering information are influenced by the stock of prior experiences that readers possess. In addition to the grammar and topics in the text, readers have an understanding of other aspects such as text genre and how texts can be considered with respect to communicative contexts (Graesser, Millis, & Zwaan, 1997). Texts are never fully explicit (and would probably be boring if they were) thus readers need to make inferences by applying their knowledge (see Fletcher et al., 1994, for a review).

Prior knowledge needs to be applied for readers to increase the amount of information they recall from the text on a topic. Specifically, readers need to understand what it is that they know and do not know and to take action to repair comprehension breakdowns, based on the unknown knowledge (for hearing students, see review in Pearson & Fielding, 1991). For some scholars, this comprehension-monitoring, metacognitive process is the hallmark of a skilled reader. Furthermore, it explains why a wealth of prior knowledge by itself is not sufficient unless it is activated and applied. It is important to inform students on how a specific metacognitive strategy can be used to improve comprehension ability. Similar to other components of literate thought, the use of metacognitive strategies is pervasively dependent on the development of a bona fide language for communication and thought. In other words, if deaf and hard-of-hearing students do not have access to or cannot effectively use the performance form of a language (i.e., speech and/or signs), it is highly unlikely that they can engage in mature metacognitive activities.

Table 8-6 provides highlights for early literacy development and includes a discussion and brief examples of word identification and comprehension components.

Table 8-6 Highlights of Early Literacy Development

- To proceed to the development of the alphabet system, including orthographic development, children need to understand that print is drastically different from pictures.

- One of the most important milestones is the understanding of the concept of a word. Children begin to realize that words are entities whose sounds are arbitrarily related to their meanings. Eventually, children make distinctions between words and the referents for words.

- Children proceed from whole sentences to smaller units such as phrases and words. Subsequently, children can attend to the internal structures of words, particularly the internal phonological structures of spoken words.

- Children develop print and book awareness (see Table 8-1 for a brief discussion of print and book awareness). They become familiar with terms associated with books and the reading process.

- As their linguistic knowledge develops, children begin to engage in more elaborate conversations with adults during book- or story-sharing events. They are able to discuss abstract ideas, including concepts that are not present and those that occurred in the past.

- An understanding of the reading process deepens with the development of written language.

Word Identification

- Word identification requires an understanding that words are composed of letters that represent sounds. In general, word identification refers to the ability to pronounce (or sign) words in a rapid, automatic, fluent manner (see Table 8-1 for additional details).

- The emerging view is that skillful word recognition involves both direct visual processing and phonological translation. However, these two routes stand not as independent alternatives to one another but as synergistic parts of the same process (Adams, 1990).

- There seems to be evidence that an awareness of morphology contributes to the learning of words, especially their spellings and meanings within the structure (syntax) of sentences. In essence, a complete mastery of the spelling system of English requires a deep sensitivity to morphology and syntax.

- According to Johnson and Pearson (1984):

    The three types of word identification skills that need to be taught are (1) phonic analysis, (2) structural analysis, and (3) contextual analysis. *Phonics* is the term used for relating letters to sounds. Phonics instruction is concerned with providing the child with the means of *pronouncing* an unfamiliar *printed* word, and consequently recognizing it from one's oral/aural vocabulary. *Structural analysis* refers to learning the meaning of a new word by discovering parts of the word that are already meaningful. *Contextual analysis* refers to learning the meaning of a new word by the way it is used in a sentence or larger passage.

    All three are very powerful word-identification skills. Good readers use all three skills regularly and almost automatically as they read new materials. As the skills are used, the child's reading vocabulary is expanded and reading efficiency increased. (p. 115)

(continues)

368 ■ LANGUAGE AND DEAFNESS

(Table 8-6 continued)

Example of an activity based on contextual analysis from Johnson and Pearson (1984):

Sample Sentences

a. A person who is fussy about what he eats is *finicky.*

   Finicky means _____.

b. A *rustic* setting is one that is simple and away from the city.

   Rustic means _____.

c. An *absurd* story is one that is foolish.

   Absurd means _____.

d. To *procrastinate* means to not to do something right away.

   Procrastinate means _____.

e. To *grasp* the meaning of the sentence means to understand what is being said.

   To *grasp* means _____. (p. 144)

Comprehension

- There is little doubt that word knowledge contributes to reading comprehension. Good readers know many words (i.e., breadth of knowledge), and they also have an in-depth knowledge of words (i.e., depth of knowledge).

- Much of readers' knowledge of words comes from varied and extensive reading experiences and reflections on words.

- Many readers, especially poor readers, do not learn much about the words that they encounter in single contextual situations (i.e., only once or twice). Poor readers are not likely to possess a range of skills that enables them to use context effectively and are not likely to read widely to benefit from multiple exposures to the words.

- Vocabulary learning is so complex that it is counterproductive to set this up as an either-or situation, that is, incidental reading versus vocabulary instruction.

- It is best to consider prior knowledge and metacognition together because prior knowledge is most effective when it is applied during the reading process, and metacognition, in one sense, addresses the application of prior knowledge via the use of strategies.

- The application of prior knowledge is critical for performing reading tasks such as drawing conclusions, finding the main idea, and relating the text information to other similar themes from other texts.

- Prior knowledge needs to be applied for readers to increase the amount of information they recall from the text on a topic. Readers also need to engage in metacognitive tasks such as comprehension monitoring (i.e., evaluating their understanding of the text) and comprehension repairs (i.e., engaging in strategies to address unknown or difficult information which impedes understanding).

Example of Prior Knowledge for Prereading Activity (Paul, 1998a)

To activate or enrich the prior knowledge of students, teachers should:

. . . consider the construction of prereading questions for an expository story entitled *Bats*.

Bats—Prereading Questions

1. This is a story about animals called bats. Have you ever seen a live bat? A picture of a bat? Tell me about it. What do you think this story will tell us?

2. Tell me what you know about bats. What do they look like? Are they big or small or both? Are bats different from birds? Why or why not? Are bats similar to birds? Why or why not?

3. What is a mammal? Are bats mammals? How do you know that? What other animals are mammals? What is a reptile? An amphibian? How are mammals different from reptiles? How are mammals and reptiles similar? Compare mammals and amphibians. Tell me about the differences. The similarities.

4. What do bats do during the day? At night?

5. Where do bats live? Why do they live in these places?

6. Do bats fly in the dark? How do bats fly in the dark? Do bats fly during the daytime? How do they do that?

7. What do bats eat? How do bats catch their food?

8. How do people feel about bats? Why? How do you feel about bats? Are bats dangerous? How do you know that? (p. 225)

Development of Literacy: A Brief Summary

It can be inferred that typical hearing children bring a wealth of information to school, particularly by the time they begin formal instruction in reading and writing. However, several scholars (Adams, 1990; Snow et al., 1998) have mentioned that a number of children are at risk and that a significant portion of the adult population (from 20% to 40%) experience difficulty in the higher level functions often associated with reading. Snow et al. (1998) provided a comprehensive treatment of at-risk factors, some of which are discussed in this chapter.

For children to be ready for formal instruction in literacy, it would be ideal if they arrive at school with a well-developed first language and a wide variety of and extensive experiences with emergent literacy. These experiences not only depend on a literacy-rich home environment but also parental interactions that proceed beyond the asking of simple controlled questions (i.e., those requiring short literal answers) and that engage children into meaningful discourses, some of which should be child directed and initiated. In short, these interactions should enable children to develop emergent metacognitive skills that provide the foundation for the subsequent mature development of literate thought.

To become independent readers (and writers), there is a need for children to develop phonological and phonemic awareness to understand the alphabet system or, specifically, to understand the connection between spoken words and their written representations. The use of a phonological recoding strategy seems to be a very productive skill for beginning readers, especially with its application for addressing unknown words. To proceed toward reading fluency—that is, the point at which word identification becomes automatic and almost effortless and the point at which most energy can be spent on comprehending and interpreting the message—children need increased experiences with print as well as deeper and more extensive growths in vocabulary, morphology, and syntax. This increase in knowledge supports the word identification process and strengthens the reciprocal relations between word identification and comprehension.

This road from beginning reading to fluency in conventional reading was described eloquently by Snow et al. (1998):

> *Children need simultaneous access to some knowledge of letter-sound relationships, some sight vocabulary, and some comprehension strategies. In each case, "some" indicates that exhaustive knowledge of these aspects is not needed to get the child reading conventionally; rather, each child seems to need varying amounts of knowledge to get started,*

but then he or she needs to build up the kind of inclusive and auto-matic knowledge that will let the fact that reading is being done fade into the background while the reasons for reading are fulfilled. (pp. 79, 84)

DEAFNESS AND LITERACY

Estimates of the reading and writing achievement levels of deaf and hard-of-hearing students have been based on the results of standardized tests, par-ticularly those that assessed general achievement with subtests pertaining to literacy (typically, reading subtests). In light of the earlier discussion, it is clear that children with deafness are members of an at-risk group. The findings of the national surveys confirm this label; that is, the overwhelming majority of children with severe to profound hearing impairment do not read above the fourth-grade level (see reviews in Allen, 1986; Paul, 1998a). More interesting, this plateau at the fourth-grade level has been in existence since the begin-ning of the formal testing movement (Quigley & Paul, 1986).

This plateau is not unique to deaf and hard-of-hearing students; in fact, it can be found in research on other populations including at-risk children, especially children in special education programs (Adams, 1990; Snow et al., 1998). The reasons for the plateau are varied and are not simple and straight-forward. It is possible that there could be artifacts associated with the type of test used. Some scholars argued that the inferential and language demands of literacy increase dramatically after the third-grade level. These demands exhibit their greatest deleterious effects on students who are at risk at the end of sec-ond or third grade. That is, students who are behind by the end of second or third grade find it difficult to deal with the demands of advanced literacy texts. Stanovich (1986) labeled this the *Matthew Effects* in which the rich get richer, but the poor either stay the same or get poorer. Thus, good readers become even better readers (i.e., grow in knowledge and understanding via reading), whereas poor readers cannot experience this growth via the use of script lit-eracy skills and thus fall further and further behind. It has been documented that many children who are behind by the end of third or fourth grade almost never catch up, at least as measured by standardized achievement measures.

There are some children with moderate to profound hearing impairment who perform better than the reported national norms associated with achieve-ment tests such as the Stanford Achievement Tests—Hearing Impaired Version. Not all of these children read on the level of their typical hearing peers; thus even within this group, there are still a number of them who are at risk for their entire mandatory education period. Nevertheless, there is some evidence to clarify the reasons for the superior performance of few of these children and adolescents with hearing impairment. For example, Luetke-Stahlman (1988a, 1988b), discussed in Chapter 6, suggested that it is important for deaf students to be exposed to either bona fide languages or manual systems that completely encode spoken English (e.g., cued language/speech, seeing essential English, and signing exact English). Setting aside the debates on the completeness of the signed systems, this finding is certainly in line with the need for the development of a language for thought and for communication that can be used for developing metalinguistic and other skills necessary for advanced literacy development, as discussed previously.

Additional perspectives have also been offered. Delaney et al. (1984) argued that academic achievement, particularly reading achievement, is not dependent solely on type of instructional or communication input. Other important factors include the skills and knowledge of the teacher, design of the curricula, involvement of parents/caregivers, and the development of oral communication skills. Geers and Moog (1989) emphasized the reciprocal relationships between the oral and written forms of a language.

In light of the work of Snow et al. (1998) and others (Adams, 1990; Anderson et al., 1985), it is possible to react to these major findings, including those from research reviews (Paul, 1996, 1997, 1998a, 1998b). Comments have already been made on the need for a language for communication and for thought, the need for phonological and phonemic awareness (not necessarily good speechreading or speech skills), and the reciprocal relations between word identification and comprehension. In addition, there have been attempts to provide insights into the parental-child interactions with book sharing or reading or emergent literacy activities that also contribute to growth in literacy (see discussion in Paul, 1998a). Although it is beyond the scope of this chapter, another possible at-risk factor, associated with teacher education, is the preparation of teachers for teaching literacy. This situation might be exacerbated by the certification process in which most teachers can become certified from kindergarten to 12th grade. Perhaps deaf education should adhere to the certification models developed for general education (e.g., early childhood, middle childhood, and secondary education).

With respect to student characteristics, one still relevant way to characterize the at-risk situation of most deaf and hard-of-hearing students is as follows:

The poor reading performance of most deaf students may be viewed within an interactive theoretical framework in which the reader uses specific skills (e.g., decoding and inference) to hypothesize at various linguistic levels (e.g., lexical, syntactic, semantic, textual) about the infor-

*mation contained in the text. . . . In relation to this, the reading diffi-
culties of deaf students may be attributed to deficits in experiential (e.g.,
world knowledge), cognitive (e.g., inferencing), and linguistic (e.g., word
knowledge) variables. Other variables of equal importance are educational and socioeconomic in nature. (Quigley & Paul, 1989, p. 5)*

Support for this passage discussing deaf children and adolescents can be
found in several sources (see the discussions in Brown & Brewer, 1996; Kelly,
1995; Paul, 1998a).

The ensuing paragraphs present a summary of the research findings associated with a few selected studies and related to some of the issues discussed
in the earlier passage. It will become obvious that there is a dearth of intervention research studies that focus on improving some of the literacy aspects
such as vocabulary knowledge, prior knowledge, and metacognition. Even more
distressing is the fact that there are few intervention efforts to address phonemic awareness or other aspects of word identification (e.g., orthography and
morphology) (see Looney & Rose, 1979, as an example of intervention with
morphology and finger spelling in Chapter 6). Much of the known information relates to a survey of basic morphological knowledge related to the use
of a signed system (the work of Raffin in Gilman et al., 1980; Raffin, 1976;
Raffin et al., 1978) or in the research on written language (Cooper, 1967). There
are a number of studies on the phonological recoding and phonics abilities
of deaf and hard-of-hearing students (see reviews in LaSasso & Metzger, 1998;
Leybaert, 1993; Paul, 1998a).

Is the development of literacy different for deaf and hard-of-hearing students? That is, is what is known about literacy for typical students also applicable to at-risk students, including students in special education programs or
who have special education labels? There are several scholars who seem to
support the qualitative similarity hypothesis or some aspects of it (Brown &
Brewer, 1996; Hanson, 1989; Hayes & Arnold, 1992; Paul, 1985, 1993, 1997,
1998a, 1998b; for orally educated students, see Daneman, Nemeth, Stainton,
& Huelsmann, 1995; also see the work of Quigley and his collaborators,
reviewed in Russell et al., 1976, and in this text). In essence, what this means
is that all children need to understand the logic of the alphabet system, and
such instruction may need to be intensive, extensive, and creative. It does not
mean, for example, that phonics is the only means by which to develop phonological and phonemic awareness. In fact, phonemic awareness training should
involve more than phonics (see Table 8-7 for some examples of phonemic
awareness activities).

Table 8-7 Examples of Phonemic Awareness Activities

Whispering Game

Objective: To exercise the children's ability to overcome distractions, pronunciation differences, and so on, while listening to language.

Activity: Seat the children in a circle. Then whisper something to the child on your left; that child then whispers something to the child on her or his left, and so on. The whispering continues, child to child, in clockwise order until it reaches the last child, who says out loud whatever she or he has heard.

Word Rhyming

Objective: To evoke the realization that almost any word can be rhymed—not just those in other people's poems.

Activity: In this game, you produced a word to be rhymed (e.g., *cat*), then signal to the children to give a rhyming word. You can increase the game's complexity by additionally challenging the children to suggest a second word that is meaningfully related to your clue word as well as a rhyme for that word. Once the game is familiar, individual children may be invited to respond and to choose the next word to be rhymed. Examples include the following:

cat—hat	dog—?
car—far	truck—?
mouse—house	rat—?
bag—rag	sack—?
chair—hair	sofa—?
talk—walk	shout—?
rose—hose	flower—?
book—hook	read—?
face—lace	smile—?
bed—red	night—?

Note: Taken from Adams, Foorman, Lundberg, and Beeler (1998, pp. 25, 33). Other activities can be found in this source.

There might also be lessons to be learned from studies on children who are severely reading disabled. For example, Lovett et al. (1994) demonstrated that word recognition skills of severely disabled readers can be substantially improved via the use of intensive supplementary training. In this project, students received training in explicit instruction in phoneme awareness and letter-sound relations and in using common orthographic patterns and analogies to identify unfamiliar words. Even more interesting, especially for those who work with deaf and hard-of-hearing students, the use of phonologically oriented training programs—albeit most effective in conjunction with other reading skills—is not the only type of intervention that can foster the development of word identification skills. It might be possible to use more orthographically oriented approaches with similar benefits for improving word identification in students with severe reading difficulties. The use of an orthographically oriented approach is not a panacea because children with severe reading difficulties, including deaf children, have deficiencies in many other areas, for example, phonological skills in both the oral (performance) and written mode. In addition, as stated previously, it is not uncommon to find difficulties in critical areas such as spoken (i.e., performance) vocabulary, language comprehension (e.g., morphology and syntax), and the extent and use of prior knowledge skills. All of these issues have to be taken into consideration when addressing the literacy difficulties of deaf and hard-of-hearing students. A sample of research on some of these issues related to deaf and hard-of-hearing students are discussed in the ensuing sections.

RESEARCH ON SELECTED TEXT-BASED FACTORS
Words and Word Meanings

The research on vocabulary and deafness has focused on determining children's knowledge of words and word meanings, including multiple meanings of words—that is, the breadth and depth of vocabulary knowledge. Researchers have shown that there is a strong relationship (i.e., correlation) between vocabulary knowledge and reading comprehension. There is also some evidence on deaf and hard-of-hearing children's ability to derive word meanings from context, that is, the incidental learning of word meanings. As mentioned previously, there are very few studies on the facilitative effects of variables for word identification skills. The discussion of phonological awareness and related aspects is presented in the section dealing with working memory (see description of this concept in Chapter 3).

There have been extensive studies on knowledge of words and word meanings of children who are deaf and hard of hearing (Fusaro & Slike, 1979; Hatcher

& Robbins, 1978; LaSasso & Davey, 1987; Paul, 1984; Paul & Gustafson, 1991; Schulze, 1965; Silverman-Dresner & Guilfoyle, 1972; also, see various surveys by the Center for Assessment and Demographic Studies reviewed in Paul, 1998a). Comparing the lexical knowledge of deaf children with that of hearing counterparts, it has been demonstrated that the vocabulary knowledge of deaf children is quantitatively reduced. In addition, if deaf and hard-of-hearing students have problems with other language variables, notably, syntax and orthographic knowledge, this tends to make it difficult for them to infer the meanings of the word via the use of adequate context clues (see discussions in Kelly, 1996; Paul & O'Rourke, 1988).

That knowledge of words is important for deaf students has been documented in the few studies that examined the relationship between lexical knowledge and reading comprehension. For example, LaSasso and Davey (1987) analyzed the performance of prelingually, profoundly hearing-impaired students. Their findings indicated that vocabulary knowledge is an effective predictor of reading comprehension performance. Their results were confirmed in a later study by Paul and Gustafson (1991), who examined the relationship between knowledge of multimeaning words and reading comprehension. These researchers noted that there is a strong correlation between knowledge of two meanings of words and reading achievement scores.

To understand better the relationship between knowledge of words and reading comprehension, several researchers attempted to study factors that contribute to the difficulty of a word (MacGinitie, 1969; Paul, 1984; Paul & Gustafson, 1991; Walter, 1978). Word difficulty is influenced by numerous factors, for example, prior knowledge, conceptual load, ability to use context clues, pronunciation, context surrounding the word, letter frequency, word frequency, and multiplicity of meanings (Anderson & Freebody, 1985; Nagy & Herman, 1987; O'Rourke, 1974; Paul & O'Rourke, 1988). In addition to the text-based and reader-based factors, there are task factors, specifically those related to the construction of vocabulary tests such as test format (e.g., multiple choice and free response) and difficulty of the items themselves (see discussion of item difficulty and vocabulary tests in Curtis, 1987).

In an early study, Walter (1978) compared the lexical knowledge of children with normal hearing and those with hearing impairment. It was reported that the gap between the two overall groups increased as the frequency of the words decreased. In light of these findings, Walter argued that previous estimates of the vocabulary knowledge of students who are deaf were spuriously high. That is, there was an overestimation of the word knowledge of deaf students, particularly on general achievement tests.

In addition to examining the relationship between vocabulary knowledge and reading comprehension, Paul and his collaborators (Paul, 1984; Paul & Gustafson, 1991; Paul, Stallman, & O'Rourke, 1990) assessed the comprehension of high-frequency words by both students with normal hearing and those with profound hearing impairment. As expected, the hearing subjects had significantly higher scores than the deaf subjects relative to selecting both single meanings and two meanings of the same words. Surprisingly, no significant effects of age on selecting two meanings of words were observed for either group. It was also found that selecting two meanings of words was significantly more difficult than selecting one meaning of the same words for both groups.

Paul and Gustafson (1991) argued that knowledge of multimeanings of words is important for reading comprehension. For example, approximately two thirds of the words that appear in the spoken and written language contexts in the primary grades are multimeaning words (Johnson, Moe, & Baumann, 1983; Searls & Klesius, 1984). Comprehension difficulties might surface if students are not aware of the secondary or other meanings of words that appear in print. There is still a need to determine which particular meanings or the number of meanings of words that are used in reading materials for these students. It is expected that the number of word meanings that appear in print might vary with the frequency of the appearance of the word itself. In other words, a high-frequency word would have more meanings expressed than a low-frequency word.

Research on Deriving Words From Context

Another area for further research is to examine the issue of acquiring word meanings from context (i.e., during reading). There are numerous factors that impact this issue—text-based (e.g., difficulty of words, syntactic structures, and the contexts surrounding the words), reader-based (e.g., knowledge of language variables and amount and variety of reading experiences), and task-based factors (e.g., type of assessment used). Because of these factors, it is not clear if deaf readers, especially poor readers, can acquire or derive many word meanings during the act of reading (see the various viewpoints and discussions in Ahn, 1996; Davey & King, 1990; de Villiers & Pomerantz, 1992; Paul & O'Rourke, 1988).

There have been a few studies that investigated the ability of students with hearing impairment to use context cues during reading to derive the meanings of words. Most of these studies focused on the effects of context on readers' comprehension of unknown words in syntactically difficult sentences (Nolen & Wilbur, 1985; Robbins & Hatcher, 1981).

In an early study, MacGinitie (1969) examined the effects of context (i.e., lists of words) and multiplicity of meanings on both students with typical hearing and those with hearing impairment. Results revealed that the scores of subjects with typical hearing were depressed by misleading contexts. Contrariwise, the scores of the deaf and hard-of-hearing subjects were not affected by the contexts. As expected, typical-hearing subjects knew more words and more meanings of words than the subjects with hearing impairment.

de Villiers and Pomerantz (1992) examined students' ability to derive word meanings from printed English sentences when students were instructed to focus on the words (i.e., words are highlighted by italics, etc.). Target words were embedded in short sentences in three different types of contexts. The contexts were labeled relative to the richness of information: *lean, rich*, and *explicit*. The lean context provided little information about the words, whereas the rich context provided substantial information. The explicit context contained sentences that described, discussed, or contrasted the meaning of the word.

Subjects were required to provide a definition; to judge the connotation of a word in terms of good or bad; to judge a grammatical category such as noun, verb, or adjective; and to evaluate the correct usage of words in the sentences. In general, the researchers found that students with hearing impairment can derive meanings of unknown words from contexts that are highly informative, namely, rich or explicit. That is, students with hearing impairment used contextual information to infer the meanings (partial meanings) of words. More important, the students' ability to derive word meanings was related to their reading comprehension level. That is, better readers gained more meanings from context than poor readers overall. More interesting, the poorer readers had great difficulty inferring the meaning of words from the highly informative contexts. The researchers hypothesized that this could be due to the difficulty with the surrounding syntax or to the use of inappropriate strategies for inferring meanings.

Ahn (1996) also examined the ability of students with hearing impairment to acquire the meanings of words from context but in an incidental situation (i.e., no explicit instructions were provided to focus on words in the stories). Words that the students did not know initially, based on their responses on the pretest, were selected as target words for a posttest. Two context conditions were used, rich (information added) and natural (story as is).

Similar to the results of the de Villiers and Promerantz study (1992), the results of the Ahn (1996) study indicated that (a) the students did learn vocabulary meanings from context during reading; (b) the more information about the words that was in the text, the easier it was for students to derive the meanings; and (c) high-ability readers learned more meaning of words through reading than low-ability readers although both ability groups of students learned significantly from context.

Table 8-8 provides highlights and additional details on selected vocabulary studies.

Table 8-8 Highlights of Selected Vocabulary Studies

Studies	Findings
MacGinitie (1969)	Examined the effects of context and multiplicity of meanings on both students with typical hearing and those with hearing impairment. Ages of the oral subjects with hearing impairment (mean of 88 dB) ranged from 9 to 20 years, inclusive. Scores were compared with a group of subjects with typical hearing in Grades 4 to 8. Results revealed that the scores of subjects with typical hearing were depressed by misleading contexts. Contrariwise, the scores of the deaf and hard-of-hearing subjects were not affected by the contexts. Hearing subjects knew more words and more meanings of words than the subjects with hearing impairment.
Silverman-Dresner & Guilfoyle (1972)	This was one of the most extensive investigations of reading vocabulary knowledge. The researchers constructed definitions for a list of 7,300 words taken from two sources (Dale & Chall, 1948; Dale & Eicholtz, 1960). The major purpose

(continues)

(Table 8-8 continued)

	of the study was to develop a set of age-graded vocabulary lists that reflected the actual reading vocabulary levels of deaf students. Tests were administered to 13,000 students from age 7 to 17 years in 89 schools for deaf students. The tests focused on single meanings of words.
Walter (1978)	Subjects were 199 children with profound hearing impairment whose ages ranged from 10 to 14 years old. Their performance was compared to 277 peers with normal hearing. The gap between the two groups increased as the frequency of the words decreased. It was argued that previous estimates of vocabulary knowledge of deaf students were spuriously high (i.e., overestimation).
LaSasso & Davey (1987)	Analyzed the performance of 50 prelingually profoundly hearing-impaired students whose ages ranged from 10 to 18 years. Findings indicated that vocabulary knowledge is an effective predictor of reading comprehension performance.
Paul & Gustafson (1991)	Studied 42 students with hearing impairment and 42 with typical hearing. The ages of subjects with hearing impairment ranged from 10 to 18 years, inclusive, and the age of the subjects with normal hearing ranged from 8 to 11 years, inclusive. As expected, the hearing subjects had significantly higher scores

than the deaf subjects. It was also found that selecting two meanings of words was significantly more difficult than selecting one meaning of the same words for both groups.

de Villiers & Pomerantz (1992)

The researchers examined students' ability to derive word meanings from printed English when students are instructed to focus on the words (i.e., words are highlighted by italics, etc.). They conducted two studies. In the first study, the researchers involved students from a high school program that used an oral communication method (72 to 117 dB with a mean of 97 dB). In the second study, they used students from a middle school using either oral communication (80 to 120 dB with a mean of 100 dB) or Total Communication (i.e., speaking and signing simultaneously) methods (71 to 110 dB with a mean of about 95 dB).

Found that students with hearing impairment can derive meanings of unknown words from contexts that are highly informative, namely, rich or explicit. The students' ability to derive word meanings was related to their reading comprehension level. That is, better readers gain more meanings from context than poor readers overall. The poorer readers had great difficulty inferring the meaning of words from the highly informative contexts. It was hypothesized that this could be due

(continues)

(Table 8-8 continued)

	to the difficulty with the surrounding syntax or to the use of inappropriate strategies for inferring meanings.
Ahn (1996)	Examined the ability of students with hearing impairment to acquire the meanings of words from context but in an incidental situation (i.e., no explicit instructions were provided to focus on words in the stories). The subjects were 18 students, with prelingual deafness from a residential school for deaf students that employed a Total Communication approach, that is, speech, signing, and finger spelling are used simultaneously. The ages of the students ranged from 12 years to about 18 years (mean age was 15). Their unaided hearing loss was between 57 and 117 dB (mean was 90 dB). Results were similar to those of the de Villiers and Promerantz (1992) study.

Summary Information on Vocabulary Development

- Studies have shown that there is a strong relationship between vocabulary knowledge and reading comprehension. In fact, knowledge of words with multiple meanings is extremely important.

- There seems to be some evidence that deaf and hard-of-hearing children have the ability to derive word meanings from context; however, this is dependent on the reading ability of the students. Specifically, problems with syntax and orthographic knowledge make it difficult to infer the meanings of words through the use of adequate context clues.

- Compared to children with typical hearing, the vocabulary knowledge of deaf students is quantitatively reduced—albeit, it seems to be qualitatively similar.

- There is little doubt that much of the learning of words and word meanings comes from wide and varied reading experiences, that is, via the efforts of students who are independent word learners.

- Given the frequency and importance of words with multiple meanings, it seems that vocabulary instruction should be focused on what is called *semantic elaboration techniques* (word maps, semantic maps, and semantic feature analysis).

Implications for Vocabulary Instruction

The research cited earlier has important implications for instructional practices. Similar to the previous discussion for hearing students, it is counterproductive to establish this as an instruction of vocabulary versus reading in context dichotomy. There is little doubt that much of the learning of words and word meanings comes from wide and varied reading experiences, that is, via the efforts of students who are independent word learners. However, all deaf and hard-of-hearing readers need periods of vocabulary instruction. This is especially true for poor readers who do not receive much benefit from contextual reading unless they can engage positively in these experiences.

Given the frequency and importance of words with multiple meanings, it seems that vocabulary instruction should be focused on what is called *semantic elaboration techniques* (word maps, semantic maps, and semantic feature analysis), as mentioned previously (see examples in Johnson & Pearson, 1984). Instead of single, often isolated meanings, and the practice of simply using words in sentences (i.e., the definition and context approach), students need to be exposed to and to work with the conceptual frameworks that surround words and need a variety of reading experiences (with rich or explicitly added contexts) that demonstrate aspects of these conceptual frameworks (e.g., multimeanings, nuances, synonyms, and metaphorical usage). These implications have also been supported by the previous work of Conway (1990) in his study of the semantic relationships in the word meanings of students with hearing impairment:

> *Traditional programs of learning definitions for lists of words should give way to learning words in semantically rich contexts. The contexts can serve as bridges to old information and as foundations for developing further conceptual interrelationships. . . . Such rich contexts should also include use of semantic mapping . . . and adaptations of networking strategies. (p. 346)*

Syntax

The research on syntax has focused on several general issues, three of which are: (a) comprehension of the structures and the frequency of structures in reading materials, (b) the effects of factors such as instructional methods and context of passages, and (c) the effects of short-term working memory on the comprehension of syntax. The more recent studies have attempted to explain students' difficulty with certain syntactic structures within the framework of Chomsky's work (e.g., universal grammar, etc.) (Berent, 1996a, 1996b; Lillo-Martin, Hanson, & Smith, 1991, 1992) and other language hypotheses (Wilbur, Goodhart, & Fuller, 1989). The selection of the studies discussed in this section is representative of much of the research in this area and serves as exemplars for major points involving the importance of syntactic knowledge for reading comprehension (for descriptions of Chomsky's UG, see Cairns, 1996; Cook & Newson, 1996).

The work of Quigley and his associates (Quigley, Power, & Steinkamp, 1977; Quigley, Smith, & Wilbur, 1974; Quigley, Wilbur, & Montanelli, 1974, 1976; also see the review in Russell et al., 1976) detailed the performance of a national stratified, random sample of students with profound hearing impairment between the ages of 10 and 19 years old on tests of comprehension of various syntactic structures presented singly in sentences. Table 8-9 depicts summary information on (a) the order of difficulty of various structures for both students with normal hearing and students who are deaf and (b) the frequency of occurrence of each structure in reading series from Houghton-Mifflin (McKee, Harrison, McCowen, Lehr, & Durr, 1966).

Table 8-9 Summary of Performance on Syntactic Structures and Their Frequency of Occurrence per 100 Sentences in the *Reading for Meaning* Series

	Deaf Students				Hearing Students
	Age				
Structure	Average Across Ages %	10 %	18 %	Increase %	Average Across Ages %
Negation					
be	79	60	86	26	92
do	71	53	82	29	92

| | Deaf Students | | | | Hearing Students |
| | Age | | | | |
Structure	Average Across Ages %	10 %	18 %	Increase %	Average Across Ages %
have	74	57	78	21	86
Modals	78	58	87	29	90
Means	76	57	83	26	90
Conjunction					
Conjunction	72	56	86	30	92
Deletion	74	59	86	27	94
Means	73	57	86	29	92
Question formation					
Wh- questions comprehension	66	44	80	36	98
Yes/No questions comprehension	74	48	90	42	99
Tag questions	57	46	63	17	98
Means	66	46	78	32	98
Pronominalization					
Personal pronouns	67	51	88	37	78
Backward pronominalization	70	49	85	36	94
Possessive adjectives	65	42	82	40	98
Possessive pronouns	48	34	64	30	99
Reflexivization	50	21	73	52	80
Means	60	39	78	39	90
Verbs					
Auxiliaries	54	52	71	19	81
Tense sequencing	63	54	72	18	78
Means	58	53	71	18	79

(continues)

(Table 8-9 continued)

| | Deaf Students | | | | Hearing Students |
| | Age | | | | |
Structure	Average Across Ages %	10 %	18 %	Increase %	Average Across Ages %
Complementation					
Infinitives and gerunds	55	50	63	13	88
Relativization					
Processing	68	59	76	17	78
Embedding	53	51	59	8	84
Relative pronoun					
Referents	42	27	56	29	82
Means	54	46	63	17	82
Disjunction and alternation	36	22	59	37	84

| **Frequency of Occurrence** | | |
Structure	Level of First Appearance	Frequency in 6th-Grade Text
Negation		
be	1st primer—13	9
Conjunction		
Conjunction	1st primer—11	36
Question formation		
Wh- questions comprehension	2nd primer—5	6
Yes/No questions comprehension	1st primer—5	3
Pronominalization		
Backward	4th grade—1	0 (4 per 1,000)
Possessive adjectives	1st grade—4	27
Possessive pronouns	3rd primer—1	0 (3 per 1,000)
Reflexivization	2nd grade—1	2

Frequency of Occurrence

Structure	Level of First Appearance	Frequency in 6th-Grade Text
Verbs Auxiliaries	1st grade—1	18
Complementation Infinitives and gerunds	2nd primer—4	32
Relativization Processing	3rd primer—2	12
Disjunction and alternation	1st grade—1	7

Note: Adapted from Quigley, Power, Steinkamp, and Jones (1978).

Inspection of Table 8-9 reveals that the average 8-year-old hearing student scored higher on the various tasks than the average 18-year-old deaf student. In addition, there exists a huge gap between the age when deaf students comprehend various syntactic structures in single sentences and the typical age level at which the same structures appear in a typical reading series. Given the fact that current reading series might also present problems for deaf students relative to vocabulary and other text features, the use of present unadapted materials might be inappropriate for most students with severe to profound hearing impairment.

Despite the quantitative delays in syntax, Quigley and his associates also demonstrated that deaf students were acquiring syntactic structures in the same manner (i.e., qualitatively similar) as younger hearing students. That is, the deaf students proceed through stages, make errors, and use some strategies that seem to be similar to those of hearing students. This qualitative similarity can also be seen in the written language productions of deaf students discussed later.

Since the extensive studies conducted by Quigley and his collaborators, there have been several studies that focused on specific syntactic structures, for example, anaphoric relationships within conjoined sentences, indefinite pronouns (Wilbur & Goodhart, 1985), modals (Wilbur et al., 1989), and relative clauses (Kelly, 1998; Lillo-Martin et al., 1992). Wilbur et al. (1989) examined students' ability to comprehend English modals (e.g., *will, won't, would, can, could, shall,* etc.). These students met the same criteria as those in the Quigley studies summarized earlier.

Wilbur et al. (1989) reported that the students' comprehension of English modals was related to the level of reading achievement. In addition, the researchers analyzed their data with respect to an order of acquisition. They discussed this order of acquisition relative to the prediction of three hypotheses: developmental, theoretical, and syntactic (e.g., use of syntactic transformations). The researchers concluded that the acquisition of English modals requires more than just a knowledge of transformational rules—there is a need to consider semantic and pragmatic aspects. As stated by these researchers:

> *To approach an adequate account of the English modals, much more than transformational rules are needed. In the last decade, the case has been made for the importance of including proper pragmatics and semantic considerations, both in the classroom and in testing situations. (p. 16)*

Several other researchers have argued that a better understanding of deaf readers' knowledge of English syntax requires an analysis that goes beyond the sentence level (Ewoldt, 1981; McGill-Franzen & Gormley, 1980; Nolen & Wilbur, 1985). For example, McGill-Franzen and Gormley (1980) examined deaf children's comprehension of truncated passive sentences (e.g., *The window was broken*) presented in context and in isolation. Results indicated that the subjects understood the structure better in context than in isolation.

In another study, Ewoldt (1981) argued that deaf students could actually bypass the specific English syntactic structure and proceed directly to meaning. Her results are based on the performances of four deaf students between the ages of about 7 years to about 17 years. The researcher claimed that deaf students did not overrely on text information; in fact, the researcher argued for a top-down approach to reading instruction. The whole language approach has been derived from top-down models, particularly a transactional-sociopsycholinguistic focus (Goodman, 1976, 1985, 1994) and is a widely used approach in the education of children with hearing impairment (see discussion in Dolman, 1992; Paul, 1998a). However, the whole language approach should not be interpreted globally because there seem to be some variations on the way this approach is used (e.g., with basals, etc.) (see discussion in LaSasso & Mobley, 1997).

Taken together, there seems to be some evidence that students with severe to profound hearing impairment can understand syntactic structures better in context than in isolation. However, there are still several issues that need to be resolved by further research. Similar to the research on context and vocabulary knowledge, the use of context to comprehend syntax is indicative of the student's ability to derive the meaning of the structure. Deriving the meaning of structure—similar to deriving word meaning—might be more indicative of reading skill. This skill, however, is also influenced by the type of context in which the structure is housed in the passage. For example, it is possible to describe the context (typically, a phrase or sentence) that surrounds a word as misdirective, directive, and nondirective (see reviews of research in Davey & King, 1990; Paul, 1996; Paul & O'Rourke, 1988). There needs to be further research on the description of context (perhaps, two sentences or a paragraph) that surround a particular syntactic structure. This research is necessary to understand the effects of context on students' comprehension of syntax.

Lillo-Martin et al. (1991, 1992) argued that deaf students' difficulty with reading is not due to specific syntactic comprehension problems. Rather, it is due to an underlying processing deficit—that is, lower level phonological processing. This seems to be a strict bottom-up perspective of reading that in the author's view, is not a complete picture of the processing issue. In all fairness, Lillo-Martin et al. remarked that their findings should not be interpreted to mean that poor deaf readers never have structural problems. Rather, researchers and educators should be open to the possibility that some syntactic problems may be related to a processing deficit. In fact, there seems to be some evidence that both phonological and syntactic deficits contribute to inefficient or inaccurate processing (see discussions in Kelly, 1996; Paul & Jackson, 1993; also see the discussion of reader-based factors, especially working memory, in this chapter).

In sum, there seems to be some evidence (de Villiers & Pomerantz, 1992; Kelly, 1996) that deaf students might have difficulty deriving word meanings, especially if they have problems with syntax. The importance of syntax and other language variables on overall reading comprehension seems to be fairly well established (see discussions in Kelly, 1995, 1996; Paul, 1996, 1998a). These results can be interpreted within the framework of a number of cognitive information processing theories (Adams, 1990; Just & Carpenter, 1987; Rumelhart, 1977; Stanovich, 1980).

In the research on students with typical hearing, there is substantial evidence that the ability (especially the speed) to recognize (or comprehend) words in isolation is indicative of reading ability (see research reviews in Adams, 1990; Snow et al., 1998). Of course, it is also important for readers to derive the meanings of words from context, especially if there is a breakdown in comprehension. However, it is critical that readers do not spend too much time on deriving word or word meanings on a conscious, repairing level.

The intent of the previous discussion is to show that the same logic might apply to syntax. There is ample evidence that knowledge of syntax in isolation is important for reading comprehension, as discussed previously in the work of Quigley and his collaborators. Additional support was provided by

Negin (1987), who reported that syntactic segmentation significantly affects the ability of students with hearing impairment to comprehend narrative and expository reading materials. It is important for readers to be able to derive the meanings of certain structures during reading, particularly if there is a breakdown in comprehension. However, good readers do not have to spend a preponderant amount of time figuring out the meaning of a specific structure. Finally, similar to the research on vocabulary knowledge, it should be clear that the mere comprehension of syntactic structures is not sufficient for building a model of what the text means—although it does seem to contribute to that meaning-building process.

The importance of syntax, especially in light of deficits in other areas of processing during reading, should not be underestimated. In his review of studies, Kelly (1996) presented several salient points:

- *Slow lexical retrieval encroaches on working memory capacity.*
- *Readers whose working memory capacity is limited by inefficient processing tend to experience difficulty making simultaneous use of important syntactic and semantic information available in a single sentence.*
- *Inefficient readers have difficulty processing sentences with complex syntax.*
- *Syntactic processing does consume working memory capacity to some extent, regardless of the efficiency of the reader. (p. 76)*

In essence, there is substantial evidence on the negative effects of limited syntactic competence on the overall reading comprehension ability of deaf and hard-of-hearing students (Kelly, 1993; see review in Russell et al., 1976). Finally, the teaching of syntax to deaf individuals, especially individuals who do not have proficiency in complex structures such as relative clauses and passive voice, still presents formidable challenges for the field of deaf education (Kelly, 1998).

Figurative Language

It is not immediately obvious that the English language contains a significant number of idiomatic and other figurative expressions. The most conspicuous examples are figures of speech such as simile (*Running around like a chicken without a head*) and metaphor (*The night was a blanket*). Examples of idiomatic expressions include *It's raining cats and dogs* and *She's out of her mind*.

The bulk of figurative expressions take the form of verb-particle phrases and multimeaning words (Paul, 1984; Payne, 1982). Examples of verb-particle phrases include *look up*, *ran into*, and *rip off*. Common examples at the word level are *head* of the class, *hands* of the clock, and *eye* of the needle. It has been argued that one of the fastest growing groups of figurative expressions is the verb-particle phrase (Payne, 1982).

Research on the comprehension of figurative language is difficult to conduct because of the interactions and influences of other language variables such as vocabulary and syntax as well as the interactions between language and thought (see Chapter 3 of this text). Nevertheless, the reader, even the beginning reader, encounters numerous instances in print (Dixon, Pearson, & Ortony, 1980). There is research showing that both deaf and hearing readers, especially second language readers, have difficulty with figurative language (see discussions in Grabe, 1988, 1991; King & Quigley, 1985; Paul, 1998a). In addition to vocabulary and syntax, the use of figurative expressions is another language variable that is often controlled for in the development of special reading series (Quigley & King, 1981, 1982, 1983, 1984; Quigley, Paul, McAnally, Rose, & Payne, 1990, 1991).

Many students with severe to profound hearing impairment have difficulty comprehending figurative expressions in printed materials (Conley, 1976; Giorcelli, 1982; Payne & Quigley, 1987). For example, Giorcelli (1982) constructed a test of figurative expressions in printed materials. Two groups of subjects, hearing and deaf, served as participants. Giorcelli reported that the hearing subjects performed significantly better than the deaf subjects on the total test and on 7 of the 10 subtests. Similar to the research of Quigley and his associates on syntax reported previously, the researcher found that the 18-year-old deaf students did not perform as well as the 9-year-old hearing students. In fact there was little improvement in the performance of deaf students beyond 13 to 14 years of age.

Payne and Quigley (1987) assessed both deaf and hearing students' comprehension of the verb-particle figurative expressions. The researchers developed a test using verb-particles at three levels of semantic difficulty (literal, e.g., *walks out*; semi-idiomatic, e.g., *washes up*; and idiomatic, e.g., *gives up*) and in five syntactic patterns (subject, verb, adverb; subject, verb, adverb, object; subject, verb, object, adverb; subject, verb, preposition, object; and subject, verb, adverb, preposition, object). Similar to Giorcelli's findings, the researchers reported that the hearing subjects performed significantly better than the deaf subjects on all levels of semantic difficulty and for all syntactic structures.

Some researchers have documented that deaf students can understand metaphorical expressions if the vocabulary and syntax are controlled (Iran-Nejad, Ortony, & Rittenhouse, 1981) or if there is sufficient context to disambiguate the meaning of the expressions (Houck, 1982; Page, 1981). It has also been suggested that deaf students may learn the expressions as a whole and that vocabulary and syntax do not present problems (Wilbur, Fraser, & Fruchter,

1981). Nevertheless, there is research showing that knowledge and explanation of figurative expressions (e.g., similes, metaphors, idioms, and proverbs) are related to the reading comprehension levels of deaf students (Fruchter, Wilbur, & Fraser, 1984; Orlando & Shulman, 1989). Thus, proficient readers, for a number of reasons, are able to deal with metaphorical expressions better than less proficient or poor readers. It should be possible for future researchers to examine the use of rich or explicit contextual additions on the understanding of figurative expressions (see the previous discussions of studies by Ahn, 1996, and de Villiers & Pomerantz, 1992).

Similar to the research on vocabulary (Paul, 1984; Paul & Gustafson, 1991), it is difficult for many readers who are deaf to derive the meaning of figurative expressions from context. This is due to major difficulties, some of which have been highlighted previously: (a) Students who are deaf and hard of hearing may not have the level of reading competence to use context clues, and (b) the context of the reading material typically does not reveal the meaning of the expression.

Table 8-10 provides a summary of the major points and findings of selected studies on syntax and figurative language.

Table 8-10 A Few Major Points of Selected Studies on Syntax and Figurative Language

---

Syntax

- The research on syntax has focused on several general issues, three of which are: (a) comprehension of the structures and the frequency of structures in reading materials, (b) the effects of factors such as instructional methods and context of passages, and (c) the effects of short-term working memory on the comprehension of syntax. More recent studies have attempted to explain students' difficulty with certain syntactic structures within the framework of Chomsky's work.

- The work of Quigley and collaborators revealed that the development of syntax knowledge in deaf students was quantitatively delayed when compared to hearing students. Quigley and his associates also demonstrated that deaf students acquired syntactic structures in the same manner (i.e., qualitatively similar) as younger hearing students. That is, the deaf students proceed through stages, make errors, and use some strategies that seem to be similar to those of hearing students.

- A number of researchers have argued that a better understanding of deaf readers' knowledge of English syntax requires an analysis that proceeds beyond the sentence level and entails perspectives that include semantics and pragmatics considerations.

- There seems to be some evidence that deaf and hard-of-hearing students can understand syntactic structures better in context than in isolation. However, similar to the research on context and vocabulary knowledge, the use of context to comprehend syntax is indicative of the students' ability to derive the meaning of the structure. Deriving the meaning of structure—like deriving word meaning—might be more indicative of reading skill. This skill, however, is also influenced by the type of context in which the structure is housed in the passage.

Figurative Language

- Research on the comprehension of figurative language is difficult to conduct because of the interactions and influences of other language variables such as vocabulary and syntax as well as the interactions between language and thought.

- Many students with severe to profound hearing impairment have difficulty comprehending figurative expressions in printed materials. It is also difficult for many readers who are deaf to derive the meaning of figurative expressions from context. Some researchers have documented that deaf students can understand metaphorical expressions if the vocabulary and syntax are controlled.

- Similar to results on other language variables, it has been reported that proficient readers, for a number of reasons, are able to deal with metaphorical expressions better than less proficient or poor readers.

RESEARCH ON SELECTED READER-BASED FACTORS AND DEAFNESS

The research on the effects of reader-based factors on the reading ability of deaf and hard-of-hearing students has not been as extensive as the research on text-based factors; however, there is a growing interest in this line of research (see reviews in King & Quigley, 1985; Paul, 1998a). The selection of studies and reviews here is representative of much of the work on certain high-level aspects such as prior knowledge and metacognition. In addition, it is important to address what should be a growing area of interest in this field—the research on working memory, particularly the relationship between phonological coding in WM and reading comprehension.

Prior Knowledge and Metacognitive Variables

The work of Wilson (1979) is illustrative of the research on the inferencing ability of students who are deaf. Based on his analysis of previous studies, this researcher hypothesized that one of the major reasons for students' difficulty with reading materials beyond the third grade was their difficulty in making inferences. The task of making inferences is predominant for the higher reading levels due to the abstract and implicit nature of the information. The researcher documented students' problems with inferences in a series of short passages in which inferencing was studied in various syntactic environments with the vocabulary controlled for level of difficulty.

The ability to make inferences in, for example, answering questions is highly related to the prior knowledge and metacognitive abilities of the students (for students who are hearing, see Baker & Brown, 1984; Fincher-Kiefer, 1992). There is some research showing that students with severe to profound hearing impairment have the ability to use their prior knowledge to comprehend aspects of the text (Kluwin, Getson, & Kluwin, 1980), to organize information for retelling a story (i.e., story grammar) (Griffith & Ripich, 1988), or to answer high-level comprehension questions (Schirmer & Woolsey, 1997). As discussed previously, the research on deriving word meanings and syntax can be interpreted as deaf students having the skill to apply prior knowledge and metacognitive aspects. However, it should be clear from these studies that students who are deaf either do not have adequate prior knowledge or metacognitive skills, do not apply these skills during reading tasks, or most interestingly, do not have opportunities to use or develop such skills (see discussions in Jackson, Paul, & Smith, 1997; King & Quigley, 1985; Paul, 1998a; Strassman, 1997; Strassman, Kretschmer, & Bilsky, 1987).

Although there is considerable debate on whether to ask questions on different levels (e.g., Question-Answer Relationships [QARs]) or whether the types of questions asked should support (i.e., scaffolding technique) readers' understanding of the difficult aspects of the text on an ongoing, dynamic basic, there is little doubt that asking questions is important (Dole, Duffy, Roehler, & Pearson, 1991; also see the review in Pearson & Fielding, 1991). The types of questions asked for understanding and assessing prior knowledge and relating this to comprehension is important (Jackson et al., 1997). However, there seems to be little evidence that it is necessary to ask questions at a lower, literal level to support the development of answering questions on a higher, inferential level.

There is some evidence that this is true also for deaf students. For example, Schirmer and Woolsey (1997) not only demonstrated that deaf children can address high-level comprehension questions and that their ability to answer these questions did not require that they answer low-level, detail-type questions about the story. For the purposes here, the researchers also reported that the children had some difficulty with the application of relevant and accurate prior knowledge and other reading tasks. This does not mean that detail-type questions should be avoided entirely; some might be important and relevant, such as in a mystery story. Nevertheless, there is a need for teachers to focus mostly on higher level inferential questions and, more importantly, as stated previously, to provide children with opportunities and support for addressing these types of reading tasks.

The notion that reading is thinking, reasoning, or essentially a higher level cognitive activity and that instruction should be based on this principle can be found in several reviews and analyses of the research literature (Erickson, 1987; Martin, 1993; Paul, 1993, 1998a; Strassman, 1997). Because of the similarity between cognition and reading, some researchers have argued that an improvement in the cognitive thinking skills of students will lead to a subsequent improvement in their reading skills (Martin, 1993; Naglieri & Das, 1988). Reading beyond the literal stage (i.e., reading for meaning) has been described as follows:

> *The evaluative, inferential reading comprehension act, among other things, is a culturally-loaded, linguistic, metacognitive response to the printed word . . . the deaf . . . [should] . . . be exposed to advanced comprehension tasks commensurate with the maturity of their thinking abilities. Inferential and critical reading should be taught as natural extensions of the thinking process. (Erickson, 1987, p. 293)*

This focus on cognition, specifically metacognition, seems to be an important, underrated, and problematic aspect in reading and deafness, at least from the few studies and reviews cited here. For example, Strassman (1992) stated the purpose of her study as a question: "What metacognitive knowledge do deaf students have about school-related reading?" (p. 327). She conducted and videotaped interviews with the students on an individual basis, using the Reading Comprehension Interview (Wixson, Bosky, Yochum, & Alvermann, 1984). Strassman interpreted the results as showing that many deaf students can be classified as passive readers. She stated that:

> *It is not clear that these adolescents had metacognitive knowledge about why they did what they did in school-related reading or what the long-term goal of reading in school was. Rather, they seemed to mechanically employ the techniques that they had been taught. (p. 328)*

Strassman (1997) provided an eloquent review of the literature on metacognition and reading for deaf students. This researcher reiterated evidence that has been documented for hearing children. For example, deaf children might not be given sufficient opportunities to engage in high-level metacognitive tasks or in appropriate metacognitive tasks. This might be due to the type of reading materials that are used, which are not sophisticated enough (i.e., low-level materials). In addition, deaf students might be engaged in instructional activities that do not foster the development of comprehension skills (e.g., use of drill sheets, focus on low-level details in stories, etc.). Finally, probably one of the most important synthesis proffered by Strassman is that the metacognitive skills of deaf students can be affected positively (i.e., improved) by good focused instruction.

Another perspective on the literacy process of deaf and hard-of-hearing students may be gleaned from recent research that employed newer models, for example, reader-response theory (Lemley, 1993; Williams, 1994; Williams & McLean, 1996). In general, reader-response theorists maintain that there is a need to understand how children transact with printed materials. This transaction may involve the reading of a text or attending to the text while it is read aloud by another person. In sharing their reactions, understandings, and so on, children may be asked to talk out loud and/or to manipulate characters (e.g., cut out posters of the story characters). With this approach, children can see similarities and differences between their responses and those of others. In addition, researchers can obtain glimpses of how children make sense of their worlds, using the information from the text as one type of input. This type of approach, including the use of literature, is a very powerful and motivating factor for children, even those who are considered poor readers (Lemley, 1993; Williams & McLean, 1996). Most interesting, it is possible to assess (albeit difficult) how much information children are using from the text in constructing their understanding of topics and issues. In fact, in the Jackson et al. (1997) study mentioned previously, it was obvious (although no formal measures were used) that many deaf subjects relayed information about a topic (i.e., bats) that was not actually in the story that they were required to read. Yet, these subjects remarked to the investigators that such information was indeed in the story although they did not offer or were extremely reluctant to show the location.

Table 8-11 provides highlights of this section on prior knowledge and metacognition, including additional information on these two major concepts in reading.

Working Memory and Reading

This section examines the relationships between working memory (WM) and reading. As mentioned in Chapter 3, WM is an aspect of short-term memory. First, the types of coding that occur in working memories of both hearing and

Table 8-11 Highlights on Prior Knowledge and Metacognition

- Research on the effects of reader-based factors, such as prior knowledge and metacognition, on the reading ability of deaf and hard-of-hearing students has not been as extensive as the research on text-based factors; however, there is a growing interest in this line of research.

- In general, it seems that a number of students who are deaf either do not have adequate prior knowledge or metacognitive skills, do not apply these skills during reading tasks, or most interestingly, do not have opportunities to use or develop such skills.

- The importance of the combination of prior knowledge and metacognition has been documented. As an example, Yamashita (1992) studied 61 students with a degree of hearing impairment ranging from 36 dB to 120 dB. Results indicated that both prior knowledge and metacognition are significantly related to reading comprehension. Further regression analyses revealed that metacognition has the strongest effect for all measures of reading comprehension, which was described as answering different levels of questions.

- The focus on cognition, specifically metacognition, seems to be an important, underrated, and problematic aspect in reading and deafness, at least from the few studies and reviews cited in this chapter.

- From Paul (1998a):

  Results of reading research . . . indicates that prior knowledge of a topic increases the amount of information that children recall from the text on that topic. Prior knowledge . . . refers to general knowledge of the story structure (e.g., story grammar) and knowledge and experiences about topics and themes in stories. . . . Readers with high prior knowledge are able to answer more questions correctly than readers with low prior knowledge in that subject area. This is especially true for inferential questions. . . .

  Metacognition is concerned with strategies readers use to monitor and repair their comprehension of written texts. . . . Metacognitive activity is related to children's reading comprehension. In addition, metacognitive status has been shown to vary with age and with reading level. Older and skilled readers know more about reading strategies, detect errors more often during reading, and have better recall of text information. [It is possible to improve the metacognitive ability of students.] It was found that trained students performed better than untrained students at evaluating types of questions and at providing correct answers. (pp. 58–59)

Note: Additional information on prior knowledge and metacognition can be found in Table 8-1.

deaf individuals are described. Next, the relationships between type of coding and verbosequential properties of a spoken language such as English (i.e., linguistic properties that are dependent on time and left-to-right, linear sequences for processing information—also known as temporal-sequential processing) are discussed. Finally, it is argued that both cognitive knowledge of the alphabetic system and the use of a phonological-based code in working memory are important for the development of reading ability. Of course, there are other important skills, for example, knowledge of language components such as syntax and vocabulary, as discussed previously. Nevertheless, it seems that the use of a phonological-based code is most efficient for handling verbosequential tasks (as required for English reading) and for facilitating cognitive awareness of the alphabetic system.

Cognitive awareness of the alphabetic system is typically connected to phonological and phonemic awareness. One of the avenues for continuing and utilizing such awareness has been the use of phonics, an instructional technique/strategy that purports to assist in developing an understanding of the relationships between phonemes and graphemes (i.e., orthography). Reviews of studies on the phonics abilities of deaf and hard-of-hearing individuals reveal that it is possible for these individuals to acquire knowledge of the phoneme-grapheme links (see review in LaSasso & Metzger, 1998). There seems to be more variability among deaf students in this area than among hearing students (Leybaert, 1993). In addition, as discussed previously, deaf students' progress with orthographic knowledge is seriously impeded by their difficulties with phonological and phonemic awareness. This difficulty seems to be related to the processes of working memory for phonetic languages such as English.

Working memory has been defined by Baddeley (1990) as the mental system responsible for the processing and temporary storage of information. Much of the research in deafness has focused on recoding strategies in WM, specifically the advantages of using a lower level phonological-based code (Hanson & Lichtenstein, 1990; Lichtenstein, 1983, 1998). For example, Harris and Beech (1998) found that phonological awareness (i.e., implicit awareness) was a good predictor of early success in reading English for both hearing and deaf children (5 year olds). Daneman et al. (1995) investigated higher level aspects, specifically those that describe working memory capacity, in a small group of orally educated students. Similar to the phonological-based findings, WM capacity was also a good predictor of reading achievement.

Descriptions of the nature of WM coding strategies are dependent on the similarities between the features of the tasks and the strategies used by individuals. By analyzing the production errors or by analyzing the manner in which individuals remember certain segments of information, it is possible to spec-ify their WM strategies. For example, the use of phonological code can be inferred if individuals produce confusion errors based on the similarities between two rhyming sounds in words such as *bill* and *mill*.

Hearing individuals use a phonological-based code in working memory for recalling both spoken and written linguistic stimuli. The use of a phono-logical-based code seems to be related to the structure of their spoken lan-guage, in this case, English. This characterization is an abstraction of the phonological and morphological structures of English. For example, it has been remarked that: "Words are composed of sequentially arranged processes, and morphological processes typically add one or more prefixes and/or suffixes (each composed of one or a series of phonemes) to a stem (Krakow & Hanson, 1985, p. 265)."

Research on deaf individuals has revealed five major types of coding (including a combination or multiple type) on either WM tasks or during reading—sign (Bellugi, Klima, & Siple, 1974/1975; Odom, Blanton, & McIntire, 1970), dactylic (Locke & Locke, 1971), phonological based (reviews in Conrad, 1979; Hanson, 1989), visual (Blanton, Nunnally, & Odom, 1967), and multi-ple (Lichtenstein, 1983, 1984, 1985, 1998; MacSweeney, Campbell, & Donlan, 1996). Table 8-12 provides a brief description of each internal coding type and additional information on verbosequential and other types of processing.

Deaf students who use predominantly a phonological-based code in WM tend to be better readers than other deaf students who use predominantly a nonphonological-based code (see reviews and discussions in Hanson, 1989; Hanson et al., 1984; LaSasso & Metzger, 1998; Tzeng, 1993; for another view, see Gibbs, 1989). As expressed in the following passage:

> *What makes phonological coding in working memory so important? In reading and listening, individual words of a sentence must be retained while the grammatical relations among words are determined. Evidence suggests that working memory is most efficient for verbal mate-rial (including written material) when the processing involves phono-logical coding. For readers suffering from impaired phonological coding in working memory, processing individual words and putting these words together into phrases and sentences can be computationally overload-ing, impairing overall reading performance. (Lillo-Martin et al., 1991, p. 147)*

The importance of phonological coding for reading and handling ver-bosequential information has been documented in a number of studies (see Hanson, 1990; Hanson & Lichtenstein, 1990; LaSasso & Metzger, 1998; Leybaert,

1993; Lichtenstein, 1983, 1984, 1985, 1998; Tzeng, 1993). The following studies are representative of this line of research, especially for older deaf adolescents.

Craig and Gordon (1988) provided a perspective on the interrelationships among verbosequential processing, working memory, and reading achievement as well as other types of academic achievement, for example, mathematics. The researchers administered a series of cognitive tasks to students who were severely to profoundly hearing impaired and between the ages of 15 and 20 years old. The sample was divided into two broad groups: high readers and low readers. The researchers were interested in assessing verbosequential skills, associated primarily with the left hemisphere, and visuospatial skills, associated primarily with the right hemisphere (see discussion in Table 8-12).

Table 8-12 Types of Internal Coding Strategies and Other Processing Information

Internal Coding Strategy	Description
Sign	Refers to the manual aspects of signs from ASL or one of the English signed systems.
Dactylic	Refers to the manual alphabet; also known as finger spelling.
Visual	Refers to the shapes of printed letters or graphemes.
Speech or phonologic	Refers to either the subvocalization or the mental representation of the auditory-articulatory process.
Multiple	Refers to combinations of the types of internal codes.
Other Terms	**Description**
Temporal-sequential	Refers to the presentation of stimuli in a serial, sequential manner, typically one item at a time. After exposure, each item is removed from sight prior to the presentation of the next item. This involves a time element. The auditory sense

seems to process input in a temporal-sequential manner predominantly. Temporal-sequential is also known as verbosequential.

Spatial-simultaneous Simultaneous (i.e., co-occurring) stimuli are presented in chunks; that is, at one time. Because the presentation involves the use of a certain amount of space, it is often referred to as spatial-simultaneous. The vision sense processes spatial-simultaneous information predominantly. Spatial-simultaneous is also known as visuospatial.

Additional Information on Temporal-Sequential and Spatial-Simultaneous Processing

Vision might be a less efficient processor of sequential information than is audition. The temporal-sequential/spatial-simultaneous distinction seems to be related to the properties of languages. For example, English and other phonetic-based languages can be characterized mainly by temporal-sequential properties, whereas ASL and other sign languages are characterized mainly by spatial-simultaneous properties (however, ASL does have sequential properties). These language properties are related to the main sense used for processing, audition, and vision, respectively.

Additional insights into the processing of information can be gleaned from studies that focus on the specialized cognitive function associated with the left or right hemisphere (e.g., see discussions in Craig & Gordon, 1988). There is evidence that the left hemisphere is specialized for language functions, particularly for analytic and temporal-sequential processes. On the other hand, the right hemisphere is specialized, or has the far greater role, for areas such as visuospatial skills and in holistic, or gestalt, processing.

Results revealed that the students with hearing impairment performed below average on tasks requiring verbosequential processing and average and above on tasks requiring visuospatial processing. In addition, there was a strong relationship between verbosequential skills (e.g., verbal fluency and serial tasks) and academic achievement, including reading. Weak relationships were found between visuospatial skills and achievement. Finally, it was noted that high readers performed significantly better than low readers on all verbosequential tasks. However, no differences between the groups were reported on the visuospatial tasks. It should be noted that the researchers recommended the teaching of strategies for using right hemisphere skills "to bridge toward and improve left hemisphere performance" (Craig & Gordon, 1988, p. 40).

Lillo-Martin et al. (1991) provided additional insights into the interrelationships among phonological coding, working memory, and syntactic comprehension. The researchers were interested in delineating factors that differentiate good deaf readers from poor deaf readers. They focused on the comprehension of one syntactic structure, relative clause, in several modes, for example, written English, signed English, and American Sign Language. The researchers also investigated a long-standing issue discussed previously: the effects of phonological coding in working memory on reading ability.

Subjects were Gallaudet University students with severe to profound hearing impairment who came from homes in which ASL was the major mode of communication. The subjects were divided into two groups: good readers and poor readers. The average reading level of the good readers was about ninth grade. No differences between IQ scores of the two groups were observed.

The test battery included the Gates-MacGinitie Reading Test—comprehension subtest, the Test of Syntactic Abilities (Quigley, Steinkamp et al., 1978)—Relativization 1: comprehension subtest (selected items), American Sign Language relative clause comprehension test, signed English relative clause comprehension test, and a serial recall test. Results revealed no significant differences between the two groups on the written English relative clause test and on all the signed tests. In addition, it was observed that the performance of the groups was similar across sentence types and that there was no group by sentence type interaction. Lillo-Martin et al. (1991) interpreted this latter result as support for their unified-processing deficit hypothesis rather than for structural deficits, for example, knowledge of grammar. This means that deaf students have adequate knowledge of syntax; thus, differences between the reading ability of the two groups in this study must be due to their processing ability (however, see previous discussion of the processing-structural issue, Kelly, 1995, 1996). Surprisingly, the researchers did not find evidence of phonological coding for either group.

One of the most important lines of research in this area is the work of Lichtenstein, reported in several publications (1983, 1984, 1985, 1998). Lichtenstein's research (1983, 1998) involved students at the National Technical Institute for the Deaf (NTID), all of whom had reading abilities considerably above the average for prelinguistic deaf students. His subjects exhibited a considerable range of competence in English skills and came from a variety of educational and communication backgrounds. Lichtenstein's goals were (a) to study their working memory processes with word and sentence memory tasks;

(b) to obtain extensive self-reports through questionnaires of their conscious coding and recoding strategies; (c) to gather extensive descriptive and performance data on their auditory, intellectual, and linguistic abilities; and (d) to analyze the relations among these data in the framework of a series of hypotheses connecting working memory to coding and recoding processes and to psycholinguistic functioning. His detailed investigations produced findings of critical importance to understanding the role of working memory in the development of primary and secondary (reading and writing) language in deaf children and adolescents.

Lichtenstein reported that individual deaf students typically used two or more codes rather than just one exclusively. The various codes were used with varying degrees of effectiveness. The most commonly used codes were sign and speech. It was also found that the better readers relied very heavily on speech (phonological-based) coding. In addition, reliance on speech coding was not confined to those deaf students who had intelligible speech. The primary relationships of working capacity and coding processes seem to be with syntactic skills. Speech coders tend to be better readers apparently because speech coding can better represent the grammatical structure of English than sign or visual coding. This allows the short-term retention of enough information to decode grammatical structures that often are not linear (e.g., relative clause: *The boy who kissed the girl ran away*; passive voice: *The dog was bit by the boy*). These findings have been confirmed by other studies (see reviews in Hanson, 1989; Paul & Jackson, 1993). The hypothesis is presented here that the findings of current and future studies conducted on younger age deaf and hard-of-hearing students will not deviate much from the major points of Lichtenstein's work.

Whether Lichtenstein's research accurately explains the working memory of deaf individuals remains to be seen. It has been argued that a model of working memory for deaf persons should include subsystems for articulatory, sign, and visual coding (Chalifoux, 1991). This model should be robust enough to explain the contributions of the combination of codes (i.e., sign, speech, etc.) that deaf persons used. It might be that the mechanisms and processes of WM of individuals who know a sign language (e.g., ASL) are essentially different from those who know a spoken language or from those who use a speech-based code in their WM (Wilson & Emmorey, 1997). These differences seem to be due to the processing demands and capacities of the sense modalities (i.e., vision vs. audition). There are similarities; however, differences do emerge in light of the processing constraints of the senses. This seems to be a confirmation of differences between the processing demands for a sign language (e.g., mostly visuospatial) and those for a spoken language (e.g., mostly temporal-sequential), discussed previously (also see Table 8-12).

Nevertheless, whether using a combination of codes (see Lichtenstein, 1983, 1998; MacSweeney et al., 1996) is as efficient as using a predominant phonological code for handling phonetic-based linguistic information is an open question. If the accumulation of evidence indicates that a combination or a predominantly sign-based code is not as efficient, then it might be feasible to talk about qualitative differences in the literacy development of those individuals who rely predominantly on visuo-spatial processing. Indeed, this once again raises the possibility of a psychology of deafness with respect to language and literacy development (Paul, 1998a; Paul & Jackson, 1993). That is, for those individuals who rely predominantly on a sign-based code in WM, the development of a language on which a speech-based code is necessary to use might be an extremely difficult, even unrealistic, goal. Finally, it has become clear (or is becoming clear) that a degree of language proficiency seems to be necessary for the sufficient operation of a memory system, particularly WM, and again, this affects the subsequent development of learned skills such as reading and writing (see the discussion in Bebko, 1998).

Table 8-13 presents a summary of the major points and findings of selected studies on working memory and reading.

Table 8-13 Summary of Major Points of Selected Studies on Working Memory and Reading

---

- Much of the research in deafness has focused on recoding strategies in working memory (WM), specifically the advantages of using a lower level phonological-based code.

- Research on deaf individuals has revealed five major types of coding on either WM tasks or during reading—sign, dactylic, visual, phonological-based, and multiple.

- Deaf students who use predominantly a phonological-based code in WM tend to be better readers than other deaf students who use predominantly a nonphonological-based code.

- Speech coders tend to be better readers apparently because speech coding can better represent the grammatical structure of English than sign or visual coding. This allows the short-term retention of enough information to decode grammatical structures that often are not linear (e.g., relative clauses and passive sentences).

- The reliance on speech coding is not confined to deaf students who have intelligible speech.

- For those individuals who rely predominantly on a sign-based code in WM, the development of a language on which a speech-based code is necessary to use might be an extremely difficult, even unrealistic, goal.

DEVELOPMENT OF WRITING

Theories and research on writing have been influenced by theories and research on reading and some that have focused only on writing. One useful framework for understanding these influences was proffered by McCarthey and Raphael (1992; also see the discussion in Paul, 1998a). McCarthey and Raphael utilized the broad themes of cognitive information processing, naturalism, and social constructivism and presented advantages and disadvantages of each mental framework (see Table 8-3). The development of writing has also been affected by the recent thinking on models of instruction—that is, whether writing can be or should be taught to students. In addition, research on writing has been discussed relative to the type of research inquiry, namely, the use of quantitative or qualitative methodologies. Implicit in all theories of both reading and writing is the notion that children are active little scientists. That is, they construct hypotheses about how the language works in both the oral and written mode (see discussion in Ruddell & Haggard, 1985).

Research on emergent literacy has revealed that some children scribble in their early attempts to write (Harste, Burke, & Woodward, 1982; Heath, 1982; Sulzby & Teale, 1987; also see the review in Snow et al., 1998). Children seem to explore the functions of print and to make progress with their understanding in a natural manner. Some children, particularly those at risk (see Snow et al., 1998), may need to learn about these roles and functions and how they are expressed conventionally via their interactions with peers and significant others.

The beginning of the chapter uses a quote by Tierney and Pearson (1983) on the relationship between reading and writing. Although there has been some discussion on this relationship, particularly similar underpinnings for both reading and writing (see McCarthey & Raphael, 1992), some scholars have opined that this line of research seems to have lost some interest (Clay, 1994). Nevertheless, with respect to this relationship, one of the most common statements that has been made is that children/adolescents need to be given numerous opportunities to write. In a national report (Snow et al., 1998), one of the major recommendations on writing for reading instruction in kindergarten through third grade is as follows:

> *Once children learn to write letters, they should be encouraged to write them, to use them to begin writing words or parts of words, and to use words to begin writing sentences. Instruction should be designed with the understanding that the use of invented spelling is not in conflict with teaching correct spelling. Beginning writing with invented spelling can be helpful for developing understanding of phoneme identity, phoneme segmentation, and sound-spelling relationships. Conventionally correct spelling should be developed through focused instruction and practice. Primary-grade children should be expected to spell previously studied words and spelling patterns correctly in their final writing products. Writing should take place on a daily basis to encourage children to become more comfortable and familiar with it. (pp. 323–324)*

One common model proffered to address the writing process, as described by Tierney and Pearson (1983), is that of Flower and Hayes (1980). The model of Flower and Hayes has been expanded to include five stages: planning or prewriting, drafting or composing, revising, editing, and sharing (see discussion in Tompkins, 1990). The stages are briefly described in Table 8-14.

Table 8-14 A Classroom Writing Model Based on the Work of Flower and Hayes

---

Stages of the Writing Model

Stage 1
- This is the prewriting stage in which students/writers need to select topics and develop a plan or outline. Students/writers identify their audiences and establish a purpose for their composition. Classroom activities during this stage are similar to those for a prereading stage. That is, teachers can assist in activating and enriching the prior knowledge of students relevant to specific topics by asking questions or using semantic maps or other elaboration techniques. Students should be encouraged to be creative or imaginative with their plan or outline and not simply follow a prescribed plan by the teacher or the class.

Stage 2
- During this stage, the students/writers produce a first draft of their papers, often called the rough draft. Students/writers use their outlines or plans to guide the structure of their composition. For example, they can focus on an introductory paragraph, supporting sentences and paragraphs, and a summary or conclusion. Teachers and peers can provide supporting comments and ask questions for clarification purposes (e.g., "Why are you saying this?" "What does this mean?" "Can you use a better word or phrase?" and "I like the way you say this."). At this point, students/writers might request assistance with the mechanics of writing, for example, spelling, punctuation, word choice or phrases, and so on. The primary focus, however, should be on the organization and overall content.

Stage 3
- In general, this is considered the revising stage; however, it is possible that revisions have been occurring throughout all previous stages of the writing process. In the act of revising, the writer becomes an active reader. The student/writer engages in the reading of his or her draft as well as the drafts of others in the classroom. There will be ample opportunities for altering, expanding, clarifying, and embellishing the written compositions based on the comments of peers and the teacher. Again, student writers should be encouraged to be as creative and imaginative as possible so that the suggestions do not lead to a writing style that is not reflective of the particular student/writer's voice. During the revising stage, much attention can and should be paid to the mechanics of writing. Teachers might decide that some students/writers need a large amount of assistance or additional instruction in troublesome areas. Individual conferences may be established periodically.

Stage 4
- In the editing stage, there is an attempt to proofread papers that have incorporated all of the suggested revisions; however, editing might have occurred previously as well. In classroom situations, students/writers proofread their own compositions as well as those of others. At this point, all mechanic issues should be resolved. There should be no major rewriting activities during this stage. Nevertheless, it is possible that some students might want or need to return to the revising stage or to proceed between revising and editing periodically.

Stage 5
- The final stage of writing is considered to be the formal sharing stage. That is, students/writers attempt to share their work by publishing or displaying it

(continues)

(Table 8-14 continued)

for others to read, review, or discuss. The discussion or reviewing aspects should focus on the interpretation or meaning of the work—there should be no discussion of mechanics or grammar. In addition, participants might wish to react by expressing their feelings of the displayed or published work. Of course, getting published might require several additional steps depending on the place of publication (i.e., magazine, newspaper, etc.).

Perhaps a useful way to discuss writing is to divide perspectives into two broad categories: product and process (Czerniewska, 1992; Laine & Schultz, 1985; Paul, 1998a). Traditional research and instruction on writing has focused on the products, whereas the more recent research emphasis is on the process of writing (Bereiter & Scardamalia, 1983; Hillocks, 1986). As argued elsewhere (Paul, 1998a), this should not be construed as an either-or situation:

> *In order for the reading and writing interaction to proceed smoothly, students need to have automatic, fluent lower-level (i.e., decoding/encoding) skills so that they can concentrate on the construction of meaning via the use of higher-level processes. In other words, teachers need to emphasize comprehension and other higher-level skills such as organization, intent, and audience along with meeting needs for lower-level skills such as grammar, spelling, and punctuation. (p. 233)*

The interplay between lower level and higher level processes is reiterated throughout the ensuing sections.

The Product View of Writing

The products of writing refer to items such as spelling, punctuation, capitalization, grammar, and legibility (Czerniewska, 1992; Laine & Schultz, 1985; Paul, 1998a). Similar to the understanding of the reading process, written English literacy is also dependent in part on knowledge of the alphabet system, or the relationship between sounds (phonemes) and their letter representations (graphemes) (see discussions in Brady & Shankweiler, 1991; Snow et al., 1998; Templeton & Bear, 1992). Thus, the acquisition and development of writing is hindered if the student does not possess automatic lower level skills such as the mechanics mentioned previously.

There are a number of studies that have demonstrated that poor readers are also poor writers (at least from a cognitive information processing point of view) (see research reviews in Adams, 1990; Chall, Jacobs, & Baldwin, 1990). This has been reported also for many students with severe to profound hearing impairment (Moores, 1996; Paul, 1998a). One assumption is that to be a good writer, one must be at least a good reader. Another assumption is that writing skills, similar to reading skills, must be taught (see discussions in Chall et al., 1990; Czerniewska, 1992; Snow et al., 1998).

Despite the linearity of the product view of writing, it is important for the writer to possess fluent lower level skills in mechanics. However, lower level skills are not sufficient. A number of good readers do not become good writers (see discussions in Bereiter & Scardamalia, 1983; Czerniewska, 1992). These findings have led some scholars to call for a paradigm shift in the view of the development of writing or at least to recognize that good writing requires the use of higher level skills that proceed beyond the mere use of mechanics.

The Process of Writing

A predominant recent view is that writing is a social process (Czerniewska, 1992). The underpinnings of this viewpoint can be found in several models, notably the work of Vygotsky (1962), whose views have also influenced theories of language development. Support for the social view of writing can be found also in the current reader response theories and even in literary critical frameworks (see discussion in Paul, 1998a).

Because writing is an aspect of language, it is a social process whose meaning, role, and value vary across contexts or communities (see Harste et al., 1982; Sulzby & Teale, 1987). Within this framework, writing is not merely or only a representation of an individual's thoughts. Similar to the use of language, a person writes to generate or create meaning. In other words, written language is not an attempt to represent or reflect reality; it is the writer's creation or construction of reality.

The social process of writing emphasizes what can be called higher level cognitive aspects, for example, organization, purpose, and audience. The lower level skills such as legibility and grammar are dealt with afterward as needed. That is, after producing or completing a draft, students might receive assistance with grammar and mechanics from other student writers or teachers.

As mentioned previously, one popular model of writing development contains stages such as planning (topic generation and organization), composing (first draft), revising (editing and rewriting), and sharing (e.g., publishing). These stages are not always mutually exclusive. For example, a writer might choose to compose and revise at the same time. During the composing stage, the writer might decide to reorganize the manuscript.

The social process of writing seems to be a predominant top-down approach. In the author's view, this approach is linear and has shortcomings similar to the product, or bottom-up, approach in reading. It is somewhat beneficial to view writing as an interactive social-cognitive process that is similar to the process of reading (Rubin & Hansen, 1986; Tierney & Leys, 1984; Tierney & Pearson, 1983; Tompkins, 1990).

The notion of similar underlying processes implies that both reading and writing involve the construction of meaning. In addition, writing, similar to reading, entails the interaction between the individual and the text that the individual is attempting to compose. There is a reciprocal relationship between the top-down (e.g., organization and intent) and bottom-up aspects (e.g., spelling and grammar) of writing. In essence, writing develops as a result of and in conjunction with reading (Adams, 1990; Anderson et al., 1985).

To understand and to research the process of writing, some scholars have argued for the use of holistic methodology (see discussions in Bereiter & Scardamalia, 1983, 1987; Czerniewska, 1992) and natural instructional approaches (see discussions in Laine & Schultz, 1985). As remarked by Bereiter and Scardamalia (1983), holistic approaches "insist on viewing natural behavior in its full context and . . . seek to break down the rigid division between observer and observed" (p. 21). Nevertheless, there is no superiority or God's eye view associated with any particular type of methodology. Consequently, a better understanding of writing, and any other phenomenon, as both a cognitive and social process entails the use of both quantitative and qualitative methodologies (Bereiter & Scardamalia, 1983, 1987).

In tandem with research methodologies and theories motivated by the framework of naturalism (see McCarthey & Raphael, 1992), there has been a push for natural instructional approaches, especially in the areas of reading and writing. Relative to writing, the natural approaches assert that writing is not something that can be taught in a linear fashion—that is, the imparting of knowledge from teachers to students. It has been stated that:

> *The emphasis of these and other contemporary approaches to writing is on generating meaning (rather than correctly recording or transmitting what already exists). . . . Teachers are doing more writing themselves and learning to discuss their own composing processes. They write in class with their students, share drafts of their own writing, and ask students to comment and make suggestions. Students see that writing isn't difficult only for kids and magic for teachers. (Laine & Schultz, 1985, p. 16)*

RESEARCH ON WRITTEN LANGUAGE
Use of Written Language Productions

Until the recent upsurge of interest in American Sign Language and manually coded English, much of the research on the language of deaf and hard-of-hearing children was conducted on their written language productions. This is in distinct contrast to hearing children, where primary spoken language is usually the focus of interest. The major reason for this situation was that the spoken language of many children with severe to profound hearing impairment is extremely limited and often unintelligible and therefore not readily available for inspection and analysis.

There is some research showing that written language productions are not completely reflective of what deaf students can do in the primary performance mode, that is, via the use of English-based signed systems or the use of sign communication in general (see Everhart & Marschark, 1988; Marschark, Mouradian, & Halas, 1994). For example, Everhart and Marschark (1988) interpreted their results as indicating that "literalness evidenced in written English need not be indicative of the more general cognitive literalness assumed from such results by previous researchers" (p. 191).

From another perspective, spontaneous written language productions are generally considered to be among the best indicators of a child's level of mastery of English. However, there are a number of problems associated with the use of written language productions. These problems are discussed in the ensuing paragraphs.

1. Typically, some external stimulus is used to elicit a written sample—a picture, picture sequence, short film, request to write a story or letter, and so forth. The validity and reliability of these techniques often are unknown. If it is found that certain vocabulary items, morphological structures, syntactic structures or other linguistic units of interest do not appear in the writing samples elicited, it is difficult to determine whether this is due to the child's inability to produce such structures or whether it is merely that the stimulus used did not elicit them.

2. Some linguistic units (e.g., infinitival complements—Mary wanted *to make a million dollars*) might appear in the written productions but in insufficient numbers or variety to allow for study and analysis.

3. Some constructions (e.g., some types of relative clauses) appear in linguistic environments such that it is difficult to understand them and their role in a sentence.

4. As probably every teacher knows, the written language productions of many children with severe to profound hearing impairment are often as unintelligible as their spoken language.

Despite these problems of eliciting and analyzing written language productions, such productions provide some valuable information about the children's understanding of English and about the internalized language structure with which the child is operating. Researchers have employed two broad methods for eliciting written productions: free response and controlled response. *Free response* methods refer to the spontaneous, freely produced samples of writing. *Controlled response* methods entail the use of techniques to control or manipulate the behavior of a subject or informant by holding certain linguistic variables constant (see discussion in Cooper & Rosenstein, 1966). The linguistic method of presenting pairs of sentences that differ on only one structure and asking subjects for judgments of the sentences' grammaticality is one example.

With a focus on the products of writing, analyses of the written language production of students with hearing impairment have been influenced by the prevailing linguistic theories, typically, structural linguistics or Chomsky's transformational generative grammar (see Chapter 3). Although dividing lines between free response and controlled response studies and traditional and generative frameworks are not always sharp, the categories are adequate for grouping the data on the written productions of deaf and hard-of-hearing students. It is also important to discuss research on the written language of students that has been influenced by the emerging paradigms associated with the process of writing, particularly the interpretation of the writings of students beyond the sentence level, that is, at the multisentence level.

Research on Written Language and Deafness

The research on the written language of deaf and hard-of-hearing students is discussed relative to two broad areas: the sentence level and the multisentence level. At the sentence level, data are presented from both free response and controlled response studies, influenced by both traditional/structural and transformational generative grammar theories. The more recent studies, focusing on the multisentence level, viewed writing as a social process.

Sentence Level—Free Response: Traditional Framework

The two predominant findings of the early traditional free response studies were: (a) Students had lower performances on written language than younger children who were hearing, and (b) the writings of deaf and hard-of-hearing students varied greatly from standard English (Heider & Heider, 1940; Stuckless & Marks, 1966; Templin, 1950). For example, Heider and Heider (1940) revealed that the students who were hearing impaired used fewer words and clauses (e.g., shorter sentences) than did students who were hearing. The students who were hearing impaired did not attain the average sentence length of 8-year-old children who were hearing until they were 17 years old (also see Myklebust, 1964). Relative to the notion of complexity, Heider and Heider reported that students who were hearing produced more complex sentences than did the students who were deaf and hard of hearing. The researchers found that the students with hearing impairment were typically 17 years old before they used the same proportion of compound and complex sentences in their compositions as 10-year-old students who were hearing did (also see Taylor, 1969).

Although the written language development of the students who were hearing impaired showed improvement with the advancement of age, it seemed to plateau at about the level of the 9- or 10-year-old student who was hearing. There was the emerging view that students with severe to profound hearing impairment did not have a command of the grammar of English, particularly in the areas of vocabulary and syntax (see Templin, 1950, for a historical perspective). This inadequate command of standard English was deemed to be the global reason for the written language performance of deaf students. This resulted in the prevalent use of, for example, stereotypic phrases (see examples in the ensuing paragraph). In addition, it was found that students with severe to profound hearing impairment use more determiners, nouns, and verbs than did hearing children and fewer adverbs, auxiliaries, and conjunctions.

With the aforementioned view in mind, several researchers described the errors and rigid writing samples of deaf and hard-of-hearing students. For example, it was noted that the students produce errors of addition (adding unnecessary words), omission (omitting words needed to make the sentence correct in standard English), substitution (substituting wrong words), and order (word order departing from that of standard English) (Myklebust, 1964). Myklebust (1964) and Simmons (1963) also documented a number of carrier phrases that were found to appear more often in the rigid writing samples of students with hearing impairment than in the writings of hearing students. Examples include: *I see a* _____ ; *There is a* _____ ; and *They had an idea*. It has been argued that the presence of stereotypical phrases might be either an artifact of the test instrument used or the structural approach to teaching language to deaf and hard-of-hearing students (see van Uden, 1977; Wilbur, 1977).

Some prominent reading researchers, concerned mainly with children who are hearing, have attempted to provide a global interpretation of these early studies on deafness. For example, it has been remarked that: "Both the Heider and Heider and the Templin studies point to a significant relationship between oral and written language development. The opportunity for oral language experience through hearing would appear to exert direct influence on performance in written language" (Ruddell & Haggard, 1985, p. 68).

It should be emphasized that these studies were descriptive in nature. This information is important; however, a better understanding of the free response data emerged with interpretations from a generative grammar framework (Chomsky, 1957, 1965; for recent discussions, also see Cook & Newson, 1996), which focused on explanatory adequacy. That is, these theories attempted to explicate the rules that children use to produce sentences at various developmental levels. The idea of language being generative refers to the fact that there is a limited number of highly abstract mechanisms used (at a subconscious level) for the processing (comprehension and production) of a theoretically infinite number of sentences. These abstract mechanisms are often described in terms of rules for sentence processing (production or interpretation).

Sentence Level—Free Response: Generative Grammar

One of the most important and seminal research studies was that of Taylor (1969), who provided information on deaf students' understanding of rules associated with, for example, morphology and transformations (e.g., for relative clauses, passive voice, etc.) (see Chapter 2 for a discussion of these terms). Taylor (1969) pioneered a new analysis for the written language of deaf and hard-of-hearing children—a transformational-generative analysis. In addition, many of Taylor's findings have been confirmed by other researchers.

The results of Taylor's research indicated that the written language productions of children with severe to profound hearing impairment vary considerably from standard English usage. In general, the 16-year-old students achieve mastery over many aspects of the production of simple active declarative sentences, particularly of the subject-verb-object order. Nevertheless, even at this age, students still have problems with morphology, especially in areas of noun and verb inflections. In addition, they have difficulties with the determiner and auxiliary systems of English. Students make relatively few mistakes in producing complex transformations; however, they rarely wrote these constructions. In essence, students know little about complex transformations such as relativization and nominalization. When they attempt to write such transformations, students produce numerous variant structures. It can be concluded that these students were not just making errors in producing English sentences; rather, they were producing correct (for them) sentences from rules that were not based on those of standard English.

Besides examining the comprehension of specific syntactic structures by the use of specific tasks discussed previously, Quigley, Wilbur, Power, Montanelli, and Steinkamp, 1976 obtained written language samples from their national sample of deaf students (i.e., students with profound hearing impairment). Similar to Taylor's findings, only limited instances of the structures studied by the Test of Syntactic Abilities (TSA) were found in the freely produced written samples. There seems to be a correlation between the limited productions and the comprehension (i.e., order of difficulty) of these structures.

Sentence Level—Controlled Response: Generative Grammar

Based on transformational generative grammar, a substantial body of research exists that used controlled presentation of stimuli. The use of controlled response tasks provides additional information on the grammatical competence of students who are deaf and hard of hearing. In many cases, the results of these studies confirmed and extended the findings of Taylor (1969). For example, some of the studies provided insights into deaf students' strategies for processing or understanding certain language transformations such as negation and the passive voice. Only one study is discussed briefly here as a representative example of this type of research. Table 8-15 presents highlights of selected studies in this area.

Table 8-15 Highlights of Selected, Representative Studies based on Transformational Generative Grammar

Studies	Findings
Cooper (1967)	Found deaf children's knowledge of inflectional morphemes to be superior to their knowledge of derivational markers. This is consistent with the difficulty the children have with derived nominals of various types, as discussed in Chapter 2 of this text. Cooper's data generally confirm and extend those found by Taylor (1969) in her free data-gathering situation.

(continues)

(Table 8-15 continued)

Schmitt (1969)

Administered comprehension and production tasks involving the selection of one of four pictures to match correctly a given sentence. He found that most of his subjects who were deaf (ages 8 to 17 years) understood the meaning of the negative marker *not* in English sentences. However, there was a number of the 8-year-old subjects who failed consistently on this task. Schmitt hypothesized that they were operating with what he called the *no negative rule*, "which specifies the ignoring of the marker 'not' and the treatment of negative sentences as equivalent to affirmative sentences" (p. 124). It might be that such a response is even more typical of the performance of children who are deaf and younger than those Schmitt tested.

O'Neill (1973)

Developed a Test of Receptive Language Competence in which deaf and hearing subjects were required to judge whether simple sentences generated by correct and incorrect rules were right or wrong. In the omission section, her deaf subjects (ages 9 to 17 years) made correct judgments on 75% (vs. 84% for children who were hearing) of the items and showed significant improvement with age. In general, the subjects who were hearing impaired did as well as the subjects who were hearing in selecting the right sentences as *right*, but they had a tendency to label wrong sentences as *right* much more often than did the children who were hearing. Specifically, the subjects with hearing impairment were more likely to accept incorrect sentences in which function words such as determiners, prepositions, and verb particles had been omitted than sentences in which nouns, verbs, and adjectives (content words) had been incorrectly omitted. These findings are in close agreement with those reported by Taylor (1969) for free written production discussed previously.

The *redundancy* category was observed to be slightly more difficult than *omission* for O'Neill's deaf subjects (73% correct overall, vs. 85% for subjects who were hearing). O'Neill found a pattern of results similar to that reported for the *omission* category previously. That is, sentences containing redundant determiners, prepositions, and verb particles were more difficult for subjects who were deaf to judge than those containing redundant content words. It was also noted that the subjects who were deaf tended to accept sentences that contained a redundant verb—for example, *The children went walked to the park.*

Relative to the lexicon category, O'Neill (1973) developed a selectional restriction subtest, which was the most difficult test for both deaf (69% correct) and hearing (82% correct) subjects. Subjects accepted as correct a wide range of sentences that violated selectional restrictions on nouns and pronouns. Examples include: *The desk serenaded Matilda* and *Milk are good for you.*

Note: Only representative studies that were not discussed in the chapter are listed.

Power and Quigley (1973) used three tasks to investigate the acquisition of the passive voice (e.g., *The ball was hit by the girl; The window was broken*). In the comprehension task, deaf children (90+ dB average PTA) were required to move toys to show the action of the passive sentence. The researchers concluded that even at ages 17 and 18, the majority of deaf children have a defective rule for the processing of passive sentences. This rule can be stated as "passive reversal of subject-object order to process meaning of such sentences is signaled only by *by*; tense markers are free to vary" (Power & Quigley, 1973, p. 76). In essence, it seems that many deaf students, including the older ones, persisted in interpreting all sentences in terms of the standard subject-verb-object order of the English simple sentence.

Recent Research on the Process of Writing

The few studies discussed in this section are a representative sample of the recent research on the process of writing with deaf individuals, especially with analyses of connected discourse (i.e., beyond the sentence level). Some of the early work in this area was conducted by Gormley and Sarachan-Deily (Gormley & Sarachan-Deily, 1987; Sarachan-Deily, 1982, 1985). Gormley and Sarachan-Deily (1987) analyzed the writing samples of high school age students with severe to profound hearing losses. The focus of the study was to examine the similarities and differences between good and poor writers.

The students' written language samples were analyzed relative to three categories: content (e.g., suggestions, reasons, and conclusions), linguistic aspects (e.g., organization and cohesion), and surface mechanics (e.g., spelling, punctuation, and capitalization). Results revealed no significant differences between the two groups on the surface mechanics and most of the linguistic aspects. It should be noted that both groups made a number of errors in these two categories. However, the major difference between good and poor writers was in the area of content. That is, the compositions of good writers were more developed, cohesive, and readable. In short, the major difference was with the use of higher level writing skills. Although the researchers argued that writing instruction should focus mainly on higher level skills, they suggested that there is also a need to encourage deaf and hard-of-hearing writers to reread and revise their manuscripts. These activities should help students to reduce their errors in surface mechanics and many linguistic aspects.

Other studies also focus on analyses beyond the sentence level or discourse processes. For example, de Villiers (1991) reported that deaf students use fewer cohesive markers than hearing students. On the other hand, Maxwell and Falick (1992) reported no difference in the number of cohesive markers; however, they noted that deaf students tended to exhibit less variation in the use of lexical (words) items to indicate or signal the act of cohesion. In a more recent study, Yoshinaga-Itano, Snyder, and Mayberry (1996) did not find any differences between deaf and hearing students on the variables such as number of propositions and cohesive markers in written language productions. However, Yoshinaga-Itano et al. (1996) noticed that deaf students tended not to elaborate on their ideas or points as much as hearing students.

Within the framework of writing as a process approach, a number of recent studies have emphasized strongly that there should be a continual focus on higher level skills such as organization, intent, and authorship and that teachers should encourage writers to engage in thinking, planning, and evaluating activities. This focus can be seen in studies that examined the free writing of children with hearing impairment in kindergarten (Andrews & Gonzales, 1991) to students in elementary and secondary grades (Kluwin & Kelly, 1991) to students in a postsecondary program (Brown & Long, 1992). The researchers reported that the quality of deaf students' written productions improved over time and that there were noticeable changes in content and syntactic complexity.

The emphasis on the process approach does not mean that it is not important to attend to lower level skills. Some researchers have provided guidelines for teachers to work on skills such as fluency, syntax, and vocabulary (Luckner & Isaacson, 1990; Paul, 1998a). In one sense, focusing on the product of writing only (particularly, lower level skills) is similar to a bottom-up approach in reading, whereas focusing on the higher level skills only (as in a process approach) can become a strict top-down model. Given the earlier discussion that reading and writing are related, that is, both lower level and higher level skills are important, it seems that viewing writing as a social-cognitive interactive process might yield productive research and instructional effects for children and adolescents with hearing impairment (cf. McCarthey & Raphael, 1992, on the limits of such approaches for instructional purposes).

The difficulties deaf individuals have with written language is certainly not limited to the writing of English but also for other spoken languages (see reviews in Conrad, 1979; Fabbretti, Volterra, & Pontecorvo, 1998). In one study, Fabbretti et al. (1998) reported similar types of writing difficulties, including morphology, for Italian deaf native signers. In the review of the literature for their study, Fabbretti et al. (1998) also reiterated major findings on written language acquisition similar to those reported previously in this section:

- *Deaf subjects produce shorter sentences and simpler syntactical structures than their hearing counterparts.*
- *They display poor vocabulary and lexical rigidity.*
- *They encounter problems with relative, subordinate, and pronominal clauses.*
- *Although they show difficulties in various aspects of written language (lexical, morphological, syntactic, and pragmatic), their problems are most striking in the area of grammatical morphology, including omissions, substitutions, and additions of various morphemes. (p. 231)*

In sum, reviews of the literature reveal that the level of the written language development of deaf students is roughly similar to that of their reading development and, for the most part, significantly below that of hearing counterparts (Paul, 1998a). This slow rate of acquisition is even slower during the adolescent years; however, it might not be uniform across all language components that affect the writing process (Musselman & Szanto, 1998; Yoshinaga-Itano & Downey, 1996; Yoshinaga-Itano et al., 1996). For example, development in semantics may be faster than syntax and may account for much of the variance in studies (Yoshinaga-Itano, et al., 1996). Higher scores may be found for measures of semantics and orthography (e.g., spelling, punctuation, capitalization, etc.) as opposed to those on measures of grammar (e.g., syntax) (Musselman & Szanto, 1998). In addition, it is possible that genre (journal writing, letters, poetry, etc.) might have an effect on the quality of writing as well as the quality of spontaneous performance (i.e., spoken and signed) interactions (Musselman & Szanto, 1998; Schick, 1997). Perhaps most interestingly these remarks reiterate the general assertion that writing, similar to reading, is not a unitary skill. Thus, it might be unrealistic to approach the improvement of writing (and reading) on a global level, especially with respect to students who are at risk or who have special needs in this area. Rather, it might be important to determine which aspects or skills cause the most or pervasive difficulty for prospective writers.

Table 8-16 provides a summary of the major points and findings of selected studies in this section.

Table 8-16 Highlights of the Recent Research on the Process of Writing

- Livingston (1989) found that writers who were deaf tended to make more additions, whereas students who were hearing tended to make more deletions in their written compositions. However, both groups were similar in their revisions on the syntactic level.

- In one study, the major difference between good and poor writers was in the area of content. That is, the compositions of good writers were more developed, cohesive, and readable. In short, the major difference was with the use of higher level writing skills. A number of more recent studies seem to emphasize the need for a focus on higher level skills such as organization, intent, and authorship and that teachers should encourage writers to engage in thinking, planning, and evaluating activities.

- Although some researchers observed no differences between deaf and hearing writers on variables such as number of propositions and cohesive markers, it was found that deaf students tended not to elaborate on their ideas or points as much as hearing students.

- The new emphasis on higher level writing skills such as organization, purpose, and audience does not mean that it is not important to attend to lower level skills such as fluency, syntax, and vocabulary.

- The difficulties deaf individuals have with written language is certainly not limited to the writing of English but is also true for other spoken languages. These difficulties have been reported to be similar those on the English language (e.g., shorter sentences, simpler syntactical structures, poor vocabulary, and problems with complex clauses, syntax, and morphology).

- Reviews of the literature reveal that the level of the written language development of deaf students is roughly similar to that of their reading development and for the most part significantly below that of hearing counterparts. The rate of acquisition is not uniform across all language components that affect the writing process. This seems to substantiate the fact that writing, similar to reading, is not a unitary skill. Thus, it might be unrealistic to approach the improvement of writing (and reading) on a global level. Rather, it is important to determine which aspects or skills cause the most or pervasive difficulty for prospective writers.

FINAL REMARKS

This chapter describes the impact of deafness on the development of reading and writing skills. Summaries and highlights of selected major studies on literacy are presented within the various sections of the chapter. Only a few comments are reiterated here.

In general, it is argued that the reading difficulties of deaf and hard-of-hearing students should be discussed within the framework of theories that address both lower level (e.g., spelling and mechanics) and higher level (e.g., organization and purpose) literacy skills. Understanding reading has led to an increased understanding of the process of writing. There seems to be similar underpinnings; that is, both readers and writers attempt to construct a working model of meaning.

It is somewhat surprising, and perhaps distressing, that researchers' cumulative knowledge of the literacy process has not resulted in a substantial improvement of the low literacy achievement of most deaf and hard-of-hearing students. Perhaps there needs to be a more concerted effort to explore the interrelations of theory, research, assessment, curriculum, and instruction. In addition, there needs to be more research on specific factors that have not been studied extensively—notably, metacognition, motivation, and the exercise of control as in self-efficacy. For sure, as indicated by research syntheses in this chapter, there is a need to move away from considering reading or writing as a unitary skill. There are numerous factors that should be considered with respect to the domains of text, reader/writer, task, and context.

With concerted, collaborative efforts, research—especially instructional research—might lead to an improvement—albeit in small increments—of the script literacy skills of many deaf and some hard-of-hearing students. On the other hand, script literacy might not be a realistic goal for many students with prelingual severe to profound hearing impairment. This possibility should be considered in light of what is known about the interrelationships among working memory, phonological coding, and literacy achievement. In addition, the development of a first language as early as possible has been a long-standing problem in the field of deafness. Deaf students' struggles with literacy are compounded because of their attempts to learn both a language and to read and write in that language. Although there is a reciprocal relation between language learning and literacy, it is extremely helpful to possess a working intuitive knowledge of the language in which one is attempting to read and write. Even typical 3-year-old hearing children who might scribble on paper know quite a bit intuitively about the language on which their scribbles are purportedly based.

These enormous difficulties with the development of English as a first language have provided support for the implementation of bilingual and second language programs for deaf students. Is English easier to develop as a second language after a first language, typically taken to mean ASL, is developed? This is one of the main topics of the next chapter.

SCRIPT LITERACY: DEVELOPMENT OF READING AND WRITING
COMPREHENSION QUESTIONS

1. The beginning of the chapter listed four categories of factors with respect to literacy: text, reader/writer, task, and context. Describe each category and provide a few examples.

2. Discuss the basic tenets of the three broad literacy frameworks listed below:
   a. cognitive information processing
   b. naturalism
   c. social constructivism

3. Discuss the basic tenets of the three cognitive information processing theories listed below:
   a. bottom-up
   b. top-down
   c. interactive

4. Describe the following terms and provide some examples:
   a. phonological awareness
   b. phonemic awareness
   c. phonics
   d. alphabetic principle

5. Discuss some of the findings from the research on the early period of literacy development. (See "A Few Remarks on Early Literacy Development.")

6. Describe word identification. Why is it important? What does this mean for deaf students who communicate via the use of a manual system or finger spelling?

7. Describe the following comprehension components: word knowledge, prior knowledge, and metacognition. What are the research findings on the relationships of each component to comprehension ability?

8. Much of the research seems to indicate that there is a plateau at the fourth-grade level with respect to the reading achievement of deaf students. What are some reasons (hypotheses) for this plateau?

9. Much of the research on reading and deafness has been conducted on text-based factors. Discuss the major findings of research in the following areas. You may cite specific studies within each area and/or present general findings for the entire area. (These areas are headings in the chapter.)
    a. words and word meanings
    b. deriving words from context
    c. syntax
    d. figurative language

10. There has been some research on reader-based factors. Discuss the major findings of research in the following areas. You may cite specific studies within each area and/or present general findings for the entire area. (These areas are headings in the chapter.)
    a. prior knowledge and metacognitive variables
    b. working memory and reading

11. List and discuss the five stages of the writing process (i.e., model of Flower & Hayes).

12. Describe the following writing terms:
    a. product view
    b. process view

13. The research on the written language development of deaf and hard-of-hearing students is discussed relative to two broad areas: the

sentence level (e.g., free response and controlled response studies) and the multisentence level (e.g., writing as a social process). Provide a summary of the major findings for each area.

14. What does it mean to say that writing is not a unitary skill? What are some instructional implications?

CHALLENGE QUESTIONS

(Note: Complete answers are not in the text. Additional research is required.)

1. There is a debate in the field of literacy concerning whether or not literacy (reading or writing) should be taught or caught. (These issues are discussed briefly in Chapter 10 of this text.) Do you think that word identification skills can be or should be taught? Can comprehension be taught? Provide some examples of comprehension instruction.

2. Consider the following question: Is reading different for deaf students? That is, is reading for deaf students different from reading for hearing students? The chapter presented a few remarks on this statement. What is your opinion? Can you provide theoretical and research support for your assertion? What are some instructional implications if the answer to this question is yes? What are some instructional implications for a no answer?

3. According to the chapter, there has been little research on what can be called the reading-writing connection (i.e., reading and writing share similar underpinnings or have reciprocal relations). Conduct a review of the literature and see if you can find specific research studies on the reading-writing connection for deaf students. Do you think this connection is important to investigate? Why or why not? What are some instructional implications?

4. Similar to the chapter on language theories, there does not seem to be a coherent comprehensive theory of reading and/or writing. Do you think that such a theory is attainable? Why or why not? What would you expect from a coherent comprehensive theory? Do you think theories on hearing children and literacy are applicable to deaf and hard-of-hearing children? Why or why not? Can you justify your answer?

FURTHER READINGS

Atwell, N. (1990). *Coming to know: Writing to learn in the intermediate grades.* Portsmouth, NH: Heinemann.

Au, K. (1993). *Literacy instruction in multicultural settings.* Fort Worth, TX: Harcourt Brace.

Cornoldi, C., & Oakhill, J. (Eds.). (1996). *Reading comprehension difficulties: Processes and intervention.* Hillsdale, NJ: Lawrence Erlbaum.

Lipson, M., & Wixson, K. (1997). *Assessment and instruction of reading and writing disability: An interactive approach* (2nd ed.). New York: Longman.

Olson, D., & Torrance, N. (Eds.). (1996). *Modes of thought: Explorations in culture and cognition.* New York: Cambridge University Press.

Bilingualism and Second Language Learning

What is the difference between first and second language learning? It cannot be the case that a language is "learnable" as a first language, but less so as a second language. Is the predisposition to acquire whatever language one is exposed to good for a one-time use only? Does this ability self-destruct after one use, or does the presence of a first language alter the conditions for language learning? Can an explanation of the variability in second language learning tell us anything about language learning in general? (Wong Fillmore, 1989, p. 313)

Since the publication of this passage, it is not surprising that researchers still do not have complete answers to the questions posed by Wong Fillmore. What has become clear is that children who are bilingual or are learning English as a second language are a group that is considered at risk for acquiring English literacy skills, according to a recent national report on reading difficulties in children and adolescents (Snow et al., 1998). Similar to the concept of reading, bilingualism is another politicized issue, resulting in, for example, the movement in California to abandon bilingual education programs because of the so-called lackluster or lack of positive effects on the acquisition of English literacy as determined by scores on statewide proficiency and other achievement tests. However, similar to other complex concepts or skills, bilingualism is not a unitary entity, and to determine its effectiveness by only using English proficiency or achievement tests may be shortsighted or even unfair given the shortcomings of the manner in which English literacy is measured or the limitations of using only this particular type of test (also see the discussion in Paul, 1998a).

Despite the rhetoric in the California debate, the merits of bilingual education programs that emphasize both languages and cultures and the positive effects of bilingualism are well documented (see reviews and discussions in Cummins, 1984, 1989; Hakuta, 1986; Hakuta & Mostafapour, 1998; Hamers, 1998). With respect to deaf and hard-of-hearing children, this issue has become even more complicated and, of course, politicized—especially when viewed within the context of sociopolitical movements (see Stone, 1998; Stuckless, 1991). The call for bilingual and second language programs for deaf students is motivated by the persistent finding of low levels of achievement in literacy, particularly on standardized achievement tests (Allen, 1986; Paul, 1998a). There have been numerous arguments for the establishment of such programs, with the use of American Sign Language and English soliciting the most attention (Ewoldt, 1996; Livingston, 1997; Luetke-Stahlman, 1983; Paul, 1990; Paul, Bernhardt, & Gramley, 1992; Reagan, 1985; Strong, 1988). It is presumed that for many deaf students, this model, involving the use of a sign language as the first language or as one of the languages, is most beneficial or more beneficial than any spoken minority language/English language model due to deaf students' difficulty with spoken languages. There is some empirical evidence, as well as theoretical evidence, for such programs (Strong & Prinz, 1997; also see the reviews in Drasgow, 1998; Mayer & Akamatsu, 1999; Paul & Quigley, 1994). Drasgow (1998) provided supporting points for the ASL/English bilingual models. These points emphasize the ease of acquisition of ASL by deaf children, an acquisition that is comparable to a spoken language by hearing children (Newport & Meier, 1985; Petitto & Marentette, 1991). More important, ASL (or any other sign language) seems to be best suited to the cognitive capacity of deaf individuals who are visually oriented to manual or sign communication (Bellugi, 1991; Poizner, Klima, & Bellugi, 1987).

Although there is no consensus on what type of bilingual or second language learning education program should be established, several models have been described in the literature (see discussions in Mayer & Akamatsu, 1999; Paul, 1998a; Paul & Quigley, 1994; Strong, 1988). There seems to be the proclivity for models that propose that deaf children be exposed to ASL and English concurrently (50/50) in infancy and early childhood or that ASL be developed first in a normal interactive manner, with English developed later as a second language. In the majority of these models, students' exposure to English is only via print. There are few opportunities or attempts for students to learn to manipulate English in the performance mode, either via speech or sign.

Consequently, the underpinnings or assumptions of these programs for developing English literacy have been questioned in light of what can be perceived as misinterpretations of existing second language learning models such as those developed by Cummins or those based on the work of Vygotsky (Mayer & Akamatsu, 1999; Mayer & Wells, 1996; Paul, 1998a). As is discussed in this chapter, there are major concerns in establishing ASL/English programs, particularly if one of the goals is the development of English literacy skills. The major basis for these concerns is the fact that ASL does not have a writing system similar to script literacy associated with languages in literacy-based societies. This does not denigrate or diminish the need for such programs; however, it does require a better understanding of how to develop second language literacy with a population whose first language is not represented using chirographic or typographic symbols in the conventional literacy sense.

Perhaps another perspective on the complexity of this issue for deaf students can be gleaned from the recommendations of a recent national report on preventing reading difficulties for children who are limited speakers of English. Snow et al. (1998) suggested that:

> *If language-minority children arrive at school with no proficiency in English but speaking a language for which there are instructional guides, learning materials, and locally available proficient teachers, these children should be taught how to read in their native language while acquiring oral proficiency in English and subsequently taught to extend their skills to reading in English.*
>
> *If language-minority children arrive at school with no proficiency in English but speak a language for which the above conditions cannot be met and for which there are insufficient numbers of children to justify the development of the local capacity to meet such conditions, the initial instructional priority should be developing the children's oral proficiency in English. Although print materials may be used to support the development of English phonology, vocabulary, and syntax, the postponement of formal reading instruction is appropriate until an adequate level of oral proficiency in English has been achieved. (p. 325)*

It should be kept in mind that these recommendations need to be couched in the nature of reading and the prevention of reading difficulties as perceived by individuals who worked on this national report. The reason for including them here is that the manipulation of the performance (or oral) mode of English is considered to be a critical goal for developing English literacy skills (see Verhoeven, 1990; also see Chapter 8 of this text). In addition, it is also worthwhile to support literacy in the first or minority language of limited speakers/users of English. Both of these recommendations are or might be unfeasible for most deaf students for whom ASL is the first or home language. That this group is at risk for developing English literacy is an understatement. More important, it might be unrealistic or difficult to use all of the principles of existing bilingual or second language programs, which are typically based on the development of spoken languages. These are just some of the issues that scholars and educators need to consider in the development and implementation of such programs for deaf and hard-of-hearing students.

A brief survey of the literature on bilingualism and English as a second language (ESL) reveals that these fields have as many and as deep differences in theory, research, and practice as does the education of deaf students (Bernhardt, 1991; Hakuta & Mostafapour, 1998; McLaughlin, 1987). This survey is important because there is still very little coherent empirical research information available on bilingualism, ESL, and deafness. In addition, it might provide a context for some of the misunderstandings and misinterpretations of models on which the few ASL/English programs have been based. Of course, as discussed in Chapters 1 and 8 of this text, misunderstandings are usually the interpretative products of proponents who ascribe to different philosophies or metatheories. Nevertheless, misunderstandings are also due to an incomplete or lack of understanding of the entire domain of a theory or model.

The plan for the chapter is as follows. First, some selective background on bilingualism and second language learning with hearing students is provided. This entails a discussion of definitions, theories, and a synthesis of a representative sample of research studies. In addition, a number of other issues are addressed relevant to bilingualism, second language learning, and deafness such as (a) similarities and differences between first and second language acquisition; (b) the nature of second language literacy, particularly reading; (c) research on bilingualism and second language learning; and (d) the debate on the nature, content, and research on ASL/English programs. This information is discussed with respect to the author's interpretation of the research on bilingual educational models for hearing minority students. Final remarks center on selective issues for future directions in bilingual education and deafness. It should become clear that the major focus is on English language proficiency, which is primarily a linguistic and psycholinguistic approach.

DESCRIPTIONS/DEFINITIONS

There is still considerable disagreement about what constitutes bilingualism and second language learning (Cook, 1991; Crystal, 1987, 1997; McLaughlin, 1984, 1987). Some of the confusion stems from the lack of making a distinction between psycholinguistic (e.g., language proficiency and use) and sociolinguistic (e.g., social participation) descriptions (e.g., Hakuta & Mostafapour, 1998). In addition, there is some confusion on what constitutes biculturalism and the relation of biculturalism to bilingualism (see discussions in Grosjean, 1998; Padden, 1998b). As noted by Grosjean, it is possible to have bilingualism without biculturalism (inhabitants of countries that have lingua francas, etc.) and biculturalism without bilingualism (members of a minority culture who no longer know or use the minority language but retain some aspects of the culture). Similar to the notion of bilingualism, there are various degrees of biculturalism.

The term *bilingualism* implies the use of two languages; however, this seemingly simple notion has engendered pervasive politicized discussions in the research and theoretical literature. Factors that contribute to controversies that are psycholinguistic oriented (i.e., proficiency and use of the languages) include the notion of language, language competency, language proficiency, and the time frame in which languages are learned. It seems clear that a bilingual individual is not two monolinguals in one but rather a person who uses one language or the other either separately or together for various purposes and functions.

There is some consensus that bilingualism is not an all or nothing phenomenon, even in the field of deafness (Grosjean, 1998; Padden, 1998b). However, even this consensus is problematic. For example, how much proficiency in a language is required before one can be considered a user of that language? If someone uses a few Spanish words and knows English, should one label this person as *bilingual?* That is, is a little knowledge of words without an understanding of the grammar and other aspects sufficient for a label of *bilingualism?* Nevertheless, the author agrees with Grosjean (1998) that: "Bilinguals are starting to be studied in terms of their total language repertoire, and the domains of use and the functions of the bilingual's various languages are being taken into account" (p. 22).

With a heavy focus on language variables, there is the problem of what constitutes a language. As discussed previously in this text (Chapter 7), ASL is a bona fide language that is different in grammar and form from English and the English-based signed systems. It is clear that English is a second language for deaf students who come to school knowing ASL or some other minority language such as Spanish or German. For example, a bilingual situation for some deaf students might consist of exposure to ASL and one of the English-based signed systems or ASL and oral English. Exposure to oral English and one of the signed systems would not constitute bilingualism but simply two coding forms of a single language—English.

Given the discussion in Chapter 6, one could make a case that exposure to a particular signed system is not sufficient for exposure to English as a language. That is, the signed systems are not adequate representations of English, and consequently, deaf students are not really exposed to English as a language. Admittedly, they are exposed to English morphology and syntax, but even this is debatable. Perhaps a stronger case can be made for cued speech/language as a representation of the English language. Or perhaps the author is splitting hairs here with the emphasis on inadequate or incomplete exposure to a language or its representations. Nevertheless, these are critical issues in discussing bilingualism and second language learning for deaf students. For example, inadequate exposures (or related descriptors) can refer to the opportunities and resources that individuals have in their attempts to learn a second language. Obviously, this situation has some effect on the degree to which an individual learns the language. Incomplete exposure (or related descriptors) refers to the fact that the signal itself (signs and cues) does not convey the complete or major components of a language or makes it difficult for individuals to acquire a language because of a mismatch between their processing capacity and the properties of the signal itself. This latter issue is quite different from the inadequacy issue for hearing bilingual individuals and renders the situation much more complex for many deaf students who are visually oriented to the use of manual and nonmanual signals for receptive and expressive communication. This certainly resonates with the scholarly voices who claim that English is always a second language for deaf individuals, and indeed, it might be difficult for many deaf students to acquire a second language that is typically spoken (see discussions in Johnson et al., 1989; Paul, 1998a). This difficulty also extends to the acquisition of the written literate forms of the languages as well.

In the larger field of hearing individuals, several scholars have attempted to clarify the distinction between bilingualism and second language learning. Lamendella (1977), for example, argued for the adoption of the following terms: *primary language acquisition, secondary language acquisition,* and *foreign language learning.* Lamendella referred to primary language acquisition as the normal language learning process occurring up to the age of about 5 years regardless of the number of languages involved and the manner in which they are introduced to the child. Secondary language acquisition, which can also involve the learning of two or more languages, is considered to occur in a naturalistic setting and manner after the period of the primary language acquisition (after about 5 years of age). Lamendella described foreign language learning as that which occurs in the formal classroom setting and is cognitively different from secondary language acquisition.

From another perspective, there seems to be little developmental difference between learning a language in either the classroom or in a naturalistic setting (McLaughlin, 1985, 1987). In addition, the time frame of Lamendella's primary language acquisition is not widely accepted. This issue, known as the critical period hypothesis, is still being debated (Crystal, 1987, 1997; LaSasso & Metzger, 1998; McLaughlin, 1984; Paul & Jackson, 1993). However, there seems to be an optimal period for learning a language or languages (from birth to about puberty), and this issue has pervasive implications for language and deafness. The proffering of an optimal or critical period should not overshadow or undermine the extreme importance of developing a bona fide conventional linguistic system as early an age as possible, especially during the first 5 or 6 years. There is a growing body of research on this issue with deafness and the acquisition of American Sign Language (see Chapter 7 of this text).

A useful chronological age distinction between bilingualism and second language learning was offered by McLaughlin (1984). This scholar stated that the presence of two languages before the age of 2 years leads to simultaneous acquisition, that is, bilingualism. The acquisition can be described as successive (i.e., second language learning) if the presence of a second language is delayed until the age of 3 years or later. There seems to be some consensus that the learning of a second language, particularly in later childhood, adolescent, or adulthood, is much more difficult than the learning of two languages in a bilingual situation in early infancy and childhood (see McLaughlin, 1984, 1985; Parasnis, 1998; Wong Fillmore, 1989).

Despite the varying views, it is safe to conclude that bilingualism and second language learning is not an all or nothing phenomenon. Rather, it is a function of degree depending on the age of the individual and the mode of the language (e.g., speaking/signing, listening/watching, and reading/writing). Deciding whether a situation is a bilingual or second language learning one is important for the establishment of programs. As is discussed later, with respect to type of bilingual program, there is some research that supports certain types of programs over others. This is dependent on an agreement on the goals of such programs. To provide a context for the various types of programs that have been proposed and implemented, it is instructive to discuss some of the prominent theoretical models and research on hearing students in bilingual and/or second language situations.

Table 9-1 provides information on descriptions/definitions and a discussion of additional terms related to bilingualism and second language learning. The intent of the discussion of additional terms is to facilitate understanding of the information in this chapter.

TABLE 9-1 Descriptions of Selected Terms Relevant to Bilingualism and Second Language Learning

- *Ambilingual:* Typically, this refers to an individual who can speak two languages equally well. It is possible that the individual also has an equal range of proficiency in the various modes—speaking (signing), listening (watching), reading, and writing—of both languages as well. A synonymous term is *balanced bilingual* or *true bilingual.* This situation most likely occurs in individuals who have been exposed to two languages prior to the age of 3 years.

- *Biculturalism:* The existence of two different cultures—often based on the influences or uses of a specific language or vocabulary (consider feminism and homosexuality). It is possible to have biculturalism without bilingualism as in the case of minority members who no longer speak their native language but have retained aspects of their culture. It is also possible to have bilingualism without biculturalism as in the case of individuals who use what is called a lingua franca for education and other formal purposes. Biculturalism is not an all or nothing phenomenon; there are degrees of biculturalism.

- *Bidialectal:* An individual who is proficient in the use of two dialects (i.e., in speaking ability). Dialects are variations (vocabulary, grammar, style, and speech qualities) of a language due to factors such as socioeconomics, geography, and education.

- *Bilingualism:* Refers to proficiency in the use of two languages by an individual (individual bilingualism) or by a society (societal bilingualism). This does not mean proficiency in all modes (speaking [signing], listening [watching], reading, and writing) in both languages or complete mastery. In essence, bilingualism is not an all or nothing phenomenon. Typically, individuals have a range of proficiency in the various modes of the two languages.

- *Code switching:* The changing or switching from one language or a variety of one language to another language or variety. This is also referred to as *language mixing.* There are several factors that contribute to the switching phenomenon, for example, ease of expressive communication, ability/characteristic of the listener, type of situation, and so on.

- *Contrastive analysis:* The identification and analysis of structural or grammatical differences between two languages. These differences are assumed to cause problems for the language learner. (Also see *interference.*)

- *Creole:* This is a pidgin that has become the mother language of a speech community. For example, children who have been exposed to a pidgin (via parents, etc.) became native users of that system, which has become a creole (i.e., the natural development of a pidgin into a bona fide linguistic system). A creole has the range and function of a language.

- *Deviance:* The use of structures (spoken or written) that do not conform to the rules of a specific language. These structures are considered to be highly idiosyncratic and cannot be explained by any general acquisitional process (cf. *interlanguage*).

- *Dominant language:* In a multilingual society or speech community, this is considered the most important or prestigious language. From another perspective, this is the language in which a bilingual individual has the most proficiency; indeed, it is the language of choice for most communication situations.

- *Foreign language:* This is a nonnative language; that is, a language that has no status in a particular country. Some scholars refer to *foreign language teaching* and *foreign language learning* as activities that occur in formal classroom settings. These activities are considered to be cognitively different from the natural processes of bilingualism and second language learning. Other scholars have argued that there are little differences between learning a language in either a formal classroom or in a naturalistic setting. (See *second language learning* and *successive acquisition*.)

- *Immersion:* In general, this term refers to bilingual programs in which children are exposed initially to a nonnative language as their major medium of instruction for the first few years. This can be labeled *majority-language immersion* because the language of instruction might be the majority language of society; however, it is also possible to have two languages that are majority languages. In a minority-language immersion program, children are immersed in instruction in their home or native language. As mentioned in this chapter, this is also known as the vernacular advantage model.

- *Interference:* This term is related to the principle of transfer. That is, transfer refers to the effects of a individual's first or home language on the acquisition of the second or target language. Positive interference refers to the facilitative effects (i.e., transfer of skills from L1 to L2), and negative interference refers to the difficulties or problems that arise from the structural differences (i.e., factors that seem to impede the acquisition of the second or target language). It was often assumed that many of the errors of second language

(continues)

(Table 9-1 continued)

learners of English, including deaf learners of English, were due to negative interference of the structure of the first or home language. However, there seems to be a consensus (or at least a majority view) that many of these errors are developmental. That is, these errors have been observed in individuals attempting to learn English as a first language.

- *Interlanguage:* This is a language system used by an individual during the acquisition of the second, target, or foreign language (see discussion of this term in the chapter). It is considered an intermediate acquisitional stage. The structures of the interlanguage are called fossilizations (i.e., frozen features), which seem to appear only in the second language productions of the second language learners—not in their first or home language productions.

- *Language maintenance:* In general, this refers to the continued use, development, and maintenance of all languages in bilingual or multilingual situations. According to some scholars, true bilingual programs are those that support and enhance both languages and cultures. There is no shifting or transition from one language to the other (see *language shift*).

- *Language planning:* The development of official policies and intentions governing or concerning the use of a language in a particular country. For example, a country might decide that English is the official language for formal institutions such as education, business, and government (i.e., spoken and used in written documents), whereas the native language(s) can be used in informal situations. In addition, some countries might have policies that dictate the use of certain vocabulary or grammar in the language (consider the work of prescriptive grammarians, who attempt to describe the correct or desired use of a language).

- *Language shift or transition:* With respect to bilingual programs, this concerns the use of instructional activities and materials that assist an individual in shifting from the use of the first or home language to the use of the second or target language. In some programs, the first language is rarely or only used to ease the transition, whereas in other programs, the first language might be used frequently. However, the use of L1 is mostly for easing the transition—there is little or no attempt to support or enhance the development of L1.

- *Multilingualism:* The use of several languages by a person or by a speech community. Proficiency is not all or nothing, similar to that of bilingualism (see *bilingualism*).

- *Pidgin:* A form of communication (i.e., symbol system; some say language) with a reduced range of structure (i.e., vocabulary and grammar) and for limited uses or purposes (trading or exchange situations or brief discussion of concrete items). A pidgin has no native users (speakers/signers). Typically, the pidgin is the communication result of two speakers, each with limited understanding of the other's language (i.e., one might know English and the other French). To develop a pidgin for communication purposes, the two languages need to be of the same form (i.e., spoken or signed). Thus, a pidgin can result from two spoken languages such as English and French or two sign languages such as ASL and CSL (Chinese Sign Language). It is not possible (or nearly impossible) to develop a pidgin from a spoken language and a sign language because there is no blending of speech and signs that is analogous to the blending or combining of, for example, English and French words or of ASL and CSL signs.

- *Second language learning:* Refers to the learning of a nonnative language—that is, a language that is not the first or home language. The learning might occur in either a formal classroom or naturalistic setting. If the second language is a language that is nonnative to a specific country or has no prestige, it can be labeled a *foreign* language (see *successive acquisition*).

- *Simultaneous acquisition:* Exposure to and learning of two (or more) languages prior to the age of 2 years. This is often considered to be true bilingualism or multilingualism.

- *Successive acquisition:* Exposure to and the learning of a language from the age of 3 years and beyond. There seems to some consensus that learning a second language in later childhood, adolescence, or adulthood is much more difficult than the learning of two languages in a bilingual situation (*simultaneous acquisition*). The varying levels of proficiency in the second language is often due in part to the age at which an individual is exposed to and learns that language.

- *Teaching Method:* There are several teaching methods often associated with second language instruction or learning. A few of the most widely known are *grammar-translation, direct method*, and *audiolingual*. The grammar-translation approach is similar to the use of the contrastive analysis (see *contrastive analysis*) discussed previously in which individuals are led to discover the manner in which the two languages are different in structure and grammar. A metacognitive awareness (see Chapter 8) of these differences is said to facilitate the acquisition of the second or target language. The direct method

(continues)

(Table 9-1 continued)

refers to the use of speaking in the target language in natural meaningful situations (albeit in classroom settings). The emphasis is on learning the language naturally without explicit conscious attention to the grammar or structure of the target language. This is similar to natural approaches to teaching language to deaf and hard-of-hearing students, as is discussed in Chapter 10. The audiolingual approach is considered to be a more formal systematic language teaching approach that focuses on the use of drills, exercises, and dialogues with respect to the development of speaking and listening skills. This approach is somewhat similar to the structured approaches for teaching language to deaf and hard-of-hearing students, as is discussed in Chapter 10. There have been several new approaches developed that seem to offer a more natural manner for learning a language similar to what one would expect in the home or in the country that actually uses that language. The effectiveness of these new methods have not been researched extensively (see discussion in Crystal, 1997).

THEORETICAL MODELS OF BILINGUALISM

There is a diversity of theoretical models in the literature on bilingualism and second language learning. There is also diversity in the classification of these theories (see Hamers, 1998; McLaughlin, 1987). Any classification framework depends on the metatheories, methodologies, and foci of the theorists and researchers. For example, there are a number of models dealing with the effects of bilingualism on cognitive and academic achievement (Cummins, 1977, 1978, 1984, 1989; Lambert, 1972; Macnamara, 1966). It is also possible to classify models according to certain disciplines such as linguistics (Krashen, 1981, 1982, 1985; Selinker, 1972), sociolinguistics (Hymes, 1974), social psychology (Lambert & Tucker, 1972), neurolinguistic (Lamendella, 1977), cognition (McLaughlin, 1987; Chapter 6), and social cognition (Hamers, 1988; Hamers & Blanc, 1989). The framework of McLaughlin (1987) is still relevant and most useful for present purposes. McLaughlin (1987) described five types of theories in second language acquisition and process: the monitor model, interlanguage theory, linguistic universals, acculturation/pidginization theory, and cognitive theory—the latter can be extended to include social aspects, which would include social-cognitive models.

Despite the preponderant amount of theoretical and research work in the area of bilingualism and second language learning, there is no coherent theory of bilingualism relative to linguistic, cognitive, and social phenomenon (see Baetens-Beardsmore, 1986; Cook, 1991; Parasnis, 1998). In addition, the classification schemes mentioned are not mutually exclusive. The approach here is to discuss a few of these models in the various categories mentioned and those that are also discussed in several reviews of the literature (Baetens-Beardsmore, 1986; Cook, 1991; McLaughlin, 1987; Parasnis, 1998). With the remarks on classification schemes in mind, two groups of models are discussed next. The first group of models seems to be most related to the effects of bilingualism on cognition and academic achievement, whereas the second group focuses mainly on the language acquisition process.

Effects of Bilingualism: Theoretical Considerations

Macnamara (1966) proposed a balance theory, sometimes termed the *genetic inferiority* or *verbal deprivation* theory. This researcher asserted that an individual has a fixed amount of language learning ability that must either be divided among two or more languages or devoted entirely to one. It is claimed that most people are unable to learn two languages simultaneously as well as monolinguals learn one by itself. There is a large body of data that demonstrates inferior performance of bilingual individuals in one language (usually, the majority or dominant language of society) (see review in McLaughlin, 1984). This suggests that the other language interferes with the learning process. The deficiency in the majority language is purported to be reflected in the lowered performance in all academic areas. The reanalysis and reinterpretation of these data have led to different explanations for the results and to different conceptualizations of models, as discussed in the ensuing paragraphs.

Lambert (1972; Lambert & Tucker, 1972) espoused an interdependence theory. He argued that under certain conditions, access to two languages can positively influence the development of some cognitive processes that can consequently lead to higher IQ scores and academic achievement levels. For these positive effects to be detected by research studies, certain confounding factors must be controlled, for example, socioeconomic status (SES), gender of subjects, and degree of bilingualism.

The contradictory findings in the literature have been addressed by Lambert (1972; Lambert & Tucker, 1972) with an additive/subtractive hypothesis, which is a corollary to his interdependence model. Lambert attributed the contradictory findings to differences between bilingual individuals in an additive environment and those in a subtractive environment. An additive educational or social environment is one that poses no threat of replacing the first (L1) or home language of the language user with a second (L2) or majority language of the culture. On the contrary, a subtractive environment aims to supplant the minority, home, or first language with the majority one.

Lambert argued that bilingual individuals in an additive environment usually possess a first language, which may be the dominant or majority language of the culture (i.e., majority-language users). These students (typically from middle or upper socioeconomic status classes) become balanced bilinguals when they add another language (either a majority or minority one). Consequently, they perform as least as well as matched monolingual users of either of the two languages involved. Contrariwise, the inferior skills of many of the bilingual subjects reported in other studies were probably due to the fact that these subjects were in a subtractive environment that posed a threat to the first language (and possibly the culture). In addition, some of the contradictory findings might be due to studies failing to (a) control for the bilingual subjects' level of competence in either L1 or L2 and (b) acknowledge that subjects might have had less than native-like skill in both their languages because they came from low SES environmental backgrounds.

A model somewhat similar to the additive/subtractive one is the societal factor model. Proponents of this model have argued that a home-school language switch results in high levels of functional bilingualism and academic achievement in majority-language children; however, it also leads to inadequate command of both languages and poor academic achievement in many minority-language children. These scholars have also argued for an emphasis on the determining role of societal factors (see discussions in Baetens-Beardsmore, 1986; Cook, 1991; Hamers, 1998; McLaughlin, 1987). In essence, the societal factor model rejects axiomatic statements regarding the medium of instruction and assigns a fundamental causal role to societal or sociocultural factors.

Development of L1 and L2

There are several models that focus on the relationship between the development of the two languages involved. Cummins (1977, 1978, 1984, 1989) proposed a threshold model, which is also offered as an explanation for the contradictory findings in the research literature. He argued that the cognitive and academic effects of bilingualism are mediated by the levels of competence attained in both languages regardless of whether the subjects possess a majority or minority language as a first language. Cummins further argued that there might be threshold levels of linguistic competence a bilingual child must attain (i.e., in the two languages) both to avoid cognitive disadvantages and to allow the potentially beneficial aspects of bilingualism to influence cognitive functioning. The threshold model assumes that those aspects of bilingualism that might positively influence cognitive growth are unlikely to come into effect until the child has attained a certain minimum or threshold level of competence in the second language.

Another of Cummins' models, termed the *developmental interdependence model* (or *linguistic interdependence*), proposed that the development of skills in a second language is a function of skills already established in the first language (Cummins, 1989; McLaughlin, 1984; Skutnabb-Kangas & Toukoman, as cited in Cummins, 1978). In situations where the first language is inadequately developed, the introduction and promotion of a second language can impede the continued development of the first. Consequently, this inadequate development of the first language limits the development of competence in the second language. Contrariwise, a highly developed L1 (prior to the introduction of L2) contributes to a high level of development in L2 at no cost to L1 competence. The developmental interdependence model emphasizes the importance of the continuing development of the first language. This model, along with the work of Vygotsky, has been used to promote the approaches to script literacy in ASL/English bilingual/bicultural programs. However, as discussed later, proponents of bilingual/bicultural programs for deaf students have misinterpreted the major tenets of Cummins' model.

There are a few models concerned with the development of L1 and the subsequent development of literacy skills, particularly reading, in the second language. The vernacular advantage model asserts that the best medium for teaching a child in a bilingual situation is in the mother language or first language (see discussions in Cummins, 1984, 1988; Modiano, 1968; Rosier & Farella, 1976). This model is specifically intended for children whose first language is a minority language. Proponents have argued that instruction through the medium of the first language or mother tongue for minority-language children in the early grades is a prerequisite for equality of educational opportunity. Furthermore, when instruction is through the medium of a second or majority language and the school makes no concessions to either the language or the culture of the minority-language child, the result is frequently low levels of competence in both languages and academic failure.

It is argued that reading should be introduced in the learner's first language (i.e., mother tongue), for which the child has already acquired the sound system, structure, and vocabulary. Subsequently, when the student achieves an independent reading level in L1, the student can then begin to read in the second language. It is reasoned that the acquisition of reading skills in the first language leads to an efficient transfer of skills and, thus, a faster acquisition of second language reading (Cummins, 1988; Gamez, 1979). The vernacular advantage model seems to be the major impetus for minority-language immersion programs, discussed later, and the salient principles of this model have been endorsed by a recent national report on preventing reading difficulties (Snow et al., 1998) as well as other reviews of second language literacy (Cummins, 1984, 1988; Paul, 1998a).

Some scholars have argued that the direct approach to reading is the most efficient approach. That is, reading should be introduced initially in the second language. Most of the evidence for this position seems to be from students whose first language or home language is the majority language or one that is equally prestigious as the second language (Cummins, 1988; Genesee, 1987; Swain & Lapkin, 1982).

The issue of the most efficient way to transfer skills from one language to another in reading is an area of intense research and much debate in the field of deafness (Drasgow, 1998; Mayer & Akamatsu, 1999; Paul, 1998a). It has brought the debate on the theories of first language reading (see Chapter 8) into the realm of research on reading in the second language. Nevertheless, there is still considerable work to be done in this area (Snow et al., 1998).

Table 9-2 presents a summary of the major highlights of the theoretical models and studies discussed in this section, including some additional points relevant to the development of reading in a second language as presented by McLaughlin (1985). These models focus specifically on the effects of bilingualism on cognitive development and academic achievement (e.g., literacy). Other views of the second language acquisition process are discussed briefly in the next section.

Table 9-2 Summary of Major Highlights of Theories and Studies That Focus on the Effects of Bilingualism on Cognition and Academic Achievement, Particularly Reading

---

Theorist/Researcher	Major Points
• Macnamara	The researcher proposes a balance theory, also known as the genetic inferiority or verbal deprivation theory. An individual has a fixed amount of language learning ability that must either be divided among two or more languages or devoted entirely to one.
• Lambert	The researcher proposes an interdependence theory. Access to two languages can positively influence the development of some cognitive processes that can consequently lead to a higher IQ and academic

achievement. An additive educational or social environment is one that poses no threat of replacing the first or home language with the second or majority language of the culture. On the contrary, a subtractive environment aims to supplant the minority or first language with the majority one.

- Cummins

  The researcher proposes a threshold model. Cognitive and academic effects of bilingualism are mediated by the levels of competence attained in both languages regardless of whether the subjects possess a majority or minority language as a first language. Aspects of bilingualism that might positively influence cognitive growth are unlikely to come into effect until the child has attained a certain minimum or threshold level of competence in the second language. In another model (developmental interdependence or linguistic interdependence), Cummins argued that development in the second or target language is related to the level of development in the first or home language. Thus, for example, inadequate development in a first language might limit the development of proficiency in a second language.

Specific Instructional Models (discussed in the section)

- Vernacular advantage model: The best medium for teaching a child in a bilingual situation is in the mother tongue or first language. The model is intended for children whose first language is a minority language. Reading should be introduced in the learner's first language (L1). Subsequently, when the student achieves an independent reading level in L1, the student can then begin to read in the second language.

- Direct approach to reading: Reading is introduced and developed in the second or target language only.

Common Bilingual Reading Models (based on McLaughlin, 1985)

- The three general types of models are labeled *first language programs, second language only programs*, and *simultaneous programs*.

(continues)

(Table 9-2 continued)

- In first language programs, individuals continue to develop skills in their home language and culture, including literacy skills. This approach is said to assist in the subsequent acquisition of the second or target language. These programs are based on the concepts of minority-language immersion, the native language approach, or the vernacular advantage model (see earlier discussion).

- In second language reading programs, there is no reading instruction in the home or first language. Individuals are taught to read only in the second or target language. Most likely, there is no use of the first or home language. This approach is similar to the use of the direct approach to reading (see earlier discussion) and transitional bilingual programs (discussed in this chapter).

- In simultaneous reading instruction programs (50/50 programs), there are attempts to use both the first and second languages throughout the school day. As an example, one language might be utilized in the morning or with certain subjects, whereas the second or target language might be used in the afternoon and with the remaining subjects. The selection of the languages and subjects varies according to the skills of the students.

Other Major Highlights

- There are a number of bilingual models in the theoretical and research literature. Any classification framework is influenced by the perspectives of individuals who attempt to perform this task.

- There is no coherent theory of bilingualism that encompasses linguistic, cognitive, and social phenomena.

- Bilingualism and second language learning is not an all or nothing phenomenon. Rather, it is a function of degree depending on the age of the individual and the mode of the language (speaking, listening or signing, watching, and reading, writing).

Theories of Second Language Learning

The models in this section focus specifically on the acquisition process involved in second language learning. Not all second language models are discussed here. Although the selection of the models is primarily subjective, it is based on several reviews of the theoretical and research literature (notably, Baetens-

Beardsmore, 1986; Cook, 1991; McLaughlin, 1987; Parasnis, 1998). As in first language acquisition, the models in this section have been influenced by the prevailing views on language development, for example, linguistic and cognitive (including cognitive-interactionist and social-interactionist). There is also some influence from the emerging field of neurolinguistics as well as from metatheories such as naturalism and social constructivism (see discussions in Bernhardt, 1991; McCarthey & Raphael, 1992; Paul, 1998a).

Interlanguage

A few models have been motivated by the linguistic thinking of Chomsky (1957, 1965; also see Cook & Newson, 1996). One of these, termed the *interlanguage theory* (Selinker, 1972), has been labeled a bottom-up approach to the problem of second language acquisition (McLaughlin, 1987). This is interpreted as an inductive approach to theorizing that attempts to deal with a restricted range of data. Initially, the interlanguage model was used to explain adult second language acquisition; however, it has also been be used to account for the acquisition of a second language by children (Davies, Criper, & Howatt, 1984; Selinker, Swain, & Dumas, 1975).

The term *interlanguage* is said "to refer to the interim grammars constructed by second language learners on their way to the target language" (McLaughlin, 1987, p. 60). Selinker (1972) proposed this notion to deal with the inadequacies that exist in the weaker language of a bilingual individual who has not achieved fluency in this language. In essence, the learner's knowledge base of the weaker language is not commensurate with that of a native speaker of the same language, especially from a transformational generative grammar perspective.

Selinker (1972) offered this hypothesis to show also that the spoken productions could not be attributed solely to interference from the first language or to the transfer of first language skills. He stated that the interlanguage is a separate linguistic system that is distinct from both the first language of the speaker and the target (or second) language that the speaker is attempting to learn. This system is the result of the user's attempts (i.e., strategies and hypothesizing) to learn the target language.

Selinker (1972) argued further that the interlanguage is a distinct system based on the occurrence of fossilized (or frozen) features in the target or second language. That is, the second language user persists in the use of certain features in the interlanguage despite the seemingly adequate input from or experiences with the second language. Fossilization may occur because the second language learner has reached communicative competency although not grammatical competency, or it may be the result of other forces (language transfer). It should be underscored that fossilized features do not appear in the development of the first language.

In essence, Selinker argued that second language learners proceed through a series of transitional stages, with the stages corresponding to the growth of the individual in understanding the second language. The individual, similar to first language learners and learning, is constructing hypotheses on how the second language works. During each stage, the individuals use a language system that is neither equivalent to L1 or to the target L2—thus, the term *interlanguage*.

The notion of interlanguage has evolved, and there are several additional models (see discussion in Bialystok & Sharwood-Smith, 1985). Interlanguage is considered to be a reaction against behaviorism because of its emphasis on the influence of internal cognitive factors (see McLaughlin, 1987). Even more striking is the fact that it is becoming increasingly difficult to separate interlanguage theory from others (e.g., Universal Grammar) (see discussion of UG in Cook & Newson, 1996) because of overlapping components (Baetens-Beardsmore, 1986; McLaughlin, 1987). Although the theoretical merits of interlanguage are open to question, one of its greatest weaknesses is its inability to explain fully why later bilingual individuals do not achieve a level of competence commensurate with early bilingual individuals (Baetens-Beardsmore, 1986). One attempt to deal with this issue has been the Monitor Model, proposed by Krashen (see 1981, 1982, 1985).

Monitor Model

Krashen's Monitor Model is considered to be mainly a deductive model on which research is based and hypotheses are derived. The model is an attempt at explanatory adequacy (see Chapter 3). In this sense, it has been labeled "the most ambitious theory of the second language learning process" (McLaughlin, 1987, p. 19). Because of Krashen's attempts to elucidate his model, it is widely known by teachers of second language.

To deal with the differences between the late and early bilingualism, Krashen sought to develop a theory that made a distinction between language acquisition and language learning. Within this perspective, acquisition is considered a natural unconscious process, whereas learning is a contrived conscious activity. Thus, the truly competent bilingual individuals are those who acquire the two languages in a natural noninstructional setting.

Krashen also hypothesized that differences can be attributed to the age of the learner, specifically if one is attempting to learn a language after the age of 12. In this view, the potential for using language acquisition processes diminishes with the onset of abstract metacognitive abilities. This is the basis of the monitor hypothesis of his overall Monitor Model. The language learner (as opposed to the language acquisitioner) makes use of monitor functions that are similar to the editing or revising functions of a reader or writer. Because of constraints and difficulties associated with time and the representation and use of language rules, the language learner is not as successful as the language acquisitioner.

In the further development of his model, Krashen proposed the notion of affective filter, which is said to account for discrepancies in the ultimate attainment of the two languages between late and early bilingual individuals (see Baetens-Beardsmore, 1986; McLaughlin, 1987). The affective filter contains emotional and other affect aspects such as motivation, anxiety, and confidence. In all, there are five hypotheses associated with Krashen's Monitor Model: monitor, acquisition/learning, affective filter, input, and natural order (see Krashen, 1981, 1982, 1985).

Despite the few merits of Krashen's model, it has been widely criticized because of its inconsistencies and its broad sweeping claims (see McLaughlin, 1987). There is no intention here to provide a point-by-point refutation of each aspect of the model. However, it is important to note that there is a growing support for the assertion that little differences exist between the notions of acquisition and learning (see reviews in McLaughlin, 1984, 1985; Parasnis, 1998).

Several statements should be made on this issue. First, it is difficult to separate these two entities; that is, an individual who achieves competency in a language probably has engaged in both processes (assuming there is a difference). In addition, it is possible to learn a language in a classroom setting with a level of proficiency commensurate with that of acquiring a language in a natural setting. Finally, this issue tends to blur somewhat the distinctions between the debates regarding the teachability versus learnability of languages and those on the natural versus structural language teaching methods (for an in-depth discussion of these issues relative to deafness, see McAnally et al., 1994; also see Chapter 10 of this text).

Other Linguistic Approaches

Several other linguistic approaches have been influenced by the work of Chomsky (1965, 1975, 1980, 1988), particularly the notion of Universal Grammar (also see Cook & Newson, 1996). Universal Grammar is mainly concerned with first language acquisition. However, this notion has also influenced research on language acquisition and deafness (Lillo-Martin et al., 1991; also see Marschark et al., 1997) and on second language learning (see reviews in Baetens-Beardsmore, 1986; Cook, 1991; Cook & Newson, 1996; McLaughlin, 1987).

Felix (1982) proffered a novel linguistic approach to account for the differences in achievement between early and late bilingual individuals. This researcher argued that differences between the two groups can be attributed to the use of different cognitive systems. Early bilingual persons, particularly children, use cognitive structures that are suited for the acquisition of language. Late bilingual persons, particularly adults, are using two systems that compete with each other: language-specific cognitive system and a cognitive system that functions for general problem-solving tasks. Felix labeled this process in adults as the *Competition Model.*

Because of the notion of separate cognitive systems in the brain, it seems that this researcher and others (notably, Fodor, 1983) ascribed to the principle of modularity (see Chapter 3 of this text). For dealing with linguistic information, the general problem-solving systems are not as efficient as the language-specific cognitive systems. The emergent of the problem-solving system occurs after puberty. Felix's hypothesis asserted the importance of the critical-age hypothesis; however, this importance is not based on physiological criteria. It seems to be related to what is considered age-determined changes in the development of the cognitive system of humans.

Other Approaches

Dissatisfaction with pure linguistic approaches have led to the use of approaches that can be termed *sociolinguistic, social psychological, neurolinguistic,* and *cognitive*—specifically information processing, social cognitive, and sociocultural (also see, Hamers, 1998). For example, the sociolinguistic framework has been influenced by the work of Labov (1972) and the social psychological view by Schumann (1978). The sociolinguistic framework has been used to explain the varieties of language used by deaf individuals (Bochner & Albertini, 1988). Even more interesting is the influence of this view on determining the nature of ASL. A number of scholars have called into question the pure linguistic descriptions of ASL (see *The Deaf American,* 1990).

Cognitive models have exerted a pervasive influence on theories of second language acquisition. Perhaps the most noticeable influence has been on second language reading, particularly via the use of interactive theories (Grabe, 1988, 1991; Paul, 1998a) and the importance of a phonological code (i.e., phonological and phonemic awareness) for second language readers (Snow et al., 1998). Similar to the situation for first language learning, there will be an ongoing strong research thrust to understand bilingualism and second language learning within a sociocultural or a social-cognitive perspective. This framework should engender a more detailed description of the influence of social interactions and social milieus on the development of intellectual functioning of individuals who are bilinguals and offer implications for developing and implementing bilingual or second language learning education programs. The reader should keep in mind (Chapter 3) that the sociocultural framework considers language and cognition as outgrowths of the social milieu, not as separate entities (see discussions of this line of research for bilingualism in Hamers & Blanc, 1982).

Despite differences among the major theoretical frameworks, there are several critical summary statements that have been made by a number of scholars. The following remarks, representing one perspective, are still relevant:

> *What does seem to be emerging from the different types of argument put forward by various scholars is that bilingual ability, by and large, seems to be affected by the age of initial* prolonged *contact with the second language, that in the process of becoming bilingual the speaker goes through several stages of interlanguage in the L2, that these are partially determined by factors like the nature of the input, interference effects from L1 and other effects independent of L1, that the acquisition of bilingual proficiency partially follows that of native-language acquisition but not completely, that strategic competence seems to play a significant role in the achievement of linguistic goals in the weaker language and that fossilization may set in at different stages of bilingual development, leading to only partial attainment in the L2. (Baetens-Beardsmore, 1986, p. 135)*

Table 9-3 provides a summary of the major highlights of the theories/models discussed in this section.

Table 9-3 Highlights of Selected Theories of Second Language Acquisition/Learning

---

Interlanguage

- This model, influenced by the linguistic thinking of Chomsky, is labeled a *bottom-up* approach to the problem of second language acquisition.

- The term *interlanguage* refers to a separate linguistic system that is distinct from both the first language of the speaker and the target or second language that the speaker is attempting to learn. It is a result of the users attempts (i.e., strategies and hypothesizing) to learn the target language.

(continues)

(Table 9-3 continued)

- The system is based on the occurrence of fossilized (or frozen) features in the target or second language. Fossilized features do not appear in the development of the first language.

- It is proposed that the interlanguage is influenced by five cognitive processes: language transfer, language teaching effects, learning strategies, communication strategies, and overgeneralization.

- One of the greatest weaknesses of the interlanguage model is its inability to explain fully why individuals who become bilingual later in life (during adolescence or adulthood) do not achieve a level of competence commensurate with individuals who become bilingual during early childhood (i.e., by the age of 4 or 5 years).

Monitor Model

- To account for differences between early and later development of bilingualism, this model makes a distinction between language acquisition and language learning.

- It was argued that major differences can be attributed to the age of the learner, specifically if one is attempting to learn a language after the age of 12. This model seems to be influenced by the critical period hypothesis (see Chapter 3 of this text).

- There are five hypotheses associated with the model: monitor, acquisition learning, affective filter, input, and natural order.

- There have been a number of criticisms against the monitor model due to its broad sweeping claims. One of the most persistent criticisms is that there seems to be little difference between the notions of acquisition and learning.

Other Approaches

- There have been other linguistic approaches influenced by the thinking of Chomsky. One of the most notable models is labeled the Competition Model, which adheres to the salient principles of modularity hypothesis (see Chapter 3; also see Fodor, 1983) and the critical-age hypothesis (similar to the Monitor Model).

- Dissatisfaction with pure linguistic approaches have led to the use of models with labels such as *sociolinguistic, social-psychological, neurolinguistic, cognitive information processing, social-cognitive,* and *sociocultural.*

- Cognitive models have exerted a marked influence on the development of theories on second language acquisition and learning.

DEVELOPMENT IN L1 AND L2: SIMILAR OR DIFFERENT?

This section discusses whether the acquisition of English as a second language by hearing individuals is qualitatively similar, at least globally, to the acquisition of English as a first language by native learners of English who are hearing. This issue is also examined relative to the acquisition of English literacy, particularly reading. These issues have wide-reaching implications for instruction and curriculum developments as well as for theoretical frameworks. Later in the chapter, the focus is on the acquisition of English by students with severe to profound hearing impairment. Some of these insights, relative to deaf and hard-of-hearing students, were discussed in Chapter 8 of this text.

Research on the development of English as a second language has been documented relative to three broad groups: preschool, school-age children, and adults (see reviews in Cziko, 1992; McLaughlin, 1984, 1985, 1987; Paul, 1985). One of the critical issues seems to be the notion of language transfer. That is, the issue is what effects, if any, does the nature of the first or native language of the individual have on the acquisition of the second or target language? This is referring to the notion of interference (McLaughlin, 1984, 1985; Paul, 1985).

In general, it has been documented and argued that the notion of interference, albeit important, does not adequately explain the acquisition process of the second language (King, 1981; McLaughlin, 1984, 1985; Paul, 1998a). For example, second language learners of English from different L1 backgrounds make similar errors, and these errors are also similar to individuals learning English as a first language. Although the acquisition process entails the interaction of both developmental and transfer factors (transfer of reading skills in L1 to the acquisition of reading in L2), the bulk of the process seems to be explained by developmental factors.

It should be highlighted that transfer (in this case, interference) results in the production of some deviant structures, that is, structures that are not typically produced by the language learner in either the first or second language development. The production of these structures might be related to the influences of social and psychological factors on language learning strategies. A greater number of deviant structures have been documented in school-age children as compared to preschool children. This has been attributed mainly to two major factors: (a) the lack of native language peer models and (b) the use of unsound instructional practices and methods (McLaughlin, 1985; Paul, 1985). Similar arguments have been made for the stilted English written language productions of deaf students (see Chapter 8). A third factor, the learning of a language in a classroom setting, has not withstood the test of time. That is, there is no substantial evidence that learning a language in a classroom setting is developmentally different from learning the same language in a natural setting (McLaughlin, 1985; Parasnis, 1998).

Similar findings have been reported for adult second language learners. The few interference errors are common in the early stages of the language acquisition process. Most of the errors are similar developmentally to individuals learning English as a first language. As is discussed later, the same seems to be true for students with hearing impairment learning English as a first or second language (King, 1981; Paul, 1998a). In essence, it has been remarked that:

> *There seems to be little evidence from studies comparing language learning in children and second language learning in adults that the two groups go through radically different processes. What evidence there is points to the conclusion that the processes involved are basically the same. (McLaughlin, 1984, p. 66)*

The issue of transfer (i.e., the skills) is not a closed issue; it is still important to understand what is transferred from the first language to the second language. In addition, although interference may play a minor role in the transfer process, there is still the possibility that it causes problems for specific second language learners, especially in the acquisition of English literacy skills (see a brief discussion in Snow et al., 1998). Finally, as discussed previously, scholars know very little about the transfer issue for individuals whose first language has no written form and/or whose phonology is not based on sound (as in sign languages).

There is increasing evidence that reading in English as a second language is similar to the process of reading in English as a first language (see reviews in Bernhardt, 1991; Grabe, 1988; Paul, 1993, 1996, 1998a). This viewpoint can be seen in the shift from the use of reading comprehension models such as bottom-up and top-down to those that are interactive on to social-cognitive models. In fact, the influences of both the social and cognitive aspects are evident in nearly all models of reading and literacy (Ruddell et al., 1994).

BILINGUAL EDUCATION MODELS

In addition to having a variety of theoretical acquisition models, the field of bilingualism has a number of program models. The descriptions and research effectiveness of these models are shrouded in controversies. This is due primarily to the philosophies and goals of specific programs (see Cummins, 1988; Hakuta & Mostafapour, 1998; Hamers, 1998; Paul, 1985; Reich, 1986). In fact, a misunderstanding of these issues probably contributes to the confusion surrounding the merits of the programs. To obtain a better understanding of some of these issues, it is necessary to discuss the type of student and language goals.

Type of Student

Bilingual education programs may vary according to the type of student who participates in the program. For example, bilingual programs may be established for majority-language students, that is, individuals who speak the majority (or main) language of society (Cummins, 1988; Genesee, 1987). In the United States, such students may typically enroll in foreign language or second language course(s).

On the other hand, one commonly accepted bilingual program model in Canada is the immersion model. This model is employed in an area in which there are two main or heritage languages such as English and French. That is, individuals in these areas who speak either English or French are considered majority-language students. These individuals are expected to acquire communicative competency in both languages and knowledge of both cultures. In an immersion program, students receive instruction in the early grades in a language that is not their native language. Instruction in their native language occurs after a reasonable level of competency is established in the nonnative language (Genesee, 1987; Swain & Lapkin, 1982).

Individuals who do not speak the majority or main language of society are labeled *minority-language students*. In the United States, most bilingual programs are established for or involve students who do not have competency in the majority language (English) and its accompanying culture. Relative to deafness, individuals may be reared in minority or non-English-using homes, for example, homes in which the native language is ASL, Spanish, or German. It is also possible to consider other deaf students as minority-language users if they have not acquired an adequate level of communicative competency in the majority language (English) by the time they begin their formal schooling. This latter group might pertain to most students with severe to profound hearing impairment (King, 1981; Paul, 1990, 1991).

Controversies that have arisen about the appropriate goals and procedures for minority-language students are similar to some of the controversies in the education of deaf and hard-of-hearing students. For example, there is disagreement as to whether the goal should be to make the minority-language student a fully participating member of the majority culture even at the expense of the student's minority culture (assimilation). Some scholars favor the preservation and maintenance of the student's native culture even if this means lessened participation in the majority culture (language and cultural separatism).

Language Goals

The various types of programs are also related to language goals. Programs vary from complete submersion in the general educational system with limited or no support in the student's native language and culture to separate education in the student's native language and culture and gradual submersion in the general educational system. There are also programs that maintain a 50/50 model throughout the school years (Cummins, 1988; Navarro, 1985; Reich, 1986).

Relative to bilingual education programs, there are three broad language goals: language shift, language maintenance, and language enrichment. The main goal of submersion or transitional programs is to enable minority-language students to learn the language and culture of the majority society. In essence, the students shift from their home language to the majority language. Submersion programs are conducted in the majority language only (English). In transitional programs, the home or native language may be used to ease the shift to the majority language. For example, students acquire content and cultural knowledge via the use of their home language while they are attempting to learn L2. It should be underscored that there is no attempt to promote competency in L1.

In general, language maintenance refers to the maintenance bilingual education programs. One type of program is labeled *static maintenance*, which is somewhat similar to the transitional model (Otheguy & Otto, 1980; Reich, 1986). Static maintenance refers to the process of preventing the loss of minority-language students' L1 skills while promoting proficiency and literacy in L2. In both static maintenance and transitional programs, reading is typically introduced in the second or majority language. Proponents of these models endorse the balance acquisition theory of bilingualism (discussed previously) (Macnamara, 1966). Four basic arguments are presented: (a) Instruction in or on L1 subtracts from instruction for developing L2 skills; (b) development of L1 competes with L2; (c) minority-language students already possess competency in their L1, thus, it is not necessary to teach L1; and (d) reading skills are best developed in L2 by employing the language of L2, not L1. In general, these proponents argue that the best way to teach English to limited-English users is simply to teach them English only (see discussions in Cummins, 1988; Troike, 1981). It appears that this idea has pervasively influenced movements to reconsider and, perhaps, abolish bilingual education programs such as that which is occurring in California in the United States.

Language enrichment can be applied to another type of maintenance program entitled *developmental maintenance* (Cummins, 1988; Otheguy & Otto, 1980; Reich, 1986). The major aim of developmental maintenance bilingual education programs is to develop a high level of competency in both the minority and majority language. These programs can refer to those involving total or partial immersion in a second language or to programs in which the two languages are employed more or less equally (50/50) for instructional purposes. In essence, developmental maintenance programs are considered to be truly bilingual programs because of the emphasis on the development and maintenance of two languages.

Synthesis of Research

The research effectiveness of the French immersion programs in Canada has been well documented (see reviews and discussions in Cummins, 1988; Genesee, 1987; Hamers, 1998; Reich, 1986; Swain & Lapkin, 1982). Because of its success, there have been attempts to establish immersion programs for students in the United States (see discussion in Cummins, 1984, 1988). One problem with the application is the neglect of considering type of student, that is, majority-language students in Canada and minority-language students in the United States. A major issue is the misinterpretation of the goals and success of bilingual educational programs in Canada. For example, the success of the French immersion programs has been used as support for English immersion (actually submersion) programs in the United States for minority-language students (Cummins, 1988).

In the United States, four types of immersion programs have been identified: L2 submersion, L2 monolingual immersion, L2 bilingual immersion, and L1 bilingual immersion (Cummins, 1988; also see Cziko, 1992). Previously, some of the tenets of submersion programs were briefly described. The only difference between submersion and L2 monolingual immersion is that the latter modifies the content and grammar of the majority language to facilitate comprehension. Both L2 bilingual immersion and L1 bilingual immersion programs offer instruction in both languages and cultures; however, L1 immersion actively promotes the language and culture of the students' home environment.

It has been argued that both L1 and L2 immersion programs are most effective for minority-language students. There is some theoretical support (Cummins, 1988, 1989) and some empirical support (for L2, see Baker & de Kanter, 1981; for L1, see reviews in Cummins, 1984, 1988; Parasnis, 1998). The reason for the research effectiveness has been attributed to the fact that there is a greater transfer of skills from L1 to L2. This transfer is facilitated by the inclusion of the students' home language and culture.

In essence, there is a growing consensus for programs that emphasize both languages and cultures of minority-language students (see discussion in Hamers, 1998; Paul, 1998a). With respect to the focus of this chapter, this consensus seems to be motivated by the necessary conditions for developing literacy in students who are attempting to learn English as a second language (Snow et al., 1998). It is important to reiterate that there are both similarities and differences between bilinguals who are hearing and those who are deaf and hard-of-hearing (including members of the Deaf culture or community) (see Grosjean, 1998; Padden, 1998b). However, with respect to the development of English literacy, much of the available theoretical and research literature seems to converge on the qualitative similarity variable, as discussed in the next section.

Table 9-4 provides a summary of major highlights on bilingual education models, including type of student, program, and research effectiveness.

Table 9-4 Major Points of Bilingual Education Models

- To understand bilingual education models, several other concepts need to be discussed, for example, type of student, language goals, and type of program. Research effectiveness needs to be considered with respect to these concepts.

- Majority-language students are individuals who speak the majority language of society. Minority-language students are individuals who come from homes in which the majority language of society is not the home or first language. Some scholars have considered some deaf students as minority-language students (i.e., limited speakers/users of the majority language) if they do not have proficiency in the majority language of society—although they may be exposed to it in the home.

- Bilingual education programs may vary according the type of student as well as language goals.

- There seems to be three broad language goals: language shift, language maintenance, and language enrichment.

- Language shift refers to the shift from the home language of the minority-language students to the target or majority language of society. In some educational programs, submersion programs, instruction is conducted in the majority language only. In transitional bilingual programs, the home or native language may be used to ease the transition to the majority or target language.

- Language maintenance is often associated with maintenance bilingual programs. The emphasis is on preventing the loss of skills in the first or home language while promoting proficiency and literacy in the second or target language. Reading is typically introduced in the second or majority language only.

- Language enrichment, associated with developmental maintenance bilingual programs, aims to develop a high level of proficiency in both the minority and majority language.

- With respect to language goals, it is possible to understand the focus of various types of bilingual programs, ranging from submersion to 50/50 to immersion, with goals such as shift/transition and maintenance/enrichment.

- In the United States, four types of immersion programs have been identified: L2 submersion, L2 monolingual immersion, L2 bilingual immersion, and L1 bilingual immersion. The major difference between the first two is that the latter, L2 monolingual immersion, permits modifications of content and grammar of L2 to facilitate comprehension. With respect to the last two types, only L1 immersion actively promotes the language and culture of the students home environment.

- Research has shown that both L1 and L2 immersion programs are most effective for minority-language students; however, it seems to be important to promote actively the language and culture of the home environment, as is the case for L1 immersion programs.

BILINGUALISM, SECOND LANGUAGE LEARNING, AND DEAFNESS

As mentioned in the second edition of this text, there has been a dearth of theoretical and research literature on the issues of bilingualism, second language learning, and deafness. In addition, bilingualism and biculturalism still remain poorly understood topics, although it is possible to find a number of publications addressing some aspects of these issues (Grosjean, 1992; Lucas & Valli, 1992; Volterra & Erting, 1990). There are also a number of anecdotal reports with descriptions of a few existing bilingual programs and proposed models for ASL/English bilingual educational programs. The information discussed in this section is selective, but contains a relevant sample of theoretical, empirical, and research synthesis publications. In addition, this section also presents the ongoing debate on the proposed nature of ASL/English programs, including the issue of how and whether English literacy can be developed. Again, the debate on the development of English literacy is the main focus and interest.

Primary Bilingual Development

There are several publications dealing with deaf and Deaf (i.e., culturally Deaf) children who were exposed to both English (speech and/or signs) and American Sign Language (see discussion in Padden, 1998a, 1998b). One recent publication (Philip, 1992) indicated the existence of a successful bilingual ASL/English program at a learning center for more than 5 years (now more than 10 years); however, little empirical information has been provided, especially with respect to the development of English literacy skills. It should be emphasized that the type of signing used by deaf parents in earlier studies, discussed next, was presumed to be ASL although an adequate description of the grammar of ASL did not emerge in the research literature until the late 1970s (see discussions in Klima & Bellugi, 1979; Lane & Grosjean, 1980; Liddell, 1980; Wilbur, 1987). Some of the studies in the ensuing paragraphs are discussed at length to show the extent and nature of the investigation.

Schlesinger and Meadow (1972) described the primary linguistic development of four deaf children, each from a different family with either deaf or hearing parents. Only one child, who had deaf parents and two sets of deaf grandparents, is reported here. The subject, a girl, was diagnosed as deaf (due to heredity) at the age of 3. Her hearing threshold averaged 85 dB across the speech frequencies in the better ear. Although no formal assessment of the parents' proficiency either in ASL or English was conducted, Meadow (1980), in reporting this study in a book, remarked that:

> *Ann's mother, also the child of deaf parents, used English syntax in her written English and alternated between English and Ameslan [i.e., now known as American Sign Language] syntax in her signed and spoken communications. Ann's father was more likely than her mother to use Ameslan syntax in all his communication. (p. 19)*

Schlesinger and Meadow (1972) observed the child from age 8 months to 22 months. At 8 months, the child engaged in vocalization and gestures to convey emphasis and emotions. By the end of 12 months, she executed (approximately) the formal adult signs for PRETTYand WRONG, and she understood the command COME HERE. By the 20th month, her sign vocabulary totaled 142, and she knew 14 letters of the finger-spelled alphabet. The researchers concluded that the subject had a sign vocabulary that "compares very favorably with the spoken vocabulary of hearing children" (p. 60).

Schlesinger and Meadow (1972) also described the use and meaning of the subject's first individual signs/words, which were similar to the one-word utterances of hearing children. A one-word/sign can have one of several functions: (a) It can express a feeling; (b) it can label or name an object; or (c) it can fuse the label with the feeling about the object. This one-word/sign can also be classified according to a single feature. For example, the deaf child appropriately used the sign DOG for pictures of dogs, real dogs, and the *Doggie Diner Restaurant*. However, the child inappropriately used the sign to refer to all animals or even to animal objects not resembling the parents. It was reported that the deaf girl did not use all aspects of a sign (i.e., shape, movement, and placement) in the adult form. This finding is similar to that observed for hearing children who must mature to reproduce the sounds of language in their more adult forms. The most interesting finding reported was that the deaf child's vocabulary of 117 signs at 19 months was greater than the typical range of hearing children's words, which has been estimated to be more than 3 and fewer than 50 (Goodluck, 1991; Ingram, 1989; Lenneberg, 1967).

Collins-Ahlgren (1974) analyzed recorded expressive language samples of a girl, deaf from heredity, from age 16 months to 44 months. The deaf girl's parents were college graduates and were informally judged to be proficient in ASL and English. It was reported that the parents used both a "native language of signs" (p. 486) and English-based signs. The girl was exposed to ASL-like signing (i.e., accompanied by speech) in the earlier months. After various grammatical and semantic functions became productive through the sign forms, the parents introduced standard English forms (articles, auxiliaries, and inflections) through the use of signed or manual English techniques.

The results indicated that the deaf girl's expressive language proceeded through several stages, ranging from invented and imaginative ASL signs to uninflected signs used in English word order to some inflected English-based signs and finally to signed standard English. An example is the manner in which the subject demonstrated awareness of the present progressive function. Initially, she used the ASL form NOW as in I GO NOW (these words are the English glosses for the ASL signs). Then, her parents presented the auxiliaries and -*ing* forms as in I AM GOING (in this case, the NOW would be dropped unless the English sentence is: *I am going now*). A transitional stage with partial omission occurred prior to the time the full form became productive.

Collins-Ahlgren (1974) concluded that the girl was developing a language equivalent to that of her hearing peers. The researcher also argued that the educational signed or manually coded English systems should be taught as a second language to children of both deaf and hearing parents. In essence, these systems can "build on a native language foundation, and it should prove helpful for English reading and for communication with the hearing world" (p. 493).

Effects of ASL on the Subsequent Development of English

There are few studies dealing with the English linguistic abilities of children who were exposed to ASL in infancy and early childhood. One of the foci here is on studies that employ the paradigm of comparing deaf children of deaf parents with deaf children of hearing parents. Some of the studies were retrospective (Brasel & Quigley, 1977; Meadow, 1968) and used various means for determining the form of language used with the deaf children in infancy and early childhood. Even the best techniques, however, leave some doubt when respondents (deaf parents) are reporting on events that occurred as much as 10 to 15 years previously.

The performance of dcdp was compared with that of dchp on a number of measures, for example, overall academic achievement, intelligence, psychosocial development, reading, vocabulary, written language, speech reading, finger spelling, and signing abilities. A consistent finding emerged across several investigations, namely, that the performance of dcdp was significantly better than that of dchp (Balow & Brill, 1975; Meadow, 1968; Quigley & Frisina, 1961; Stuckless & Birch, 1966; also see the reviews in Drasgow, 1998; Paul & Jackson, 1993). Relative to reading, it was observed in some studies that the mean reading level of dcdp was almost two grades higher than that of dchp. In addition, even having one deaf parent was sufficient—that is, this condition correlated with higher achievement scores.

There have been numerous debates on the interpretations of this line of research (see discussions in Drasgow, 1998; Paul & Jackson, 1993). The differences between the two groups of deaf children have been attributed to broad variables such as parental acceptance, early use of manual communication (presumably ASL), and the early development of a bona fide language. There is little doubt that a high level of parental acceptance is an important factor (see discussions in Levine, 1981; Marschark, 1993; Meadow, 1980; Paul & Jackson, 1993); however, it is not only present in deaf parents or in deaf parents who sign. Some researchers have reported a high level of acceptance in homes where deaf parents used speech with their children and in homes in which the parents were hearing (Corson, 1973; Messerly & Aram, 1980).

Another common assumption in some of these studies was that the language input was relatively homogeneous—specifically, it was primarily American Sign Language. Obviously, the research cited earlier on parental acceptance presents contradictory evidence. In addition, interpreting the form of manual communication as ASL must be done with caution because a grammar of ASL has only recently been written. Furthermore, as discussed in Chapter 6, Brasel and Quigley (1977) demonstrated that the type of manual communication was important, especially if it corresponds to the structure of English. Brasel and Quigley's findings were supported in a recent study by Luetke-Stahlman (1988a; also discussed in Chapter 6). Luetke-Stahlman asserted that the most important issue was how well or how complete English was represented (as in the SEE systems and cued speech/language) and whether a particular symbol system was a language (as in the use of ASL). Finally, as discussed in the previous chapter, the development of English is such a complex activity that it should not and cannot be attributed to one all-encompassing factor such as ASL or any other manual communication form or even to one global factor such as parental acceptance. There should be studies that employ what can be called a multivariable approach. That is, researchers should look at the various contributions of a number of variables such as parental and child satisfaction, parental acceptance, signed and oral communication, and so on, including how these variables interact with each other.

The comparison of dcdp with dchp still seems to capture the attention of researchers and theorists (see discussions in Drasgow, 1998; Paul & Jackson, 1993). Although such studies are instructive, they are quite limited in advancing the understanding of how deaf or Deaf children acquire or deal with English. An interesting, and perhaps fruitful, line of research has been done within an emergent literacy framework (Erting, 1992; Maxwell, 1984; Padden, 1991, 1998a, 1998b). Among other insights, this line of research might shed some light on the manner in which some Deaf children acquire an understanding of a few aspects of English (see Grushkin, 1998a). For example, it has been argued that Deaf children's spelling development does not seem to proceed via the invented spelling to conventional spelling route, as noted for hearing children (Padden, 1991). This is interpreted to mean that these children are not utilizing phonemic processes. Because the errors seem to involve the positions of letters, it is argued that young Deaf children (4 to 10 years old) seemed more aware of orthographic structures rather than morphological ones (also see Chapter 7). There needs to be additional studies in this area, especially in light of what is known about the importance of both phonemic and morphological awareness and the move into more conventional spelling and writing (Snow et al., 1998). Perhaps there are indeed some qualitative differences between culturally Deaf acquisition of spelling and typical hearing or other deaf and hard-of-hearing students. Perhaps the emphasis on a visual modality (see Grushkin, 1998a) is the major defining issue.

There is some evidence of a correlational relationship between proficiency in American Sign Language and that of English script literacy skills (Strong & Prinz, 1997; also see Prinz, 1998). Strong and Prinz (1997) showed that the level of ASL proficiency is correlated with the level of English literacy skills. That is, a higher level of proficiency in ASL is associated with a higher level of proficiency in English. This seems to support the beneficial effects of ASL for the development of English for some deaf children. Keeping in mind that this is a correlational relationship, there is a great need to understand the extent and nature of how a bridge can be constructed from ASL to English (see discussion in Drasgow, 1998). Not only is the nature of the bridge in dispute but also whether it follows theoretical second languages principles similar to those for hearing second language learners. This issue is discussed later.

Table 9-5 presents a summary of major highlights of the sections addressing primary bilingual development and the effects of ASL on the subsequent development of English.

Table 9-5 Highlights of Primary Bilingual Development and Effects of ASL on English

Early Studies on Primary Bilingual Development

- In the early studies, it was presumed that the type of signing used by parents was American Sign Language; however, a published description of ASL grammar was not available until the late 1970s.

- Schlesinger and Meadow (1972) described the primary linguistic development of four deaf children—the focus here is on the child with deaf parents (and grandparents). The researchers reported that the child's signing vocabulary (observed from 8 months to 22 months) was roughly commensurate (at the 20-month level) with the spoken vocabulary of hearing children.

- Collins-Ahlgren (1974) recorded and analyzed expressive language samples of a young deaf girl, from age 16 months to 44 months. The researcher concluded that the girl was developing a language equivalent to that of her hearing peers. It was also argued that manually coded English systems should be taught as a second language to children of both deaf and hearing parents.

Effects of ASL on English Development

- One of the main foci of the studies in this area has been on comparing deaf children of deaf parents with deaf children of hearing parents.

- The consistent finding of the early studies was that the performance of dcdp was significantly better than that of dchp. Differences were also observed in families that had one deaf parent.

- There have been numerous debates on the interpretations of these findings, which have been clarified somewhat by subsequent research studies.

- The differences between the two groups of deaf children have been attributed to broad variables such as parental acceptance, early use of manual communication (presumably ASL), and the early development of a bona fide language.

- The factor of parental acceptance has been clarified. It is not uniquely attributed to deaf parents or to deaf parents who sign. Some researchers have reported a high level of acceptance in homes where parents are hearing and where deaf parents used speech with their children.

- The contributions of the language factor still remains contentious. In one study, it was argued that it is the type of manual communication that is important, especially if it corresponds to the structure of English. In another study, it was argued that (a) one critical issue is how well English is represented and (b) whether a particular symbol system was a language (as in the use of ASL).

- Despite the lingering debates, it is argued that the development of English is such a complex activity that it should not be attributed to one all-encompassing factor such as the use of ASL, a particular signed system, or even to a global factor such as parental acceptance.

- There is evidence of a correlational relationship between proficiency in American Sign Language and that of English script literacy skills. Nevertheless, there is a great need to understand the extent and nature of how a bridge can be constructed from ASL to English.

ASL/English Instructional Programs

The focus of this section is on instructional activities and programs that incorporated the use of ASL and English in either ESL or bilingual situations. Despite the theoretical and philosophical support for these types of programs, little empirical evidence is available on their use and effectiveness. Nevertheless, some insights can be gleaned from these few early studies and descriptions for the future implementation of such programs for students with severe to profound hearing impairment. It should be underscored that many of the more recent studies are only slight variations of the earlier investigations. Because of this situation, the discussion focuses on some of the earlier studies in depth. In addition, it appears that several of the existing programs have been influenced markedly by the findings of these earlier studies.

Early Investigations

Within the framework of error (i.e., contrastive) analysis, Crutchfield (1972) developed some procedures for teaching English as a second language through the use of ASL. For example, this researcher emphasized count features of both ASL and English. The count features refer to words similar to *much, many, few*, and so on. If the count features in ASL are different from those in English, the first step is to bring the ASL-like features to the students' attention. Consider the following example: MUCH BOY LEFT SCHOOL. Even with ASL-like signing, this sentence should be rejected by the ASL-using students. The students should be required to correct these unacceptable utterances using ASL. Thus, students might sign: MANY BOY LEAVE FINISH SCHOOL. The English gloss for this is: *Many boy left school.* Next, the teacher can write this sentence on the board and explain that some utterances that are unacceptable in ASL may also be unacceptable in English. In addition, some acceptable utterances in ASL may also be acceptable in English—providing *boy* is given a plural inflection (which is another lesson). Crutchfield remarked that the main purpose of this lesson (and all initial lessons) is to demonstrate similarities of acceptability and unacceptability in ASL and English. Subsequently, the instructor can proceed to those structures in English that are different from those in ASL and those in ASL that are different from English.

Goldberg and Bordman (1975) described an ESL program offered for deaf students at Gallaudet College (now Gallaudet University). It was argued that the samples of written language indicated that most students had reached adulthood without a command of English. The deaf students had difficulties in expressing themselves; these difficulties were similar to those of speakers of other languages in ESL classes.

These scholars made two major modifications in their ESL procedures. One, they conducted all language practices in writing (i.e., on the chalkboard, overhead projector, and paper). Two, they invented steps to compel students to express the concept involved. Goldberg and Bordman (1975) argued that English needs to be presented exclusively in the written form to ensure that the students know the words that are being addressed. The signed system or communication mode preferred by the students was used to communicate with the student, not to teach the students written English.

These scholars suggested also that the serious English structure problems of the deaf students are interwoven with the deeper problem of not knowing the concepts these structures expressed and not knowing when to use them. Thus, in their attempts to learn English, the deaf students are in a situation similar to that of hearing ESL speakers who do not make certain concept distinctions fundamental to English. For example, the ESL students may feel no need to distinguish between: *They eat sandwiches* and *They are eating sandwiches*. In sum, Goldberg and Bordman (1975) stated that there is a need to design materials that consider these issues.

Jones (1979) attempted to delineate the interference aspects of a signed language for the purpose of incorporating them in the teaching of written English. The researcher argued that ASL has both nonmanual and manual aspects (see Wilbur, 1987; also see Chapter 7 of this text). In writing nontechnical prose, Jones hypothesized that students who are deaf tend to translate into English only the manual signs of ASL that they would use if rendering the same passage in their use of English-based signing. The nonmanual aspects, which supply very important linguistic information, are not signed and thus are omitted in the writing of English. Consequently, the written productions of the students do not express enough of the intended message to be comprehensible to a fluent native speaker of English.

Jones (1979) further argued that the written language productions of deaf students would become more comprehensible if these productions included information from both manual and nonmanual aspects. To resolve this condition, the students need to become aware that some signed information is absent in their writing. Informal interviews with native and nonnative users of ASL by the investigator indicated that both manual and nonmanual signs are important; neither is of primary importance. This is unlike spoken communication (English) in which nonoral activity (hand movements) is secondary to oral activity.

Jones (1979) hypothesized that the influence of English has caused deaf students to feel that their native language must have only a primary channel. As a result, their writing of English must reflect the fact that English has a primary channel. Thus, the students write only English glosses of the manual signs. This writing style is described as one that is very similar to that of foreign students who are hearing and who have less than adequate proficiency in English.

In conclusion, Jones (1979) proposed two techniques for resolving this problem. One, inform the students that they are translating manual signals only and are ignoring the other nonmanual aspects of a sign that contain important linguistic information. Two, demonstrate to the students that a signed version of what they have written contains much more information. It is suggested that the second part of this technique might be more beneficial in helping the students to include the nonmanual information "without making them overly self-conscious about either language" (p. 278).

Some Recent Investigations

There have been a few bilingual or ASL/English programs and other research projects that focused on the development of both ASL and English (Philip, 1992; Strong, 1988). Relative to English, most of the programs emphasize the development of written English. The assumption is that it is possible to proceed from ASL to the written form of English.

One example is the representative work by Marbury and Mackinson-Smyth (1986), who described the performance of elementary-age ASL-using students. Using an ESL technique known as *grammar-translation* (see McLaughlin, 1985, for a detailed explanation of this technique), the students attempted to translate grammatical features of ASL into English. The content of the translation was taken from an ASL-signed story in which both students and teacher discussed certain aspects such as characters and events. The students were required to focus on the ASL features in the story and to translate these features into English equivalents. Both teachers and students produced a final draft of the story in English.

A number of researchers/educators believe it is important for students who are deaf to be able to develop an awareness of ASL and English as separate languages. This perception of differences between the two languages is a metalinguistic ability. One of the major goals of Strong's (1988) project was to develop students' ability to perceive differences between ASL-signed stories and the English-based signed stories.

The development of this metalinguistic ability might lead to an improvement in the development of English writing skills. For example, Akamatsu and Armour (1987) examined the performance of students who received grammatical instruction in both ASL and English. The researchers reported that there was some improvement in the English written language productions of the students, particularly at the grammatical level. As discussed in Chapter 8, the grammatical level involves the lower level skills of writing. Lower level skills need to become automatic so that students can use or improve higher level skills such as organization and intent.

A good model for programs using ASL and written English is the project of Neuroth-Gimbrone and Logiodice (1992). To participate, students who are deaf needed to have communicative competency in American Sign Language. One of the goals of the project was to enable students to improve their competency in ASL. This is deemed necessary for the development of metalinguistic skills—specifically, the ability to reflect on ASL. Subsequently, the students should be able to develop skills relative to translating/code-switching and English literacy. The eventual goal was an adequate development of metalinguistic skills in both ASL and English.

Development of English as L1 and L2

The question posed here is: Is the development of English as a second language similar to the development of English as a first language for deaf and hard-of-hearing students? As discussed previously, the answer to a similar question is yes, relative to hearing first and second language learners. Much of the work on this similarity issue has been investigated by Quigley and his collaborators on deaf (i.e., profoundly hearing impaired) students learning English as a first language, as discussed in Chapter 8 on literacy. The common finding has been that the English language development of deaf students is quantitatively reduced, albeit qualitatively similar, to that of hearing students. Chapter 8 also presented similar evidence for vocabulary development (Paul, 1984; Paul & Gustafson, 1991) and for the acquisition of reading (Hanson, 1989; Hayes & Arnold, 1992). Given the overall implications for teaching reading/writing to hearing students who are learning English as a second language (Snow et al., 1998), it is expected that these findings also apply to deaf and hard-of-hearing students. In fact, this can be inferred, up to a point, from the Snow et al. (1998) report, discussed in Chapter 8.

There have been a few empirical studies conducted on the qualitative status of the acquisition of English as a second language by deaf students, and there are also several reviews of this issue (Paul, 1993, 1997). One line of research has been to show that English is a second language for many deaf students by comparing their performances to second language hearing learners (Charrow & Fletcher, 1974). One researcher also examined the qualitative issue in-depth with deaf students learning English as a first language and Spanish deaf students learning English as a second language (King, 1981). These early studies are discussed at length here because they served as exemplars for this type of research. In addition, King's (1981) findings are still relevant.

Charrow and Fletcher (1974) explored the possibility that deaf children learn English as a second language. They compared the performance of two groups of deaf students, deaf children of deaf parents and deaf children of hearing parents, with each other and with a group of hearing students learning English as a second language. Three hypotheses were tested: (a) dcdp should outperformed dchp; (b) the performance of the hearing students learning English as a second language should resemble the performance of the dcdp group more than it resembled that of the dchp group; and (c) the performance by the dcdp group on a test of English as a second language and on a standard test of English skills should resemble each other less than should performances by the dchp group on the same tests. The two tests used were the Test of English as a Foreign Language (TOEFL) and the Stanford Achievement Test (SAT).

Results supported the first hypothesis: dcdp performed significantly better than dchp on most of the subtests and on the total score on the TOEFL. In addition, dcdp performed significantly better than dchp on the Paragraph Meaning and Language subtests of the SAT. Ambiguous results were reported, however, for the second and third hypotheses. Relative to the second hypothesis, it was found, as predicted, that the performances of the dcdp group resembled those of the foreign hearing students more than the dchp group did on two of the TOEFL subtests, namely, English structure and Writing Ability. This result was not observed on the other two subtests—Vocabulary and Reading Comprehension. Findings were similar for the third hypothesis. The hypothesis was supported by performances on only some subtests of the SAT.

Charrow and Fletcher (1974) concluded that the issue of whether deaf children typically are learning English similar to a second language might be too broad to investigate. Based on the mixed results for the second and third hypotheses, they argued that some aspects of English are learned by deaf students as a second language and some are not. In the absence of logical or research support for such differences among various aspects of English, the interpretation should be treated with caution.

In another study, Charrow (1975) attempted to identify and provide normative data for the nonstandard features of English language usage by deaf persons. These features were labeled as *Deaf English* (DE). This term implied that deaf persons might have a dialect of English that is different from standard English. It was argued that deaf individuals have typical patterns of variant structures in their use of English that are consistent (also see the discussion in Quigley, Wilbur, Power, et al., 1976; Chapter 8 of this text). Charrow argued further that the variances alternated with some standard English features to produce a simplification or pidginization of standard English. In essence, the range of grammatical forms, standard English and nonstandard English, appears to parallel the pidgin continuum found in the speech of pidgin English speakers.

Charrow (1975) examined this issue by comparing the responses of three groups—dcdp, dchp, and hearing subjects—to 50 Deaf English sentences written by deaf teenagers and 50 standard English sentences. The researcher presented the sentences in random order to the subjects individually. Subjects were required to write the sentences on an answer sheet from memory, one sentence at a time. Results indicated that the deaf subjects found the DE sentences easier to remember and recall than did the hearing subjects. In addition, there was no significant difference in the recall of DE and standard English sentences for the deaf subjects. Finally, there were no significant differences between the two deaf groups—dcdp and dchp.

Charrow (1975) concluded that deaf students acquire most, if not all, the rules of standard English syntax; however, they apply them in an inconsistent manner. The researcher reasoned further that many of the variances from standard English, such as omission of articles and past tense markers, that are found in the written language of students (also see Chapter 8) are not the results of interference from ASL. Rather, these errors reflect redundant nonessential features of English that are difficult to learn and easy to overlook. In sum, this study and the one by Charrow and Fletcher (1974) found little evidence that deaf children are learning English as a second language. These are indirect studies of the problem, however, and certainly do not settle the issue.

A more direct study of the issue was conducted by King (1981). Specifically, King was interested in whether the acquisition of English by deaf students is different from or similar to that of hearing children learning English as a first language. The investigation also provided some insights for bilingual education because the researcher used deaf students who were exposed to Spanish as a first language. King examined one component of language (syntax) and one mode of language (reading). The instruments used in the study were the screening test and four individual diagnostic tests of the Test of Syntactic Abilities (TSA).

Forty deaf subjects between the ages of 8 and 13 and 40 hearing subjects between the ages of 8 and 11 years old participated in the study. Twenty deaf and 20 hearing subjects were classified as L1 learners—that is, learning English as a first language. The remaining deaf and hearing subjects were classified as L2 learners, that is, learning English as a second language. The L1 subjects were exposed to English in the home and had no formal foreign or second language instruction. The L2 subjects were Puerto Rican Americans of Spanish descent. The subjects were matched on language, type of school attended, amount of exposure to English, and type of instruction received. That is, all subjects attended schools in which English was the primary language and had received English instruction in content areas.

Results indicated that the order of difficulty on the syntactic tasks were similar for both groups of deaf and hearing subjects. The researcher concluded that deaf children acquire syntactic structures in the same order as hearing children. In addition, analyses of errors revealed tentatively that the types of errors were similar for both groups. Table 9-6 illustrates the types of errors in this study and in a selection of others.

Table 9-6 Distinctive Structures in the Language of Deaf Students

Distinctive Structure	Environment	Example
Negative outside sentence	Negation	No Daddy see baby.
Negative inside sentence but not correctly marked	Negation	Daddy no see baby.
Nonrecognition of negative marker	Negation	Reads negative sentence as positive
Object-object deletion	Conjunction	John chased the girl and he scared. (her)
Object-subject deletion	Conjunction	The boy hit the girl and (the girl) ran home.
No inversion in questions	Questions	What I did this morning? The kitten is black?
Inversion of object and verb	Questions	Who TV watched?
Overgeneralization— contraction rule	Questions/negation	Amn't I tired? Bill willn't go.
Noun copying	Questions/ relativization	Who the boy saw the girl? The boy saw the girl who the girl ran home.
Pronoun copying	Questions/ relativization	Who he saw the girl? The boy saw the girl who she ran home.
By deletion	Verbs	The boy was kissed the girl.
Unmarked verb in sequence	Verbs	The boy saw the girl and the girl kiss the boy.

Be + unmarked verb	Verbs	The boy is kiss the girl. The sky is cover with clouds.
Confusion of tense markers	Verbs	Tom has pushing the wagon.
Omission of verbs	Verbs	The cat under the table.
Be/have confusion	Verbs	The boy have sick. This boy is a sweater.
Omission of be or have	Verbs	John sick. The girl a ball.
Third person marker missing	Verbs	The boy say "hi."
Omission of conjunction	Conjunction	Bob saw liked the bike.
Omission of determiners	Determiners	Boy is sick.
Confusion of determiners (Nonrecognition of definite indefinite distinctions)	Determiners	The some apples. . . . A best friend. . . . He was the bad boy.
Confusion of case pronouns	Pronominalization	Her is going home. This he friend.
Wrong gender	Pronominalization	They packed our lunch. (their) Sue is wearing his new dress today.
Object-subject deletion	Relativization	The dog chased the girl had on a red dress.
Relative pronoun + possessive pronoun	Relativization	The boy helped the girl who her mother was sick.
Noun phrases	Relativization	The boy helped the girl's mother was sick.
Extra for	Complementation	For to play baseball is fun.

(continues)

(Table 9-6 continued)

Extra *for*	Complementation	For to play baseball is fun.
Extra *to* in *-ing*	Complementation	Joe went to fishing.
Infinitive in place of gerund	Complementation	Joe goes to fish.
Omission of *to* before second verb	Complementation	Chad wanted go.
Inflection of infinitive	Complementation	Bill like to played baseball.
Adjective following noun	Relativization	The barn red burned.
For + Ving or *For + V* for infinitive	Complementation	The boy likes for fishing.
Surface reading order strategy[a]	Verbs	*The boy* was *kissed* by *the girl.*
	Relativization	The boy who hit the *girl ran home.*
	Complementation	That the boy hit *the girl surprised me.*
	Nominalization	The discussion of *the party bored Bob.*

Note: Adapted from King (1981) and Quigley, Steinkamp, Power, and Jones (1978).
[a] *Only italicized words are read.*

The most interesting finding of the King (1981) study was the effects of knowing more than one language for both hearing and deaf students. King reported that knowing Spanish as a first language appeared to have no effects on the English language abilities of hearing children on a quantitative level. This seems to suggest no positive advantages for bilingual students, at least linguistically in the area of syntax. Contrariwise, the effects of another language on the abilities of deaf children were reported to be equivocal. King proffered two explanations: (a) One of the two deaf L2 groups might have been atypical, and (b) deafness overrides any effect (positive or negative) of being exposed to two languages. It should be pointed out that these students were not in a bilingual education program per se, and this might have also influenced the results. Finally, King (1981) remarked that all deaf subjects used little or no English on entering school.

Some support for King's second explanation can be found in a study by Luetke-Stahlman and Weiner (1982). These researchers conducted a study using Spanish deaf students to determine whether there is a first language that should be used to teach language concepts. They were also interested in determining if the children were homogeneous with respect to their first language (Spanish) and thus could be grouped together in the same classroom using similar teaching methods. Five languages/systems (L/S) were delineated: (a) oral English, (b) English and signs, (c) oral Spanish, (d) Spanish and English, and (e) signs only.

Three Spanish deaf females participated in the investigation. Subject 1 was 4 years, 4 months old with a bilateral profound sensorineural hearing impairment. Subject 2 was 3 years, 5 months old and had a bilateral moderate to severe sensorineural hearing impairment. Subject 3 was 4 years, 11 months old and had a moderate to severe hearing impairment. The subjects were taught a receptive vocabulary of nouns, verbs, and adjectives in each of the five L/S. Acquisition curves were constructed for each subject's performance on each of the form class of vocabulary words.

Results indicated that Subject 1 performed best in English and signs, Spanish and English signs, and signs only. The greatest improvement was reported to be in the use of signs. Subject 2 performed best in oral English and signs only. Subject 3 had mixed results. For the noun category, the greatest improvement occurred in Spanish and English signs and signs only. For the verb category, the greatest improvement occurred in English and signs, Spanish and English signs, and signs only. For the adjective category, the greatest gain was observed using the signs only L/S. Similar to the others, these gains were determined to be due to the effects of training.

The researchers concluded that the choice of a language in educating Spanish deaf children should not be based solely on either heritage or etiological classification. They proposed that the choice of language is dependent on a combination of factors: (a) the language and/or communication system of the principal caregiver, (b) the amount of exposure to sign language and/or systems, (c) the degree of usable aided hearing ability, and (d) the language and/or system demonstrated to be most effective for learning.

Although the issue of qualitative similarity or difference is certainly not resolved, no compelling evidence was found to indicate that the acquisition of English as a second language for deaf and hard-of-hearing students is different from that of hearing students who have acquired English as a first language (also see Paul, 1997, 1998a). This does not mean that researchers do not need to be concerned about the influences of the first language (or first symbol system) on the acquisition of English as a second language (see Mayer & Akamatsu, 1999; McLaughlin, 1987; Snow et al., 1998). More important, the evidence is also strong for the acquisition of English literacy in either English as a first language or second language. As discussed in the next section, this qualitative similarity issue has caused some concerns for proponents of ASL/English bilingual models. Of course, another issue is the misinterpretation of existing second language literacy models or that some of these second language models cannot be applied directly to the situation for deaf and hard-of-hearing students.

Table 9-7 provides major highlights of this section on ASL/English instructional programs.

Table 9-7 Highlights of ASL/English Instructional Programs

- There seems to be little available scientific evidence on activities and programs that incorporate the use of ASL and English in either ESL or bilingual programs.

- One of the most common foci of early investigations was to encourage students to notice differences in the structures of ASL and English. This was to facilitate their understanding of utterances—spoken, signed, or written—that were unacceptable or acceptable in either ASL, English, or both. It was argued that students need to be aware of ASL and English as separate languages. This technique is a form of contrastive analysis and involves metalinguistic skills.

- In one study (Jones, 1979), it was argued that deaf students tended to translate into English writing (and sometimes English signing) only the manual signs of ASL. Thus, the students neglected to include nonmanual cues in the translation of ASL to English, particularly English writing. In essence, students need to become aware that some signed information is absent in their English written language productions.

- Most of the recent ASL/English programs emphasize the development of written English only. It is assumed that it is possible to proceed from ASL to the written form of English. No understanding or use of the primary performance form of English, either via speech and/or signs, is deemed necessary.

- One of the most interesting and contentious research questions has been: Is the development of English as a second language similar to the development of English as a first language for deaf and hard-of-hearing students? The answer to this question has important implications for theory, research, and instruction—many of which are discussed in Chapter 8 on literacy.

- Keeping in mind the issue of individual differences, the author of this text argues that there is no compelling evidence that the acquisition of English as a second language for deaf and hard-of-hearing students is different from that of hearing students who have acquired English as a first language. This finding is similar to that found for hearing second language learners.

- This issue of qualitative similarity is certainly not completely resolved; however, it seems to have caused difficulties for many proponents of ASL/English bilingual/bicultural programs. For example, there has been the tendency to reject mainstream theories of second language acquisition as they apply to hearing students or to misinterpret the major tenets of such theories to fit what appear to be unique needs of deaf and hard-of-hearing students with respect to learning English as a second language.

THE ASL/ENGLISH DEBATE

This section summarizes briefly some of the major points in debates on the relationships between American Sign Language and English (Drasgow, 1998; Drasgow & Paul, 1995; Livingston, 1997; Mason & Ewoldt, 1996; Mayer & Akamatsu, 1999; Mayer & Wells, 1996; Paul, 1998a; Paul & Drasgow, 1998; also see a special issue edited by Prinz, 1998). By no means is the selection of publications exhaustive; however, they do serve as guidelines for future research and debates. Furthermore, they highlight the highly political nature of this issue in the field of education and deafness.

One of the most contentious issues in these debates involves the notion of transfer. As indicated previously, this is not a well understood notion in the larger field of second language learning, and it is even less clear for students whose first language is based on a nonspoken phonology and/or does not have a written language system similar to that of literacy-based cultures. On one hand, the issue of transfer has been misinterpreted grossly by proponents of ASL/English bilingual programs, who have attempted to apply the principles of scholars such as Cummins and Vygotsky (see discussions in Mayer & Wells, 1996; Mayer & Akamatsu, 1999; Paul, 1998a). It is assumed that skills acquired in one language transfer (i.e., a wholesale transfer) to the second language, especially in an additive bilingual education program. This assumption is purportedly based on Cummins' (1989) developmental/linguistic interdependence model. In addition, these proponents have attempted to find support via Vygotsky's notion of inner speech (see Mayer & Akamatsu, 1999; Paul, 1998a for a summary). In essence, they argued that it is possible to bypass the spoken (performance) form of the written language and still learn to read and write that language.

There are several problems with these assumptions (Mayer & Akamatsu, 1999; Mayer & Wells, 1996; Paul, 1998a). In general, Cummins' model concerns two spoken languages with written literate forms. (It could certainly be applicable to the performance forms of two signed languages.) One popular interpretation of Cummins' model is that good readers in one language have the potential to become good readers in a second language (of course, possible interference and other factors need to be considered) (see Bernhardt, 1991). However, this correlation may be tenuous if the orthographies of the two languages are vastly dissimilar.

Given the obvious differences in modality between ASL (signed) and English (spoken), the transfer from the performance form of a sign language (ASL) to the literacy form of a spoken language (English) is neither automatic nor clear-cut. Paul (1998a) argued that second language learners can use the knowledge of the first language in acquiring information (grammar, etc.) about the second language; however, acquiring adequate independent literacy skills in a second language such as English requires at least an understanding of the alphabetic principle, which is, in turn, dependent on access to phonology and morphology of English. These points, and others discussed in Chapter 8 of this text, seem to have been ignored by proponents of ASL/English bilingual programs. Based on their interpretations of theoretical models such as Cummins' (1989) and Vygotsky (1962, 1978), a number of ASL/English proponents have argued that it is possible for deaf students to use their knowledge of ASL to acquire adequate independent English literacy skills without ever manipulating or having exposure to the performance form of the language (English) of print. Mayer and Wells (1996) argued convincingly that this situation does not adhere to the conditions of Cummins' (see 1989) theory of linguistic independence. To state this another way: There is little or no evidence of a correlation between proficiency in the performance (i.e., oral or signed) of one language and the proficiency in script literacy of another language, at least in research generated by the work of Cummins and others in second language literacy (see discussions in Mayer & Akamatsu, 1999; Paul, 1998a).

Apparently, Mayer and Wells' (1996) position has also been misinterpreted, most likely because of emotional-laden political issues that surround the development and implementation of ASL/English bilingual programs. These scholars are not arguing against the juxtaposition of ASL and English in bilingual/

bicultural programs. Rather, they argued that ASL by itself cannot account for the development of English literacy skills. In essence, any first language by itself is not sufficient for the development of literacy skills in a second language.

This chapter and elsewhere argues repeatedly that achieving a high independent literacy level in English as a second language requires much more than just a knowledge of the first language and transfer principles. Admittedly, much of the present reasoning is based on the author's interpretation of first language literacy, which seems to have a substantial amount of support, at least for hearing students learning English as a second language (see Snow et al., 1998). Drasgow (1998) wondered how Mayer and Wells' (1996) conclusions can be tenable in light of the high positive correlation between ASL and English in the Strong and Prinz (1997) study. Scholars are still left without empirical data to explicate fully the notion of transfer. The correlation found in the Strong and Prinz study is a good start; subsequently, it is important to examine the reasons behind the correlation and to move into experimental research paradigms for exploring the causes.

In essence, the author is in agreement with Mayer and Wells regarding the misinterpretations of or inaccurate analogies made from the work of both Cummins and Vygotsky by proponents of ASL/English bilingual programs. Ironically, this position might prevent these proponents from taking a serious and interesting look at the notion of transfer from ASL to the signed systems and, subsequently, to English literacy (Fischer, 1998). Of course, this is not without problems. As argued in Chapter 6 of this text and elsewhere (Akamatsu & Stewart, 1998; Drasgow & Paul, 1995; Mayer & Akamatsu, 1999; Paul & Drasgow, 1998), the signed systems might only be able to provide support for English literacy at the morphological and syntactical levels. This might not be sufficient, given the current understanding of the importance of lexemes and of the relationships between phonemes and graphemes. However, despite all the vituperative remarks about the inefficiency of the signed systems, it might be (all things considered) that the more representative models of English (e.g., SEE I and SEE II) are better suited to assist in English literacy development than is American Sign Language simply because they represent another avenue for deaf students to learn about English—albeit, in an imperfect manner. In addition, researchers should see some future studies on the effects of incorporating ASL-like features in English signing, which should make the systems more feasible for the visual processing abilities of deaf students (Akamatsu & Stewart, 1998). The manner in which this approach will affect script literacy skills remains to be seen.

In essence, this debate should not be set up as an either-or situation—in this case, ASL versus the signed systems, to bypass or not to bypass the performance mode of the written language, and so on. Clearly, there is more work for theorists and researchers with respect to the relationships among American Sign Language, English signed systems, and English literacy skills. To increase the understanding of the ASL/English situation or the ASL/English bridge, Drasgow (1998) offered some important recommendations:

- *Determine the amount of time and quality of exposure necessary for a deaf child to become fluent in ASL.*
- *Examine the relationship between the real-world knowledge and literacy levels in deaf students fluent in ASL.*
- *Assess exactly which, if any, ASL linguistic skills transfer to English literacy at the grammatical level.*
- *Develop a curriculum to teach deaf students about the structure of ASL after they have acquired its conversational form.*
- *Create a structured curriculum for teaching English to deaf students that is based on solid second language acquisition principles. (p. 338)*

Table 9-8 summarizes the major points of the ASL/English debate.

Table 9-8 Major Points of the ASL/English Debates

- One of the most misunderstood concepts in these debates is the notion of transfer. This concept is not well understood in the larger field of second language learning, and it is even less clear for students whose first language is based on a nonspoken phonology and/or does not possess a written language system per se.

- Some proponents of ASL/English bilingualism/biculturalism argued that skills acquired in one language transfer (most likely in a wholesale fashion) to the second language, especially in bilingual programs that facilitate the development of both L1 and L2. In essence, they reasoned that it is possible to bypass the performance form (i.e., spoken and/or signed) of the target language and still learn to read and write that language.

- There has been a misinterpretation of Cummins model by many ASL/English proponents. Given two spoken languages with written forms, Cummins hypothesized that good readers in one language have the potential to become good readers in the second language. This hypothesis becomes problematic if the orthographies of the two languages are vastly dissimilar or if one of the languages, particularly L1, does not possess an orthography per se.

- Second language learners can use their knowledge of their first language to acquire information about English. Nevertheless, the acquisition of adequate independent English literacy skills requires at least an understanding of the alphabetic principle, which is in turn dependent on access to phonology and morphology of English and is facilitated by the use and understanding of the performance (i.e., speech or its equivalent) form of English. This is a major point that has been ignored by ASL/English proponents.

- There is little or no evidence of a correlation between proficiency in the performance (i.e., oral or signed) of one language and the proficiency in script literacy of another language.

- There is a need for ASL/English proponents to consider the merits of using the performance form of English, particularly via the use of English sign systems, despite the imperfections of such systems. In short, the trend of transfer might be from ASL to English sign to English literacy.

- The ASL/English debates should not be construed as an either-or phenomenon—that is, ASL versus the English signed systems, to bypass or not to bypass the performance mode of the written language, and so on.

BILINGUAL EDUCATION PROGRAM FOR DEAF STUDENTS: BRIEF DESCRIPTION OF ONE MODEL

In advocating bilingual education programs for deaf students, there are a number of questions that need to be addressed and researched. Indeed, differences between proposed models are due to the varying perspectives on these questions. Some unanswered questions include:

1. *Should ASL and English be developed (or taught) concurrently in infancy and early childhood as in a bilingual environment?*

2. *Should ASL be taught as a first language to all deaf students with English taught as a second language?*

3. *Should English be taught as a second language only to students who know ASL as a first language or to all deaf students?*

4. *If ASL is taught as the first language, at what grade or age level should English be introduced?*

5. *When both ASL and English are used, how much exposure should be allotted to each language? (Paul & Quigley, 1994, p. 220)*

To these questions can be added others:

1. Who should participate in a bilingual education program?
2. How should the program be evaluated?
3. What are the roles of Deaf adults in these programs?

With these questions in mind, several bilingual models, or discussions of what models should focus on, have been proposed for deaf students (see Ewoldt, 1996; Livingston, 1997; Luetke-Stahlman, 1983; Neuroth-Gimbrone & Logiodice, 1992; Paul, 1990, 1991; Paul & Quigley, 1994; Strong, 1988). In the author's view, a L1 immersion model (i.e., immersion in ASL) offers the most promise because (a) deaf students have enormous difficulty in acquiring English, and (b) ASL does not have the same level of prestige as English in the education of deaf students. This model, however, is not without its difficulties (the lack of an early use of speech and other oral skills). Because of pragmatic difficulties (children with hearing parents), there is some support (mostly pragmatic, not scholarly) for using both ASL and English simultaneously, as in 50/50 programs (this seems to be similar to the model briefly discussed by Philip, 1992).

For the 50/50 models to work effectively, there needs to be an adequate quantity and quality of human interactions with both languages in both the performance and literacy modes. The use of technology might be a reasonable supplement; however, it cannot supplant these important interactions between the child and significant others. Regardless of the model used, it seems that one of the most important issues—perhaps the most important—is the development of a first language at as early an age as possible. This is clearly not the case for most deaf children of hearing parents. The late onset of a first language has pervasive negative effects on the subsequent development of academic achievement. For this reason, it seems that L1 (ASL) immersion programs might have the greatest potential for most students with severe to profound impairment despite its pragmatic difficulties. However, any educational program must be based on the needs of parents and their children at the absolute minimum.

One L1 immersion model using ASL as L1 has been described in several publications (Paul, 1990, 1991; Paul et al., 1992; Paul & Quigley, 1987b, 1994). This model has been suggested based on the theoretical and research data available for hearing minority-language students in L1 immersion programs (Baker & de Kanter, 1981; Cummins, 1984, 1988) and on reading research (i.e., interactive theory) on both L1 and L2 students (Bernhardt, 1991; Grabe, 1988).

The L1 immersion model described here has been labeled as a minority-language immersion program for deaf students. The following principles serve as guidelines for implementing this minority-language immersion model (based on Paul & Quigley, 1994):

1. A reasonable level of communicative and grammatical proficiency is established in American Sign Language; a minimum of 3 academic years is recommended.
2. ASL is used as the medium of instruction for academic content areas.
3. A reasonable level of communicative and grammatical proficiency is established in English via a form of English-based signing; modifications of English input are necessary to match the motivational and cognitive capacities of the students.
4. Development of English literacy skills and use of English to teach academic content areas.
5. Eventually, the amount of instructional time devoted to the use of ASL and English should be more or less equal, depending on the progress and proclivity of students.

Similar to other L1 immersion models, this model is constructed so that both L1 and L2 are promoted and developed. Although the acquisition of L2 (i.e., English, specifically English script literacy) is a main goal, it is not an all-encompassing goal. That is, this model recognizes that not all deaf students will be able to achieve a high level of competency in English signing or English script literacy. Nevertheless, it is hypothesized that many students will at least achieve a high level of literate thought in ASL, especially via the performance mode. Specifically, this proficiency in ASL (i.e., communicative proficiency) can be used to enable students to acquire knowledge of the educational curriculum, including that of mainstream society.

It cannot be overemphasized that any bilingual program for deaf students, including the proposed L1 immersion model, needs to be evaluated periodically. This evaluation should take several forms, for example, quantitative, qualitative, and critical (critical theory). The evaluation of any bilingual program should consider but not be limited to the following areas:

1. *Identification of deaf students for placement in a bilingual program.*
2. *Evaluation of teachers' proficiency in both ASL and English* and *in the teaching of both ASL and English.*
3. *Assessment of students' grammatical and communicative proficiency in ASL.*
4. *Assessment of students' achievement in academic subjects and socio-cultural knowledge via the use of ASL.*
5. *Evaluation of students' grammatical and communicative proficiency in English.*

6. *Assessment of students' achievement in academic subjects and socio-cultural knowledge via the use of English (i.e., in both the signing and print modes).*

7. *Evaluation of cognitive and psychosocial developments. (Paul & Quigley, 1994, p. 252)*

Table 9-9 provides major points for the bilingual education program model discussed in this section.

Table 9-9 Summary of Major Points of a Proposed Bilingual Education Program

---

• There have been several bilingual education programs proposed for deaf students. The one espoused in this chapter is labeled a *L1 immersion model* with ASL as L1.

• The L1 immersion model is proposed because of its research effectiveness with hearing minority-language students. In addition, it might be the best model for ensuring that ASL is used equitably in a program because ASL does not enjoy the same level of prestige as English in the education of deaf and hard-of-hearing students.

• The L1 immersion model has several problematic issues. Given the importance of the early development of auditory and articulatory aspects, one of the major concerns is the use and development of oral skills—such as speech, speechreading, and residual hearing.

• Similar to other L1 models, this L1 immersion model is designed to promote and develop both L1 and L2. In addition, it is recognized that not all deaf students will achieve a high level of proficiency in English signing or English literacy. It is hoped that many deaf students will achieve a high level of thought in one language—most likely, this might be ASL, especially via the performance mode.

• This L1 model, similar to any other model, needs to be evaluated periodically. Evaluation may entail grammatical and communicative proficiency in both languages, academic achievement in both languages, and cognitive and psychosocial developments.

FINAL REMARKS

The growing advocacy for the establishment of bilingual and/or second language programs for deaf and hard-of-hearing students has been motivated in part by the growing dissatisfaction with the language, literacy, and educational achievement of most of these students. Not surprisingly, there is much resistance to bilingualism and second language learning because such programs seem to be based mostly on sociopolitical goals rather than on educational goals (see Stuckless, 1991). The sociopolitical goals seem to be influenced by the thinking of critical theorists and some of their fundamental concepts such as enlightenment, emancipation, and empowerment (Gibson, 1986). For example, one interpretation of these concepts, particularly emancipation and empowerment, can be seen in the assertion that ASL should be the first language for all deaf children regardless of degree of hearing loss and family background (Johnson et al., 1989).

The present author is sympathetic to sociopolitical goals; in fact, it can be argued that all educational goals are sociopolitical goals—at least according to the basic tenets of critical theory. Nevertheless, the establishment of bilingual and second language learning programs needs to consider also the outcomes of theory and research based on the scientific method. This chapter summarizes what the author considered to be a representative sample of current thinking on bilingualism and second language learning. Based on this synthesis, it is suggested that bilingual minority-language immersion models (with some variations) might be most beneficial for some deaf and hard-of-hearing students.

Throughout the chapter, summaries of major highlights for the various sections were provided; the intention here is to select a few general remarks with respect to areas such as descriptions/definitions, theories/models of bilingualism, bilingual education models, and the ASL/English debate.

- It should be clear that both bilingualism and biculturalism are not all or nothing phenomena; rather, there are degrees of proficiency and enculturation. However, a widely accepted description/definition of bilingualism or biculturalism does not exist.

- It is possible to have bilingualism without biculturalism and vice versa.

- For some, perhaps many, scholars, true bilingualism (or multilingualism) exists when individuals are exposed to the relevant languages prior to the age of 3 years. This early exposure is most likely to lead to, for bilingualism, equal facility in both languages.

- There seems to be two broad groups of theories/models on bilingualism. One group is concerned with the effects of bilingualism on cognition and academic achievement, whereas the other group focuses on the second language acquisition process.

- Similar to language models for first language acquisition, the bilingual theories/models have been influenced by broad metatheories such as behaviorism, cognitivism, and those motivated by sociocultural aspects. The influence of behaviorism seems to be diminishing. In addition, second language literacy has been influenced by models of first language literacy—notably, social-cognitive theories.

- Despite the contentious debates, there is some consensus that the development of English as L2 is similar to that of English as L1. That is, second language learners of English proceed through stages, produce errors, and use strategies that are roughly similar to those of individuals learning English as a first or native language. There are several implications of this assertion. One of which is that the concept of negative interference (i.e., difficulties caused by the structure of the first language) does not adequately explain the second language acquisition process.

- Although the second language acquisition process is still not completely understood, there seems to be some consensus that second language learners proceed through transitional stages that correspond to their growth of understanding of the second or target language. These transitional stages have been referred to as the interlanguage.

- One of the major findings from the ASL/English debates is that proponents of ASL/English bilingualism/biculturalism have grossly misinterpreted the basic tenets of both Cummins and Vygotsky works. This misinterpretation has caused these proponents to ignore the salient findings from the research on second language literacy and hearing children.

- There is little or no evidence of a correlation between proficiency in the performance (i.e., oral or signed) of one language and the proficiency in script literacy (reading/writing) of another language. Thus, ASL/English proponents should consider the merits of using the performance form of English, particularly via the use of English sign systems, despite the imperfections of such systems.

- The ASL/English debates should not be construed as an either-or phenomenon—that is, ASL versus the English signed systems, to bypass or not to bypass the performance mode of the written language, and so on.

In sum, it should be highlighted that any proposed bilingual education program needs to be subjected to a comprehensive evaluation that entails quantitative, qualitative, and critical analyses. However, an evaluation is not possible without the establishment and implementation of programs and a concerted diligent effort to keep records on instructional and curricular activities. It still seems to be the case that the use of ASL in a bilingual or English as a second language program for some students has not been widely accepted or available in only a few places. Furthermore, although some programs have been in existence for a while, there have been few published evaluations conducted by independent researchers with little or no vested interest in the project.

This chapter provides support for bilingual programs for some deaf and hard-of-hearing students, especially L1 minority-language immersion programs with ASL as L1. There also needs to be information collected on deaf and hard-of-hearing students whose first or home language is a spoken language other than English. Much of the emphasis has been placed on the ASL/English situation. Nevertheless, the ASL/English situation might be applicable to many, if not most, deaf students who have extreme difficulty in acquiring a first spoken language (or its purported signed equivalent) if it is accepted that a first language (i.e., any language) should be developed at as early an age as possible. That is, it might be that a very strong case can be made for the use of ASL as the first language for a large number of these students.

BILINGUALISM AND SECOND-LANGUAGE LEARNING
COMPREHENSION QUESTIONS

1. There is still considerable disagreement about what constitutes bilingualism and second language learning. Discuss the various reasons for this assertion. (You should focus on psycholinguistic and sociolinguistic issues as well as definitions of bilingualism/biculturalism. In addition, consider the situation of bilingualism/biculturalism for deaf students who use sign.)

2. Describe the following terms, offered by McLaughlin (1984):
    a. simultaneous acquisition
    b. successive acquisition

3. The chapter covered two broad groups of theoretical models on bilingualism/second language learning. What are the two broad groups?

4. Discuss briefly the major highlights of the following models:

   a. balance theory

   b. interdependence theory (including the additive/subtractive hypothesis)

   c. societal factor model

   d. threshold model

   e. developmental interdependence model (or linguistic interdependence)

   f. vernacular advantage model

   g. direct approach to reading

5. Discuss the major tenets of the following second language acquisition models:

   a. interlanguage

   b. Monitor Model

   c. Competition Model

6. Discuss the perspectives on the following question: Is the development of L1 by first language hearing learners similar to or different from the development of L2 by second language hearing learners? (L1 and L2 represent the same language, for example, English.)

7. Discuss the major points in the section on:

   a. type of student

   b. language goals

8. Describe the four types of immersion programs that have been identified for students in the United States. Which type(s) seem(s) to be most effective for minority-language students? Why?

9. Provide a summary of major points in the following sections (all are headings) on bilingualism, second language learning, and deafness:

   a. Primary bilingual development

   b. Effects of ASL on the subsequent development of English

   c. ASL/English instructional programs

10. What is the chapter's position on the following question: Is the development of English as a second language similar to the development of English as a first language for deaf and hard-of-hearing students? (This question is similar to the one posed in Question 6.)

11. According to the author, the issue of transfer has been misinterpreted grossly by proponents of ASL/English bilingual programs. Discuss the notion of transfer and then describe why the author feels that it has been misinterpreted.

12. What type of bilingual education program does the author advocate for relevant deaf students? What are some of the major tenets? Does the author advocate this program for all deaf and hard-of-hearing students? Why or why not?

CHALLENGE QUESTIONS

(Note: Complete answers are not in the text. Additional research is required.)

1. The chapter mentioned a movement in California to abandon bilingual education programs because of the so-called lackluster or lack of positive effects on the acquisition of English literacy as determined by scores on statewide proficiency and other achievement tests. Find out the latest information on this event. Is it happening in other states as well? Do you agree with the movement? Why or why not? Did the information in this chapter assist you in forming an opinion? Why or why not?

2. In this chapter, the author seems to argue that development of L1 by first language learners is similar to the development of L2 by second language learners. In fact, the argument was extended to deaf students learning English as a second language. What are some possible specific educational (instructional and curricular) implications of this finding? Does this finding have implications for teacher education programs, especially those that are concerned with deaf and hard-of-hearing students? Why or why not? Do you think this finding sheds more light on the question of whether or not there is a psychology of deafness? In what way?

   Do you agree that L1 development is similar to L2 development? Why or why not? If not, can you support your assertion with research data?

3. In this chapter, it has been argued that a high independent literacy level in English as a second language requires much more than just a knowledge of the first language and transfer.

   What does this statement mean?

   Do you agree or disagree? Can you support your assertions with theoretical or research data?

If this statement is true, what are the implications for teacher education/deaf education programs (i.e., what are the implications for university programs that work with students who want to become teachers of deaf and hard-of-hearing children)?

(Some information on literacy can be gleaned from Chapter 8 of this text.)

4. Consider the bilingual education program advocated by the author in light of what you understand about the need for the early development of articulatory-auditory experiences (see Chapter 5). Do you see theoretical or research issues with respect to the author's proposed program? Are there any pragmatic issues? If you do not agree with this proposed program, what do you propose? Can you support your proposal with theoretical and research data?

FURTHER READINGS

Christensen, K., & Delgado, G. (Eds.). (1993). *Multicultural issues in deafness.* White Plains, NY: Longman.

Eckman, F., Highland, D., Lee, P., Mileham, J., & Weber, R. (Eds.). (1995). *Second language acquisition theory and pedagogy.* Hillsdale, NJ: Lawrence Erlbaum.

Flynn, S., Martohardjono, G., & O'Neil, W. (Eds.). (1997). *The generative study of second language acquisition.* Hillsdale, NJ: Lawrence Erlbaum.

Lewis, W., Kjaer-Sorensen, R., Ravn, T., Lutz, H., & Madsen, J. (1995). *Bilingual teaching of deaf children in Denmark: Description of a project—1982–1992.* Aalborg, Denmark: Doveskolernes Materialecenter

McCormick, K. (1994). *The culture of reading and the teaching of English.* New York: Manchester University Press.

10

Language
Instruction

Y*oung children have an unusual faculty for learning language and . . .
we expect them to learn far more than we could self-consciously teach
them. In order to learn it, they must become apprentices. This appren-
ticeship they accept spontaneously and with enthusiasm, in a spirit of learning
all too rare in more formal educational situations. If any deeper wisdom can
be garnered from a study of children's language learning, it would probably
be how to learn as a spontaneous apprentice. (G. Miller, 1977, p. xxvii)*

The issue of whether language, specifically a first language, can be taught
or whether it is only learned or acquired is a critical one in the field of deaf
education and also in other areas of special education. It has been the focus
of ongoing scholarly debates, especially those concerned with the acquisition
of language in children (Rice & Schiefelbusch, 1989; also see Lightfoot, 1999)
and can even be found in analyses of the philosophies of Plato and Aristotle
(Snyder, 1984). That this issue is not merely an academic one should be obvious. There are enormous implications based on the outcomes, or possible outcomes, for the establishment and implementation of research and practice. If
language can be taught, then one might ask a number of questions, for example, is there a best method or are there effective methods for language instruction? What exactly is taught with respect to language? If a language must be
learned or acquired, there are other questions, for example, what conditions

are necessary to foster this learning? What exactly is learned? Individuals who are skeptical of the conceptualization of this issue as a dichotomous one might inquire: Is there a middle ground in this debate? Is the debate really necessary? Is it possible to create both natural and structured situations to fit the needs of the learner at various stages in the language acquisition process?

The main purpose of this chapter is to provide a brief overview of language teaching methods and practices that have been used or can be used with deaf children and adolescents. The notion, language instruction, is interpreted broadly. That is, it refers to the teaching of a first or second language, although much of the focus in this chapter is on first language acquisition of English. Chapter 8 of this text provides remarks on the teaching of English literacy (reading and writing). Chapter 7 presents a brief discussion of instructional issues relevant to ASL, whereas a general discussion of bilingualism and second language learning was undertaken in Chapter 9.

In addition to providing definitional and historical perspectives, this chapter illustrates a few examples of prototypical language teaching procedures. Many of these procedures have been influenced by the broad language theories discussed in Chapter 3 and in Chapter 9 on bilingualism and second language learning. The reader is reminded that this chapter provides only a brief introduction to language instruction—a concept that is not fully understood or even widely accepted. More detailed information on the teaching of (and assessing) language and literacy with respect to deaf individuals can be found elsewhere (French, 1999; King & Quigley, 1985; Kretschmer & Kretschmer, 1988; Luetke-Stahlman, 1998, 1999; McAnally et al., 1994; Paul, 1998a; Schirmer, 1994).

It might be wondered why there are two separate chapters in this text, one addressing language instruction and one on language assessment. That is, there is or should be a close relationship between instruction and assessment (see discussions in French, 1999; Lipson & Wixson, 1997). Obviously, the closeness of the relationship is related to the type of assessment used—formal versus informal, norm-referenced versus criterion-referenced, and so on. The complexities involved in assessing language merit a chapter by itself, and that is the focus of the next chapter (Chapter 11). In any case, the separation of instruction and assessment is a matter of convenience for discussion purposes; it is not based on a theoretical or philosophical position on the author's part. Despite the growing call for instruction/assessment links in the larger field of language, literacy, and children who are typically hearing, there is a great need for this concept to be systematically applied in the field of deaf education (also see French, 1999).

REPRESENTATION AND TEACHING/LEARNING ISSUES: A BRIEF REVISIT

Prior to addressing the issues relevant to language instruction, it is important to reiterate briefly a topic that was raised in the beginning chapter of this text, namely, representation of a language versus the teaching/learning of a language. There still seems to be some confusion on this topic in the field of deaf education. The crux of the matter is this: Approaches used to represent the English language are not the same as approaches used to teach English or those used to establish meaningful language learning situations. Representation and instruction reflect two different, albeit related, lines of theory, research, and practice.

In general, representation refers to the various communication modes or approaches that have been used and discussed in this text—for example, cued speech/language in Chapter 5 and signing exact English (SEE II) in Chapter 6. Strictly speaking, the notion of representation can be easily applied to the use of English-based signed systems, most likely to cued speech/language, and probably not at all to oral methods—if the focus is on the representation of speech. Oral methods attempt to improve the reception and production of speech, which functions both as a medium and a manifestation of spoken language. Of course, what aspects of speech that are represented in the other communication modes/systems vary from the phoneme (as in cued speech/language) to parts of words or whole words (as in the various English-based signed systems).

Part of the confusion stems from the manner in which the communication modes are discussed. For example, it is not uncommon to find some writers stating that the purpose of a specific signed system is to enable deaf and hard-of-hearing students to see the grammar of English so that they can learn or acquire it (see Gustason & Zawolkow, 1993). In the research literature, especially in a number of early studies, there seems to be the assumption that exposure to an adequate representation of English is sufficient for learning English and even for learning to read and write in English (for a good critique of this line of thinking, see Moores, 1996; Paul, 1998a; Paul & Quigley, 1994). Setting aside the problems of representation, the first part of this statement is tenable, especially within a context of natural methods for learning English (discussed later). However, the latter part, referring to literacy, is definitely contentious because English literacy involves much more than an intuitive understanding of the primary (or performance) form of the language.

In any case, the various methods of communication (excluding ASL) are examples of representation or conveyance of English. A specific mode is used as a medium of instruction or for exchanging information within social situations. This is not what is meant by language teaching approaches or methods that are discussed and exemplified later in this chapter.

THE TEACHABILITY/LEARNABILITY OF LANGUAGE

To provide some context for the methods and materials used to teach language or to foster its development, it is important to present a few highlights of the ongoing debate between the learnability of language versus the teachability of language (Ingram, 1989; Lightfoot, 1999; Piattelli-Palmarini, 1980, 1994; Rice & Schiefelbusch, 1989). In essence, the debate revolves around the question of whether language can be taught. It is possible to conceptualize this issue as a debate between the nativist (e. g., Chomsky's work) and the empiricist (e.g., Skinner's model) (see Chapter 3 of this text). Consequently, this often leads to the assumption that natural methods of teaching language flow from the learnability hypothesis, whereas structural methods are reflective of the teachability hypothesis. Table 10-1 provides brief descriptions of language teaching approaches based on the work of King (1984).

Table 10-1 Brief Descriptions of Language Teaching Approaches

---

Structural approaches:	These approaches require that students engage in meta-linguistic behaviors such as the explicit study and discussion of syntax and grammar. In most approaches, the structure of language is represented by the use of a symbol system. Other labels used to describe structured approaches include *scientific, formal, logical, analytical,* and *systematic.*
Natural approaches:	The focus of these approaches is on the acquisition of language in meaningful real-life situations involving the development of colloquial and idiomatic expressions. Natural approaches do not employ symbol systems or other explicit labeling of language structures. Other labels used to describe natural approaches include *mother tongue, informal, synthetic,* and *developmental.*

Combined approaches: These approaches combine aspects of the structural and natural approaches. The relative use and combination of structural or natural aspects vary from program to program or, more likely, from teacher to teacher. One common example of a combined approach is the use of a structured approach in natural meaningful situations.

Eclectic approaches: In general, the content of an eclectic approach is determined by the individual teacher. The type of approach or combination of approaches may vary from classroom to classroom within the same program. This approach can be described as anything and everything that works. The effectiveness of the approach is also decided by the individual teacher.

Note: Based on the work of King (1984).

It is also not uncommon to encounter such debates in the field of literacy, including second language literacy (Bernhardt, 1991; Dechant, 1991; King & Quigley, 1985; Paul, 1998a). For example, King and Quigley (1985) characterized this issue relative to reading in English as a first language—that is, can reading be taught or must it be caught? The notion caught is taken to mean that a child typically can acquire reading skills by engaging in meaningful, natural reading-related activities such as reading alone, reading in groups, or listening to stories that are being read to them. The dichotomous situation of taught/caught seems to be applicable to all components of reading, for example, word identification, vocabulary, and comprehension. However, this issue seems to be most contentious when the focus is on the development of reading comprehension skills. As noted quite some time ago by Pearson and Johnson (1978):

> *At the one extreme, there is a position that contends that in teaching reading, we can only teach word identification processes. After that it is up to native intelligence and experience to aid children in understanding what we have taught them to read. A middle position argues that while we may not be able to teach comprehension per se, we can arrange instructional and practice conditions in such a way as to increase the likelihood that children will understand what they read. Then there are those, ourselves included, who contend that comprehension can be taught directly—that we can model comprehension processes for students, provide cues to help them understand what they*

are reading, guide discussions to help children know what they know, ask pointed, penetrating, or directional questions, offer feedback (both informational and reinforcing) at the appropriate time, and generate useful independent practice activities. (p. 4)

Relative to students with severe to profound hearing impairment, the teaching of language is a critical issue because it is often remarked that many of these students come to school not knowing any social-conventional language. As noted in Chapter 9, additional concerns include (a) whether English or ASL should be the first or second language, (b) if and how ASL can be used to teach English as a second language, and (c) whether English can be taught at all as either a first or second language either in the primary or performance mode (speech and/or sign) or in the secondary mode (print).

The notion of learnability—most notably, the learnability hypothesis in linguistics—refers to the specification of conditions and constraints that contribute to or enable the learning of a first or second language (see discussions in Lightfoot, 1999; Pinker, 1989). Despite their influences on the development of language methods and materials, the linguistic theories, specifically those motivated by Chomsky's (1975, 1988) thinking, ascribe to the condition of learnability (also see the discussion in Chapter 3 of this text). Chomsky viewed language as an innate process within a maturational framework. That is, the linguist attempts to arrive at explanatory adequacy in describing how and what is acquired, not how and what should be taught. This is primarily a mentalistic, rationalistic view of language development. It should be recalled that this view of language purports that language acquisition can be examined and understood independent of or apart from the social milieu. This does not mean that no social environment is necessary; however, the focus is on the development of language as a biological or maturation process. Just as no one teaches a child to walk, the same can be said for the development of a language—that is, no one, not even the child's parents, really teaches the child to speak (or sign).

At the other end of the continuum are the behavioristic theories, which view language as a verbal, observable, empirical behavior (see Chapter 3). Within this framework, the teaching of language depends on the specification of conditioning, specifically operant conditioning within a stimulus-response paradigm. The behaviorist's approach epitomizes the teachability of language, indeed the teachability of all observed behaviors. This approach, along with logical positivism in philosophy, has influenced descriptive language views, for example, structural linguistics. The most extreme position contends that a child can be or must be taught all features of language ranging from the simplest element such as word parts to more complex ones such as whole words, phrases, and sentences. The assumption is that language is composed of features that can be arranged and taught in a hierarchy from easy to most difficult. Although it is possible and feasible to focus on problematic language structures (some aspects of vocabulary or syntax) for many children, the assumption that all or even most of language is or can be taught is gravely flawed. Some evidence for this was presented in Chapter 3. The best evidence, or rather the most interesting evidence, is the fact that people can produce or understand sentences that they have never heard or read.

The following examples should illustrate this point eloquently and painfully, given the arduous efforts of teachers of deaf and hard-of-hearing students. Keep in mind that a deep understanding of these passages do require some background knowledge. Nevertheless, some understanding is possible although many were not explicitly taught the sentence structures of or even the juxtaposition of some of words in the passages. Readers will understand because of their intuitive knowledge of English buttressed by their experiences and knowledge of their own culture and those of others.

Examples

True, I talk of dreams,

Which are the children of an idle brain,

Begot of nothing but vain fantasy. (Shakespeare, Romeo & Juliet*)*

We cannot tell the precise moment when friendship is formed. As in filling a vessel drop by drop, there is at last a drop which makes it run over; so in a series of kindnesses there is at last one which makes the heart run over. (James Boswell, Life of Samuel Johnson*)*

Another broad group of language theories—interactionist, particularly social-interactionist—seems to represent a balanced view of language development with a focus on interactions among language, cognition, and the social-environmental conditions (see Chapter 3). A few interactionists place more emphasis on innate, or nature, factors, whereas others favor nurture, or social-environmental, factors. A similar analogy can be made relative to the continuum of interactionists' views on the teachability/learnability dichotomy. For example, some proponents stress the teachability notion, whereas others emphasize learnability. If teachability is emphasized, then this can be interpreted to mean that a great deal of language can be taught. On the contrary, if learnability is emphasized, then only some aspects of language can be taught. Nevertheless, it seems that interactionists are influenced by constructivist views of learning, which means that the teacher functions as a catalyst or facilitator who establishes conditions or milieus that enable children to acquire or learn language (and other areas) in naturally occurring, meaningful situations. Within this framework, it is permissible to establish situations that encourage children to use or address the use of specific language structures such as the specific and poetic use of words, the asking of questions with *wh-* words such as *what, why,* and *where,* and so on.

As is discussed later, any type of language intervention—natural, structural, combined, or eclectic (see Table 10-1)—can be viewed as favoring teachability. However, as mentioned previously, there might be a tendency to view natural approaches as those that leaned toward the notion of learnability, especially because these approaches do not advocate any explicit teaching of language features such as sounds, vocabulary, or grammar. Taking an absolute position might be problematic if despite one's best implementation of learnability conditions, many deaf and hard-of-hearing students do not learn English as a first language. In addition, as discussed in Chapters 5 ("Orality") and 6 ("Signed Systems"), there are other areas to consider besides environmental conditions if progress has not been made in language acquisition. In essence, language acquisition might involve more than what is known about teachability and learnability issues. As has been argued analogously, for the area of literacy (Paul, 1998a), the learning of a language entails not only what the individual does in social situations or interactions but also what she or he does independently or alone (e.g., thinking, reading, and writing).

This chapter is limited to the focus of language teaching approaches. Overall, the author tends to favor the learnability position with respect to language and literacy (also see Paul, 1998a). However, it is important to teach (perhaps *model* is the better word) some aspects of language and literacy or at least to construct exemplary situations in which individuals can acquire or develop proficiency in certain areas (Quigley & Paul, 1994). The real goal is to enable the learner to continue his or her growth in language in an independent manner as well as in social interactive situations. Whatever position is espoused, the issue that needs to be addressed is the difficulty that many students with severe to profound hearing impairment have in acquiring or developing a competent level in English language and literacy.

From another perspective, perhaps the question is: When should language be taught? Polloway and Smith (1992) proffered remarks on this issue for students with disabilities—these remarks are applicable to students who are deaf and hard of hearing:

> *Language intervention programs should be implemented as early as possible. Programming for children identified as having a language delay or disorder prior to their entering school should be a priority. Children*

identified after entry into school programs should receive programming as soon as possible after referral and identification.

Early intervention is recommended for several reasons. First, the longer inappropriate language is used, the more habitual it becomes. This makes successful intervention more difficult. Further, inappropriate language may result in negative self concepts, poor school performance, and limited social interactions. The longer these negative consequences are allowed to continue, the greater is the risk of permanent damage to the child's psychological status. (pp. 202–203)

If it is accepted that all children who are deaf or hard of hearing with deaf or hearing parents are at risk for learning English as a first or second language (Snow et al., 1998, as discussed in Chapter 8), then language intervention programs should begin immediately after the identification of the hearing impairment. Ideas for establishing programs for children from the prelinguistic to linguistic periods can be found in several sources (see discussion in Bochner et al., 1997; for deafness, see for example Luetke-Stahlman, 1998, 1999). Some of the highlights from these sources are presented later.

Table 10-2 presents a summary of points in this section on issues such as representation, language teaching approaches, and the teachability/learnability dichotomy.

Table 10-2 Summary of Major Points on Issues such as Representation, Language Teaching Approaches, and the Teachability/Learnability Dichotomy

Representation and Language Teaching Approaches

- There seems to be some confusion between the concept of representation and that of language teaching approaches. It should be clear that these two entities are not the same—albeit, they could be related.

- *Representation* refers to the use of various communication modes or approaches with deaf and hard-of-hearing children—for example, the English signed systems and cued speech/language. A specific mode may be utilized as the medium of instruction or as a means for receiving and expressing information within social situations. Strictly speaking, representation does not refer to the oral approaches or methods.

(continues)

(Table 10-2 continued)

- The theoretical and research debate on the issue of representation concerns the quantity and quality of representing English. It is still not clear how much of English needs to be represented for it to be acquired in a manner similar to that of typical hearing children via the auditory-articulatory mode.

Teachability/Learnability Dichotomy

- In essence, the teachability/learnability dichotomy revolves around the question of whether language can be taught.

- Proponents of the teachability hypothesis argue that language can be and should be taught, especially to students who experience difficulty in the acquisition process. It is possible to argue that for the most part, structured language teaching methods are based on the teachability hypothesis. However, it is possible to state that any type of language intervention— natural, structured, combined, or eclectic—can be viewed as supporting the teachability position.

- The notion of learnability refers to the specification of conditions and constraints that contribute to or enable the learning of a first or second language. In general, it is argued that language, especially a first language, is never taught to children. Children learn a language, analogously, in the same way they learn to walk. It is assumed that natural methods for the most part are based on the learnability hypothesis.

- With respect to language theories, there has been a tendency to associate behavior theories with teachability and linguistic theories, particularly those influenced by Chomsky, with learnability. In fact, Chomsky's work has led to several learnability models. Social-interactionism—another group of theories—seems to reflect a balanced position, and the support of teachability or learnability issues depends on the emphasis of the theorist or researcher.

APPROACHES TO LANGUAGE INSTRUCTION

Historically, there have been two major approaches to language instruction, structural and natural, as well as combinations of these approaches (see McAnally et al., 1994). Relative to deafness, the teachability/learnability distinction has become blurred due to the fact that many deaf children come to school not knowing a social-conventional language or they have not acquired a first language under natural, typical circumstances. Thus, the natural approaches in school might involve constraints and conditions (intensive and extensive exposure to linguistic stimuli within a planned format) that are different from those that exist in the homes for typical, first language or bilingual language learners.

The ensuing sections present information on the two broad language teaching approaches: structural and natural. The reader is reminded that these approaches are broad and that there have been attempts to clarify and refine the meaning of terms such as *approach* and *strategy* within the language learning/teaching framework (Marton, 1988; McAnally et al., 1994). In general, instructional strategies used with deaf and hard-of-hearing individuals are often associated with or categorized as being structured, natural, or a combination of these two categories. McAnally et al. (1994) stated that teaching strategies associated with the structured or combined (structural and natural) approach include correct-incorrect, completion, replacement, combination, scrambled sentences, and revision. The focus here is to adopt and describe the general terms *structured* and *natural* because they are most familiar to researchers and teachers of deaf and hard-of-hearing students (see discussions in King, 1984; Luetke-Stahlman & Luckner, 1991; McAnally et al., 1994; Moores, 1996; Schirmer, 1994).

It should become apparent that there is no magic bullet in either group of approaches or their combinations for assisting deaf and hard-of-hearing children in the development of language. That these approaches have engendered contentious, confusing debates is an understatement. McAnally et al. (1994) provided eloquent descriptions of the approaches as well as detailed historical backgrounds. An example of these descriptions follows:

> For the beginning professional educator, a walk through the history of the development of methods to teach language to children with hearing impairments must be confusing. The historical pendulum has swung through eras of oralism, manualism, oral-auralism, oral-aural-manualism, oral-plus, bilingualism, and multiculturalism. Instructional developments have focused on the recurring themes of natural approaches and structured approaches. With each swing of the pendulum, theorists and teachers hope that an improved method of instruction will advance the ability of the deaf child to access and acquire language for the purpose of communication. The methods of instruction selected by teachers for use with deaf students usually reflect the social trends and prevailing theories of language. The early educational approaches . . . used structured methods involving rules of syntax and parts of speech. Through the process of direct imitation, memorization, drill, and practice, the deaf child was expected to reproduce language using correct grammatical forms.

The natural and whole language approaches to language development of deaf children represent the opposite end of the spectrum. These are based on the theory that the capacity to develop language is an innate characteristic for every human being, and that deaf children are exposed to language in the same manner as are hearing children. Rules of language are not taught explicitly; instead, proponents assume that the deaf child will acquire the rules unconsciously, through exposure, imitation, expansion, and expression, without the need for rote memorization or contrived language drills. (p. 74)

Descriptions and Historical Perspectives: Structured Approaches

Advocates of structured (or structural) approaches assert that language can and needs to be taught to students with hearing impairment. Students are required to analyze and categorize the grammatical aspects of the language, for example, parts of speech such as nouns, verbs, and objects. The grammatical aspects are typically represented by patterns via a metalinguistic symbol system. Metalinguistic symbols refer to symbols such as noun phrase, verb phrase, subject, or other symbols and words used to describe the language. Students demonstrate their understanding by writing sentences that correspond to previously taught patterns. As noted by McAnally et al. (1987):

Structured methods treat language analytically and prescriptively, emphasizing knowledge of structure as embodied in rules of grammar. Through processes of direct imitation, memorization, and drill, usually within the framework of a strictly sequenced curriculum, the deaf child is expected to acquire a grammatically accurate version of the general language of the society. Examples of users of structured approaches to language development have been de l'Epee and Sicard in France in the second half of the 18th century, Clerc and Gallaudet in the United States in the early to late 19th century, and Barry and Fitzgerald in the United States in the first half of the 20th century. (p. 78)

Historically in the United States, the use of structured approaches and the language of signs occurred simultaneously, as evident in the first residential school for the deaf in Hartford, Connecticut. Influenced by the work of de l'Epee and Sicard, teachers constructed diagrams, or line drawings, to represent the various grammatical features of English. Subsequently, a number of metalinguistic symbol systems were developed during the late 19th and early

20th centuries. Examples include Barnard (straight-line and curved-line symbols), Jacobs (primary lessons), Storrs (symbols above words), and Barry (five slates or tablets of materials used for writing only, similar to the approach used by Sicard).

There are several themes that are common to most or all of these approaches used, formerly and presently, with deaf and hard-of-hearing students. For example, there seems to be the belief that drills in language aspects such as vocabulary and syntax are necessary for children to acquire or internalize the rules of grammar, leading to the development of communicative or conversational language ability. A great deal of emphasis is placed on practice and rehearsal of the various language principles. These principles are to be worked on one at a time and in a sequential, hierarchical fashion. Children need to have opportunities to be exposed to and to use the various or targeted language patterns or features in a variety of meaningful situations. One of the major problems with these earlier approaches, and indeed with many structural approaches, is that there were few provisions for the application of these principles to other more natural situations. Obviously, rote learning and memorization of language skills do not equal language proficiency. As a result, structural approaches that have been used in recent years recognized the need for the application of learned principles to novel situations (i.e., outside of the structured planned ones) to ensure generalizations of language used in a variety of situations. As is discussed later, some scholars who favor pure naturalistic approaches believe that generalization is a misused concept, especially given the unique situational uses of language. Nevertheless, the major impetus for the use of structured approaches (often in combined programs with natural approaches) is that many deaf and some hard-of-hearing children have difficulty acquiring or internalizing English solely via communicative and social interactions with parents, teachers, and significant others.

Two examples of structured approaches (and materials) are highlighted here: the Fitzgerald Key, developed during the early 20th century, and APPLE TREE, developed during the late 20th century. It is permissible to consider these two approaches as exemplars of most structured programs used with deaf and hard-of-hearing children. It is also important to remember that these two approaches, especially APPLE TREE, have been or can be used in combined situations involving structural and natural aspects. In fact, the APPLE TREE program is often categorized as a combined approach (McAnally et al., 1994).

As with any language teaching method or approach, there tend to be variations or adaptations of the approaches although practitioners might be aware of the general principles and recommended uses of the programs. The adaptations reflect issues such as teacher interpretations of the programs or the focus on individual needs of particular students. That there are adaptations can be indirectly gleaned from the discussion of the results of survey studies on the use of methods and materials (see King, 1984; LaSasso & Mobley, 1997).

The Fitzgerald Key

The Fitzgerald Key is probably the most widely known structural approach, and although rarely used at present, a few principles based on the Key are still probably used fully or partly in a few programs. In any case, the Key was one of the most popular methods until the 1960s (see discussion in McAnally et al., 1994). Russell et al. (1976) remarked that the highly structured approach of the Key was typical of "the tenets of the structuralist linguists that words are the basic building blocks of sentences and that sentences are formed by left-to-right combinations of words into strings" (p. 7).

The Key was developed by Edith Fitzgerald (1929), who was a deaf teacher at the Wisconsin School for the Deaf. With some modifications and refinement, the Key was based on the Barry Five Slate System, which entailed the use of five slates for representing visually the grammatical structures of English in a structured manner. It is often forgotten, however, that Fitzgerald intended for her Key to be used in natural meaningful situations. For many educators, this might seem to be an oxymoron; nevertheless, it is possible to find examples of natural situations in which the teacher or clinician have attempted to provide some structure or control to facilitate the acquisition and use of specific language structures.

The Key consists of six columns. Each column is headed by words or symbols as follows: subject (who and what), verb and predicate words, indirect and direct objects (what and whom), phrases and words denoting place (where), other phrases and word modifiers (how often and how much), and words concerning the concept of time (when). Examples of complex sentences that can be developed within this structure (i.e., complete Key) are as follows:

1. The professor (Column 1) will write (Column 2) a text (Column 3) in his office (Column 4) tomorrow night (Column 6).
2. My father (Column 1) is a mechanic (Column 2).
3. My doctor (Column 1) went (Column 2) to the bookstore (Column 4).

The structure of the Key is illustrated in Table 10-3.

Table 10-3 A Sample of the Fitzgerald Key

Column 1	Column 2	Column 3	Column 4
Who:		What: Whom:	
Whose:		( ) Whose:	Where:
What:		Whom: What:	

Column 5		Column 6
How much:	For:	
How often:	From:	When:
How long:	How:	

Note: Adapted from Pugh (1955).

- Column 1 contains subjects such as noun phrases and is labeled with the interrogative terms *who* and *what.*

- Column 2 contains verb phrases, subject complements, predicate nouns, predicate adjectives, and predicate pronouns. There is no heading for this column; it uses symbols that are placed below the words.

- Column 3 contains the direct and indirect objects and is marked by the interrogatives *whom, what,* and *whose* for direct objects. The *what* and *whom* with the parentheses indicate indirect object.

- Columns 4, 5, and 6 contain adverbials or phrases modifying the main verb. Column 4 represents adverbials of place and is marked by the term *where.* Column 5 contains frequency and causal modifiers of the main verb and is marked by terms such as *how much, how often, how long, for, from,* and *how.* Column 6 represents adverbials of time and is represented by the heading *when.*

It is not practical or even beneficial to expose children to the entire Key initially. To build confidence, children should begin working with the concepts of who and what, again, in meaningful, naturally occurring language situations. For example, deaf and hard-of-hearing children should receive practice in classifying pictures, objects, and so on in their environment within these two broad categories. After a reasonable foundation with the use of nouns and adjectives, children are introduced to the verb column. Exposure to simple sentence patterns (e.g., *I see a bird*; *I laughed*; etc.) in meaningful situations (i.e., opportunities for use) leads to expansions, which include complex concepts such as the production and use of intransitive verbs, transitive verbs, and adverbial phrases. After considerable practice and use, children should proceed across the entire six columns of the Key. Symbols are often used to represent the various structures in each column—a feature that is common across many structural systems.

In general, Fitzgerald (1929) asserted that the purpose of this approach is to help deaf children learn some of the English structures and to construct and evaluate their own written compositions. The use of and emphasis on reading and writing as a strategy to enhance the acquisition of English has a long illustrious history in the education of deaf and hard-of-hearing students. It is even the primary strategy for several proposed and existing ASL/English bilingual programs (see Chapter 9). With respect to the Key, the learning process was thought to be facilitated by the graphic display of syntactic and other grammatical relationships. In addition, this graphic display was purported to allow children to correct their composition (i.e., written) errors. A good discussion of the development and implementation of the Key can be found in Pugh (1955; also see McAnally et al., 1994).

As with most other predominantly structural approaches, it is easy to find and discuss flaws. For example, Wilbur (1977, 1987) was highly critical of these approaches, claiming that the teaching of certain structures were out of developmental sequence (i.e., did not follow the natural development of language structures by hearing children). In addition, Wilbur (1977, 1987) remarked that these structured approaches are responsible for the stilted written language productions of deaf and hard-of-hearing students (see discussion of written language in Chapter 8). That is, deaf and hard-of-hearing children tended to use certain stereotypic phrases and sentences (e.g., *I see a cat*; and *The cat is black*) and had difficulty learning to use creative, figurative, or metaphorical expressions (e.g., *I was so angry that I felt like climbing the walls*).

Perhaps one of the biggest flaws of the Key was that the approach might have indirectly contributed to deaf children's attempt to overuse linear (e.g., subject-verb-object) strategies in understanding English sentences. This type of strategy works effectively for sentences such as: *I hit the ball* and *The dog bit the woman*. However, it can cause misinterpretations or misunderstandings for complex hierarchical syntactical structures such as: *The dog was bit by the woman* and *The light on the blue car turned* (see discussion of research in W. Russell et al., 1976). In fact, with the use of the Key, it was and still is extremely difficult to address some of these complex syntactical structures of

English, a problem often encountered by all programs influenced mostly or mainly by structural linguistics principles (see Chapter 3). In all fairness, to place all or most of the blame for the stilted unimaginative written language productions of many deaf and hard-of-hearing students on the Key or on any other specific language approach is simply shortsighted. This assumes that all of language is learned, and in the author's view, this is simply not tenable. It can be argued that the stilted unimaginative use of language is reflective of someone's understanding of that language as well as other factors such as habit, exposure, teaching approaches, and so on. The uncovering of a single all-encompassing factor to explain (or blame!) language acquisition and use does not exist.

The Apple Tree Program

The APPLE TREE is an acronym for *A Patterned Program of Linguistic Expansion Through Reinforced Experiences and Evaluations* (M. Anderson, Boren, Caniglia, Howard, & Krohn, 1980). This program consists of pre- and posttests, workbooks, and a teacher manual designed to teach 10 basic sentence patterns as shown in Table 10-4.

Table 10-4 Sentence Patterns for APPLE TREE with Possible Examples

---

Sentence Pattern	Example
N1 + V (be) + Adjective	The boy is short.
N1 + V (be) + Where	The girls are in school.
N1 + V (be) + N1	I am a student.
N1 + V	The boy is running.
N1 + V + Where	The children are running to school.
N1 + V + Where + When	Mother went to work this morning.
N1 + V + N2	The woman bought a car.
N1 + V + N2 + Where	The boys took their bats to the game.

(continues)

(Table 10-4 continued)

N1 + V + N2 + Where + When	I will take my wife to the doctor tonight.
N1 + V + N3 + N2	Jill gave me a toy.

NOTE:
N1 = noun phrase one (i.e., subject or predicate nominative)
N2 = noun phrase two (i.e., direct object)
N3 = noun phrase three (i.e., indirect object)
Adjective = word or words that describe the noun phrase
V = verb phrase
V (be) = be verb (i.e., linking verb or copula)
Where = adverbial phrase of place
When = adverbial phrase of time

The exercises in the workbooks consist of comprehension, manipulation, substitution, production, and transformation activities. Transformations include only negation and question forms. These exercises are considered fundamental steps and part of instructional procedures (Caniglia, Cole, Howard, Krohn, & Rice, 1975). For example, the first step, comprehension, refers to the development of vocabulary, concepts, and form of the structure. The APPLE TREE program was designed to introduce the sentence patterns in a sequenced spiraling manner, that is, proceeding from the easiest to the hardest structure. It is recommended that children have a working vocabulary knowledge of common words (i.e., nouns, verbs, and adjectives).

As a supplement to the basic APPLE TREE materials, a series of short story books have been developed, using only the sentence patterns depicted in Table 10-4. Supplementary activities in the form of additional workbooks are also available. It should be obvious that this language approach is structural, but again, it can be used as part of a combined approach—involving both structured and natural activities. To complete the exercises in the workbooks successfully, the students need to know and understand the metalinguistic terminology used throughout the materials.

Examples of Lessons Using APPLE TREE

In addition to the offering of a prescribed sequence of syntactic structures, the APPLE TREE proffers instructional procedures that include five steps: comprehension, manipulation, substitution, production, and transformation. The description of these steps are as follows (M. Anderson et al. as cited in McAnally et al., 1994).

1. *Comprehension—A procedure to develop the child's understanding of the vocabulary, concepts, and form of the structure.*

2. *Manipulation—A procedure to help the child understand the structure of the language.*

3. *Substitution—A teaching procedure that allows the child to use the known to explore the unknown.*

4. *Production—A procedure to help the child reproduce the structure form spontaneously.*

5. *Transformations—A procedure to help the child make rearrangements in the simple sentence patterns. (pp. 126–127)*

After the first step (comprehension), the child has acquired or learned a number of vocabulary words and concepts. During the second step, manipulation, deaf and hard-of-hearing children attempt to apply the knowledge of words and concepts. Children are exposed to a variety of visual patterns relative to the structures of the program. In essence, the goal is to enable children to understand when the specific words can be used in the specific structures and when they cannot be used. For example, students might be required to arrange words into patterns such as the following (McAnally et al., 1994):

/Mary /	/is/	/happy./
/John/	/is/	/sad./
/Harry/	/is/	/lazy./ (p. 128)

Subsequently, the students manipulate the following word-phrase cards:

/John and Mary/	/went/	/to their grandmother's house./
/Did John and Mary/	/go/	/to their grandmother's house?/
/Where/	/did/	/John and Mary go?/ (p. 128)

The third phase is substitution. The lesson looks similar to the following:

John wants to work.

Mary wants to stay home.

I want to watch TV. (p. 129)

With these exercises, the students gain an understanding of the relationships of words within the sentences and across sentences, particularly the notion of pronominalization or pronoun reference.

During the fourth phase of the process, students are required to produce or write spontaneously using their knowledge of sentence patterns and vocabulary. The impetus for these activities might be pictures, objects, field trips, and so on. Reinforcement and enrichment exercises are also present in the workbooks that accompany the program.

The last phase deals with the transformation of the basic kernel sentences. As mentioned previously, there are two transformations: negation (i.e., the word *not*) and the question form. An example of each activity is as follows (McAnally et al., 1987; also see examples in McAnally et al., 1994, pp. 129–130):

Negation

The apple is red.

The apple is not red.

John is sad.

John is not sad.

We will go to the store this afternoon.

We will not go to the store this afternoon.

Ms. Pat sang a song at the party.

Did Ms. Pat sing a song at the party?

Ms. Pat did not sing a song at the party.

Question Form

Mr. Brown ran in the Boston Marathon.

Mr. Brown did run in the Boston Marathon.

Did Mr. Brown run in the Boston Marathon? (p. 124)

Other examples of instructional strategies and activities associated with APPLE TREE and other structural approaches can be found elsewhere (McAnally et al., 1994).

Table 10-5 provides highlights of structured approaches, including some remarks and basic tenets about the Fitzgerald Key and APPLE TREE.

Table 10-5 Highlights of Structured Approaches

Highlights of Structured Approaches

- One of the basic tenets of structured approaches is that language must be taught systematically and consistently. Rules need to be explicit for students to analyze and internalize them. Much emphasis is placed on practice and rehearsal of the various language principles.

- Structured approaches utilize a visual coding or symbol system—which requires metalinguistic skills on the students' part. That is, students need skills to think and talk about a language. Examples of metalinguistic symbols include the use of terms such as *nouns, adjectives*, and *noun phrases* or symbols such as *NP, NP + VP =*, and *[ ]*.

- Students should have ample opportunities to be exposed to and to use the various or targeted language patterns in a variety of meaningful situations.

- Two structured approaches served as exemplars for the 20th century: the Fitzgerald Key and APPLE TREE. Although both are structured approaches, they have been used in combined situations.

Fitzgerald Key

- The Key is probably the most widely known structural approach and was meant to be used in natural meaningful situations.

- In general, the Key displays graphically the syntactic relationships of words in sentences. The goal is to facilitate children's writing of acceptable sentences—that is, sentences that adhere to the English rules of syntax. Children are encouraged to use the Key to correct composition errors.

- The Key consists of six columns, with each column headed by words or symbols. Parts of a sentence that are represented include subject, verb (and predicate words), indirect and direct objects, terms denoting location and time, and word modifiers.

- Children are not exposed to the entire Key initially. Exposure is gradual, beginning with simple noun and adjective items, proceeding to simple sentence patterns and then to more complex syntactic sentences until the entire six columns are covered.

APPLE TREE

- APPLE TREE is an acronym for *A Patterned Program of Linguistic Expansion Through Reinforced Experiences and Evaluations.* The focus is on instruction of 10 basic sentence patterns. The only major transformations included in the program are negation and question forms.

- The program is designed to introduce the sentence patterns in a sequenced spiraling manner, proceeding from the easiest to the most difficult structure.

(continues)

(Table 10-5 continued)

Children need to have a working vocabulary of common words such as nouns, verbs, and adjectives.

- To participate in the lessons and activities, children need to be able to use and understand the metalinguistic terminology used throughout the program.

- In addition to the prescribed sequence of syntactic structures, the program suggests specific instructional procedures presented in five steps. The names of the steps are comprehension, manipulation, substitution, production, and transformation (see text of chapter for descriptions).

Descriptions and Historical Perspectives: Natural Approaches

Advocates of natural approaches assert that language should be acquired in a holistic manner. With intensive and extensive exposure to a language-rich environment, students with hearing impairment should be able to discover and internalize rules and principles associated with the grammar of English. It is not necessary—indeed, it is counterproductive and unnatural—to teach specific grammatical features. As remarked by McAnally et al. (1987; also see 1994):

> *Development is planned to parallel the sequence of language acquisition in hearing children. The deaf child is expected to acquire language principles inductively and unconsciously through constant exposure to appropriate language patterns in situations that are designed on the basis of the child's needs and interests. . . . Some of the foremost proponents of natural approaches have been Hill in Germany in the early and mid-1800s, Greenberger and Groht in the United States from the late 19th to the mid-20th century, and many individuals in many countries in the present era. (p. 78)*

The natural approach commanded a substantial amount of attention with the publication of *Natural Language for Deaf Children* by Groht (1958). As stated previously (also see Chapters 8 and 9), the natural approach has been heavily influenced by the concepts of psycholinguistics and, more recently, socioculturalism. With the subsequent influence of constructivist learning theory, the natural approach has led to the whole language approach in reading. All of these influences can be seen in current debates on ASL/English bilingual bicultural programs (also see Paul, 1998a).

If the structured approach is synonymous or nearly synonymous with direct instruction, then the natural approach is often associated with the inquiry method (see discussions in McAnally et al., 1994; Paul, 1998a; Schirmer, 1994). Synonymous labels for the inquiry method include *holistic teaching*, *holistic constructionism*, and even the *scientific approach* (Bateman, 1990; Schirmer, 1994; with respect to literacy, see Paul, 1998a). The teacher is often viewed as a facilitator or consultant rather than an expert who imparts knowledge. Much of the theoretical support for this approach comes from Piaget's work on the cognitive development of children and adolescents as well as the work of Vygotsky on the influences of culture on cognitive and language development (see Chapter 3).

Some of the natural language teaching models, which adhere to the inquiry method, utilize some of the basic steps of the scientific method. Although there are several variations, some possible steps are as follows:

1. Identification and definition of the problem.
2. Formulation of hypotheses.
3. Gathering of data via the use of experimentation or observation.
4. Analysis and interpretation of the data.
5. Formulation of conclusions and generalizations.

The reader should keep in mind that the student is not taught or exposed to these steps in a didactic manner. Rather, the teacher establishes situations in which to lead the student to the discovery of language principles. For example, in a beginning exercise on plurality, the teacher can introduce and lead students on a discussion of identifying and labeling multiple objects in the classroom environment—such as chalkboards, pencils, pens, desks, girls, boys, and so on. The teacher does not say that the *s* is used to mark plurality; rather, the children are led to discover this principle. Later, the teacher can work on variations of *s* as in *es* and other variations of plurality as words such as *men, women, oxen*, and *deer*. Again, children are led to discover these variations; they are not explicitly taught the various ways plurality is marked in English or the association of plural markers with groups of words.

It is also possible to have a step that deals with a reflection on the inquiry process, that is, metacognition. This is considered to be an analysis of the inquiry process itself (Joyce, Weil, & Showers, 1992) and is similar to other activities that involve thinking about language (metalinguistic) or thinking about comprehension in reading (metacomprehension and metamemory). In essence, the focus is on the use of a method that is similar to that used by scientists and researchers in attempting to understand and solve a problem or condition. This approach emphasizes strongly that science is not merely the accumulation of knowledge; rather, it is a process that involves critical and reflective inquiry in which there is little separation between the knower and the knowledge attained, as is evident in most constructivist orientations (for an interesting perspective, see Piaget, 1971; for a discussion related to literacy, see Paul, 1998a).

The natural approach seems to have a great deal of appeal to educators, possibly due to the growing movement of constructivism and also to the general trends of language intervention programs. These trends have also been observed in programs for children with language disorders. McCormick (1986) proffered descriptions of three trends: (a) development of natural language learning situations, (b) focus on functions (e.g., use) rather than forms (e.g., structure), and (c) integrated use throughout the school day. There are a number of implications associated with these trends; only a few are mentioned here. First, models based on these trends recognize that language learning is not the responsibility of one person—a number of individuals in the child's educational life can and should be involved, for example, teacher, parent, aide, speech pathologist, and so on. Activities should focus on the pragmatic function of language rather than the learning of specific structures such as vocabulary and syntax in isolated drill-like situations. More important, the focus should be on how effectively an individual uses his or her language rather than on the how well or the competence aspect. Finally, with respect to integrated use, or to use McCormick's phrase—*training across activities*—it is recognized that language learning is not or should not be restricted to a specific time frame or period during the school day. Interesting, using language all day long does not imply the generalization of skills. Rather, as within a constructivist spirit, language is to be learned and used within specific environments or situations. Making generalizations is not necessary or even feasible; the goal is to use language appropriately within the desired social milieu. A rendition of this description can be found also in the whole language philosophy, which has been influential in both language and literacy programs in deafness (see review in Paul, 1998a).

Examples of Lessons Using Natural Approaches

It should be recalled that natural approaches focus on developing language in meaningful, natural, communicative situations. The development of language is not divided into parts such as form (e.g., vocabulary and syntax), content (e.g., meaning), and use (e.g., pragmatics). Rather, these components of language are an integral part of every lesson (McAnally et al., 1994; Schirmer, 1994).

Another perspective on the natural approach is the use of a language experience activity or the LEA. In general, the LEA incorporates language from a meaningful activity (visit to zoo, museum, factory, and so on). Teachers are supposed to elicit such language from children and record their statements on a language experience chart or on the chalkboard. There are, of course, variations of the LEA. Table 10-6 provides examples taken from McAnally et al. (1994), which are still representative of instructional activities within any natural approach (also see McAnally et al., 1987). This is intended for children at the preschool level, and it is a type of language experience activity, which is also used as an approach in some reading programs.

Table 10-6 **Example of Lesson Based on Natural Language Teaching Approaches**

PRESCHOOL LEVEL

Sample goal: To develop the concept of apple.

Subunit 1: Field trip to orchard.

Lesson 1: Previsit preparation.

Objective:

- Prepare children for field trip.

Strategy:

- Planned situation as opposed to "teaching to the movement."
- Develop and/or activate prior knowledge.
- Communicative interaction between teacher and learners in speech/sign.
- Questioning.
- Discourse.

Procedure:

- Teacher reads primary version of *Johnny Appleseed*.
- After the story, teacher and children discuss a picture of the trees and apples.
- Teacher shows children a real apple and compares it with apples on the tree in the picture. Teacher: "Tomorrow, we will go somewhere. You will come to school in the morning. Then we will ride a bus. We will see many apple trees. We will buy some apples and bring them back to school. Maybe we will eat apples tomorrow. Do you like to eat apples?"
- All children have an opportunity to respond.
- Teacher and children find *tomorrow* on calendar and mark by drawing an apple on calendar.

(continues)

(Table 10-6 continued)

- Children go to a reading table to look at several books about apples and discuss them with their classmates.

Lesson 2: Trip to orchard.

Objectives:

- See apple trees.

- Pick apples off the trees.

- Buy apples in the orchard store.

- Buy apple juice.

Strategy:

- Field experience.

- Communication.

- Discourse.

- Questioning.

Procedure:

- Teacher or teacher aide should take instant-developing photographs during the trip so children see the pictures together with the real thing.

- When the children are approaching the orchard, the teacher should comment about what they see (many trees, apples on the trees, and size and colors of apples). Each child could pick an apple and the teacher could discuss "good" and "bad" apples.

- Teacher and children go into the orchard store and see and discuss the apples.

- Most orchard stores offer samples of different kinds of apples so the children can taste the different ones.

- Teacher and children buy apples and juice to take back to school.

Lesson 3: Teacher and children develop written experience story by discussing each photograph, which they make into a book. They eat apples and drink juice.

Subunit 2: Field trip to grocery store produce department.

Lesson 1: Prepare children for trip (walking trip).

Lesson 2: Trip to grocery store.

- Note different kinds of apples.

- Buy apples at store.

- Teacher and children develop a story about their trip and make it into a book.

Subunit 3: Make fruit salad.

Lesson 1: Preparation of salad.

- Teacher aide takes instant-developing photographs.

- Class discusses size, shape, and colors of apples.

- Teacher peels apple and children can inspect the inside (color is different, there is a core, and there are seeds).

- Teacher chops up apple.

- Teacher aide cuts up oranges.

- Each child peels and cuts up banana (with plastic knife). Add sugar and apple juice, and all can eat fresh fruit salad. Develop a story and make a book.

Lesson 2: Teacher and children develop experience story by discussing each photograph taken. Children can add their own artwork to the story and produce a book.

Subunit 4: Make caramel apples.

Subunit 5: Make applesauce, apple pies, or apple juice.

Note: Based on McAnally, Rose, and Quigley (1994, pp. 102–104).

Additional examples of instructional activities for elementary and older children related to natural approaches can be found elsewhere (Luetke-Stahlman, 1998; Luetke-Stahlman & Luckner, 1991; McAnally et al., 1994; Schirmer, 1994).

Table 10-7 presents some highlights of the natural approaches, including a few general principles based on the work of Groht (1958).

Table 10-7 Highlights of Natural Approaches

- One of the major tenets of natural approaches is that language should be acquired in a natural, meaningful, holistic manner. Situations should be designed to meet the child's needs and interests. Acquisition is facilitated by exposure to a language-rich environment.

- Children should discover rules and principles of language in an inductive manner. There is no need for explicit systematic instruction or drills of the grammar or exercises that require children to rehearse or analyze the grammatical features.

- The natural approach is often associated with the inquiry method or the scientific method.

- The natural approach seems to appeal strongly to educators, possibly due to the growing movement of constructivism and also to the general trends of language intervention programs.

- Groht (1958) stated several principles that seem to be common across all natural approaches. These include:

  1. Content of language lessons should be dictated by the needs of the child rather than by lists of vocabulary words or specific rules of language.

  2. Child learns natural language via meaningful situations rather than by mechanical drills and exercises.

  3. Functions of language can be taught best through conversations, discussions, writing, and the academic subjects.

  4. Language principles should be introduced incidentally in natural situations, possibly explained by the teacher in real meaningful situations, and practiced by the children in numerous activities such as games, stories, and conversations.

COMBINED APPROACHES

In the second half of the 20th century, several special language materials were developed and a number of combined approaches advocated. The combined approaches entail the teaching of language in a natural manner via the use of a structured approach (King, 1984; McAnally et al., 1994; also see the examples in Luetke-Stahlman, 1998, 1999). This type of approach seems to be a balanced approach, combining the best features of both natural and structured approaches (see materials and procedures in Blackwell et al., 1978; Quigley & Power, 1979; van Uden, 1977).

Only three representative approaches are highlighted here. van Uden (1977) developed a method called the *maternal reflective method*. It contains a natural component because of its emphasis on the development of the mother tongue—"the language first learnt by the speaker as a child" (van Uden, 1977, p. 93)—via oral conversational methods based on the experiences of the children. van Uden argued that contrived experiences and language patterning are not successful. Children do not learn questioning techniques by being presented isolated sentences such as *The box is on the table* and by being requested to produce a *wh-* question based on these sentences. van Uden also asserted that children learn language by participating in dialogue that is meaningful and by listening to the conversation of others. Thus, it is reasoned that teachers of deaf children should not only engage in meaningful dialogue with their students but should also direct the attention of their students to the conversations of others in the classroom. The influence of social-interactionist theories can be seen in this method, particularly within the framework of pragmatics (see Chapters 1 and 3 of this text).

Rhode Island Curriculum

Blackwell et al. (1978) developed the Rhode Island Curriculum designed for students at the Rhode Island School for the Deaf. This approach is primarily structural and is based on the assumptions of early transformational-generative grammar theory (Chomsky, 1957). However, it does incorporate naturalistic principles, influenced in part by Piaget's stages of cognitive development (see Chapter 3; also see Phillips, 1981, for an accessible account). Its combined approach is due to the emphasis on both linguistic knowledge and spontaneous language development.

The Curriculum is influenced by the work of Streng (1972) and contains three major components. The first component describes the major language framework and instructional procedures. The developers listed what they considered to be basic steps in the language acquisition process of deaf and hard-of-hearing children, for example, exposure, recognition, comprehension, and production. Production includes literacy skills such as reading and writing.

The second major component concerns the curriculum, which is divided into three levels. The first level is designed for children in preschool and kindergarten. This level consists of activities for the basic acquisition steps, that is, exposure, recognition, comprehension, and production of the linguistic principles. The second level is labeled the *simple sentence stage*, whereas the third level is the *complex sentence stage*. These latter two levels include activities for each of the areas identified for Level 1 with the addition of activities for sentence analysis. Although syntax serves as the unifying factor of the linguistic portion of the curriculum, it should be stressed that Blackwell et al. (1978) included provisions in their approach for the development of cognition, semantics, and pragmatics. For example, children at the preschool level are introduced to the functional use of language via the use of materials such as storybooks, experience charts, interactive games, and classroom dialogues (teacher-student and so on).

It is important to describe briefly the basic acquisition process (i.e., first step) of Level 1, mentioned previously. During the first step, preschool and kindergarten children are exposed to both the structure and function of language. Exposure to structure includes features such as basic sentence patterns, prepositional phrases, personal pronouns, and transformations (e.g., negation and question form) (see discussion of structures in Chapter 2 of this text). Functional aspects include turn-taking activities, language-play scenarios, and use of sentence types such as declarative and interrogative.

For the second step, recognition, children attempt to identify language features (word, phrase, question, and longer discourse). The act of recognition does not entail comprehension (meaning) of the form. In essence, children's responses, albeit appropriate, are influenced by the pattern of the form. Comprehension of the language form, content, and function is considered during the third step. Whether children recognize or comprehend language features is purported to be judged by their performance during the fourth step—production.

During the second level, children (preschool to about 7 years old) are introduced to five basic sentence patterns, kernel sentences—as illustrated in Table 10-8.

Table 10-8 Sentence Patterns for the Rhode Island Curriculum with Possible Examples

Sentence Pattern	Example		
NP1 + V	The bat	flew.	
NP1 + V + NP2	The bat	ate	insects.
NP1 + LV + Adjective	The bat	is	small.
NP1 + LV + NP2	The bat	is	a vampire bat.
NP1 + LV + Adverbial	The bat	is	in the cave.

Note: Based on Blackwell, Engen, Fischgrund, and Zarcadoolas (1978).
NP = noun phrase
NP1 = noun phrase one
NP2 = noun phrase two
V = verb
LV = linking verb or copula
Adjective = word or words that describes noun phrase
Adverbial = phrase of time or place

When children are competent with the kernel sentences, they should be able to handle complex ones (simple and complex sentences involving transformations), especially those constructed from the basic sentence patterns. For example, after exposure to the following sentences, *The girl hit the ball* and *The girl ran to first base*, the child is ready for *The girl hit the ball and ran to first base*.

It should be mentioned that the basic sentence patterns (e.g., one to five) do not represent a specific order of progression. Instruction of these patterns should not emphasize simple rote memorization. Activities should be developed that enable children to internalize both the form of the structures and the semantic relations as expressed in the word order. In addition, these activities reflect meaningful natural situations of the children. An excellent discussion of this program supported by examples can also be found in McAnally et al. (1994).

The Blackwell et al. (1978) curriculum also contains the coordination of the language goals with the content area goals (i.e., the third component). Thus, language is not to be taught in isolation (for a recent perspective on this issue, see Luetke-Stahlman, 1999). Because language should be used to convey information in content areas such as social studies and mathematics, it is important for teachers to consider not only their students' abilities to understand the content but also their abilities to understand the language through which the information is conveyed.

Test of Syntactic Abilities Syntax Program

The Test of Syntactic Abilities Syntax Program was designed to assist deaf and hard-of-hearing students in the comprehension and production of the nine major syntactic structures, discussed in Chapter 2. For each major structure, there is a teacher's manual, which provides descriptions of the structures, information on the acquisition of the structures by both deaf and hearing students, objectives for teaching the nine structures, diagnostic guides for assessing students' performances on the TSA, and suggestions for additional activities to reinforce the students' learning of the structures. There is also a set of 20 workbooks that correspond to the linguistic components assessed by the TSA and consist of programmed activities related to each major structure. It is not necessary for students to know metalinguistic terminology to complete the activities.

The TSA Syntax Program is based on a large body of information gained by research conducted by Quigley and his associates between 1968 and 1978. The research was motivated by the linguistic thinking of Chomsky (1957, 1965) and its variations. As with any structured program, one of the weaknesses might be that students cannot generalize their understanding to spontaneous productions. As a result, the authors suggested the use of more natural activities in the teachers' guides to assist students in the generalization process. It should be remembered that the materials covered only the syntactic component of English. Thus, Quigley and Power (1979) remarked that this program should be used as part of a language program that includes all major components of English. It is implied that any language program should be well supported by theory and research.

A good discussion of other combined approaches, including multimedia ones, can be found in McAnally et al. (1994).

Table 10-9 provides some highlights of the combined approaches.

Table 10-9 Highlights of Combined Approaches

Highlights of Combined Approaches

- In general, combined approaches involve the teaching of language in natural meaningful situations with structured symbol systems. A combined approach is considered to be a balanced position because of the use of features—the best features—of both natural and structured methods.

- Three representative combined approaches discussed in the chapter are the maternal reflective method, Rhode Island Curriculum, and the Test of Syntactic Abilities Syntax Program.

- In general, the maternal reflective method focuses on the development of the mother tongue (i.e., native home language) through the use of communicative dialogues similar to those advocated by social-interactionists. Children should also be made aware of the conversations of other classmates.

Rhode Island Curriculum (RIC)

- The theoretical basis for the Rhode Island Curriculum is the early work of Chomsky with respect to transformational generative grammar theory. There is also some influence from the work of Piaget.

- The Rhode Island Curriculum is considered a combined approach because of its focus on linguistic knowledge and spontaneous language development.

- The RIC contains three major components: language framework and instructional procedures, the curriculum, and content area goals.

- The curriculum component has three levels. The first level consists of activities for the basic acquisition steps; the second level contains simple sentences; and the third level is the complex sentence stage.

- During the first step of the first level, students are exposed to the structures (e.g., words and phrases) and functions (e.g., turn-taking activities) of language. During the second step of the first level, children engage in recognizing language features such as words, phrases, and questions. Comprehension of the language form, content, and function occurs during the third step.

- During the second level, children are introduced to the five sentence patterns—kernel sentences—and address complex sentences (i.e., some transformations of kernel sentences) during the third level.

- For the content area goals, teachers are encouraged to evaluate and work on students' abilities to understand content subjects (e.g., science and social studies), including the language (e.g., metalanguage) used to convey such information.

Test of Syntactic Abilities Syntax Program

- The TSA Syntax Program is a set of programmed materials (i.e., systematic, reinforced, and sequential) that provides exercises and activities for specific syntactic structures. The TSA Syntax Program can be used with the Test of Syntactic Abilities or with other language assessment programs.

- The program consists of 20 workbooks, divided into nine sets, focusing on the following nine structures: negation, conjunction, determiners, question formation, verb processes, pronominalization, relativization, complementation, and nominalization (discussed in Chapter 2). The program should be considered as supplemental instructional materials—not as a complete curriculum for language development.

- The program materials were designed for deaf and hard-of-hearing children 10 years old and older who are experiencing difficulties with the nine syntactic structures emphasized. It can also be used with children learning English as a second language.

(continues)

(Table 10-9 continued)

- The teacher needs to develop situations that provide opportunities for generalization and application of the language principles.

Brief Synthesis of Structured and Natural Approaches and Materials

In sum, the structured approaches epitomize the teachability of language, especially via the use of written language. There are numerous principles associated with the use of structured approaches in both first and second language teaching (see discussions in McLaughlin, 1985; Rice & Schiefelbusch, 1989; Wiig & Semel, 1984). With a focus on skills such as morphology and syntax, McAnally et al. (1994) highlighted some of these principles, taken from Wiig and Semel (1984):

- *Unfamiliar words and sentence formation rules should be presented according to normal language developmental sequences or established orders of difficulty.*
- *The words featured in the phrases, clauses, and sentences used for intervention should be highly familiar. They may be selected from vocabulary lists for age or grade levels at least 3 years or grades below the child's current vocabulary age or grade level.*
- *Sentence length in number of words should be kept to an absolute minimum. This may be achieved by limiting sentence length to 5 to 10 words and phrase and clause length to 2 to 4 words. Minimum sentence length will depend upon the syntactic complexity of the units for which the rules apply.*
- *Pictorial or printed representation of words, phrases, or clauses should be given for all spoken sentences. Pictures or referents for content words with referential meaning may be used in association with printed representations of nonreferential or function words.*
- *Unfamiliar words or sentence formation rules should be introduced in at least 10 illustrated examples. The examples should feature different word selections.*
- *Knowledge of word or sentence formation rules should be established first in recognition and comprehension tasks and then in formulation tasks.*
- *The knowledge and control of word and sentence formation rules should be established first with highly familiar word choices. It should then be extended to contexts with higher level or less familiar vocabulary or with unfamiliar concepts.*

- *The knowledge and use of words and sentence formation rules should be tested in at least 10 examples that feature vocabulary not previously used. (pp. 436–437)*

The structured approach is also associated with the concept of direct instruction or precision teaching (McAnally et al., 1987, 1994; Schirmer, 1994). Some of the basic tenets of direct instruction include: explicit teaching of rules and strategies, selection of examples, sequencing of examples, and the principle of covertization (i.e., internalizing the rules and principles). The beginning stages of direct instruction require explicit instruction of the application of rules. The thinking process is made overt and observable (Carnine, Silbert, & Kameenui, 1990). Next, a series of examples are used for guided practice and the teaching of the rule. The examples are similar enough to foster generalization to future similar examples. The use of leading questions and overt steps enable the teacher to know whether students are following specific thinking processes.

There are many descriptions of direct instruction or precision teaching. With respect to these, it should be emphasized that with adequate systematic practice and review, students are expected to demonstrate mastery at every step of the way, motivated by positive teacher feedback. The ultimate goal is for the student to proceed from a dependence on teacher-directed activities toward independent work.

It is often difficult to separate structured strategies from natural strategies—in fact, there appears to be general strategies that can be found across many approaches. For example, there are broad strategies such as modeling, role playing, prompting, coaching, and scripting (Luetke-Stahlman, 1998, 1999; McAnally et al., 1994; Polloway & Smith, 1992; Schirmer, 1994). Via modeling, teachers demonstrate the appropriate use of language in any situation. Role playing provides opportunities for students to practice or develop further the newly acquired skills. The other three strategies—prompting, coaching, and scripting (i.e., writing)—require extensive efforts on the part of the teacher.

Other instructional strategies often associated with direct instruction are similar to those discussed previously for structured approaches (e.g., correct-incorrect, completion, replacement, and so on). For example, there are a variety of methods that can be used for working on morphology and syntax. McAnally et al. (1994) described a few of these models and provided examples. In my view, the work of Muma (1971) is most reflective of the various approaches, including subsequent variations and extensions, and can be used in either structured or natural approaches. Muma (1971) delineated 10 broad techniques that focus on both syntax and semantics. Table 10-10 presents a few of these techniques.

Table 10-10 Broad Techniques That Focus on Syntax and Semantics (Muma, 1971)

- Correction: The teacher identifies and corrects students' errors. It is recommended that this approach be used judiciously because of the negative effects associated with overuse. One possible example: Child says or writes *The woman writed a book*; teacher responds with *The woman wrote a book*.

- Expansion: The teacher adds to a child's short utterance. This procedure can help children learn syntax if they pay attention to the newly added features, which have been omitted in their utterances. Example: The child says *Boy run to store*; teacher responds *The boy is running to the store*.

- Expatiation: Here, the teacher adds semantic features in response to the statements of children. This is different from expansion and may be confusing. The child says an utterance such as *A pencil*; the teacher might expand this to *Yes, this is a long, skinny, yellow pencil.*

- Completion: With this approach, the child is exposed to a stimulus in an attempt to elicit a syntactically correct form. One example is the use of a cloze procedure. Teacher utters *The girl is _____ a book*; child might respond with *reading* or *writing*, depending on the pictured stimulus.

- Combination: Presented with a series of short sentences, the child is required to combine them into one. Possible example: Teacher utters *The man is writing a book* and *The man is in his office*; child responds *The man is writing a book in his office*. A more simple variation of this approach is also possible.

Teacher:	Dad is working.
Child:	Dad is in the office.
Teacher:	Dad is busy.
Child:	Dad is busy working in the office.
	(McAnally, Rose, and Quigley, 1994, p. 143)

- Revision: With this approach, the child is required to retell a story in his or her own words after hearing the story by an adult. This is similar to the retelling technique used in reading lessons. In general, the retelling technique compels the child to paraphrase or to use his or her own language. It is also possible for the child to use some of the other strategies, described earlier, in his or her retelling rendition. In some cases, this results in the use of additional vocabulary or even syntactic transformations, creating more complex syntactic structures.

Example:

Teacher: Professors teach classes. Professors serve on committees. Professors also write articles and books. Professors need to do these activities well in order to obtain tenure in the university.

Student: To obtain tenure in a college or university, professors need to demonstrate excellent work in a number of activities within three general domains—instruction, scholarship, and service.

The next section discusses the notion of best method or approach. By now, some understanding of this issue can be gleaned from what was presented thus far in this chapter. That both natural and structured approaches have a place in language instruction can also be seen in the extensive review and examples by the recent work of Luetke-Stahlman (1998, 1999). Luetke-Stahlman (1998) provided examples to facilitate development of language form (structure), content (meaning), and use (function). Based on her synthesis, Luetke-Stahlman seemed to argue that there is no such thing as one best language method for all of each area—that is, for all of form or content or use.

LANGUAGE INSTRUCTION AND BEST METHOD

One of the most controversial and long-standing issues in the teaching of language to deaf and hard-of-hearing children and adolescents is the notion of best method (Moores, 1996; Paul, 1998a). To illustrate the major tenets of this issue, the exemplary survey research of King (1984) is discussed, and some principles discussed by Prabhu (1990) are conveyed.

King (1984) sent questionnaires to 576 programs for deaf and hard-of-hearing students throughout the United States. The questionnaires requested information on the materials and techniques teachers used in their language programs. The focus was on use, not effectiveness. This survey was considered the first generally available rendition of this issue since 1949. A survey on literacy materials was conducted by LaSasso and Mobley (1997) and is discussed in Chapter 8.

The respondents in the King (1984) study were requested to describe the language program as structural, natural, combined, or eclectic (see Table 10-1, presented previously). Results reveal that at all education levels (preschool, primary, intermediate, junior high, and high school), the combined approaches were the most frequently used approaches. Percentages of use range from 36% at the preschool level to about 56% at the intermediate level. In addition, at the preschool level, 34% of the respondents indicated the use of natural approaches. The use of the natural approaches at other levels ranged from 1.5% at the junior high level to 6.2% at the primary level. With the exclusion of the preschool level, the second most frequently reported approach, was the eclectic approach with percentages ranging from a little more than 27% at the primary level to more than 39% at the high school level.

King (1984) reported that a majority of the programs used some type of metalinguistic symbol system in the teaching of English. As discussed previously, the use of metalinguistic symbol systems is often observed for structural and combined approaches. The various language teaching systems ranged from those based on traditional/structural views to those based on transformational generative grammar. Many educational programs employed more than one symbol system.

In essence, it was reported that preschool programs classified their language curricula as natural or combined whereas those for older students (i.e., primary through high school levels) described their programs as combined and eclectic. In addition, it was stated that most respondents felt that it is better to combine several methods rather than rely exclusively on a single all-encompassing approach.

The works of King (1984), McAnally et al. (1994), and others (Luetke-Stahlman, 1998, 1999; Luetke-Stahlman & Luckner, 1991; Paul, 1998a; Schirmer, 1994) seem to indicate that there is no overall best method or that it might be counterproductive to even to continue to search for one that can be applied to all or even most students in a predominant manner. For many teachers, including those who work with deaf and hard-of-hearing children, this might not be an earth-shaking conclusion. Perhaps the notion of an objective best method has always caused skepticism in the field of deaf education.

With respect to the objectivity of a best method, it might be that teachers have a right to be skeptical. There have been three broad interpretations of this issue:

1. *Different methods are best for different teaching contexts;*

2. *All methods are partially true or valid; and,*

3. *The notion of good and bad methods is itself misguided. (Prabhu, 1990, p. 161)*

Some theorists and researchers have argued that it is nearly impossible to use objective experimental (i.e., positivistic and quantitative) research to evaluate

Items 1 and 2 from Prabhu. The assumption is that there is a complex web of interactions within the teaching/learning situation that causes the results of experimental or clinical research to be limited or impractical. That is, the success of a method in a laboratory-like setting with extraneous variables controlled may not be applicable to a classroom setting where it is nearly impossible to duplicate the conditions.

The traditional definition of a method has been considered to be too limited because it fails to consider the complex array of interactions between teachers and students. Delineating a series of steps or procedures for a particular method to be rendered in a research-controlled situation is quite different from what actually happens in a classroom. Depending on the students' needs, teachers might need to develop (i.e., ad lib) additional steps or procedures—even additional probes or modeling techniques, as in scaffolding—to assist the student in understanding a particular topic or even to encourage the student to respond to a question or task. This series of procedures might vary from student to student and even varies across the time of the school day or year.

It is not difficult to provide examples. Suppose students have read a story about bats and are required to answer comprehension questions. Some students might provide complete answers to questions such as: *What do bats look like?* and *How do people feel about bats?* However, other students might need probes or additional information to assist or encourage them to respond to these questions. Some examples for *What do bats look like?* include *What is on the bodies of bats? Are bats similar to birds? Are bats big or small or both? Do bats have fur on their bodies? What does the skin of bat feel like, according to the story?* and *Tell me about the wingspan of bats.* These probes not only differ in application from student to student, but they also might be used as strategies to assist students in remembering details about the size and appearance of bats (examples based on the work of Jackson et al., 1997).

The notion of method has been the subject of a long-standing argument by qualitative researchers (see discussion in Brumfit, 1984; Prabhu, 1990). At best, the research-controlled descriptions of best methods should be used as guidelines not in a cookbook style, as is often the case. In essence, the notion of best method is misguided; the best one can hope for is an understanding of the teacher-learner situation via the use of qualitative (and possibly critical) research approaches (Brumfit, 1984; Prabhu, 1990). This situation is not unique to language teaching situations. For example, in literacy, the pursuit of a best method of teaching vocabulary has been relatively unproductive (see reviews in Paul, 1996, 1998a). The tentative conclusion is that vocabulary learning is so incredibly complex (e.g., words are similar to little universes) that a variety of methods might need to be used for various purposes (also see Chapter 8 of this text). This explains why the relationship between vocabulary knowledge and reading comprehension is still not completely understood; some scholars say it will never be completely understood. In addition, as with language teaching methods, it is often difficult to explain what is meant by a vocabulary teaching method.

Reflecting on the either-or dichotomy that exists in deaf education, that is, the selection of either natural or structural methods, Quigley and Paul (1994) reasoned:

> *A combination of natural and more structured language development practices relative to the involvement and skill of the teacher and the reactions and responses of the students seems to be the most productive approach. As in communication approaches, the field in theory, although perhaps not in practice, keeps swinging from one approach to the other, from natural to structured and back again. This alone is usually a strong indication that each approach, by itself, holds only part of the answer. (p. 271)*

Brief Remarks on Language Intervention Approaches and Strategies

It is not difficult to find texts that focus on language instruction for students who are deaf and hard-of-hearing (Luetke-Stahlman, 1998, 1999; Luetke-Stahlman & Luckner, 1991; McAnally et al., 1994; Schirmer, 1994), students with disabilities (Polloway & Smith, 1992), or for typical and other types of children (e.g., at risk and second language learners) (Bochner et al., 1997; Budwig, 1995). In most of the texts, there are discussions of language intervention activities for children at particular age or grade levels—for example, preschool, elementary, middle school, and secondary. Nearly all of the texts mentioned here stress natural, meaningful language use and, occasionally, the use of structured approaches in naturally occurring language situations. The point here is that language development, especially for students who are experiencing difficulty is very labor intensive, and success may be incremental for many individuals.

Although there is no magic bullet, three previously mentioned issues are discussed here: language-enrichment environment, intervention activities, and the personnel involved in language intervention programs. No matter what language teaching approach is used, it is important for the teacher/practitioner to ensure that the environment is conducive—actually enriching—for language development. For example, Dudley-Marling and Searle (1988) proffered four guidelines for establishing such an environment. First, the milieu should be one that encourages speaking (or signing). One of the major problems in many classrooms is that teachers do too much talking (signing), directing, and so on. To stimulate student talk, teachers (and others) should plan activities in which students work and discuss together to solve problems, answer questions, and perform tasks. The second guideline is that the teacher should provide numerous opportunities for students to use language. Providing students opportunities to lead discussions, teach a portion of the class, report on experiences, and so on are examples. The third guideline is to establish situations for students to use language for a variety of purposes and with different audiences. It should be clear that the language people use varies according to one's purposes and audiences. This is a major axiom for developing writing skills (see Chapter 8); indeed, skills such as identifying the audience, the purpose of writing, and the use of specific vocabulary and grammatical structures are considered higher level skills. The fourth and last guideline is that the teacher should strongly encourage students to use speech (or signs). This is obviously very difficult because if students have difficulty with expressing themselves, they are likely to avoid answering questions or responding to language-generating tasks. Even more problematic, such students tend to avoid social situations, which will be detrimental not only for their language growth but also for their social development (see discussion in Ninio & Snow, 1996).

With respect to language intervention, there are a number of activities that teachers (and others) can use to develop receptive and expressive performance (speech and/or sign) language skills. Some of these examples can be found in the texts mentioned earlier. One of the most popular activities is to use a language experience approach. Another is to create meaningful tasks within classroom settings. For example, students can proceed with a walk around and near the school building and list the names of plants, trees, flowers, and animals. This can be the basis of a classroom activity in which they can develop (paint, draw, etc.) pictures. Each student can require a classmate to name and describe the picture and relate it to the outside experience—that is, the walk. This activity can be extended to include the use of adjectives such as *rough, soft, beautiful, ugly, tall, short,* and so on. Depending on the skills of the students, the teacher can develop phonemic awareness activities (see Chapter 8) and others involving close attention to the sounds or parts of words. There are numerous exercises that have been developed with the use of a tape recorder for developing listening and identification skills and for fostering conversations and discussions (Glazzard, 1982; Leverentz & Garman, 1987). Similar activities can be developed using signs and videotapes. In essence, one of the major goals is to enrich both the receptive and expressive skills of students using meaningful language stimuli and to encourage students to become active participants and conversation partners (role play as teachers and so on).

Previously, it was mentioned that language development should not be the responsibility of only the classroom teacher. Other personnel should also be involved. With respect to deaf and hard-of-hearing students, this includes at least speech pathologists and parents—although it may include other school personnel as well as significant others in the child's life. Whoever is involved should participate in a collaborative manner to ensure continuity and reinforcement. There is no question that parents (or caregivers) have a major role. Language intervention can be beneficial without the support of parents but should be more so with their involvement. Professionals need to make a concerted attempt to involve parents in this process, especially parents of children with hearing impairment (Luetke-Stahlman, 1998, 1999). Parents need to be encouraged to stimulate and respond to their children's communicative efforts. Children need to have numerous opportunities to use their language skills. It has been argued that the generalization and use of language skills are strengthened if children are encouraged to participate in all relevant settings, for example, in school, the home, and in the community.

Finally, Bochner et al. (1997) strongly emphasized the importance of involving others in the child's language program, especially other typical young children who are siblings and friends:

> *Make sure that everyone who has contact with the child, including parents, siblings, other family members, teachers, the babysitter and other carers know about your current goals. Encourage them to practise these goals with the child if there is an appropriate opportunity. Use a communication or language book to let others know what you are doing and encourage them to keep you informed about anything relevant. Put notes on the fridge and family or staff notice-boards to remind relevant adults about your current goals.*
>
> *If the child has interested siblings or friends, encourage them to become involved. It is amazing what a child can learn from another more competent child. This also helps overcome the difficulties that are sometimes encountered when one child appears to get more adult attention than others. The "helper" will be rewarded by the attention given to his or her "helpfulness." (p. 55)*

FINAL REMARKS

One of the most controversial long-standing issues in the education of deaf and hard-of-hearing children and adolescents is the manner in which English can be taught most effectively. Stating the issue in this way presumes that language can be taught and that there are methods of teaching that are better than others. Indeed, it is sometime assumed that there might be a best method.

On the other side of the coin is the assertion that language cannot be taught; the best that one can do is to facilitate its development. This chapter describes this situation as the teachability/learnability dichotomy. In one sense, the teachability/learnability dichotomy is also applicable to the question of whether instruction is necessary for literacy development—that is, the development of reading and writing skills.

The use of the teachability/learnability framework seems to have influenced the treatment of much of the content of this chapter. This was intentional and is not merely academic. How one understands and interprets this framework affects one's view on the use of language teaching methods and strategies. It also affects what type of research in which individuals will engage, for example, quantitative and/or qualitative. Ultimately, it determines the nature of the language intervention program for deaf and hard-of-hearing students.

Nevertheless, it is hoped that the reader has concluded that an either-or position is counterproductive—in any case, that is the author's interpretation of the theoretical and research literature. Focusing on the teachability/learnability issue provided the impetus for clarifying and discussing information in several selected areas, for example, representation and teaching/learning, approaches to language instruction, the notion of best method, and the use of language intervention programs and strategies. For each area, a summary of selective major points is presented.

With respect to representation and teaching/learning

- There has been some confusion caused by the terms *representation* and *language teaching*. Representation refers to the manner in which English is represented and includes the so-called invented systems such as cued speech/language and all of the English-based signed systems or manually coded English systems.

- Strictly speaking, representation does not refer to the use of oral methods, which involve the use of speech as the major mode of communication and information exchange.

- What is represented can vary from phonemes to letters to parts of words and whole words.

- The assumption that exposure to an adequate representation of English is sufficient for learning the performance form (speech and/or sign) of a language is tenable—at least from a naturalistic point of view.

Whether this holds true also for developing English literacy skills is debatable.

With respect to the approaches to language instruction

- In general, there are two major approaches to language instruction—structured and natural. When aspects of these major approaches are utilized in a conjoined manner, this is often referred to as a combined approach.

- Structured approaches seem to be motivated by the teachability hypothesis, whereas the natural approaches tend to be influenced by the learnability hypothesis. However, this distinction is not always clear-cut, as evident in the combined approaches. In addition, there are general language strategies (modeling) that can be found in the literature on both broad approaches.

- Within the structured framework, it is asserted that language must be taught. Students are required to engage in attempts to analyze certain grammatical aspects such as noun phrases and verb phrases. Often, programs utilize some type of metalinguistic symbols to mark the grammatical aspects. The structured approach is also associated with direct instruction or precision teaching concepts.

- Major criticisms of the structured approaches include few provisions for generalization of the language principles and the production of stilted written sentences. These criticisms might be shortsighted because there is more to language learning than simply being exposed to language instruction methods or approaches.

- Naturalistic proponents argue that language should be acquired in a holistic natural manner; it should not be taught. In an inquiry manner and within a language-rich social milieu, students can be led to discover and internalize language principles.

- Natural approaches have been influenced by the philosophy of constructivism in which the teacher is considered to be a facilitator or a catalyst—not an individual who is an expert or in control of the classroom situation.

- In general, the combined approach refers to the teaching of language in a natural environment or manner via the use of structured methods.

- A synthesis of the research literature on the use of the various language teaching approaches revealed that there is no superior approach.

In many instances, practitioners either used a combined approach or thought it was best to use more than one approach.

With respect to the notion of best method

- The interpretation of the concept of best method is influenced pervasively by the research or theoretical orientation of the individual.

- If an individual believes that there is such an entity as a best method or even effective methods, that person is likely to hold a philosophical position similar to the one held by quantitative researchers.

- If an individual believes that there is no such entity as a best method, that person is likely to hold a philosophical position similar to the one held by qualitative researchers.

- In essence, when quantitative researchers provide methods, these should be considered guidelines—not as a cookbook for all students for all time.

- Qualitative proponents argue that the best researchers can do is to investigate the teaching-learning situations and avoid wholesale generalizations of findings.

With respect to language intervention programs and strategies

- Three important issues discussed in this chapter were language-enrichment environment, intervention activities, and personnel involved in language intervention programs.

- There is no magic bullet with respect to language development. For deaf and hard-of-hearing children, the development of language requires enormous labor-intensive efforts, and learning occurs in small increments.

- As much as possible, language development should involve all educators and significant others who have a vested interest in the child.

In sum, it should be highlighted that there is a great need for teachers of deaf and hard-of-hearing students to improve their knowledge of the processes of language and literacy. This should not be taken as a denigrating remark; language and literacy are difficult concepts and require constant study. The application of this knowledge is no small feat either. On the basis of research syntheses, the author recommends that teachers become familiar with a wide variety of theory-based instructional strategies, including those that have been used with children who have typical hearing. More important, teachers and educators should avoid what can be construed as either-or instructional decisions.

Language instruction should be evaluated systematically. Typically, evaluation is the domain of language assessment. One of the most problematic issues in deaf education is the lack of or relative lack of an instruction-assessment link. Of course, language assessment is a complicated issue, and this issue is examined in detail in the next chapter.

LANGUAGE INSTRUCTION COMPREHENSION QUESTIONS

1. According to the author, there seems to be some confusion surrounding issues such as the representation of a language versus the teaching/learning of a language. Describe this confusion.

2. There seems to be an ongoing debate between the learnability of language versus the teachability of language. What is learnability? Teachability? Why is there a debate? What are the underpinnings (theoretical, metatheoretical, etc.) of the learnability hypothesis? The teachability hypothesis?

3. There also seems to be a learnability/teachability debate in the field of literacy. What are the issues relative to the teaching of reading (i.e., the major points of Pearson & Johnson, 1978)?

4. Provide some historical perspectives and descriptions of the structured approaches. What are some major tenets of the Fitzgerald Key and APPLE TREE? What are the underpinnings (theories, metatheories, etc.) of these approaches?

5. Provide some historical perspectives and descriptions of the natural approaches. How are these approaches different from the structured approaches (i.e., compare and contrast the two types)? How is the natural approach similar to the use of the scientific method? What are the underpinnings (theories, metatheories, etc.) of the natural approaches?

6. Describe the combined approaches, including the major tenets of the three representative approaches discussed in the chapter.

7. Why is the notion of best method controversial? Is this concept influenced pervasively by a specific metatheory/philosophy or research paradigm (e.g., quantitative or qualitative)?

8. In the last section of the chapter, the author provides his views on three issues: language-enrichment environment, intervention activities, and personnel involvement in language intervention programs. What are some of the major points?

CHALLENGE QUESTIONS

(Note: Complete answers are not in the text. Additional research is required.)

1. The author posed a number of questions/comments at the beginning of the chapter. Consider: "If language can be taught, then one might ask a number of questions, for example, is there a best method or are there effective methods for language instruction? What exactly is taught with respect to language? If a language must be learned or acquired, there are other questions, for example, what conditions are necessary to foster this learning? What exactly is learned? Individuals who are skeptical of the conceptualization of this issue as a dichotomous one might inquire: Is there a middle ground in this debate? Is the debate really necessary? Is it possible to create both natural and structured situations to fit the needs of the learner at various stages in the language acquisition process?"

   Do you feel that the author answered these questions adequately in the chapter? Why or why not? Which questions need more attention? Do you think that there are answers to these questions? If so, select one or more and conduct your own review of the literature. Share your perspectives with your classmates and instructor.

2. In this chapter, you were exposed to several either-or dichotomies, for example, learnability/teachability, natural versus structured methods, and best method versus effective methods.

   What are your perspectives on these either-or dichotomies? Do you favor one side or the other? Have you developed another position? If so, how did you do it? Do you think that there are really scientific answers (now or in the future) to these dichotomies? Why or why not? Are there other questions that should be asked?

3. The author argued that "Historically, there have been two major approaches to language instruction, structural and natural, as well as combinations of these approaches."

   Do you think that this is reflective of what occurs in classroom settings for deaf and hard-of-hearing students? Why or why not? Is it possible to argue that the statement is influenced pervasively by a specific metatheory or research paradigm, for example, positivistic quantitative approaches? Why or why not?

4. In this chapter, much of the emphasis seems to be on what language teaching approaches have been used with deaf and hard-of-hearing students. There does not seem to be much research on the effectiveness of these approaches. In your view, what types of research need to be conducted? Is your answer influenced by a particular philosophy or research paradigm? Is it really possible to assess the merits of teaching—whether it be the teaching of language, reading, or some other content area? Why or why not?

FURTHER READINGS

Cazden, C. (1988). *Classroom discourse: The language of teaching and learning*. Portsmouth, NH: Heinemann.

Duncan, D. (Ed.). (1989). *Working with bilingual language disability: Therapy in practice*. London: Chapman & Hall.

Herriot, P. (1971). *Language and teaching: A psychological view*. London: Methuen.

Locke, J. (1993). *The child's path to spoken language*. Cambridge, MA: Harvard University Press.

Oller, J., & Richard-Amato, P. (Eds.). (1983). *Methods that work: A smorgasbord of ideas for language teachers*. Rowley, MA: Newbury House.

Wells, G. (1985). *Language development in the preschool years*. Cambridge, UK: Cambridge University Press.

CHAPTER 1

Language Assessment

Assessment of students who are not making adequate educational progress is difficult and time-consuming. This task is even more challenging if a student has a physical handicap. Assessment results need to be educationally important, comprehensive, and obtained from tests, and procedures that are reliable, valid and appropriate for the student being tested. If these conditions are met, then the assessment results will contribute valuable information for developing programs that facilitate academic progress. If, however, assessments are not carried out well, then use of inadequate results can further hinder the progress of students. For professionals whose charge it is to conduct psychoeducational assessments, this is a tremendous responsibility. (Bradley-Johnson & Evans, 1991, p. xi)

If language instruction emphasizes the how (e.g., the manner in which language should be taught), then it can be stated that language assessment emphasizes the why (e.g., the reason for teaching language as well as the specific areas of focus). From one perspective, language assessment can be compared to the cornerstone of a building. Relative to the total structure of a building, the cornerstone occupies a limited amount of space. However, in light of its function, the cornerstone can be viewed as an extremely critical component of the building. This analogy applies to the notion of language assessment, which is a critical aspect for the broad area of language instruction or language intervention.

A carefully constructed language assessment program should occupy only a small portion of the designated time for classroom instruction or clinical therapy. For assessment to be effective, at least for instructional purposes, it is important for teachers and others to utilize results from a range of sources, for example, formal and informal tests, observations of student's performance in a variety of situations, and curriculum-based information. The findings of these various measures should also provide teachers and clinicians with sufficient information on students' language skills and progress toward the achievement of instructional or clinical goals. Without assessment, there is no barometer on whether students' language needs are being met. In addition, there is no way to determine the efficiency of instructional or clinical methods.

This chapter provides a brief introductory survey of several important issues in the area of language assessment. For additional specific details on the focus and content of initial and ongoing assessments and establishing relations between instruction and assessment, the reader is referred to other sources (Bradley-Johnson & Evans, 1991; French, 1999; Luetke-Stahlman, 1998). After presenting some general principles on the relation of language and assessment, the purposes and types of assessment are discussed, including some influences from the areas of language development and measurement. Subsequently, some qualities of a good formal test, namely, reliability, validity, and the characteristics of the norming sample are addressed. Some consideration is also given to other critical issues such as selection, administration, interpretation, and the use of informal measures. Also included in this chapter is a brief discussion and synthesis of several methods of assessment as well as selected assessments that are used or can be used with individuals who are deaf and hard of hearing. The selection of the samples is meant to be illustrative and hopefully representative of the types of assessments used. It is hoped that the information in this chapter can assist current and future professionals in obtaining a better understanding of the complexities of language assessment.

The importance of and issues related to language assessment have been expressed:

> To obtain useful assessment results, an examiner must thoroughly understand the type of information that various tests and assessment procedures can provide, as well as the limitations of the information that is obtained. Furthermore, with students who have a physical impairment, such as a hearing loss, one must be familiar with procedures that can circumvent a handicapping condition and understand how the handicap may affect a student's behavior. This knowledge is necessary to

ensure that results accurately reflect a student's aptitude and achievement (Bradley-Johnson & Evans, 1991, p. xi)

Because of the growing support for American Sign Language/English programs, a brief background on the language evaluation of students in bilingual or second language learning programs is provided. Finally, the chapter ends with some reflections on further developments in the area of language assessment as well as a summary of major points.

LANGUAGE AND ASSESSMENT

In assessing and explaining language acquisition, one common area of agreement across several theoretical models (see Chapter 3) is the distinction between knowledge possession and its use, that is, from the learning and the performance points of view (also see Cairns, 1996; de Jong & Verhoeven, 1992; Ingram, 1989). This is analogous to other terms, for example, the competence and performance notions of Chomsky (1957, 1965), the linguistic knowledge and channel control notions of Carroll (1961), or the notions of language as action versus language as system (D. Baker, 1989). These views should be kept in mind relative to the four skills or domains often used to discuss language development: listening (or observing, in the case of signs), speaking (or signing), reading, and writing. Listening (observing) and reading are considered to be *receptive skills,* whereas speaking (signing) and writing are labeled *expressive skills.* These two groups of skills present different types of assessment problems. For example, it is not possible to observe receptive skills directly. In addition, although expressive skills are observable, they may not be indicative of underlying competence. It has also been argued that "all that is observed in performance data is not necessarily skill related" (de Jong & Verhoeven, 1992, p. 8).

Relative to language assessment, several dichotomous models or assessment perspectives have been discussed in the literature, and these frameworks have influenced the development and use of language tests (D. Baker, 1989; Davies, 1990; de Jong & Verhoeven, 1992; Duchan, 1984; Harrison, 1983). The interest here is in those viewpoints that not only have exemplified the distinction between language knowledge and language performance but also have influenced the development and use of controlled and free methods with deaf and hard-of-hearing individuals. In addition, this information is also relevant to the discussion of language assessment and bilingualism (Baetens-Beardsmore, 1986; Cummins, 1984; McLaughlin, 1985). Pertinent to the present purposes, two dichotomies are discussed: direct versus indirect procedures and discrete-point versus integrative measures.

Direct Versus Indirect Procedures

Direct procedures refer to the emphasis on the use of language to communicate or convey information in a natural manner. The language user is presumed to use language rules intuitively to express a message, for example, in spontaneous speech. One of the main goals of this method is to obtain a language sample, either spoken or written, that can be subsequently analyzed. Direct procedures are related to the use of free methods for assessing language performance, as discussed later. Table 11-1 contains a scenario that provides one example of the use of this procedure (see the discussion of free methods later in this chapter).

Table 11-1 Scenario as an Example for the Use of Direct Procedures

---

The examiner sets up a picture that contains a few trees and birds. There are birds (sparrows) on the ground and some resting in the various trees. There are also birds captured in the act of flying toward the trees. The examiner may say to the child/student (Directions may vary given the skill/understanding level of the child/student): "Tell me what you see in this picture. You can name things, count them, and describe them. You can even tell me what is happening or going to happen." The language sample may contain several structures as well as vocabulary items. For example, the child might name, describe, and count the objects/animals such as *trees*, *birds*, *sky*, *grass*, or *ground*. He or she might indicate that there are 10 or 20 birds on the ground, 5 flying in the air, 10 in one tree, and so on. The focus might be on plurality (e.g., *tree, trees*; and *bird, birds*), present progressive (e.g., *A few (or Ten) birds are flying to the tree*), past tense (*A few birds flew to the trees*), and other aspects such as noun-verb agreement, the use of prepositions, and determiners. The language sample may be rich in that it contains a number of features to be analyzed, including target features.

Indirect procedures refer to the conscious reflections of the language user on the language rules that are required to perform or complete a particular linguistic task. These procedures often are indicative of actual testing situations such as paper-and-pencil tasks. The focus is on gathering information about the individual's language proficiency without specific reference to use or purpose. Most language tests fall into this category via the use of test formats such as fill-in-the-blanks or multiple-choice items. Indirect procedures are related to the controlled methods for assessing language performance, which is discussed later. Table 11-2 provides one example of this type.

Table 11-2 Assessing Language Performance: Example of Indirect Procedures (also Controlled Methods)

Language Test Using Indirect Procedures (or Controlled Methods)

Directions: For each item below, underline the right word to complete the sentence.

More than One!

1. The two (womans//women) are sitting on the bench.

2. Yesterday, I saw three (oxes//oxen) in the pasture.

3. How many (potatoes//potatos) did you eat?

4. We saw many (deer//deers) in the forest.

5. Those (ladys//ladies) like to drink tea and eat cookies.

It happened in the past . . .

1. My Dad's car (breaked//broke) down two days ago.

2. Mary (ran//runned) to the store about 5 minutes ago.

3. That woman (swam//swimmed) for 5 miles.

4. My mother (walkt//walked) to the mall.

5. The bird (flied//flew) for a long time.

A more detailed discussion of this dichotomy (i.e., direct vs. indirect procedures) and related issues, such as reliability and validity, can be found elsewhere (D. Baker, 1989; Davies, 1990; de Jong & Verhoeven, 1992). It should be added that both direct and indirect procedures can be used to assess language knowledge and language use. In essence, as with any kind of testing program, it is recommended that more than one type of test be used—that is, an assessment battery. Given the scope and complexity of the domain of language proficiency (form, content, and use), it is also unrealistic to collect data from only a single administration or testing period and expect that information to be reflective of a child's understanding of English or some other language.

Discrete-Point Versus Integrative Measures

Discrete-point measures focus on the evaluation of certain important language elements or skills (e.g., vocabulary, syntax, and distinctive features). In conjunction with a test format such as multiple choice, these measures are termed *objective* and *analytic* (see the earlier example under indirect method) (D. Baker, 1989; de Jong & Verhoeven, 1992). Relative to the test formats of these measures, it has been remarked that:

> *The kind of questions (usually termed "items") which were used included:*
>
> *Multiple choice items*
>
> *Sentences with gaps to be filled*
>
> *Sentences to be transformed in various ways*
>
> *All of these items types have the following characteristics:*
> 1. *There is usually only one possible correct answer for each item.*
> 2. *Each item samples a particular element through the use of one skill.*
> 3. *Items are not dependent on one another—changing one item does not change the testee's performance on the other items of the test—cf. cloze testing. (D. Baker, 1989, p. 34)*

Integrative measures were developed because of debates on the validity of the discrete-point measures—for example, the superficial, unnatural, decontextualized, and mechanical foci of language use (D. Baker, 1989; de Jong & Verhoeven, 1992). The goal of integrative measures is to obtain a global understanding of the language performance of the individual. This involves the use of holistic scoring methods and the focus on the use of language in natural meaningful situations (similar to the earlier example in the direct method). One strong influence of these measures can be seen in the emerging paradigm of writing as a process approach (Bereiter & Scardamalia, 1987; also see the discussion in Chapter 8). That is, instead of focusing on issues such as mechanics, children are encouraged to reflect on issues such as organization, purpose, and audience. Subsequently, they can go back and work on the mechanics, especially if these aspects make it difficult for their audience to understand what they (the authors) are attempting to convey. Besides being time-consuming, integrative measures are subject to problems of reliability and validity (discussed later).

GENERAL ISSUES OF ASSESSMENT AND DEAFNESS

There are several general issues that should be considered prior to, during, and after the testing situation (Anastasi, 1982; Salvia & Ysseldyke, 1991). These issues impact the selection, administration, and interpretation of a test, especially a formal test. The examiner should be well informed on the characteristics of both the test and the subject who is planning to take the test.

Relative to deafness, there are certain background demographics that are important to obtain, such as degree of hearing impairment, age at onset of impairment, etiology (cause), mode of communication, family background information, use of audition and vision, ethnic and cultural status, and the presence of additional disabilities (Bradley-Johnson & Evans, 1991; Paul & Jackson, 1993; Vernon & Andrews, 1990). These characteristics are important in determining whether a particular test is appropriate for the deaf individual. That is, it needs to be determined whether the characteristics of the sample (on normed tests) reflect the characteristics of the individual taking the test. The use and interpretation of a formal test that has not been normed on the specific sample of test-takers need to proceed with caution. It is possible, of course, to use the items as part of an informal, teacher-made, or teacher-adapted test; however, this definitely changes the interpretative function associated with that item on the original test.

Paul and Jackson (1993) listed several variables that should be considered to ensure that formal (and in many cases informal) evaluations are fair, objective, and useful: "background information on the client or test taker; ethical considerations; definition and purpose of the test; standardization of procedures; technical quality—reliability and validity; and representativeness of the sample" (p. 240). It is also important to utilize information from other sources to supplement the results of the test (Moores, 1987, 1996; Vernon & Andrews, 1990). Such sources can include files, results of interviews, and data from observations.

Within this line of thinking, it is critical to emphasize the need for considering informal and other alternative measurements in conjunction with formal tests. Despite the shortcomings of these informal methods, they do provide diagnostic information; that is, it is possible to assess a student's performance on specific language tasks or skills that are often stated in the curriculum. There are a number of informal assessment strategies, for example, self-evaluation checklists, portfolios, and observations of student's classroom performance (debates, answering questions, storytelling, role playing, etc.). In many cases, the use of alternative assessment provides more in-depth information on the child's language use than the use of formal tests alone.

Observation of performance is probably the most frequently used strategy with infants and young children; however, it can be and should be used with older children who are deaf and hard of hearing. Of course in many cases, this type of information on young deaf and hard-of-children may be more reliable and valid than that resulting from the use of standardized assessments, which are difficult to use and interpret with such children. The use of observation strategies for data collection is more time-consuming than utilizing a standardized formal measure. The examiner should gather information on the culture and values of the family. Other sources of information include observations of the child and others in both school and family environments. This can involve settings such as the classroom, playground, and the home. Observation is considered a type of ecological assessment (for a discussion of this strategy in literacy, see Paul, 1998a). In sum, a number of strategies have been suggested for conducting observations (Luckasson et al, 1992; Tierney, Carter, & Desai, 1991):

1. Observe students in a variety of natural meaningful settings.
2. Obtain in-depth information from interviewing significant others in these settings.
3. Utilize case histories, individualized educational plans, teacher reports, and other paperwork on the student.

And, as a reminder of the limitations of using only one assessment:

4. Use several types of assessments to collect information on the desired academic and social behaviors. Involve other professionals in administering and participating in the assessment process so that findings from several sources can be compared.

Finally, the use of behavior observation is important for obtaining a language sample of the deaf and hard-of-hearing child. This issue is discussed in the section on free methods.

The aforementioned information can also be presented in a portfolio approach, an approach that seems to be gaining in use in education. The portfolio can document language development in an individualized manner. It is a collection of representative, ongoing samples of a student's performance. The portfolio contains descriptive data, including samples of writing and recorded observations on language performance. This is a labor-intensive process; thus, a systematic plan for collecting and evaluating data needs to be implemented. In addition, the portfolio should not simply be a scrapbook of performance items. There should be a diagnostic function based on the interpretation of the collected data.

As much as possible, the student should participate in the collection and evaluation of information. In conferences with the teacher (or even significant others such as parents), the student can conduct a self-evaluation of the portfolio. This evaluation should include decisions on the types of products that can be placed in the portfolio as well as a discussion of the current progress and future goals. It is best for the teacher to play the role of facilitator; that is, the teacher should assist the student in becoming skilled at identifying his or her needs and establishing and implementing a plan for addressing these areas. Obviously, the role of the student in the portfolio depends on the maturity and skills of the respective student. It might be helpful for parents or significant others to play this role—that is, be the student's advocate or voice.

Table 11-3 presents a few points about the portfolio. Keep in mind that these points are suggestive in nature.

Table 11-3 A Few Points on the Use of Portfolios

- The data for the portfolio can be organized with respect to school's subjects or content areas, for example, language, literacy, mathematics, science and so on.

- For each category or area, information can be subdivided in response to questions such as: What do I (or the parent or, if possible, the child) know about the child's performance in this area? How do I know that? Do I have sufficient information to plan and/or continue to plan instruction, especially with respect to instructional strategies? Am I (or the parent or, if appropriate, the child) clear on the areas that are in need of improvement?

- For each category or area, it might be helpful to develop a checklist for collecting or interpreting information. For example, with respect to performance (i.e., oral, sign, or both), the teacher might want to observe or collect data relative to a pragmatic skills checklist (the use of Halliday's functions) or a syntax checklist (e.g., the Test of Syntactic Abilities). In the area of reading, some possible items for young children include print awareness, book concepts, the concept of a word, phonemic segmentation, speech-to-print match, and answering different levels of questions.

- Other questions/items relative to reading might include:

  Can the student identify words automatically and fluently?

  When reading orally (or with signs), does the student correct reading errors? What type of clues does the student use (graphic, meaning, and others)?

  Can a student successfully comprehend both narrative and informational (i.e., expository) material?

(continues)

(Table 11-3 continued)

What is the quality of the student's comprehension?

Can the student organize and recall information from texts?

Can the student answer different types of questions (i.e., literal and inferential)?

- It is also important to include information about the child's interests with respect to, for example, topics for reading and writing, desire to read and write outside the classroom, and so on. These interests are critical for motivational purposes in planning instruction for that child. There are a number of questions that can be asked in an interview (with parent present) based on the skill level of the child. Some possible questions include: What is reading (or writing)? What do people read or write? Describe yourself as a reader or writer. Do you like to read or write? Why or why not? Would you like to become a better reader or writer? Why or why not? What is it about reading or writing you do not understand? What would you like to read or write about? and so on.

- It is possible to utilize checklists that have been used for informal language and literacy inventories and other diagnostic measures; however, one of the major reasons for checklists or other information in the portfolio is to provide diagnostic information. Not only is it critical to know what the student can do and is interested in, it is also important to plan for further development of the student's skills.

Note: For additional details on what can be placed in a portfolio for deaf and hard-of-hearing students, see French (1999) and Luetke-Stahlman (1998).

CHARACTERISTICS OF ASSESSMENT

Three of the most important characteristics of assessment, particularly for formal measures, are reliability, validity, and practicality (Anastasi, 1982; Borg & Gall, 1983; Harrison, 1983; Salvia & Ysseldyke, 1991). In essence, these concepts can be applied to all measures: formal, informal, and unobtrusive observational assessment (i.e., alternative measures). Although alternative measures (observations, etc.) can and should be used to validate or complement formal data, the reliability and validity of alternative measures themselves should be and can be ascertained (via the use of interrater procedures, conferences, etc.). It is important for teachers and clinicians to seek objective information about the reliability and validity of a particular formal test. The criteria used for evaluating practicality depends on the needs of teachers, clinicians, and administrators.

Reliability

Reliability is concerned with the consistency of test results regarding the performances of students (Anastasi, 1982; Borg & Gall, 1983; Salvia & Ysseldyke, 1991). That is, reliability refers to the consistency or stability of test scores. There needs to be some confidence that the test scores are reflective of a student's performance even if the student retook the test a short time later. For formal, norm-referenced tests, the most common procedures for determining reliability are alternate (or parallel) forms, test-retest, and internal consistency. For informal assessment, the commonly used procedures are interexaminer and intraexaminer procedures.

Validity

The concept of validity refers to the question of whether a test measures what it is designed to measure (Anastasi, 1982; Borg & Gall, 1983; Salvia & Ysseldyke, 1991). It is also possible to assess validity by comparing the findings of a test with those from observational and clinical situations. There are several types of validity, for example, face, content, construct, concurrent, and predictive.

Highlights and additional details on the concepts of reliability and validity are presented in Table 11-4. The reader should consult other sources for examples involving computation procedures (Anastasi, 1982; Borg & Gall, 1983; Salvia & Ysseldyke, 1991).

Table 11-4 Highlights and Additional Information on the Concepts of Reliability and Validity

Reliability

- The concept is concerned with the consistency or stability of test results. Reliability refers to the degree to which test scores are representative of students' actual performances.

- For formal, norm-referenced tests, the most common procedures are alternate (or parallel) form, test-retest, and internal consistency. Alternate form involves the computation of a correlation coefficient between the two equivalent forms of the test. This is the most commonly used estimate of reliability for standardized tests. Test-retest refers to the administration of the same test. Internal consistency includes the use of analysis of variance computations, for example, the method of rational equivalence involving the Kuder-Richardson 20 and 21 formulas and the use of Cronbach's (1960) coefficient alpha.

(continues)

(Table 11-4 continued)

- The concept of equivalent or parallel forms is not without its difficulties. The two tests might differ significantly in content to such an extent that the concept of equivalence would not be valid. In this case, the reliability coefficient might be underestimated. On the other hand, the two forms might be so closely matched in content that the estimated correlation coefficient might represent an overestimation of reliability. Thus, teachers and clinicians should seek the test developer's justification of equivalency. In addition, it should be ensured that a sufficient amount of time has elapsed between the administration of the first and second parallel forms.

- Test-retest procedure refers to the administration of the same test (i.e., the same form) twice. The correlation coefficient for this procedure is typically higher than that obtained for alternate form procedure. One reason for the higher correlation might be the students' recall of their answers to specific items. On the other hand, a lower correlation might result if test takers become annoyed by the familiarity of the test. Thus, it is important to ensure that a sufficient time has elapsed between the two administrations. However, this does not guarantee an accurate correlation score.

- To save time and to minimize the problems associated with repeated testing, several methods can be used to determine the reliability of a test based on a single administration. These measures are considered internal consistency measures. Typically, the procedures entail the dividing of a test into two equal parts and comparing the students' performance on both parts. In this case, it must be ensured that both parts of the tests are equivalent in some fashion.

- For informal assessments, the commonly used procedures are interexaminer and intraexaminer procedures. Interexaminer procedure refers to the degree of agreement between different evaluators' judgments of the same data. In the intraexaminer procedure, the evaluator judges either two sets of highly similar or identical data after a period of time has elapsed.

- Relative to informal assessments, including direct, integrative, or spontaneous language samples, it might be necessary to assess reliability based on the extent to which independent analyses concur relative to the students' responses or levels of achievement. Because these evaluations are exposed to the same training procedures, it is expected that there will be a high correlation between their conclusions. This agreement aids in the interpretation of the results. Interexaminer procedures are analogous to the notion of internal consistency procedures for standardized tests discussed previously.

Intraexaminer procedures are analogous to the test-retest procedures for standardized test discussed previously.

Validity

- This concept refers to the question of whether a test measures what it is designed to measure.

- Validity can be assessed by comparing the findings of a test with those from observational and clinical situations.

- There are several types of validity—face, content, construct, concurrent, and predictive.

- Face validity is concerned with the appropriateness of a specific test for the individual. For example, the test takers should understand the purpose of the test and the manner in which they should respond (i.e., directions). One of the most important aspect of face validity is students' attitude toward the test. As discussed previously in test-retest procedures, this aspect can affect the reliability of the test.

- Content validity is also known as rational or logical validity. It is important to be aware of the assumptions of the test developers and the literature that is relevant to the variables of interest. Thus, content validity involves a comparison of the representativeness and appropriateness of the content of the test in question with the content of other similar tests that have been used.

- Construct validity refers to the degree to which the test in question is representative of a specific theoretical construct. For example, suppose that a theory maintains that the syntactic development of deaf students is qualitatively similar (i.e., manner of acquisition is similar) to that of hearing students. If a particular measurement verifies this similarity for structures such as negation and relative clauses, then construct validity has been established for hearing status relative to these two syntactic variables.

- Concurrent validity can be ascertained via the evaluation of one measure by another one that represents the same criterion. This type of validity is important for the adoption of new assessments. In essence, the scores on the new test are compared to the scores on another older test that contains different items but is said to measure the same behavior.

(continues)

(Table 11-4 continued)

- Predictive validity refers to the degree to which a test can predict an individual's performance in a future situation. This type of validity is critical for assessments that are employed to classify or select persons for specific areas, for example, entrance into college or a special education program.

Note: Adapted from Borg and Gall (1983) and Salvia and Ysseldyke (1991).

Practicality

There are several issues relative to practicality, such as the amount of time for test administration, special equipment needs, costs of test materials and scoring procedures, and special arrangement needs (for individual testing and for individuals with special needs). The issues of practicality should not be underestimated. For example, test developers might have a highly reliable and valid test, but it might be impractical for instructional environments because of the amount of time required to administer it. In essence, practicality is important for the marketability of a specific test. It has been stated:

> *In brief, tests should be economical as possible in time (preparation, sitting and marketing) and in cost (materials and hidden costs of time spent). This sounds a very obvious statement to make, but it is easy to lose sight of overall efficiency in the detailed work required to prepare appropriate and useful tests. (Harrison, 1983, p. 13)*

PURPOSES AND TYPES OF ASSESSMENT

With the brief introductory background on the theoretical foundations and characteristics of good tests, one can proceed with a discussion of purposes and types of assessments. The selection of a test or a battery of tests is influenced markedly by several factors. For example, the important factors of reliability, validity, and practicality have been discussed. Test examiners also have to decide whether they are interested in assessing only one component of language, for example, syntax, or all of language, that is, the four or five major components. In addition, they need to decide how language should be assessed; this was the focus of the information discussed previously in models of language assessment. Another area of concern is whether the test or battery of tests is appropriate for the population being assessed, in this case, individuals with severe to profound hearing impairment. It is obvious that there is no cookbook for the selection of a test or a battery of tests; however, the information presented thus far should be considered guidelines.

Perhaps one of the most important factors to consider in the selection of a test or a battery of tests is the purpose of the evaluation. This issue in turn affects the type of assessment. Type of assessment also determines the method that will be employed to collect the data. For example, norm-referenced and criterion-referenced tests typically employed the use of controlled methods (discussed in the next section). The use of observations might entail the use of free methods (also discussed later); it is also a type of informal assessment.

Several conceptualizations exist relative to types (i.e., functions) of assessment (D. Baker, 1989; Davies, 1990; Harrison, 1983). For example, Davies (1990) categorized test types as *achievement, proficiency, aptitude,* and *diagnostic.* Harrison (1983) used the terms *placement, achievement, proficiency,* and *diagnostic.* This chapter focuses on three labels: *achievement, diagnostic,* and *proficiency.* The differences among these types can be discussed relative to the variables of time and content (Davies, 1990; Harrison, 1983).

Achievement

An achievement test can also be labeled as an *attainment* or *summative test* (Harrison, 1983). The achievement test is typically used at the end of a particular period of time or of learning. The information on the test is supposed to be a representative sample of the content covered during that time frame. The time frame might be associated with a school year, an academic course, or high school or college career.

The achievement test is typically manifested as a standardized (i.e., norm-referenced) test (Anastasi, 1982; Borg & Gall, 1983; Salvia & Ysseldyke, 1991). Borg and Gall (1983) described the standardized test as:

> One . . . *that produces very similar results when different persons administer and score the measure following the instructions given and . . . for which normative data are present to describe how subjects from specified populations perform. (p. 272)*

In essence, the student's overall performance is compared with other students at the same age or grade level.

The use and development of standardized tests for deaf students have been long-standing controversial issues in the education of these students (Moores, 1987, 1996; Paul, 1998a; Paul & Jackson, 1993; Vernon & Andrews, 1990). One major problem has been the accuracy (i.e., validity) of the norms—particularly as they relate to the content of the test and the type of student taking the test. As described by Harrison (1983):

*The conditions for setting an achievement test . . . brings up problems
of sampling, since what has been learnt in a year (for example) cannot be assessed in one day, yet the test must reflect the content of the
whole course. Decisions therefore have to be made about what should
be included in the test, and whether assessing one thing can be assumed
to include another. For example, if a student can cope with the form
and meaning of the past perfect tense, does that imply a similar mastery of the present perfect, since the normal sequence of learning deals
with the second of these before the first? (p. 7)*

Diagnostic

An achievement test attempts to indicate the overall achievement of the student
(compared to other students); however, to obtain information about specific
strengths and weaknesses, a diagnostic test should be used (Anastasi, 1982; Borg
& Gall, 1983; Salvia & Ysseldyke, 1991). Davies (1990) remarked that a diagnostic test can be considered the flip or reverse side of an achievement test.
That is, an achievement test is concerned with the success of a student whereas
a diagnostic test is concerned with the failure so that it can be remedied.

A diagnostic test can be labeled as a *progress* or *formative* test (Harrison,
1983; Salvia & Ysseldyke, 1991). The test typically focuses on an individual's
performance in a particular domain or area, such as language, reading, or mathematics. The diagnostic test is manifested as a criterion-referenced test. Students'
scores are not compared with those of other students; rather, they are compared to an absolute standard, which is arbitrarily determined. In other words,
the test score purports to reflect the extent to which a student has mastered
the content of a particular domain.

It should be kept in mind that many tests are both norm-referenced (i.e.,
achievement oriented) and criterion-referenced (i.e., diagnostic oriented). It
has been argued that the distinction between the types is often misleading,
causing problems with the interpretations of the results (Carver, 1974). Carver
(1974) maintained that "all tests, to a certain extent, reflect both between-
individual differences, and within-individual growth. Because of their design
and development, however, most tests will do a better job in one area than
the other" (p. 512).

Proficiency

A number of theorists and researchers have argued for the assessment of language proficiency as opposed to language competence as defined by Chomsky,
especially for bilingual or second language students (see discussions in

Cummins, 1984; McLaughlin, 1985; Verhoeven, 1992). In one sense, proficiency is related to the performance or use of language (and other skills). The goal of a proficiency test is to ascertain the ability of an individual to apply what he or she has learned in real, meaningful situations. Unlike the achievement test, a proficiency test does not constrain the time frame or exhibit control over the previous learning experiences of the individual (Davies, 1990). Although the test is not specifically concerned with the individual's present level of competence, it is interested in the future performance of the individual in similar real-life situations. These conditions of a proficiency test might contribute to what is often called the vagueness of the test with respect to prior learning or knowledge. Proficiency tests can be related to the use of free methods in language assessment.

CONTROLLED METHODS

As mentioned previously, it is possible to categorize two broad methods of collecting language assessment data: controlled and free methods. As the reader proceeds through these descriptions, it should be possible to relate them to other categories discussed earlier, for example, direct versus indirect and discrete-point versus integrative. Again, it should not be a case of controlled or free methods; in essence, both types can be administered to obtain a more complete picture of the child's language development. There are, of course, advantages and disadvantages associated with each broad type.

There are a number of advantages to using controlled methods in the assessment of language. For example, with controlled methods, language researchers can examine certain linguistic structures that might appear infrequently or never appear in a spontaneous language sample. Without a sufficient number of examples, it is not possible to determine whether an individual has acquired or has competency in specific language structures such as in the use and understanding of relative clauses, pronouns, verb processes, and so on. Of course, the converse is true; it cannot be ascertained that an individual does not have knowledge of a particular grammatical structure. These problems have been discussed in the earlier works of L. Taylor (1969) and Quigley and his collaborators (Quigley, Wilbur, Power, Montanelli, & Steinkamp, 1976) and are still applicable today. In any case, with the use of controlled methods, investigators can construct test items that permit the study of an individual's use or understanding of specific linguistic units.

Another advantage of controlled procedures is that they permit investigators to develop tests that address specific language domains such as phonology, syntax, and semantics. It is obvious that the information from such tests would be of great assistance to teachers and clinicians. Because of the nature of language, test makers need to concentrate on developing an adequate assessment of one domain. That is, it is not possible to construct a test that would provide sufficient information on all language components. Thus, to provide detailed evaluation of a student's skill, it is best to concentrate on one language domain per assessment. This necessitates that students take several language tests.

One of the biggest advantages of controlled methods is the degree of objectivity in the analyses of test results compared to the analyses of data using free methods. Relative to the characteristics of standardized tests discussed previously, this objectivity is due to uniform procedures for administering, scoring, and interpreting the tests (Anastasi, 1982; Borg & Gall, 1983; Salvia & Ysseldyke, 1991). In addition, the interpretation of the tests also depends heavily on whether the characteristics of students taking the test are similar to those who were part of the norming procedures.

Because of standardized procedures, it is easy to compare the obtained results from controlled measures to other results of students or clients with similar characteristics. It cannot be overemphasized that test developers should specify and teachers/clincians should be aware of the characteristics of the population on whom the tests were normed. Perhaps it is not possible to develop a test for all students with hearing impairment due to the discrepancies in achievement across the various subgroups (see discussions in Moores, 1996; Paul & Jackson, 1993; Vernon & Andrews, 1990).

Another advantage associated with controlled methods is that the conditions of reliability and validity can be satisfied without much difficulty. By controlling the test stimuli, the available responses, and the characteristics of the normative sample, the amount of variance related to external factors can be reduced. The reduction of the variance should result in the enhancement of reliability and validity for the particular test (Anastasi, 1982; Salvia & Ysseldyke, 1991).

Controlled methods are not above criticism; they do have several limitations or disadvantages. Although it is possible to obtain detailed information on a specific domain of language, it might be difficult to obtain an evaluation of an individual's overall language ability. For example, a test on syntax does not yield information on an individual's understanding of pragmatics. To obtain a comprehensive evaluation of language, it is important not only to use several controlled assessments but also to use spontaneous language samples.

Another major limitation of controlled procedures can be seen in the nature of the test. For example, in a test-taking situation or a laboratory situation, the examiner attempts to control several areas such as test stimuli, test environment, and the test responses. Due to this nature of control, the investigator cannot assume that the results are reflective of an individual's language behaviors in more naturalistic settings (see discussions in D. Baker, 1989; Davies, 1990; Lipson & Wixson, 1997). Thus, it is important to compare the results obtained from the controlled measures with those obtained in a more naturalistic manner as in free methods.

Test Instruments: A Selection

This section discusses a few tests and a set of procedures that have been used with individuals with hearing impairment. It is still true that most tests and procedures used with deaf and hard-of-hearing students have been normed on or adapted from those used with typically hearing students (see discussions in Bradley-Johnson & Evans, 1991; Luetke-Stahlman, 1998; McAnally et al., 1994; Paul, 1998a; Paul & Jackson, 1993; Vernon & Andrews, 1990). It should be kept in mind that the current selection is meant to be representative, not exhaustive, of the type of method employed, that is, controlled and decontextualized. Relative to the characteristics of good assessments discussed previously, the kind of information that the selected test is purported to convey is discussed. To ensure that readers obtain an adequate understanding, some details on the content and analysis of the specific test have been included. A more detailed recent discussion of the strengths and weaknesses of a number of tests and good discussions of the selection and use of tests and procedures with deaf and hard-of-hearing students can be found elsewhere (Bradley-Johnson & Evans, 1991; Luetke-Stahlman, 1998; Luetke-Stahlman & Luckner, 1991; Thompson et al., 1987).

Berko Morphology Test

The Berko Morphology Test (Berko, 1958) was designed to evaluate children's knowledge of the morphological structure of English. The sample included 56 children who were unevenly divided across seven age levels ranging from 4 to 7 years in 6-month increments. For example, there were 14 subjects between the ages of 4 years and 5 years, 6 months (preschool) and 42 subjects between the ages of 6 and 7 years (first-grade age). No norms are available; however, it is possible to compare a student's score with the respective correct percentage scores for preschool and first-grade children in Berko's study.

The test contains 27 picture cards with accompanying sentences. The morphological structures assessed include plurals, singular and plural possessives, past tense, present progressive, and derivational morphemes. For example, there is one item that shows a picture of an animal with bird-like characteristics. Underneath this picture is another picture with two of these creatures.

The examiner remarks "This is a wug. Now there is another one. There are two of them. There are two _____." Although the test stimuli were closely controlled, the subjects' responses were not constrained.

Subjects were also required to explain (i.e., describe, define, etc.) 14 compound words. For example, given the following item: "A birthday is called a birthday because _____", the subjects were expected to provide an explanation.

Modifications of the Berko Test of Morphology resulted in the development of the Exploratory Test of Grammar (Berry & Talbot, 1966). Modifications include an increase in the number of pictorial stimuli from 27 to 30 and a change in the age range from 4 to 7 years to 5 to 8 years. Nevertheless, the limitations associated with the original test remained. For example, approximately 60% of the items on the newer test assess plural nouns and past-tense verb forms whereas only 40% of the items assess structures such as third-person singulars, possessives, derived adjectives, comparatives and superlatives, and the progressive aspect.

With adaptations of the procedures, the morphology test has been used to assess deaf and hard-of-hearing children's knowledge of the morphological rules of English. Adaptations consist of presenting language stimuli in visual modes such as writing and forms of manual communication instead of the oral form. Results have been reported by R. Cooper (1967; also see the discussion in Chapter 8) and Raffin (1976; also see the discussion in Chapter 6).

Northwestern Syntax Screening Test

Lee (1969) developed the Northwestern Syntax Screening Test (NSST) to assess the receptive and expressive skills of children between the ages of 3 years and 7 years, 11 months. The NSST contains items that focus on prepositions, personal pronouns, noun-verb agreement, tense, possessives, present progressives, active and passive voice, and *wh-* questions. There are two parts, receptive and expressive.

The receptive portion of the NSST contains 20 items. Each item has four pictures with stimulus sentences designed to assess the structure under consideration. For example, if the focus is on prepositions, the examiner would hold the appropriate pictures and remark: "On one of these pictures the cat is behind the chair, on another, the cat is under the chair. Now show me the cat is behind the chair." The subject is expected to point to the picture that represented the second stimulus sentence, namely, "behind the chair."

The expressive portion of the NSST is based on an imitation task. The subject is shown 20 pairs of contrasting pictures with accompanying sentences. Consider an item that contains two pictures of babies, one is awake and the other is sleeping. The examiner would remark: "The baby is sleeping. The baby is not sleeping. Now what's this picture?" Subsequently, the examiner points to one of the two pictures and the subject is expected to say (imitate) the previous sentence associated with that picture. Failures to imitate the stimulus sentences are counted as errors for the expressive portion of the NSST.

Norms are available for children between the ages of 3 years and 7 years, 11 months. However, nearly half of the subjects are in the 5-year-old range whereas the other 1-year spans (e.g., 3 to 4 years, 4 to 5 years, etc.) only contain from 10% to 18% of the total sample. These subjects were from middle- to upper-income families from the Midwest. Despite these norms, the test developer did not report reliability and validity scores. In all fairness, Lee (1969) remarked that the test should be used primarily as a screening assessment. To obtain a more detailed assessment of the syntactic development of young children, Lee recommended the use of additional assessments.

The use of the NSST with children who are deaf and hard of hearing was reported in a study by Pressnell (1973; also see the discussion in Chapter 5). Pressnell studied children with moderate hearing impairment and greater. Analyzing spontaneous language samples and the results of the NSST, it was concluded that the performance of the students were qualitatively similar but quantitatively reduced when compared to hearing norms. The predictability or explanatory adequacy of the NSST was questioned by Wilbur et al. (1989; also see the discussion in Chapter 8).

Carrow Elicited Language Inventory (CELI)

Carrow (1974) stated that the purpose of the elicited imitation task of the CELI is to measure "a child's productive control of grammar" (p. 4). It is assumed that children's imitations of adult utterances reflect their grammatical competence, especially if there is sufficient emphasis on the use of immediate memory capabilities (see Ingram, 1989; Menyuk, 1977).

The CELI consists of 51 sentences and one phrase ranging from 2 to 10 words. Forty-seven of the 51 sentences are presented in the active voice whereas the other 4 sentences are presented in the passive voice. Sentences can be classified as affirmative, negative, declarative, interrogative, and imperative. Among the grammatical features assessed are articles, adjectives, nouns, pronouns, verbs, negatives, contractions, adverbs, prepositions, demonstratives, and conjunctions. The test task requires the examiner to present the stimulus sentences and the test taker to imitate the items. The examiner records the deviations from the test items. Errors can be categorized into five types: substitutions, omissions, additions, transpositions, and reversals.

The CELI was standardized on 475 children between the ages of 3 years and 7 years, 11 months. The children came from middle-class homes and attended daycare centers and church schools in Houston, Texas. The reliability of the CELI has been demonstrated using test-retest and interexaminer techniques. The test-retest procedure was conducted on 25 children, five each at the ages of 3, 4, 5, 6, and 7, who were administered the test after a 2-week interval. Carrow (1974) reported a correlation coefficient of .98. The two interexaminer tests resulted in coefficients of .98 and .99.

The CELI was shown to have both concurrent and congruent validity. Relative to concurrent validity, it was found that the scores of the standardization (norming) sample increased significantly with age. In addition, the results of the CELI differentiated between children with typical language development from those with atypical or delayed language development. Relative to congruent validity, Carrow found that there was a significant correlation between the CELI and the Developmental Sentence Scoring techniques (Lee & Canter, 1971).

Test of Syntactic Abilities

The Test of Syntactic Abilities (Quigley, Steinkamp, Power, & Jones, 1978) is a comprehensive battery of 20 diagnostic tests and two forms of a screening test that assesses deaf students' ability to either select or comprehend grammatically correct English sentences, involving nine syntactic structures (see discussion in Chapter 8). The 20 diagnostic tests of the TSA were normed on a sample of 411 students who met the following criteria:

1. Between the ages of 10 years and 18 years, 11 months.
2. Had at least an average IQ score on the performance scale of tests typically used with deaf and hard-of-hearing students.
3. Possessed a hearing impairment of 90 dB in the better ear averaged across the speech frequencies (see discussion of hearing impairment in Chapter 1).
4. Acquired the hearing impairment prior to or at the age of 2 years.
5. Had no other educational disabilities.

Data have also been collected on students with typical hearing, Australian deaf children, college-level deaf students, and students with hearing impairment from Canada.

Table 11-5 depicts the nine structures assessed by the TSA, the type of task associated with each of the 20 diagnostic tests, and the internal consistency reliability coefficients for 19 of the 20 tests. Table 11-5 also shows that the internal consistency reliability scores range from .94 to .98. Because these coefficients are higher than the sufficient criterion of .80, it is possible to provide specific diagnostic information regarding the student's performance on the tests. In addition, content validity has also been demonstrated (Owens, Haney, Giesow, Dooley, & Kelly, 1983; Quigley, Steinkamp, Power, & Jones, 1978).

Table 11-5 Structures, Types of Tasks, and Internal Reliabilities for the Test of Syntactic Abilities

Structure	Type of Task	K-R 20
Negation	Recognition and comprehension	.98
Conjunction		
Conjunction	Recognition and comprehension	.97
Disjunction and alternation	Recognition and comprehension	.96
Determiners	Recognition	.96
Question formation		
Wh- questions	Recognition	.96
Answer environments	Comprehension	.96
Yes/no questions	Recognition	.97
Verb Processes		
Verb sequence in conjoined structures	Recognition	.97
Main verbs, linking verbs, and auxiliaries	Recognition	.95
Passive voice	Recognition and comprehension	.97
Pronominalization		
Possessive adjectives	Recognition	.96
Reflexives	Recognition	.96

(continues)

(Table 11-5 continued)

Possessive pronouns	Recognition	.96
Forward and backward pronominalization	Recognition	.97
Relativization		
Comprehension	Comprehension	.94
Relative pronouns and adverbs	Recognition	.93
Embedding	Recognition	.96
Complementation		
That-complements	Recognition and comprehension	.94
Infinitives and gerunds	Recognition	.94
Nominalization	Recognition and comprehension	—

Note: Adapted from Quigley, Steinkamp, Power, and Jones (1978).

Each of the 20 diagnostic tests of the TSA contains 70 multiple-choice items written, in terms of vocabulary, at approximately the first-grade level. The time required for administering a single test ranges from about 35 minutes to 1 hour. Because administering the total battery would take about 10 to 20 hours, the TSA developers constructed two forms of a screening test that requires about 1 hour to administer.

Each screening test contains 120 items, which is representative of the nine syntactic structures contained in the diagnostic tests. The internal consistency reliability coefficients (KR-20) for the two tests are .98, and the coefficients for each of the nine structures ranged from .80 to .87. The reliability indices for each of the nine structures on the screening tests are sufficient for that purpose only—screening. It is suggested that the screening test be administered initially to determine those structures with which test takers have difficulty. On the basis of these results, the examiner can select the relevant diagnostic tests to administer to obtain detailed data on a particular structure.

After administering the diagnostic battery, it is possible to engage in both formal and informal interpretation procedures. Relative to formal procedures, the examiner can determine the student's percentile rank, percentile range, and age-equivalent scores. Informally, the investigator can calculate the percentage of correct responses for the types of tasks associated with each structure, that is, recognition and comprehension. The same can be done for the types of substructures associated with each of the nine major syntactic structures. For example, the examiner can determine the percentage of correct responses on the Question Formation test for yes/no questions (e.g., *You ate the cookie, didn't you?*) and *wh-* questions (e.g., *What is your name?*).

There is another interpretation feature of the TSA that provides additional information on deaf students' understanding of syntax. The distractors (incorrect responses in terms of standard English usage) are representative of structures found to appear consistently in the language production of deaf individuals. Thus, by analyzing the incorrect responses, the investigator can ascertain if a particular student consistently selects a deviation from standard English usage that is commonly found among deaf students of comparable age. Along with other diagnostic information on the specific syntactic structure, information on the use of common deviant usages is important for developing remediation instructional programs.

Grammatical Analysis of Elicited Language

The Grammatical Analysis of Elicited Language (GAEL) was developed at the Central Institute for the Deaf in St. Louis, Missouri. The GAEL has three different levels: the presentence level (GAEL-P) (Moog, Kozak, & Geers, 1983), the simple sentence level (GAEL-S) (Moog & Geers, 1979), and the complex sentence level (GAEL-C) (Moog & Geers, 1980).

With GAEL-P, the investigator can assess the language readiness skill of the student. In addition, it is also possible to assess up to three-word combinations in comprehension, production, and imitation tasks with the use of adequate prompts. The GAEL-P was administered to hearing children between the ages of 2 years, 6 months and 3 years, 11 months. It was administered and normed on 150 children with hearing impairment between the ages of 3 years and 5 years, 11 months. Based on the results of 20 students with hearing impairment, the test developers reported test-retest reliability coefficients as follows: .97 for the comprehension task, .95 for the prompted production task, and .93 for the imitation task. The subjects with hearing impairment were identified as educationally hearing impaired; that is, the subjects were too young to provide reliable audiological data reflective of a particular degree of hearing impairment.

With 94 pairs of identical sentences, the purpose of the GAEL-S is to assess the student's ability to produce and imitate specific syntactic structures given adequate prompts. The structures for the GAEL-S were selected from Lee

Developmental Sentence Scoring (Lee, 1974) and from Language Sampling and Analysis (Tyack & Gottesleben, 1974). Among the structures included were articles, adjectives, quantifiers, possessives, demonstratives, conjunctions, pronouns, nouns in subject and object positions, *wh-* questions, verbs and verb inflections, copulas and their inflections, prepositions, and negatives.

The GAEL-S was normed on both children with typical hearing and those with hearing impairment. The hearing sample included 200 children between the ages of 2 years, 6 months and 5 years old who resided in the St. Louis, Missouri, area. The sample of children with hearing impairment included 200 children between the ages of 5 and 9 years from 13 oral programs for children with hearing impairment in the United States. The children with hearing impairment met the following criteria:

1. Had a hearing impairment greater than 70 dB in the better ear across the speech frequencies (see Chapter 1).
2. Incurred the hearing impairment prior to the age of 2 years.
3. Possessed no additional educational disabilities.

The test developers reported high reliability and validity scores. To establish validity, the test developers use statistical analyses to substantiate the effects of age on the specific language variables that were assessed. They also reported a test-retest reliability coefficient of .96 for both the prompted and imitated tasks. The test-retest procedures involved 20 subjects with hearing impairment who were retested after a 30-month interval.

With 88 pairs of identical sentences, the purpose of the GAEL-C is to assess students' production and imitation of complex sentences with the use of adequate prompts. The GAEL-C contains structures such as articles, noun modifiers, nouns in subject and object position, noun plurals, personal pronouns, indefinite and reflexive pronouns, conjunctions, auxiliary verbs, other verbs and verb inflections, infinitives and participles, prepositions, negatives, and *wh-* questions.

The norming sample of the GAEL-C involved three groups of children. One group was 240 hearing subjects between the ages of 3 years and 5 years, 11 months. There were two groups of children with hearing impairment. One group had 120 children who had hearing losses between 70 and 95 dB and who were between the ages of 8 years and 11 years, 11 months. The second group included 150 children who had hearing losses greater than 95 dB and who were also between the ages of 8 years and 11 years, 11 months.

Using test-retest procedures, 20 children with hearing impairment were retested after a 2-month interval. The test developers reported reliability coefficients of .96 for the prompted (or production) task and .95 for the imitation task. A sample of 26 hearing children were also retested. The coefficients were .82 for the prompted task and .81 for the imitation task. The test developers also established statistical validity by correlating the scores with those of other tests that assess both receptive and expressive skills. The test developers used the subtests of the Illinois Test of Psycholinguistic Abilities, the Northwestern Syntax Screening Test, the Peabody Picture Vocabulary Test, and the Test for Auditory Comprehension of Language. Correlations with the subtests of tests assessing receptive skills ranged from .45 to .68. The correlation of the GAEL-C with the tests assessing expressive ability ranged from .83 to .87.

There have been a few tests used to assess the communicative skills (e.g., oral, manual, and simultaneous) and achievement areas (e.g., reading and written language) of students with hearing impairment. A good discussion of the strengths and weaknesses of these tests can be found elsewhere (Bradley-Johnson & Evans, 1991). There is a need for more research and development in the assessment of communication skills, specifically as they relate to certain signed systems such as signed English, signing exact English, and seeing essential English. At present, there is no standardized assessment for a specific English signed system.

Other Instruments

As mentioned previously, the earlier discussion on the selected instruments was meant to be illustrative, not exhaustive of all the instruments that have been or can be used with deaf and hard-of-hearing students. Additional excellent discussions of instruments (formal and informal) can be found in Luetke-Stahlman (1998) and Moeller (1988), for example. Luetke-Stahlman (1998) provided a discussion of formal tests, including reliability and validity information. A few tests for vocabulary and other areas of semantics mentioned in her review include:

- Comprehensive Receptive and Expressive Vocabulary Test (CREVT)
- Test of Language Development—Primary (TOLD-P)
- Test of Word Knowledge
- The Word Test—Adolescent
- The Word Test-R: Elementary
- Assessing Semantic Skills Through Everyday Themes (ASSET)
- The Clinical Evaluation of Language Fundamentals—Preschool (CELF-Preschool)
- The Clinical Evaluation of Language Fundamentals—Revised (CELF-R)

The reader should bear in mind that many of these tests and others have not been normed on students who are deaf and hard-of-hearing. Their usefulness and validity for this population still need to be investigated.

FREE METHODS

In general, the use of free methods entails the collection of a language sample for analysis. There are of course various procedures that have been proposed for analyzing the sample. It is important to obtain information on children's spontaneous use of language through the use of elicitation or prompting procedures such as pictures or videotapes. The goal is to record a large corpus of utterances, typically about 50 to 100. The utterances should be collected in as naturalistic a setting as possible. Several researchers have provided guidelines for collecting informal language samples (Luetke-Stahlman, 1998; Luetke-Stahlman & Luckner, 1991; Thompson et al., 1987). For example, some suggestions offered are as follows:

- *Obtain a sample of each student's language at least two times per year, at the beginning and end of the year.*
- *Obtain eight to ten utterances of each student's language for 5 days, for a total of 40 to 50 utterances. Make every effort to obtain samples of running discourse.*
- *Each day obtain the eight to ten utterances at different times when the student is communicating with different people in different circumstances so that you sample use of language in different contexts.*
- *Always record some continuous dialogue because this will help you to evaluate discourse strategies the student is using.*
- *Don't talk too much yourself. The goal is to get the student to do the talking.*
- *Use questions like "What happened next?" "What do you think will happen?" or "That's interesting. What else can you tell me?"*
- *Be sure to use the Pragmatic Checklist, the Kendall Communicative Scale, or any other scale, checklist, etc. that will supplement your grammatical analyses of the language sample and assist you in reviewing how your student uses language. (Thompson et al., 1987, pp. 103–105)*

In obtaining a language sample for young children, it is suggested that the examiner use toys, objects, pictures, or activities that are familiar and interesting to the child. The language sample should be transcribed as soon as possible after it is collected. It is best to have at least two individuals evaluate the sample and to collaborate to resolve differences of opinion. Another perspective on obtaining a language sample can be found in Table 11-6.

Table 11-6 Tips for Obtaining a Language Sample

- Establish situations in which you and the child can play with toys or use books that are of interest to the child. As the session begins, do not say anything for a few minutes or only say a few words to encourage the child to talk. If you are playing with toys with the child, engage in parallel play, following the child's lead, and letting the child tell you how to play. After a little while, the play session can take an interactive turn in which you can discuss with the child what you and she or he are doing. The child may respond with her or his version.

- Record the play session for about 5 to 10 minutes using both video and audiotape.

- In transcribing the tape, you and another individual should:

  1. Write down all utterances produced by the investigator and child, even those that are not complete sentences. In the event of a long pause, present the next set of words as a new utterance.

  2. Use a new line for each utterance.

  3. To facilitate analysis, code the investigator's and child's utterances in different colors or typeset (i.e., font, size, bold, etc.).

  4. Record any meaningful signs or gestures that accompany the utterances. (Those that are associated with a sign language or signed system should be recorded as utterances. See Luetke-Stahlman, 1998.)

  5. Ensure that you only record what was said or seen. If the child's speech is unclear—mark it with a question or some other indicator.

  6. Conduct an interrater reliability check. Resolve differences.

Note: Adapted from information presented in Appendix A of Bochner, Price, and Jones (1997).

Strengths and Weaknesses

Perhaps the greatest advantage of free method procedures is the assumption that if a child consistently produces a specific structure, then she or he must have knowledge or competency of that structure. Another advantage is that the interpretation of the data is based on the student's own linguistic features in comparison with other student's language productions rather than with norms (e.g., percentile, age, or grade equivalent scores).

There are a number of limitations associated with the use of free methods. These limitations should be interpreted from the framework of the scientific method, which strives for the condition of objectivity. For example, one limitation is the amount of subjectivity or idiosyncrasy. There is a danger of reading into the data those factors that are of interest to the examiner; this is much more evident than with the use of more controlled methods. To limit the effects of subjectivity, it is recommended that the examiner who performs the analyses undergo extensive training.

Another difficulty involves the notion of reliability. With the small number of subjects, it is impossible statistically to assess reliability using test-retest, equivalent forms, or internal consistency coefficients. Examiners must rely on the concepts of inter- and intrarater reliability coefficients, which are often used in single-subject designs.

The use of free methods with children with hearing impairment presents additional difficulties. For example, it is difficult to record the utterances of children with severe to profound impairment. There is the likelihood that their speech would be unintelligible, rendering the data difficult to analyze. It is possible to record the signing utterances of the individuals. However, because of the nature and use of signing in the home and schools (also see Chapter 6 of this text), the analysis of this phenomenon is no less problematic (also see Luetke-Stahlman, 1998).

The substitution of written language samples for spoken or signed utterances does not resolve this difficulty. Although useful information can be gleaned from analyses of written language productions, this information is not the same as that obtained from spoken or signed utterances. There are major differences in the linguistic and cognitive demands for each domain, although it is possible for one to attain a similar level of literate thought in either one despite the modality difference (see Chapters 1 and 12). Finally, the written language samples of both hearing and deaf individuals are typically more limited in scope than the conversational or performance mode utterances (i.e., spoken and/or signed).

Analysis Procedures

There are several analysis procedures that can be used for written language productions. It is possible to use terms that have been employed to describe the written language of deaf students, specifically within the paradigm of the products of writing (R. Cooper & Rosenstein, 1966; also see Chapter 8). These terms include *productivity, complexity, flexibility, distribution of parts of speech*, and *grammatical correctness*. Other analysis procedures designed for analyzing spoken utterances include mean length of utterance, developmental sentence types (Lee, 1966, 1974), developmental sentence scoring (Lee, 1974), and others (Bloom and Lahey approach and Kretschmer spontaneous language analysis procedure).

Traditional grammar analysis procedures relative to written language productions were briefly discussed in Chapter 8. For example, productivity (Heider & Heider, 1940; Myklebust, 1964) refers to two measures: the average number of words written in a sample and the mean length of the sentences in the sample. The notion of complexity has three measures: (a) ratio of simple sentences to compound, complex, and compound-complex sentences (division procedures); (b) the number of subordinate clauses per main clause; and (c) the T-unit—defined as "one main clause plus all subordinate clauses attached or embedded in it" (Hunt, 1965, p. 141; see discussion of the works of Marshall & Quigley, 1970; L. Taylor, 1969 in Chapter 8; also see the brief discussion of language terms in Chapter 2).

Another example is flexibility, which involves the use of a type-token ratio for assessing vocabulary diversity. This ratio is calculated by dividing the total number of different words by the total number of words in a 50-utterance sample. The distribution of parts of speech refers to the use of different parts of speech, obtained by dividing the number of occurrences of a part of speech (verbs) by the total number of words in the sample (see discussion of a few parts of speech in Chapter 2).

The last category to be discussed is correctness. This category refers to the errors or deviations from standard English usage. Two approaches have been developed. The first approach entails the use of frequency counts for the types of errors found in the written language samples of children with hearing impairment (Myklebust, 1964). This approach does not have much theoretical or educational significance.

The second approach is an extension of the first one and is more informative and useful because of the attempt to describe the type of errors. For example, L. Taylor (1969; also see the discussion in Chapter 8) described the "rules violated in the production of any deviant or non-grammatical structures"

(p. 45). The researcher noted that deaf students frequently omitted direct objects. However, Taylor also analyzed this phenomenon relative to the linguistic environments in which the omissions occurred at different grade levels. She reported the omissions at the third-grade level appeared primarily in simple sentences containing transitive verbs. At the fifth- and seventh-grade levels, however, the omissions of direct objects occurred most frequently in conjoined sentences. At the ninth-grade level, the deaf students produced omissions in complementized sentences, which are more complex structures. Thus, it was found that the frequency of occurrence of direct-object omissions did not decrease as the students advanced in school grades. Nevertheless, the analysis of the linguistic environments in which the omissions occurred did indicate that the students' levels of syntactic complexity were increasing and this contributed to the errors.

Mean Length of Utterance (MLU)

The MLU refers to the average number of morphemes per utterance in a sample of 100 utterances (see R. Brown, 1973). A morpheme is the minimal unit of meaning in language. For example, the word *cat* contains one morpheme, whereas the word *cats* contains two morphemes—*cat* and the plural *-s*. Some guidelines for calculating the MLU include (see further discussion in R. Brown, 1973):

1. Compound words (e.g., bluebird and hot dog) and proper names (e.g., Joe, Jane, and Jeremiah) count as single morphemes.
2. Irregular past tense verbs (e.g., ran and saw) count as one morpheme.
3. Auxiliaries (e.g., can, must, and should) and inflectional morphemes (e.g., possessives, plural, third-person singulars, regular past-tense verb endings, and progressive aspect endings) count as separate morphemes.

R. Brown's (1973) suggestions/rules have been adapted for use with deaf and hard-of-hearing students. Luetke-Stahlman and Luckner (1991), also repeated in Luetke-Stahlman (1998), provided several recommendations, which are listed in Table 11-7.

Table 11-7 Guidelines for Computing Mean Length of Utterances (MLUs) for Deaf and Hard-of-Hearing Students

---

1. Use transcription that does not involve a recitation of some kind. Do not use utterances that have been read or sung.

2. Use only fully transcribed utterances. If a word in an utterance is unintelligible or the user does not complete an idea, do not use the utterance.

3. Do not use exact repetition of immediately prior utterances.

4. In a case in which a word is repeated for emphasis ("*No, no, no*") count only the initial use of a word.

5. Do not count fillers such as "*mm*" or "*ah ha*" but do count "*oh no,*" "*yeah,*" and "*hi.*"

6. All compound words (two or more free morphemes), proper names, and reduplications count as single words (*birthday, highway, Mary Pat, quack-quack, night-night, pocketbook,* and *see-saw*).

7. Count as two morphemes all irregular verb tenses (*get, did, went,* and *saw*).

8. Count as multiple morphemes all words with affixes (*exactly, happiness,* and *replace*). If the word with a prefix or a suffix is signed as one sign in a particular system, it is credited as the multiple spoken morphemes it represents (*wonderful* in signed English).

9. Count as separate morphemes all auxiliary verbs (*is, have, will, can, must,* and *would*). All catenatives (*gonna, wanna,* and *hafta*) are counted as two morphemes. Count as separate morphemes all inflections, for example, possessive, plural, third person singular, regular past, and progressive.

10. Count as multiple morphemes signs that conform to spoken English grammar but might be signed with a single sign (HAVE TO = 2; DON'T KNOW = 3; A LITTLE BIT = 3).

11. If the sign system uses several signs to represent a single English word (as in SEE I, MOTORCYCLE = 3 signs; in ASL and signed English, TODAY = 2 signs), count it as one morpheme.

Note: Based on Luetke-Stahlman (1998).

For calculating the MLU, Luetke-Stahlman (1998) proposed the following equation (p. 159):

total # of spoken morphemes/total # of utterances per transcript = VMLU

total # of signed morphemes/total # of utterances per transcript = SMLU

A few of her examples are (p. 160):

| 1. *The boys* | *ran* | *up the hill.* | *(VMLU = 8)* |
| *BOY BOY BOY RUN + past* | | *UP   HILL* | *(SMLU = 6)* |

2. I DON'T CARE   HOW THEY DO IT.   (VMLU = 8)

* I   CARE   HOW   DO IT.   (SMLU = 6)*

For children with MLUs of five or less, this procedure is a good index of syntactic development. For example, J. Miller (1981) reported on predicted chronological ages from the MLU for hearing children. Thus, it is possible to compare the MLUs of children with disabilities, including deafness, with those provided by Miller.

There are several problems, however, with using the MLU procedure in other situations. For example, it is not a reliable index of syntax for children with MLU over five. With the emergence and frequency of conjoined structures, it is possible to overestimate children's MLUs relative to their language development. Blackwell, Engen, Fischgrund, and Zarcadoolas (1978) reported additional difficulties. One, the length of the utterance measures obscures differences in syntactic and semantic complexity. Two, the MLU does not provide information regarding children's functional use of the language. Three, relative to children with hearing impairment, it is debatable to assume that a deaf child with a MLU of 2.3 (Brown's Stage II) displays the same linguistic features as a hearing child at the same stage of development.

Developmental Sentence Types (DST)

The DST is used to assess the presentence stage of language development (Lee, 1966, 1974). It should be used when less than 50% of the child's utterances contain both a subject and a predicate. After collecting a language sample consisting of at least 50 utterances, the utterances can be described relative to a chart that contains three horizontal dimensions and five vertical dimensions. The three horizontal dimensions are single words, two-word combinations, and multiword constructions. The five vertical dimensions are noun phrases, designative phrases, predicative sentences, subject-verb sentences, and fragments. The DST is based on the debatable assumption that children first learn simple active, affirmative, declarative sentences and then learn to apply transformations to these sentences (see discussion in Kretschmer & Kretschmer, 1978).

Developmental Sentence Scoring (DSS)

The DSS is used when more than 50% of the child's utterances contain both a subject and a predicate (Lee, 1974; Lee & Canter, 1971). In general, the utterances are rated relative to eight grammatical categories: indefinite pronouns or noun modifiers, personal pronouns, main verbs, secondary verbs, negatives, conjunctions, interrogative reversals, and *wh-* questions. The test developers constructed a scale of 1 to 8 for the categories. For example, the examiner assigns 1 point for first- and second-person pronouns. For pronouns such as *oneself*, the examiner assigns 7 points. The total number of points for the utterances are divided by 50 (number of utterances). This score can be compared with the norms available for children between the ages of 2 to 6 years. Similar to the DST, the DSS does not consider semantic and pragmatic aspects.

Bloom and Lahey Approach

L. Bloom and Lahey (1978) developed procedures that focus on both syntactic (form) and semantic (content) features. The researchers identified 21 semantic features that interact in a hierarchical manner with eight syntactic features within a phase framework. For example, Phases 1 and 2, which correspond approximately to one- and two-word utterances, contain the semantic features of existence, nonexistence, recurrence, rejection, denial, attribution, possession, action, and locative action (mentioned in Chapter 2). Phase 3 utterances include the semantic features in Phases 1 and 2 as well as locative state, state, and quantity. Phase 4 utterances include the semantic features of notice and time, and Phase 5 includes the features of coordinate, causality, dative, and specifier. Phases 6 to 8 contained complex sentences, syntactic connectives, modal verbs, and relative clauses in this order. The semantic features of these phases include epistemic, mood, and antithesis. For complete descriptions of all categories, the reader should consult L. Bloom and Lahey (1978).

With this procedure, it is possible to obtain a fairly complete picture of the child's language development (pragmatics included). Nevertheless, this procedure demands a great deal of time because of the number of utterances required (200).

Kretschmer Spontaneous Language Analysis

Kretschmer and Kretschmer (1978) developed a very extensive and comprehensive procedure for studying the free spontaneous language samples of children who are deaf and hard-of-hearing. The procedures can be used for both spoken and signed utterances as well as for written language samples. Although similar in many respects to Bloom and Lahey's procedure, there are three notable differences: (a) This technique is not dependent on the quantitative measures of MLU; (b) there is a more extensive treatment of semantic categories in Kretschmer's procedure; and (c) there are strategies for describing the atypical language performance of children with hearing impairment.

There are six sections of the Kretschmer and Kretschmer (1978) analysis protocol. Each section is described as follows:

1. Descriptive information on the preverbal level of the student.
2. Tallying syntactic and semantic features for the one- and two-word stage.
3. Syntactic and semantic descriptions for single prepositions.
4. Syntactic descriptions for complex sentences.
5. Communication competence of the child.
6. Isolation of structures that differ from standard English.

Similar to the Bloom and Lahey procedure, the procedure by Kretschmer and Kretschmer can be used to obtain a fairly complete description of the language development of children who are deaf and hard-of-hearing. The two main limitations are (a) the amount of time required to complete the assessment and (b) the amount of linguistic knowledge required of the examiner.

Teacher Assessment of Grammatical Structures (TAGS)

To accompany the GAEL tests, discussed earlier, Moog and Kozak (1983) developed procedures for analyzing the spontaneous language productions of children with hearing impairment. Thus, there is a protocol for each of the three GAEL tests. The analysis protocol indicates whether the student has acquired or is in the process of acquiring a particular structure under consideration, relative to specified levels of competence. With the exception of the presentence level, each rating form (i.e., analysis protocol) contains levels of imitated, prompted, and spontaneous productions.

The TAGS procedures for each level (i.e., TAGS-P, TAGS-S, and TAGS-C) consist of analyses of six grammatical categories described as follows: TAGS-P, single words, two-word combinations, three-word combinations, *wh-* questions, pronouns, and tense markers; TAGS-S, noun modifiers, pronouns, prepositions, adverbs, verbs, and questions; and TAGS-C, nouns, pronouns, verb inflections, secondary verbs, conjunctions, and questions. The six categories of each TAGS procedure are also divided into six levels, indicating increasing syntactic complexity.

Other Procedures

Relative to elicited and spontaneous language samples, a number of investigators have described procedures that focus on the widely quoted Bloom and Lahey terms, namely, *form, content,* and *use* (Luetke-Stahlman, 1998; Luetke-

Stahlman & Luckner, 1991; Thompson et al., 1987). Despite attempts to use both formal and informal assessments in describing the language performance of students who are deaf or hard-of-hearing (Luetke-Stahlman, 1998; Moeller, 1988), there seems to be a strong movement toward the use of informal, context-bound pragmatics assessments. As eloquently described by Duchan (1984):

> *Like Buffalo chicken wings, pragmatics can be bought in its mild, medium, or hot versions. The mild version takes pragmatics as a new aspect of language which needs to be assessed along with our traditional assessment approaches. . . .*
>
> *Those with medium tastes . . . will willingly abandon their standardized procedures and look at the child's language in light of its intentions, and listener and situational appropriateness. However, they still hold to the idea that language is what they are studying, and context is what is influencing it.*
>
> *The hot version . . . opt for overthrowing our previous conceptions that language is what we are assessing, and propose that we move toward a new conceptualization which examines communication and context, and if called for, the language within it. The hot view is the one that must be embraced if we are to take seriously what the literature in pragmatics has to tell us. (pp. 177–178)*

ASSESSMENT ISSUES FOR BILINGUALISM AND SECOND LANGUAGE LEARNING

This section provides a brief overview of a few assessment issues for students in bilingual or second language learning programs. The author attempted to adhere to extant theories, especially those based on research with hearing individuals (Baetens-Beardsmore, 1986; Cummins, 1984; McLaughlin, 1985, 1987; Verhoeven, 1992). As indicated in Chapter 9, there is a compelling need to develop language assessments for deaf and hard-of-hearing children, particularly those students who might be candidates for a bilingual and/or English as a second language learning program. It is also important to develop an assessment for individuals who desire to become teachers in bilingual programs. Relative to deaf students and interested teachers, the major focus has been on the development and implementation of programs that entail the use of ASL and English. There is a need to consider the establishment of programs for other types of minority-language deaf and hard-of-hearing students, for example, students who reside in homes in which Spanish or German is the native language.

APPROACHES TO THE ASSESSMENT OF BILINGUALISM

Similar to the approaches to language assessment in the first language, second language or bilingual assessment has also been influenced by theories of language acquisition (see Chapter 9). These influences have engendered a number of controversies regarding the types, purposes, and methods of assessment, for example, the use of discrete-point versus integrative measures (Cummins, 1984; McLaughlin, 1985).

A number of tests have been developed to determine degree of bilingualism in hearing individuals (see Cummins, 1984; McLaughlin, 1985, 1987). These tests can be described according to the categories used previously for first language assessment, for example, direct versus indirect measures. Nevertheless, research reviews reveal that many of these tests suffer from difficulties in reliability and validity (Baetens-Beardsmore, 1986; Cummins, 1984; McLaughlin, 1985).

A good example of these ongoing difficulties was provided previously by McLaughlin (1985). This description refers to tests designed to measure language dominance:

> *For example, the Crane Oral Dominance Test consists of a memory task in which children are given 8 words, 4 in English and 4 in Spanish. The children are to recall the words, and if they recall more Spanish words, they are regarded as Spanish-dominant; if they recall more English words, they are thought to be English-dominant. However, it is questionable to assert that recall for vocabulary items measures language dominance. (p. 204)*

In essence, the passage by McLaughlin indicates that there is a continuing debate on the notions of language dominance and language proficiency. These concepts are discussed in the ensuing paragraphs.

Language Dominance

Much of the debate has focused on the distinction between language dominance and language proficiency (Cummins, 1984; McLaughlin, 1985; Verhoeven, 1992). There seems to be no wide agreement on what constitutes language dominance and language proficiency.

The concept of language dominance seems to be concerned with the degree of bilingualism. That is, researchers attempted to compare the individual's levels of skills in two or more languages. As illustrated in the example by McLaughlin (1985) discussed previously, one goal is to determine which language is dominant. The overall goal is to ascertain degree of bilingualism based on an assessment of the individual's ability on certain language elements in the languages involved.

Historically, the preoccupation with the notion of language dominance was considered to be important for the development and implementation of bilingual programs (see McLaughlin, 1985). Ascertaining language dominance was critical for identification of students and faculty for bilingual programs, the initial language for further testing and possibly instruction, and the requirements for funding, such as program evaluation and needs assessment.

In addition to the general characteristics of tests used, a number of theorists and researchers have proffered several criticisms of the concept of language dominance (see Cummins, 1984; McLaughlin, 1985; Verhoeven, 1992). The notion of dominance is not a one-language-or-the-other-only phenomenon (also see the discussion in Chapter 9 for ASL and English). For example, consider the case in which an individual is exposed to both English and French. It is possible for the individual to be English dominant in some situations and French dominant in others. In addition, the individual might be English dominant in the use of syntax but French dominant in the area of pronunciation. This major criticism has led to the growing use of the term *language proficiency* and the development of more pragmatic-oriented assessment (see Cummins, 1984).

Language Proficiency

As with language dominance, there is little consensus regarding the nature of language proficiency (McLaughlin, 1985, 1987; Verhoeven, 1992). In general, language proficiency refers to the individual's degree of competence in one language, that is, the relative proficiency in both languages (Cummins, 1984). The current debate on language proficiency is centered on the question of whether language proficiency is a unitary concept.

Oller and his collaborators (Oller, 1979; Oller & Perkins, 1978, 1980) argued for a global language proficiency factor, analogous to Spearman's *g* factor in intelligence testing. This global factor is said to account for the variance in a wide variety of language measures. It can be measured via the use of tasks that involve listening, speaking, reading, and writing and is correlated with measures of academic achievement and IQ tests, both verbal and nonverbal measures. Most of Oller's data come from literacy-related tasks, for example, written cloze tests.

A number of theorists and researchers have argued against the global language proficiency model (see Cummins, 1984; Verhoeven, 1992). A widely cited dichotomous model has been the one developed by Cummins (1984). This model has been used also in discussions of bilingual programs for deaf students (Luetke-Stahlman, 1998; Luetke-Stahlman & Luckner, 1991).

Cummins categorized the performances of language learners into two groups, which were originally labeled as *cognitive/academic language proficiency* (CALP) and *basic interpersonal communicative skills* (BICS). CALP refers to general cognitive or academic skills, for example, knowledge of vocabulary and syntax. BICS refers to the use of language and interpersonal communication. This dichotomous model is the basis for the theoretical foundation of Cummins' interdependence hypothesis, discussed in Chapter 9. In essence, Cummins argued that surface features developed separately in the two languages; however, there is an underlying cognitive/academic proficiency that is common across the languages.

Cummins' CALP/BICS distinction has been misinterpreted as a distinction between cognitive and communicative aspects of language proficiency. This misinterpretation has led to Cummins' disuse of the terminology (see McLaughlin, 1985). The intent of Cummins' model was to make a distinction between proficiency in communicative-related tasks (as in face-to-face contextualized conversations) and proficiency in literacy-related tasks as in reading, writing, and academic subjects.

Cummins' thinking on language proficiency, particularly the dichotomous model, is applicable not only to the establishment of bilingual programs for deaf students but also to account in part for their low academic achievement levels. For example, most students with severe to profound hearing impairment do not possess an adequate level of language proficiency in English on entering school and, in many cases, on graduation from high school (King & Quigley, 1985; Moores, 1996; Paul, 1998a). Deaf students are expected to acquire academic knowledge via the use of a language of instruction (i.e., English) in which they might have little or no communicative competence. That is, they are expected to engage in the extremely difficult task of learning the academic language and acquiring academic content simultaneously (also see Chapter 9 of this text). Luetke-Stahlman (1998) provided a readable, accessible rendition of Cummins' work with possible applications to the field of deaf education.

In sum, despite the lack of a general consensus on the nature of language proficiency, this concept has engendered changes in the field of second language instruction and assessment. It has become clear that assessing the language of bilingual children is much more difficult than assessing that of monolingual children. Whether the new conceptual framework for assessing language proficiency is on the right track is currently being debated. In addition, as in first language testing, the field of second language research is also grappling with the various issues of language assessment as discussed in this chapter—for example, the use of formal versus informal measures, controlled versus free methods, direct versus indirect methods, or discrete-point versus integrative formats. Most scholars do not view this as either-or; however, there seems to be much support for naturalistic and integrative measures. The increased support for informal, alternative, and naturalistic measures is due mainly to the argument against the sole use of standardized assessments, which are considered to be unfair, biased, and incomplete when used with students from minority-language speaking (and signing) homes (see Cummins, 1984).

The remarks by McLaughlin (1985) provided an eloquent brief summary of this movement and are still relevant today (also see Verhoeven & de Jong, 1992).

The point was made earlier that the increased interest in integrative tests, the development of communicative competence models, and the influence of sociolinguists and ethnographers on language assessment all reflect a common Zeitgeist. In the last decade or so, many researchers and teachers have become convinced that traditional approaches to measuring language proficiency are not fair to many children, especially those from minority-language backgrounds. Whether these developments in assessment will provide practitioners with the tools they need to assess minority-language children fairly remains to be seen. (p. 223)

FINAL REMARKS

This chapter attempts to establish the importance of language assessment to both language instruction and curriculum. Although the instruction-assessment link depends on the type of assessment used, it is a link that needs to be seriously considered in the field of deaf education. Specifically, teachers and clinicians should ensure that there is a strong interrelationship among theory, assessment, instruction, and curriculum. It is also important for teachers and clinicians to be well educated about the types and purposes of assessment so that they can effectively evaluate the merits of their practices and materials.

Admittedly, the concept of assessment is complex and controversial, as evident by the various issues discussed in this chapter with respect to first language and second language learning. As was discussed in the chapter on language instruction, a number of these issues are often presented in a dichotomous, either-or fashion. The reader should have noted that this is a counterproductive situation for language assessment, just as it was for language instruction.

The following paragraphs provide the author's interpretation of selective salient points associated with the major headings of the chapter: assessment perspectives, assessment and deafness, characteristics of assessment, purposes and types of assessment, controlled and free methods, and assessment for bilingualism and second language learning.

With respect to assessment perspectives

- Two major dichotomous frameworks were discussed: direct versus indirect and discrete-point versus integrative.

- Direct procedures refer to assessing the use of language in communicative, natural situations and are related to the use of free methods. One of the most important tasks is the collection of an adequate language sample—either spoken (signed) or written.

- Indirect procedures are often indicative of actual formal testing situations, utilizing paper-and-pencil tasks and objective formats such as multiple choice or fill in the blanks. Typically, there is no collection of information on the use or purpose of language. Indirect procedures are related to controlled methods for analyzing language development.

- Discrete-point measures focus on the testing of certain linguistic features such as vocabulary or syntax knowledge. They tend to be labeled *objective* and *analytic*.

- Integrative measures focus on a global understanding of the language performance of the individual. This involves the use of holistic scoring methods (or rubrics) with a focus on the use of the language in natural meaningful situations.

With respect to assessment and deafness

- In selecting and using an assessment with deaf and hard-of-hearing individuals, the investigator should consider certain background demographics such as degree of impairment, age at onset, family and culture information, and so on.

- There is a need to consider the use of informal and other alternative assessments in conjunction with the formal tests.

- The use of informal or alternative assessments may be critical for the younger student to supplement the unstable results of standardized formal tests.

- Observation of performance seems to be one of the most promising strategies and one of the most effective ways to organize the information is the use of a portfolio.

With respect to characteristics of assessment

- Three general characteristics were described—reliability, validity, and practicality.
- Reliability is concerned with the consistency of test results regarding the performance of students. Common procedures for determining reliability were discussed.
- Validity refers to the question of whether the test measures what it was designed to measure. The types of validity discussed were face, content, construct, concurrent, and predictive.
- Practicality refers to issues such as administration time, special equipment needs, costs of materials, scoring procedures, and special arrangements for individuals with disabilities or specific conditions.

With respect to purposes and types of assessment

- Three concepts were discussed—achievement, diagnostic, and proficiency.
- The achievement test is a summative test used at the end of a particular period of time or of learning. It is typically manifested as a standardized test and is purported to assess a representative sample of the information covered during a specified period of time.
- Diagnostic assessments reveal strengths and weaknesses of a particular student as compared to an arbitrarily decided standard. Students' scores are not compared to those of other students. The focus is on an individual's performance in a particular domain or area.
- The goal of a proficiency test is to ascertain the ability of an individual to apply what he or she has learned in real, meaningful situations. There is no time frame. This test is concerned with the individual's performance in similar real-life situations. Proficiency tests are related to the use of free methods in language assessment.

With respect to controlled and free methods

- There are advantages and disadvantages to the use of both controlled and free methods of language assessment. This should not be construed as an either-or situation; both types are necessary and useful.

- Controlled methods permit the language researcher to examine in an objective manner certain linguistic structures that might appear infrequently or never appear in a spontaneous language sample. It is possible to examine specific language domains such as phonology, syntax, and semantics.

- One major disadvantage of controlled methods is that it is not possible to obtain a comprehensive evaluation of language. Not only must one use several controlled assessments, but also, the use of spontaneous language samples is critical.

- Another major disadvantage of controlled methods is that it is difficult to generalize the results from laboratory-clinical situations to situations that resemble more naturalistic settings.

- Free methods entail the collection of a language sample for analysis—typically, a corpus of 50 to 100 utterances is required.

- Several procedures for analyzing language samples have been proposed and discussed, for example, mean length of utterance, developmental sentence type, developmental sentence scoring, the Bloom and Lahey approach, and the Kretschmer spontaneous language analysis.

- The greatest advantage of the use of free methods is the assumption that if a child consistently produces a specific structure, then he or she must have knowledge or competency of that structure.

- One of the greatest disadvantages is the problem of objectivity. It is difficult to interpret the data without imposing one's perspectives or expectations. This leads to reliability and validity problems.

With respect to assessment for bilingualism and second language learning

- There has been an ongoing debate between the notion of language dominance and that of language proficiency.

- Language dominance is concerned with a particular level of achievement, whereas language proficiency is concerned with the use of the language. However, there is no widespread consensus on the descriptions of these terms.

- The trend in bilingualism and second language learning seems to favor language proficiency, given the increased support for informal, alternative, and naturalistic measures.

- There is a great need to develop language assessments for deaf and hard-of-hearing students and teachers who might be candidates for a bilingual education program. Such tests are useful not only for evaluating the languages used but also for evaluating the effectiveness of a program.

In sum, this chapter also underscores the need for the development of tests that are normed on deaf and hard-of-hearing children and adolescents. The construction of such tests is not an easy matter given the fact that this population contains a number of subgroups with varying characteristics. Concurrently, there is a need for educators to supplement the results of formal tests with those from the use of informal and alternative measures to ensure a complete picture (or as complete as possible) of language development. The goal of these efforts has been stated eloquently: "It is hoped that significant improvements will be made in the psychoeducational assessment of hearing-impaired students so that it will be possible to make a more helpful contribution to the education of these students" (Bradley-Johnson & Evans, 1991, p. 218).

LANGUAGE ASSESSMENT COMPREHENSION QUESTIONS

1. In this chapter, there was a discussion of direct versus indirect procedures. Describe the major tenets of both approaches. Create an example of each approach based on the prototypes presented in the chapter. How do these procedures relate to the use of controlled and free methods?

2. There was a discussion of discrete-point versus integrative measures. Describe the major tenets of both measures. Create an example of each measure based on the information presented in the chapter. Do these measures shed any additional light on the discrete-point versus indirect procedures? Describe the major points.

3. It is highly recommended that informal as well as formal assessment tools be used with deaf and hard-of-hearing students. What are some types of informal assessment strategies that can be or have been used?

4. Three of the most important characteristics of assessment, particularly for formal measures, are reliability, validity, and practicality. Describe each characteristic, including the specific types of reliability and validity.

5. Describe the major tenets of the following types of assessment:
   a. achievement
   b. diagnostic
   c. proficiency

6. The selection of a test or a battery of tests for language is influenced markedly by several factors. Describe the factors mentioned in the chapter.

7. Discuss the major principles of controlled methods. What are the advantages and disadvantages of these methods? Provide some examples of test instruments that reflect the use of controlled methods.

8. Discuss the major principles of free methods. What are the advantages and disadvantages of these methods? Provide some examples (tests, etc.) that reflect the use of free methods. What analysis procedures can be used for free method language-sampling data?

9. Describe the following terms relevant to assessment of bilingualism:
   a. language dominance
   b. language proficiency

CHALLENGE QUESTIONS

(Note: Complete answers are not in the text. Additional research is required.)

1. Consider the following passage from the chapter:

   To obtain useful assessment results, an examiner must thoroughly understand the type of information that various tests and assessment procedures can provide, as well as the limitations of the information that is obtained. Furthermore, with students who have a physical impairment, such as a hearing loss, one must be familiar with procedures that can circumvent a handicapping condition and understand how the handicap may affect a student's behavior. This knowledge is necessary to ensure that results accurately reflect a student's aptitude and achievement. (Bradley-Johnson & Evans, 1991, p. xi)

   In your opinion, did the author of the chapter provide evidence to support the passage by Bradley-Johnson and Evans? If not, what are some areas of need? With respect to language assessment, does this passage omit anything that you feel is important and relevant? What?

2. As a type of informal assessment, the portfolio seems to be a highly popular instrument. Conduct a review of the literature on the use of this tool. What are the advantages and disadvantages? Is this tool used with deaf and hard-of-hearing students? Why or why not?

   Create a personal portfolio that focuses on your understanding of language and deafness. What would be your headings? What sources did you use to create the headings or to decide on the contents of the portfolio? Do you have a systematic plan for collecting information and for assessing progress? Why or why not?

3. With respect to controlled and free methods, the chapter only presented a few representative examples. Conduct a review of the literature on hearing children who have been tested for either language or literacy in their first language. What type of method is used? Can these tests be used with deaf and hard-of-hearing students? Why or why not?

4. One of the themes of this chapter and the previous one (Chapter 10) was the instruction-assessment link. After reading both chapters, do you have a better understanding of this link? Why or why not? What else should have been discussed or presented? Is this link restricted to the use of informal measures only? Why or why not? Does the use of proficiency tests—such as those for obtaining high school diplomas—support the major tenets of the instruction-assessment link, as you understand it? Why or why not?

FURTHER READINGS

Carroll, B., & Hall, P. (1985). *Make your own language tests: A practical guide to writing language performance tests.* New York: Pergamon.

Cummins, J. (1989). *Empowering minority students.* Sacramento, CA: California Association for Bilingual Education.

Gallagher, T., & Prutting, C. (1983). *Pragmatic assessment and intervention issues in language.* San Diego, CA: College-Hill Press.

Lincoln, Y., & Guba, E. (1985). *Naturalistic inquiry.* Beverly Hills, CA: Sage.

Oller, J. (Ed.). (1983). *Issues in language testing research.* Rowley, MA: Newbury House.

Worthen, B., & Sanders, J. (1987). *Educational evaluation: Alternative approaches and practical guidelines.* White Plains, NY: Longman.

CHAPTER 12

A Brief Synthesis

But what are these fundamentals? One and one only! Language, and then language—spoken, spelled, or written—and the power to read, and the power to understand what is read. Other requirements will then follow more easily and with greater results than now attained. (R. Johnson, 1916, p. 95)

There are several interpretations of this passage with respect to the various issues that have been discussed in this text. Each interpretation can be the topic of a full-length book. For example, it is possible to focus on the relationship(s) between language and thought. Despite the controversies in this area, it seems clear that high-level advances in one domain are dependent on concomitant levels of advances in the other. Language is also important for developing the skills of reading and writing. Of course, literacy is much more than knowing a language—in this case, the ability to speak and/or sign the performance form of the language in which one is trying to learn to read and write. This text also argued (as have others) that with respect to learning to read and write in a phonetic language such as English, educators need to address the issue and implications of phonemic awareness. Clearly, this presents difficulty for many deaf and some hard-of-hearing students; however, it also emphasizes the importance of words and word parts as an integral component of the word identification process in reading. In essence, there seems to be reciprocal relations between word identification and comprehension in literacy activities.

Perhaps, the most critical—and for the author the most interesting—interpretation of the earlier passage is the implications for literate thought. The author of the aforementioned passage and many educators today still believe not only in the importance of developing script-literacy skills in English but also that such skills are critical for the development of literate thought. In this text, literate thought has been defined as the ability to think critically, logically, creatively, and reflectively. Hopefully, this text demonstrates that literate thought is mode independent. In short, script-literacy skills represent only one mode for developing literate thought. Controversies in this area notwithstanding, there seems to be little doubt that the development of literate thought or critical thinking skills is dependent on a high level of proficiency in the performance form of any language at as early an age as possible. To learn to read or write in a language does require additional skills; however, the author remains unconvinced that difficulty or failure in this domain reflects the inability to engage in literate thought. Nevertheless, the early development of the performance form of a language is critical due to the pervasive effects of language on all subsequent aspects of emotional, social, and cognitive development.

This text addresses these interpretations relative to students with severe to profound hearing impairment, with some attention to students with slight to moderate levels of hearing impairment. Students with severe to profound hearing impairment represent the subgroups of the population of deaf and hard-of-hearing students who have had the most difficulty in acquiring a spoken language such as English—the language of mainstream society in the United States. As stated in Chapter 1, it is important to define the sample under consideration to avoid overgeneralizations of research results and to develop relevant and effective instructional practices and curricular materials.

This concluding chapter presents reflections on three broad questions, two of which were motivated by the ones posed by King (1981):

1. How do deaf students learn the performance form of a language?

2. How well do deaf students learn both (a) the performance forms of English and American Sign Language and (b) the written form of English?

3. Is literate thought dependent on the development of script-literacy skills? What are the implications of this answer?

The *How do* question refers to both the acquisition of the performance (or conversational) form of English (speech and/or sign) and of ASL. In the

How well question, this text attempts to chart and compare the development of English literacy in deaf and hard-of-hearing students (including those learning English as a second language) to that of hearing students. There seems to be the implicit assumption that there is a critical period for learning a language. This also applies to the development of literacy skills. Again, for the author, the most critical issue is whether individuals have the opportunity to develop a high level of literate thought. This presents the greatest challenge for educators of deaf and hard-of-hearing students—one that has enormous social, legal, and political ramifications. One rendition of literate thought has been the debate on whether English or ASL should be the first language for most, perhaps all, deaf students. This is an oversimplification of a complex problem—as will be reiterated and elaborated on in this chapter.

THE HOW DO QUESTION

The *How do* question refers to the development and use of language intervention systems with deaf and hard-of-hearing students in infancy, early childhood, and during the school years. This pertains to the representation of English in some performance form (i.e., that speech and/or signs) or to the use of American Sign Language, including the use of ASL to teach English as a second language. It should be clear that this does not refer to the use of language teaching methods, for example, natural, structured, and eclectic (McAnally et al., 1987, 1994; Quigley & Paul, 1994). The main goal of the language intervention systems is to enable fluent and intelligible communication to occur between deaf and hard-of-hearing students and significant others. This in turn leads to the internalization of a language for communication, thought, and identity. In the United States, there is the explicit assumption that this language should be, at least, the language of mainstream society—that is, English.

LANGUAGE AND COMMUNICATION INTERVENTION SYSTEMS

The merits of the various language and communication intervention systems were discussed in several chapters in this text. The use of ASL as an intervention system is evident when the topic is bilingualism or second language acquisition. Regardless of the type of intervention, there needs to be a common goal of developing English, either as a first or second language. There are other important, legitimate benefits associated with the implementation of bilingual and/or second language programs—literate thought, for example. However, the litmus test of most educational innovations is the success in developing the ability to use English in both the performance (speaking and/or signing) and script-literacy (reading and writing) modes. Whether the performance mode is or should be as prestigious and is equivalent to the script-literacy mode is discussed later in this chapter.

With this in mind, there appears to be three general ways to enable deaf and hard-of-hearing students to develop a self-controlling communication/thought system (a system with a feedback loop such as that which exists for articulation and audition or the hearing-speech link). Quigley and Paul (1994) provided their descriptions of the three ways, which are based primarily on a clinical perspective of hearing impairment:

> *The first way would be to have the defective auditory component repaired to the extent that the auditory-articulatory mechanisms would be a functional communication system. The second way would be to use the auditory-articulatory mechanisms as much as possible and to supplement them with the visual-manual mechanisms. The third way would be to substitute other physiological mechanisms for the auditory-articulatory mechanisms, such as visual mechanisms for audition and manual mechanisms for articulation; this would result in a communication system based on visual-motor mechanisms. Each of these three ways is the basis for a major category of approaches to educating deaf children—oral-aural, total communication, and American Sign Language—with the main objective for all being to produce as normal and adequate development of language as is possible. (pp. 257–258)*

Both the oral and total communication methods are concerned with the representation and development of the performance (i.e., conversational) form of English. Oral methods employ the use of speech, speechreading, and residual hearing and can be grouped into two broad categories: unisensory and multisensory. In general, unisensory refers to the use of and reliance on one sense, typically audition, whereas multisensory approaches employ the use of two or more senses, which include at least audition and vision. Cued speech/language can be labeled as a *multisensory oral approach*. The manual system of cued speech was designed to represent the phonological system of a language (i.e., vowels and consonants); suprasegmental aspects (rhythm and intonation) are also conveyed. The manual component of the English signed systems was designed to represent the morphosyntactic aspects of written standard English with the phonological aspects to be received by the listener/watcher via the use of speechreading skills.

Although many public school programs employ the use of oral methods, the exemplary oral programs, as reported in previous editions of this text, still seem to be those that exist at comprehensive, intensive oral education schools such as the Central Institute for the Deaf and the St. Joseph School for the Deaf, both in St. Louis, Missouri (Connor, 1986). It has been hypothesized that the oral components of these programs—that is, speech training, speechreading training, and the exploitation of residual hearing—are much more focused, extensive, and comprehensive than those that have been reported in typical oral education programs in regular public schools. It might also be that students who attend these exemplary oral programs represent a select group, with higher than average IQs, come from high socioeconomic backgrounds, and have highly motivated and involved parents. This is a controversial and debatable issue.

Most educational programs for deaf and hard-of-hearing students adhere to the philosophy of Total Communication, which has been the dominant philosophy since the early 1970s (Moores, 1996). TC approaches entail the use of two forms, oral and manual, and aspects of two languages, English and ASL. These forms and languages can be combined in various ways to produce manually coded English systems such as the Rochester method, the SEE systems, and signed English. The various signed systems are supposed to be used in conjunction with speech. Despite the elements common across the systems, each system operates according to its own set of rules for forming and using signs. Although the signed systems use signs from ASL, the ASL syntactic and semantic constraints of these signs are violated to represent the written language structure of English in the performance signed mode. As discussed later, the critical issues are how well English can be represented manually and the quality of this representation as compared with the use of speech.

There is a sign communication system that does not specifically adhere to a set of rules: English-like signing, also known as contact signing, conceptually accurate signed English, manual English, Pidgin sign English (archaic), sign English, signed English, and simultaneous communication (SimCom). Essentially, the main thrust of English-like signing (and its synonyms) is the use of ASL in an English word order, using few invented inflectional sign markers and, as much as possible, adhering to the correct grammatical use of the sign as it is used in ASL. English-like signing is claimed to be the most prevalent form of sign communication in the schools; however, it is still not possible to describe the patterns or rules of this mode due to wide variations in its use. Based on the manual form alone, this type of sign communication does not, and neither was it intended to, represent the complete grammatical structure of the two languages on which it is based: English and American Sign Language.

With respect to English, English-like signing, similar to the other name brands (SEE I, SEE II, etc.), needs to be used simultaneously with speech to provide a complete representation of the form of English—including phonology, morphology, syntax, and semantics. Because phonology is essentially conveyed via the use of speech, the debate on the English signed systems seems to be on the most efficient and feasible way to represent the rest of the form of English. Again, the goal is for students to develop an internalization model of the structure of English in the same intuitive manner as typically hearing students do for spoken English. Nevertheless, the litmus test for success—albeit a limited or indirect one—is the performance of the students on written English language measures such as literacy and academic achievement.

The third way refers to the use of ASL as a language intervention system, particularly in a bilingual or English as a second language program. Some deaf students are reared in homes in which ASL is either the mother tongue or is used as one of the primary conversational languages as in bilingual homes. However, it is suspected that most students with severe to profound hearing impairment acquire ASL via interactions with other native or near-native student users. This is most likely to occur at residential schools, which are the bastion of Deaf culture and ASL. In any case, there is some evidence that residential deaf students are more proficient in ASL than are their public school peers (Luetke-Stahlman, 1984).

There is no question that some deaf (i.e., profoundly hearing impaired) students know ASL as their primary performance language and that many others, perhaps most, acquire ASL by the time they reach adulthood. The debate centers on whether ASL-using deaf students can learn English as a second language or can achieve a higher proficiency in English than non-ASL-using deaf students. Even more debatable is the radical position espoused by some researchers (R. Johnson et al., 1989) that ASL should be the first language developed in all deaf students—that is, *deaf* is defined as all students with hearing impairment. The focus of Johnson et al. and others is on the notion of accessibility. In other words, the school curriculum is argued to be inaccessible to deaf students because of their difficulty with the conversational and written forms of English—the mode in which the curriculum is typically presented and discussed. Via the use and development of ASL, it is argued that deaf students can access the school curriculum and develop English as a second language primarily by learning to read and write it (not speak or sign it). Due to the lion's share of the attention on ASL/English bilingualism/biculturalism, it is often forgotten that some students come from other minority homes such as Spanish and German and that this presents even more challenges for educators. Nevertheless, there is the implicit assumption that students from spoken-language homes, in which English is either a first or second language, will benefit mostly from the use of American Sign Language, the sign language that is used predominantly by Deaf persons in the Northern Hemisphere, particularly in the United States. The basis of this assumption is that most deaf individuals do not learn adequately the spoken languages of their home environments. These issues, and others, are discussed in the *How well* section of this concluding chapter.

OTHER ISSUES

Before leaving the *How do* issue, one additional concept needs to be discussed—world of vision versus the world of audition (see further discussion in Paul & Jackson, 1993). Educational and clinical experiences have shown that beyond some level of hearing impairment (qualified by the interactions of other critical factors such as IQ and SES) even the best amplification and utilization of residual hearing provide only extremely limited feedback in speech production. Hearing impairment can certainly be represented on a continuum as measured on a decibel scale. However, at some point on that continuum an individual ceases to be linked to the world of communication, to any useful extent, primarily by hearing and becomes linked to it primarily by vision. At this point, the term *deaf* can be usefully applied to individuals who must process the language by eye. This term should distinguish this particular group from the vast majority of individuals with hearing impairment who can with appropriate amplification and training process language by ear.

That the distinction between world of vision and world of audition is critical is not always made or even accepted by some educators and researchers. Furthermore, this distinction begs the question of whether a spoken language such as English can be processed adequately by the eye—that is, by visual-manual mechanisms. For example, given the research on the manner in which some deaf students process the signs of the signed systems, it seems clear that there are visual constraints in processing these contrived signs as opposed to processing the signs of a sign language. In addition, given the limitations of the signed systems, as discussed in Chapter 6, it can be asked whether it is possible to represent English completely via the use of visual-manual mechanisms. This is especially true if deaf individuals do not have adequate speechreading skills, which seem to be necessary for important phonological information, including both segmental and suprasegmental aspects. It has been argued that cued speech/language, a type of manual system, has the potential to convey the building blocks (i.e., phonology) of English (and any other spoken language). More empirical research is still needed, as discussed in the next section.

Paul and Jackson (1993) provided some remarks on the two broad worlds:

Whether an individual is linked predominantly to the world of audition or to that of vision may be instrumental in explaining many of the research findings on language, cognition, and academic achievement. For example, one of the most important educational questions . . . is: Can students connected predominantly to the world of vision learn a spoken language in any form—that is, in the primary (speech and/or sign) and/or secondary literacy modes?. . . . Does the type of linkage, audition or vision, have important implications for the acquisition of a particular form of language at as early an age as possible? (p. 29)

Finally, to shed more light on this distinction between world of vision versus world of audition, it seems critical for future researchers to focus on providing an explanation (i.e., explanatory adequacy) of the language development of deaf and hard-of-hearing students and of the representativeness of the language intervention systems. Much of the research on language and deafness still tends to be focused on a description of language development relative to a specific language/communication system. This global approach has many shortcomings, as discussed in Chapter 6. Although this type of information is important, it is not sufficient for developing sound instructional practices and curricular materials.

The world of audition versus the world of vision has been presented as an all-or-nothing dichotomy. That is, either one is connected to the world of audition (via amplification and/or speechreading skills) or one is connected to the world of vision (via the use of a sign language). This might not be an accurate picture or a situation that fits the majority of deaf students in education programs. It is theoretically possible to observe combinations of these two worlds; meaning, for example, some students might have some skills in speechreading to connect them to the world of audition but not enough for an adequate mastery of the English language. These same students might have other skills that are conducive for being connected to a world of vision. Indeed, there seems to be direct and indirect evidence of these combinations, considering the research on ASL-using deaf individuals who are also good readers of English (see discussion in Chapter 8).

Perhaps it is misleading to present this as an either-or phenomenon, especially because the author has written much against this type of rendition in other areas, for example, literacy (Paul, 1998a). Of this, the following seems certain: If an individual has limited access to the phonology of a language, he or she will have extreme difficulty learning adequately that language in either the performance mode (speaking and/or signing) or in the script-literacy mode (reading and writing). In this case, it is argued that the individual is linked predominantly to the world of vision—a mode that is conducive to learning a sign language, not a spoken language. It is certainly possible to be linked (or have possible links) to the world of audition (i.e., being able to understand aspects of a spoken language) without having the ability to hear adequately as long as such knowledge is cognitively developed. Obviously, being able to hear or to possess an auditory-articulatory link facilitates the cognitive development of this knowledge. However, as argued in the section on cued speech (Chapter 5), the phonology of a spoken language does not need to be rendered via a sound medium. The point (also stated by others) is that phonology needs to be rendered in some adequate, clear fashion to learn a language.

A challenge is issued here to future researchers/scholars to clarify this world of audition versus world of vision phenomenon. It might also be that clarification of this concept is pervasively contingent on continued advances in technology, for example, in the area of cochlear implants. In essence, the future research effects of cochlear implants should provide another perspective on not only the *How do* question, but also the *How well* question, discussed in the next section.

Table 12-1 provides a summary of major points for the *How do* section.

Table 12-1 Summary of Major Points for the *How Do* Section

- *How do* refers to the development and use of language intervention systems with deaf and hard-of-hearing students. This entails the representation of English in some performance form or to the use of ASL, including the use of ASL to teach English as a second language.

- There are three general ways to enable deaf and hard-of-hearing students to develop a self-controlling communication/thought system. Each of these three ways is the basis for a major category of approaches to educating deaf children—oral-aural, Total Communication, and American Sign Language.

- Oral methods employ the use of speech, speechreading, and residual hearing and can be grouped into two broad categories: unisensory and multisensory. Unisensory refers to the use of and reliance on one sense, typically audition, whereas multisensory approaches employ the use of two or more senses, which include at least audition and vision. Cued speech/language is a multisensory oral approach.

(continues)

(Table 12-1 contiinued)

- Total communication approaches entail the use of two forms, oral and manual, and aspects of two languages, English and ASL. These forms and languages can be combined in various ways to produce manually coded English systems such as the Rochester method, the SEE systems, and signed English. The various signed systems are supposed to be used in conjunction with speech. Each system operates according to its own set of rules for forming and using signs.

- The debate on the English signed systems seems to be on the most efficient and feasible way to represent the form of English. Phonology, the building block of a language, is essentially conveyed via the use of speech—not via the manual forms of the signed systems.

- The third way refers to the use of ASL as a language intervention system, particularly in a bilingual or English as a second language program. Some deaf students are reared in homes in which ASL is either the mother tongue or is used as one of the primary conversational languages as in bilingual homes. One important debate is on whether ASL-using deaf students can learn English as a second language or can achieve a higher proficiency in English than non-ASL-using deaf students.

- With respect to *How do*, there is a need for future research to clarify the concept of world of vision versus the world of audition—which concerns the processing of language primarily by ear (audition) or by eye (vision).

- If an individual has limited access to the phonology of a language, he or she will have extreme difficulty learning adequately that language in either the performance or script-literacy mode. This is the litmus test for all language/communication systems.

HOW WELL

A synthesis of the information discussed in Chapters 5 to 9 provides the bulk of the insights for the *How well* issue. These insights can be presented relative to the development of the performance form of English via the use of oral and TC approaches and via the use of ASL. A summary is also presented on the acquisition of English literacy skills, either in English as a first language or English as a second language—which is an indirect reflection of the *How well* issue.

LANGUAGE AND COMMUNICATION APPROACHES

One of the themes of this book has been that the primary language development of deaf and hard-of-hearing children should be considered in terms of the communication form by which it is developed and through which it finds expression. This means that the primary (or performance) language development should be considered in terms of oral English, manually coded English, including English signing (e.g., archaic PSE, contact signing, etc.), and American Sign Language. Much of the information in Chapters 5 and 6 was organized in this manner, with Chapter 7 focusing on ASL. As was the case for the previous edition of this text, there continues to be very limited amount of data on the effectiveness of these communication forms. In addition, there is still limited information on the use of these forms by members of different ethnic groups—which constitutes either bilingualism or multiculturalism (see Chapter 9). Nevertheless, it is believed that there is now a clearer picture of the issue of representation of English via the use of manual modes. That is, for any communication form to be effective, it has to represent as adequately as possible the phonologic component of a language. This seems to be a major problem for all of the English signed systems, at least.

Oral English

The studies cited in the OE chapter (Chapter 5), including cued speech/language, involved those deaf and hard-of-hearing students in indisputably oral programs or those integrated in the general education classrooms. In general, it was found that the performance (or conversational) and written language developments of these students are qualitatively similar to albeit quantitatively slower than those of students with typical hearing. However, a number of these students do perform on grade level when compared to hearing peers. At the very least, with respect to literacy development, research on these students seems to substantiate the importance of phonemic awareness for the development of English literacy skills. Whether students exposed to cued speech/language can develop adequate phonemic awareness without having much residual hearing or traditional speechreading skills is in need of additional research; however, theoretically, the author is convinced of the potential benefits of cued speech/language (see review in Paul, 1999). The reader is reminded that there is more to English literacy than the possession of phonemic awareness—an issue discussed again later in this chapter.

It might be difficult to generalize the results of students exposed to OE, including cued speech/language, to other deaf students on two counts, at least: (a) An active, comprehensive oral approach to language development might be present only in a few educational programs, and (b) deaf students in these programs might be members of a more select group, especially in relation to IQ, SES, and highly educated and involved parents than deaf students in other programs. Despite these two points, these studies indicate that deaf students in incontestably oral programs or those select few integrated in general education classrooms do develop superior language and academic skills compared to most other deaf students in the general school population, especially those in special education programs. It should be underscored, however, that very few deaf students can acquire a high level of English proficiency in oral programs. It seems that this language intervention approach does not enable most deaf students to develop and use an automatic, self-controlling auditory-articulatory system similar to that of students with typical hearing (Quigley & Paul, 1994). Whether more deaf students can benefit from oral English approaches remains to be seen. It might be that improvements in instructional techniques need to occur in tandem with improvements in technology for the perception of speech stimuli. Nevertheless, the advances in technology are encouraging, especially in light of the research on cochlear implants with or without other aids (e.g., tactile), as discussed in Chapter 5.

Manually Coded English

Most of the MCE approaches, including English signing (archaic PSE, contact signing, SimCom, etc.), discussed in this text have been in use for 25 years or longer. Very little educational success has been reported, especially for a majority of deaf and hard-of-hearing students on the development of literacy skills on graduation from high school. In many cases, there has been reports that certain aspects of English grammar, for example, morphology, can be taught through a particular approach. This does not mean—neither has it been shown—that students can master the morphological component of English. Studies demonstrating the most success (Babb, 1979; Brasel & Quigley, 1977; Luetke-Stahlman, 1988a; Washburn, 1983; also see Stewart & Luetke-Stahlman, 1998) indicate that certain conditions are necessary for this level of achievement, for example: (a) active involvement in the home and school by parents/caregivers, (b) instruction that adheres to the developmental patterns of hearing children, and (c) the use of a manual form that is considered a more complete representation of English, such as the SEE systems—seeing essential English and signing exact English.

Relative to the third condition, it seems that educational programs should consider the adoption of systems such as seeing essential English (SEE I) and signing exact English (SEE II) because these seem to be most representative of English in the manual mode. In addition, there have been some impressive results from students exposed to these systems. Given the shortcomings of all signed systems, as discussed in Chapter 6, the success of students still needs to be investigated further. That is, it is still not clear why some students are successful with a system that does not convey adequately the phonological component of English. It is suspected that the successful students are internalizing or developing phonological knowledge via existing speechreading skills or via other mechanisms (exposure to print).

Nevertheless, it is surprising that most programs for students with hearing impairment use a form of signing that does not adhere to an established set of rules or principles, such as contact signing, signed English, sign English, SimCom, and so on. It is possible to find some students who are successful within this loosely defined mode. However, it seems that the performance of students in this mode is inferior compared with that of students exposed to other systems—notably SEE I or SEE II. The use of this mode of communication might be based on reasons other than research effectiveness—perhaps ease of use is a strong factor.

From another perspective, it has been difficult to evaluate the usefulness of approaches most representative of English (e.g., SEE I and SEE II) because of the difficulty that many practitioners have had in adhering faithfully to the rules of these systems for forming and using signs (Kluwin, 1981; Marmor & Petitto, 1979; Strong & Charlson, 1987). This situation is said to be due to the incompatibility of signing and speaking simultaneously, resulting in the omission of signs and/or sign markers. This results in an impoverished language model for deaf and hard-of-hearing students and calls into question the usefulness of the MCE systems or any form of English signing (Drasgow, 1998; Drasgow & Paul, 1995; Maxwell, 1990; Paul & Drasgow, 1998).

A number of other criticisms have been made concerning the English signed systems, many of which were discussed in Chapters 6 and 8. For example, it has been argued that there is a lack of a community of users outside the school system, making it difficult for students to continue to grow in the use of the language behind the system. As mentioned previously, one of the strongest criticisms has been the presence of processing constraints the cumbersome systems present for many deaf and hard-of-hearing students. For example, Gee and Goodhart (1988) reported that their deaf subjects alter the grammatical (morphological and syntactic) elements of the various MCE systems. These alternations occur because the rate of sign execution within the MCE systems is much slower than both the expressive and receptive capacities of deaf students. This phenomenon has been reported and discussed in a number of deaf students (see review in Drasgow, 1998).

In essence, these criticisms seem to suggest that the acquisition of American Sign Language (or any sign language) is easier (and more feasible) than the acquisition of any signed system based on a spoken language such as English. In addition, they seem to call into question whether English can be acquired at a proficient level by many students with severe to profound hearing impairment. The issue of accessibility, as argued by R. Johnson et al. (1989), clearly is a critical one. There needs to be a better understanding of how much and what deaf and hard-of-hearing children and adolescents are accessing (or acquiring) when they are exposed to either the oral or manual forms of English.

Developing models of accessibility might be the next progressive step in obtaining a more comprehensive picture of the language acquisition process. Insights gained from the accessibility models should complement what is known about language development based on the language acquisition models. Relative to individuals with hearing impairment, the accessibility issue is concerned with specific types of linguistic information that is or can be captured by the ear or the eye and what is meant by the perception of linguistic information presented simultaneously in different modes (i.e., speaking and signing simultaneously).

The work of Maxwell and others seems to imply that the presentation of English via a simultaneous mode is complete when it is analyzed at the semantic or meaning level although there are gaps at the morphologic and syntactic levels. Fleetwood and Metzger (1998) showed that without access to accompanying speech stimuli (or adequate representations of abstract phonemes), all signed systems do not convey phonological information—the building blocks of a language. The gaps at the morphologic and syntactic levels are due mostly to the omissions of information by practitioners while they attempt to adhere to the rules for forming and using signs.

It is still not clear what deaf and hard-of-hearing students perceive when they are exposed to simultaneous presentations. Much of the research has been on the comparisons of the sign systems on a global level (e.g., reading and educational achievement). For example, it is still not known how much and what information deaf and hard-of-hearing students acquire relative to major components of English such as phonology, morphology, and syntax via the use of the signed systems. Are deaf and hard-of-hearing students acquiring or internalizing the necessary suprasegmental features such as intonation and stress? It is often forgotten that an intuitive knowledge of phonology of English means an intuitive knowledge of both segmentals (vowels and consonants) and suprasegmentals. This knowledge seems to be important—perhaps critical—for acquiring high-level literacy skills. Similar analogies can be made about deaf and hard-of-hearing students' intuitive knowledge of the other major English components.

One of the most important inferences that can be drawn from these criticisms of the signed systems is the need for an ongoing assessment of the language development of deaf and hard-of-hearing students. In essence, this is another reference to the acquisition of a language at as early an age as possible. There is substantial evidence indicating that children with typical hearing develop a first language by the age of 5 or 6 years (see Chapter 4). If English is the first language of choice, the goal should be to develop proficiency as soon as possible. It is true that proficiency has levels and that it is difficult to ascertain a certain level of proficiency, especially in young deaf and hard-of-hearing children. Nevertheless, for those deaf and hard-of-hearing children for whom English is the first language of choice, parents and educators might need to consider alternative routes such as bilingualism (English and ASL) if these children seem to have persistent low proficiency levels, based on best estimates. Proceeding to a bilingual route based on a failure or difficulty in acquiring a first language is not what bilingual or second language proponents have in mind and might not even be acceptable to most of these proponents. Political disagreements notwithstanding, it is unacceptable to the author to require 10 to 15 years for a high-level development of a first social-conventional language. Or, as is the case for many deaf children, no adequately developed social-conventional language by the time they graduate from high school. The lack of an adequate language for communication and thought clearly has pervasive negative effects on the subsequent development of literate thought in any form, as discussed later in this chapter.

American Sign Language

If English (or any spoken language) is a very difficult, or perhaps impossible, language for most deaf students to acquire, it might be best to consider the use of a bona fide sign language such as American Sign Language. Clearly, if ASL is the first language for some deaf students, then English should be approached as a second language. In any case, developing proficiency in two languages in which one is the majority language of the culture would be optimal; developing proficiency in any language is a necessity.

Only a representative sample of research studies on the acquisition of ASL was presented in this text (Chapter 7). It is clear that ASL is a bona fide language with a grammar different from that of English (Klima & Bellugi, 1979; C. Lucas, 1990; Wilbur, 1987). Psycholinguistic research indicates that the acquisition of ASL is essentially similar to and parallel to that of spoken language acquisition (see review in Bonvillian, 1999). For example, strategies and features such as overgeneralization and markedness have been observed in both

ASL and English. Another example is that certain semantic relations and pragmatic functions observed in hearing children have also been reported in the early acquisition stages of deaf children. Certain areas of syntactic development need further investigation, for example, sign order and nonmanual cues. One interesting finding on ASL development has been the documentation of manual babbling in deaf infants (Petitto & Marentette, 1991).

As discussed in Chapter 9, there seems to be a growing consensus for the development and implementation of ASL/English bilingual programs. The impetus for this approach is that it should be easier for deaf students to learn English if teachers use ASL as the medium of instruction for content courses as well as for teaching English as a second language. Nevertheless, as argued in Chapter 9, knowledge of ASL is not sufficient for the acquisition of English literacy skills any more than knowledge of French is. Most of the bilingual models discussed in Chapter 9 seem to overlook the major tenets of reading comprehension theories or have misinterpreted some of the major principles of second language theorists such as those of Cummins or Vygotsky. A better understanding of this issue can be gleaned from the synopsis of the major tenets of the development of English literacy skills in the ensuing section.

ENGLISH LITERACY

Since the beginning of formal testing procedures, most of the literature reviews have reported that the English literacy achievement of many students with severe to profound hearing impairment who graduate from high school is at about a fourth-grade level. Without oversimplifying, it is possible to discuss deaf students' difficulty with respect to two broad areas: processing and knowledge. Processing refers to the ability to use a phonological code in short-term memory (actually, working memory). Knowledge refers to an understanding of the various aspects of English, for example, phonology, morphology, syntax, semantics, and pragmatics. It might be that a high proficiency level of the form of English—that is, phonology, morphology, and syntax—is dependent on the processing strategies. This is another way of saying that there seems to be a strong interrelation among phonological coding, word identification, and comprehension. Not surprisingly, this interrelation is also important for the development of adequate literacy skills in deaf students learning English as a second language.

One framework for understanding this interrelation is to consider that literacy, particularly reading, incorporates both bottom-up and top-down processing skills (Adams, 1990; R. Anderson et al., 1985; Snow et al., 1998). Bottom-up, or decoding, skills pertain to the perception of linguistic aspects of a text such as letters, syllables, and words. Top-down, or comprehension, skills involve the knowledge-based aspects associated with the reader such as prior (topic or world) knowledge, use of metacognitive skills, and knowledge of the language of print. Adequate bottom-up skills lead to the development of rapid automatic word identification (decoding) skills, and well-developed top-down processing facilitates the understanding of the text.

As discussed in Chapter 8, there are two other groups of factors that have been proffered as part of the literacy process: task factors and context factors. However, the focus here is on text-based and reader-based factors because in the author's view, these are most directly related to the process of literacy— especially with respect to accessing the print on the page. To state this another way: The author believes the access issue requires a better understanding of the relationship between the text (i.e., words that are captured in print) and the reader (knowledge in the readers' minds). Contributions from task and context factors are important; however, the earlier mentioned relationship is typically underscored by the reciprocal influences of word identification and comprehension.

Word identification facilitates comprehension, and comprehension facilitates word identification. This reciprocal relationship for reading and writing activities is dependent on the overall reciprocal relationship between the performance (conversational) and written form, which is activated by the association between phonology and orthography (Brady & Shankweiler, 1991; Snow et al., 1998; Templeton & Bear, 1992). Understanding the link between the phonemes of speech of a phonetic language (i.e., phonological knowledge) and the graphemes of print (i.e., orthographical knowledge) is critical for reading an alphabetic system such as English. That is, there needs to be an awareness that speech can be segmented into phonemes, which are represented by an alphabetic orthography. This is not a natural unconscious process; it is a learned behavior.

Fluent word reading, which is a by-product of rapid word identification skills, also seems to be dependent on the use of a phonological-based code in short-term memory (or working memory). The efficient use of WM is dependent on the use of this code, and this efficiency allows the reader to expend more energy on the important top-down processes. The use of a phonological-based code in WM is best for processing verbosequential (or temporal-sequential) information that characterized primarily the structure of a phonetic language such as English.

The use of a phonological code—albeit critical—is not the only skill needed for developing adequate reading comprehension ability. In addition, the inability or difficulty of deaf students in using a phonological-based code in WM does not mean that their memory is deficient per se. It means that deaf students will not perform well on tasks requiring this type of code. As noted by Paul and Jackson (1993):

> *It should not be inferred that the nature of short-term memory is the only factor accounting for the English language and literacy difficulty of these students. However, it may be a major one, especially if the tasks or materials require verbal (i.e., phonological) encoding. Within this perspective, the problem seems to be a task- or material-specific one. The problem does not indicate a memory impairment. (p. 270)*

The use of a phonological code or, perhaps, the ability to abstract phonological information is related to the development of phonemic awareness. Phonemic awareness leads to an understanding of the link between the performance and written forms of English, as discussed in Chapter 8. In Chapter 9, it was argued that phonemic awareness is also important for learning to read and write in English as a second language. This factor seems to be overlooked by many proponents of ASL/English bilingual/bicultural programs.

Second language students, including ASL-using deaf students, typically do not begin the reading of English with the same level of English language and cultural knowledge as native first language learners (Bernhardt, 1991; Paul, 1998a; Snow et al., 1998). These students also do not possess adequate knowledge about the written language of English, for example, vocabulary, syntax, and the alphabetic principle. It is possible for second language students to learn about English culture for the purpose of reading via instruction in their native language. This seems to be the major impetus for some minority-language immersion programs, as discussed in Chapter 9. Nevertheless, both hearing and deaf second language learners still need a deep understanding of the alphabetic principle of English, which facilitates and permits the effective use of higher level comprehension processes during literacy tasks. In essence, this deep understanding of the alphabetic principle is facilitated by phonological and phonemic awareness; however, it might be possible to utilize other routes—albeit less efficient—such as the use of morphology (in structural analysis programs). Use of morphology in conjunction with phonemic awareness, however, is more effective in developing knowledge of orthography, including conventional spelling skills, than the use of morphology alone.

Similar to deaf students learning English as a first language, it is possible to characterize the difficulty of ASL-using deaf students as a processing problem. This processing issue might entail one or two conditions: (a) difficulty in accessing segmentals and suprasegmentals of the phonology of English as well as its other grammatical components and/or (b) difficulty in processing phonological information in WM as evident in poor readers who are fairly adequate speakers-listeners of English. Both of these conditions are related to the overall development of the phonological component of English, a phonetic language. This text has attempted to show that difficulty in accessing the phonological component of any language leads to an incomplete or inadequate internalization of the form of that language because phonology is considered the building block. This lack of internalization leads to problems in developing both phonological and phonemic awareness, which are important for the subsequent development of reading and writing skills.

It is possible to use ASL to teach the necessary school curricula and other content knowledge that are critical for understanding the language of print. However, ASL-using deaf students—as well as other second language users—still need a high-level understanding of English, particularly of the alphabetic code. Without this knowledge and relying predominantly on their first language (i.e., not English), ASL-using deaf students will depend too heavily on the use of top-down skills (e.g., prior knowledge via ASL), which can lead to misinterpretation of the texts (see Kelly, 1995; Paul, 1998a, 1998b). It should be emphasized there is no compelling evidence that second language students can learn to read in the second language via exposure to the print of that target language and explanations in their native or first language (Bernhardt, 1991; Paul 1998a).

Because of deaf children's difficulty with phonology and the use of a phonological-based code in WM, a few scholars have argued for the use of visual-based strategies such as the sight word approach or the use of a predominant orthographic approach (see review in Paul, 1998a, 1998b). In fact, this is a major impetus for several ASL/English bilingual programs in which English is taught via the written mode only. Paul (1998b) provided one interpretative synopsis of this position:

> *Some scholars, including those who advocate ASL/English bilingual programs, seem to favor the perception that reading is primarily a "visual" process (i.e., mostly orthographic) in which deaf students can access words and larger structures (e.g., syntax) and, subsequently, understand their meanings (i.e., a semantic process) without the use of a phonological "recoding" or "mediating" process. . . . That is, there is little or no need for deaf students to be taught or even apply letter-sound relationships, which requires, at least, the integration of phonological and morphological knowledge and orthography (e.g., graphemes, spelling, etc.). In general, there is the perception that deaf students can proceed directly from "print" (i.e., letters, words, phrases, sentences) to meaning. (p. 261)*

This position is misleading at best and inaccurate at worst. First, for hearing students, it has been argued that word identification entails the use of both visual processing and a phonological translation. This phonological translation is not possible without phonological and phonemic awareness. Even more interesting, visual processing (i.e., orthography) and phonological translation are not independent entities; rather, they are synergistic parts of the same process (Adams, 1990; also see the discussion in Snow et al., 1998). At the very least, educators and researchers should consider the role of both phonology and orthography in the literacy acquisition process of deaf and hard-of-hearing students.

Difficulties with phonology might provide the bulk of the explanation for many deaf and some hard-of-hearing students' struggles with the development of adequate literacy skills. It seems clear that the role of phonology cannot be ignored. It might be quite astonishing to many educators of deaf students to accept that "sight word reading is not necessarily a rote memorization process that ignores letter-sound relations" (Ehri, 1991, p. 383). In essence, the "evidence suggests that phonological recoding skill is not a mere facilitator but a necessity for reading words by sight" (Ehri, 1991, p. 402). It still remains to be seen whether these assertions are applicable to most deaf and hard-of-hearing students. With the author's proclivity for the qualitative similarity hypothesis (Paul, 1998a, 1998b), he believes that future research will substantiate this issue overwhelmingly for deaf and hard-of-hearing students.

If both phonological and phonemic awareness are critical for the development of high-level literacy skills, it might be wondered whether the development of English script literacy is a realistic goal for many deaf students. As discussed briefly in Chapter 1, the ability to read and write is important for success in society. But, is literacy really necessary for the development of literate thought, that is, the ability to think rationally, critically, logically, and creatively? Is it an epiphenomenon or a by-product? This represents the third group of questions posed at the beginning of this chapter. The answers to these questions and others have pervasive educational and ethical implications.

Table 12-2 provides a summary of major points for the *How well* section.

Table 12-2 Summary of Major Points for the *How Well* Section

---

- With respect to oral approaches, it was found that the performance and written language developments of students are qualitatively similar to albeit quantitatively slower than those of students with typical hearing. A number of students do perform on grade level when compared to hearing peers.

- Research seems to substantiate the importance of phonemic awareness for the development of English literacy skills. With respect to phonemic awareness, additional research is needed on all students, particularly students who are exposed to cued speech/language.

- It is difficult to generalize the results of students exposed to oral English, including cued speech/language, to other deaf and hard-of-hearing students. Nevertheless, the few deaf students in incontestably oral programs or those select few integrated in general education classrooms do develop superior language and academic skills compared to most other deaf students in the general school population, especially those in special education programs.

- Despite 25 or more years of use of various signed systems, very little educational success has been reported, especially for a majority of deaf and hard-of-hearing students on the development of literacy skills on graduation from high school.

- Studies demonstrating the most success indicate that certain conditions are necessary for this level of achievement. These include the active involvement of parents/caregivers, instruction that matches the developmental patterns of typical children, and the use of a manual form (signed system) that is considered a more complete representation of English, such as the SEE systems.

- It is still not clear why some students are successful with signed systems that do not convey adequately the phonological component of English. It is suspected that successful students are internalizing or developing phonological knowledge via existing speechreading skills or other mechanisms such as exposure to print.

- Most programs seem to use English signing (sign English, contact signing, etc.), which is a loosely defined entity, making it difficult to describe and to evaluate.

- One of the strongest criticisms of all signed systems, particularly the more cumbersome systems, has been the presence of processing constraints for many deaf and hard-of-hearing students. Students tend to alter the grammatical elements of the systems to match their capacities. This seems to call into question whether English can be acquired at a proficient level by many students with severe to profound hearing impairment.

(continues)

(Table 12-2 continued)

- It is still not clear what deaf and hard-of-hearing students perceive when they are exposed to simultaneous presentations (speaking and signing simultaneously).

- There is a need for an ongoing assessment of the language development of deaf and hard-of-hearing students.

- If English is a very difficult, or perhaps impossible, language for most deaf students to acquire, it might be best to consider the use of a bona fide sign language such as ASL.

- Psycholinguistic research indicates that the acquisition of ASL is essentially similar to and parallel to that of spoken language acquisition.

- There seems to be a growing consensus for ASL/English bilingual/bicultural programs. However, most of the bilingual models seem to overlook the major tenets of reading comprehension theories or have misinterpreted some of the major principles of second language theorists.

- Since the beginning of formal testing procedures, most of the literature reviews have reported that the English literacy achievement of many students with severe to profound hearing impairment who graduate from high school is at about a fourth-grade level.

- There seems to be two broad areas of difficulty: processing and knowledge. Processing refers to the ability to use a phonological code in working memory. Knowledge refers to an understanding of the various aspects of English.

- The development of adequate literacy skills requires at least the use of both bottom-up (i.e., decoding) and top-down (i.e., comprehension) processing skills.

- Understanding the link between the phonemes of speech of a phonetic language (i.e., phonological knowledge) and the graphemes of print (i.e., orthographical knowledge) is critical for reading an alphabetic system such as English.

- Phonemic awareness is also important for learning to read and write in English as a second language. In essence, ASL-using deaf students—as well as other second language users—still need a high level of understanding of English, particularly of the alphabetic code. Without this knowledge and relying predominantly on their first language, ASL-using deaf students will depend too heavily on the use of top-down skills (e.g., via ASL), which can lead to misinterpretation of the texts.

- There is no compelling evidence that second language students can learn to read in the second language via exposure to the print of that target language and explanations in their native or first language.

A PERSPECTIVE ON LITERATE THOUGHT

This section elaborates on the concept of literate thought, which was introduced in Chapter 1. First, historical and traditional views of literacy are described, including its importance for a technologically driven society such as the United States. Then, it is argued that current thinking and current metaphors of literacy are reflective of the notion of literate thought. In short, script literacy, as one type of literacy, is seen as one manifestation or form of literate thought. Additional information is provided on the related concepts of performance and performance literacy, which were also mentioned in Chapter 1. Research support for performance and the more recent phrase, *performance literacy*, comes mostly from historical research on orality—that is, the oral tradition or the use of the spoken mode. On the basis of historical research and current views on literacy, it is argued that literate thought is mode independent—although it is critical for an individual to possess a bona fide language, in the performance form at least, at as early an age as possible.

If it is accepted that literate thought is mode independent, then the heavy reliance on script literacy—especially for diplomas, degrees, and other prestigious conditions—might be seen as an example of oppression. For many deaf students, including other students who are poor readers, the pervasive emphasis on script literacy might prevent or preclude the high-level development of literate thought. A perspective on this assertion can be gleaned from the discussion of Stanovich's Matthew Effects (Stanovich, 1986). The last part of this section provides questions for further research endeavors.

Background on the Importance of Script Literacy

Why is script literacy (i.e., reading and writing) so valuable and important? Consider the value of reading as stated in the following passage.

Reading is important for the society as well as the individual. Economics research has established that schooling is an investment that forms human capital—that is, knowledge, skill, and problem-solving ability that have enduring value. While a country receives a good return on investment in education at all levels from nursery school and kindergarten through college, the research reveals that the returns are highest from the early years of schooling when children are first learning to read. The Commission on Excellence warned of the risk for America from shortcomings in secondary education. Yet the early years set the stage for later learning. Without the ability to read, excellence in high school and beyond is unattainable. (R. Anderson et al., 1985, p. 1)

Now, consider the value of possessing writing skills as discussed in the ensuing passages:

Olson (1986) . . . Ong (1982), and others claim, roughly, that writing is necessary for the forms of consciousness found in modern Western thought. (C. Feldman, 1991, p. 47)

Even if there was no agreed theory on the role of literacy in social and cognitive change, there was and continues to be a general agreement that literacy, printing, and the alphabet, however they did it, were fundamental to those changes. (Olson, 1986, p. 111)

Oral cultures indeed produce powerful and beautiful verbal performances of high artistic and human worth, which are no longer even possible once writing has taken possession of the psyche. Nevertheless, without writing, human consciousness cannot achieve its fuller potentials, cannot produce other beautiful and powerful creations. In this sense, orality needs to produce and is destined to produce writing. Literacy, as will be seen, is absolutely necessary for the development not only of science but also of history, philosophy, explicative understanding of literature and of any art, and indeed for the explanation of language (including oral speech) itself. (Ong, 1982, p. 15)

There is no question that reading and writing skills are highly valued and important in a scientific, technological society such as that which exists in the United States. Based on the aforementioned passages, particularly the ones on writing, there seems to be the perception that high-level writing skills are reflective of the ability to think at high levels; that is, the ability to think in a rational, logical, complex, reflective manner often associated with Western world consciousness or in societies that have written languages. In addition, giving the availability and widespread use of the written word, one needs to read and perhaps write to continue to learn and, perhaps, survive in literate societies. In other words, reading and writing skills contribute to and are examples of the literate mind as well as tools that might be necessary for participating in and reaping the benefits of the social, economic, and political realms of mainstream society in the United States.

From another perspective, it can be asked: Are reading and writing skills really necessary or important for the high-level development of literate thought?

If the answer is no, then it can be argued that the strong emphasis on reading and writing skills in educational settings is an oppressive situation for many, perhaps all, individuals who may be poor readers and writers according to the results of standardized tests but nevertheless are good thinkers otherwise in the performance mode (e.g., speaking or signing) of a language. In other words, if there are equally viable roads to literate thought besides the script literacy ones, then this becomes an equity and diversity issue. Similar to what has been argued by some critical theorists (see discussion in Gibson, 1986), one should be asking questions such as: Whose values are being served? Why should diplomas, degrees, a big slice of the economic pie, and so on be available to only those who can read and write well? Should one value and respect all forms of literate thought, not just those that are manifested by script literacy skills?

What is Literacy?

A better understanding of literate thought may be obtained by a discussion of the current views of literacy, particularly script literacy. In other words, what is literacy? At the very least, it has been argued that reading and possibly writing is an entity involving an array of processes such as linguistics, cognitive, social, and even political (Pearson & Stephens, 1994). Perhaps the better question that needs to be answered is: What is a literate thinker? Another question is: How is this concept related to forms of literacy, for example, performance, reading/writing, mathematics, computer, and so on?

The pursuit of a so-called multidisciplinary approach to script literacy has led—among other things—to the use of different metaphors to answer the question what is reading (or writing). On a surface level, when some, perhaps many, educators think of reading (or writing), what comes to mind is the reading or writing of print. It seems that some of the debate is centered on accessibility, specifically the accessibility of English print. Access can have at least two broad components: access to the language of print and access to the information captured in print. These two components can be separated for discussion purposes. Think of the possibilities: It is possible to access the language of print but not be able to use the information (i.e., understanding and applying information). It is equally possible to access and use information through the performance-based mode (speech and/or signs) of one's native language but not understand the language of English print. There are of course other possibilities. Before proceeding, it should be stated that there is probably no broad consensus on what the word *access* means. The main point here is that the use of the word *access* is not really synonymous with the interpretation or the meaning associated with a passage or even the application of that interpretation or meaning. Of course, access to print helps the individual in this process, especially if she or he is required to perform tasks in the printed mode only.

Consider the following metaphors, which represent some of the currently used ideas to describe reading. Readers should get the impression that these metaphors seem to almost bypass or downplay the access part of the process of reading. There is no question that access is important; however, it is not reading according to these metaphors. It should also be clear that the existence of numerous metaphors for reading is reflective of the position that reading, similar to other concepts involving the human mind, is an ill-defined construct. Theoretically, reading has been labeled as an *ill-structured domain* (see Spiro's metaphor next).

Metaphors for 'Reading'

1. John Downing's theory of cognitive clarity: Downing has asserted that the salient goal of all instructional activities—such as phonics, vocabulary, comprehension, studying, thinking, or mathematical problem solving—should be to promote cognitive clarity (Downing, 1979).

2. Rand Spiro's theory of cognitive flexibility: Spiro and his colleagues have used this idea as a way to explain a variety of learning in domains that are considered dynamic and, more specifically, domains that are referred to as ill-structured domains. Cognitive flexibility theory has been evoked to account for such complex, diverse, and dynamic events as learning to read, learning to teach, and learning to diagnose medical problems. Spiro has invoked one of Wittgenstein's metaphors: crisscrossing the landscape from multiple directions—a metaphor that is apt for the ongoing thrust of developing multidisciplinary models (Spiro et al., 1987).

3. Rosenblatt's metaphor of a poem: Rosenblatt has argued that meaning is not on the printed page, or in the head of the reader, or a result of the task or context. Instead, meaning is created in the transaction between reader and text. Rosenblatt has used the metaphor of a poem to refer to the meaning, which resides above the reader-text plane. Meaning is neither subject (reader) nor object (text) but transaction (Rosenblatt, 1978). It should be highlighted that transaction is different from interaction. Transaction views the reader and text as a whole; that is, there is no separation of the reader and the information as the notion of interaction implies. Interaction is compared to the notion of Cartesian dualism—which was learned from Decartes and

Newton—or a separation of the knower from the knowledge, whereas transaction is somewhat similar to constructivism and also to phenomenology—which was learned from Hegel and Kant among others (for a readable discussion of these philosophies, see Copleston, 1985; B. Russell, 1972).

4. And, there are of course other views—inspired by sociolinguists, post-structuralists, and critical literary theorists (see discussions in Paul, 1998a; Pearson & Stephens, 1994).

Implicit in all these metaphors on script literacy is the focus on cognition. There seems to be an emphasis on concepts such as thinking, reasoning, reflecting, and so on. This focus also seems to suggest that developing script-literacy skills, particularly with the captured information in print, requires the use of critical thinking skills and the understanding and use of a metalanguage (i.e., specific terminology) for discussion purposes. Metalanguage is a broad term that can refer to what is often labeled metacognitive skills in reading and writing; however, metalanguage is not confined to script-literacy modes. It can be extended to any captured mode of information—print, videotapes, audiotapes, pictures and graphs, and so on. In addition, it is the study of and reflection on each captured mode of information that contributes to the development of literate thought. The focus here is on the captured mode of verbal information—in essence, the manner in which this information is captured is merely a matter of convenience rather than the road to literate thought.

If this is accepted, then one of the roads to literate thought is via the use and development of performance literacy skills.

Performance Literacy: Background and Research

As mentioned in Chapter 1, *performance* is a term that refers to information presented in the oral or conversational form of the language. For much of the world, this refers to the use of speech; however, it can also refer to the use of signs as in signed systems and sign languages used with deaf and hard-of-hearing students. Performance can also refer to other areas such as music, art, and drama, but here it is confined to spoken and/or signed languages or signed systems and other nonscript-based symbol systems that individuals use to express thoughts and feelings.

Traditionally, the notion of performance has been influenced by the research on orality and the oral tradition (Denny, 1991; C. Feldman, 1991; Olson, 1989, 1991). With the advent of sign languages and signed systems, there is a need to update the thinking about orality; more important, it is the research on orality plus the current views on literacy that have provided an emerging, perhaps better, understanding of what it means to be literate (for a discussion of some current views on literacy, see Beach, 1994; Tierney, 1994; Weaver, 1994). The capture of information in the performance mode can be labeled *performance literacy*; information captured in the print or written mode is the traditional script literacy.

It should be inquired whether performance or performance literacy is as complex, rational, and logical as script literacy. To do this, several assumptions about script literacy can be addressed briefly. As mentioned previously, it is often claimed that script literacy, particularly writing, is responsible for the complexity and abstractness of thought in the Western world. This seems to be due mainly to the decontextualization and the capture of the spoken word in print (Denny, 1991; C. Feldman, 1991; Olson, 1991).

On the contrary, there is an emerging idea that reading or writing might not be the main issue, but rather, they are the outcomes of literate thought. Succinctly stated, reading and writing skills are part of the overall language comprehension process. As a decontextualized process, writing has led to the separation of text and its interpretation. That is, with the invention of writing and then the printing press, there now is a separation of the text and reader's interpretation that permits a discussion of the meanings of texts to be manifested by the various interpretations of the readers. In other words, the text contains information that is separate from a reader's comprehension and interpretation of it. More important, the capture of the information permits individuals to engage in a deeper, more rational and critical reflection on and organization of this information. It is the decontextualization process that leads to or facilitates the production of highly abstract, complex thought because of the ease of refinement and elaboration on the captured text and on thoughts in a mind that is intensely engaged in reflection.

Despite the separation of text and interpretation, the process of writing does not lead to a specific development of consciousness but to the realization that a person can recognize his or her interpretations as interpretations (Denny, 1991; C. Feldman, 1991). In essence, writing is an avenue—similar to mathematics, speaking, or signing—that can be used to reflect or represent the cognitive products of literate thought. Of course, writing and reading can be used as tools for developing further one's abstract, complex thinking skills; however, they are not the only tools for these purposes.

It is not difficult to find support for these remarks, especially from historical and current research. That is, there is support for the ability to engage in literate thought through the use of the performance mode and without accessing printed materials. For example, historical researchers have reported numerous accounts of individuals who participated in the discussions of texts or printed documents that were read or orally presented to them. These events were quite common during earlier periods (and even later) after the invention of the printing press. Script-literacy skills were not common, and in many cases, there were few copies of texts or materials available. Basically, the reader or speaker was a person whose major role was to read or present the information to a group of individuals. The reader or speaker did not actively engage in discussing the information. It was the responsibility of members of the group to participate in the debate of the merits of the information, particularly when some documents required a vote or an action to be taken (Olson, 1989).

Even more interesting, based on anthropological data, it can be argued that—similar to script literacy—there are oral genres and that these genres also represent a separation of text and interpretation, thus inviting reflection and abstraction (Feldman, 1991). For example, in societies with no competing written forms, there are distinctive oral forms that proceed beyond those associated with ordinary conversation.

Perhaps the most convincing case for the possible benefits of performance literacy can be made with the use of technology in which people now have the ability to capture the performance utterances electronically. The content of presenting or delivering information in the performance mode can be as complex and as difficult as information presented in the written mode. Furthermore, it can closely resemble the vocabulary and grammar of script literacy, depending on the purpose for delivering the information. Consider the example of talking books for individuals with visual impairment and others (audiobooks) that are commercially made and focused on popular books or classics. Analogously, it is possible to capture all script-literacy information electronically from newspapers or other printed materials such as legal documents and textbooks—that is, to capture this information in a performance literacy mode.

In essence, literate thought develops when individuals have opportunities to reflect on and study captured information—the mode of the captured information is not critical. To proceed to high levels of literate thought, individuals need to become familiar with the metalanguage (specialized vocabulary) of the topics or subjects. Finally, as with any other learned activity, it is necessary to acquire and use a bona fide first language at as early an age as possible. In other words, given what is known about thought-language relations, there seems to be a reciprocal relationship between a high level of development in thought and a high level of development in the use of a language.

Equity, Diversity, and the Matthew Effects

For individuals with so-called script-literacy problems, the availability and use of information might be an accessibility issue. Specifically, it might even be an oppression issue, especially if it is clear that the same individuals could have reached or can reach a high level of literate thought through the predominant use and application of performance-based information and other script-based information captured by electronic media.

It might be wondered how literate thought through the performance mode or performance literacy mode can be sufficient for living in a scientific technological society—one that depends on the values of the larger mainstream society. Admittedly, it might be difficult to participate in such a society without script-literacy skills because of the general lack of accessibility and of educational programs that are not oriented to using predominantly electronic media. Nevertheless, there is still a need to investigate whether the development of high-level script-literacy skills is the hallmark or an epiphenomenon of an advanced civilization (see Olson, 1989).

Perhaps a better understanding of the notions of accessibility and oppression can be obtained through a discussion of the Matthew Effects. There is some support for the idea that there is a critical or optimal period for developing script-literacy ability, due to what is called the Matthew Effects (Stanovich, 1986). The Matthew Effects is interpreted mainly as the rich get richer—for example, good readers are bound to become better and more advanced readers because of their ability to read widely and voraciously. Conversely, a secondary interpretation is that the poor stay the same or become poorer. That is, poor readers do not read extensively and cannot experience much growth and learning solely by engaging in print-related tasks. In addition, as poor readers advance in age, the more difficult it is to improve their script-reading ability and the greater the lag between their achievement levels and those of good readers, at least according to standardized comparison milestones.

These remarks seem to provide support for the idea that an equal amount of emphasis should be placed on the development of both performance and performance literacy skills so as not to impede the typical overall cognitive and language development of students who are labeled as *poor* readers and writers. Performance literacy skills might support the script acquisition process; however, its main value lies in facilitating the development of literate thought.

Implementation of Performance Literacy

With respect to the implementation of performance literacy, there are many factors that need to be considered. Only two broad ones are mentioned here:

the need for (a) fixated, captured, decontextualized texts representing all varieties of performance literacy genres, including academic subjects and literature books; and (b) the development and use of a metalanguage—that is, the language often associated with the study and discussion of learned academic topics in learned institutions.

In essence, recorded electronic materials can be used to perform the same or similar functions as books and other printed materials, and learned debates, discussions, and instruction can be organized around these materials. Individuals should be able to take all texts home for review and study and to become engaged in meaningful discussions in the classrooms and other locations. Many current instructional activities for script literacy can be used or adapted for performance literacy—specifically, prior knowledge and metacognitive activities, possibly some vocabulary activities, and even assessment activities. Even classroom discussions can be videotaped and used as texts for additional discussion purposes. It should be possible to develop both standardized versions and individualized supplements to match the communication and cognitive levels of the students.

A few final comments should be made about the idea of performance literacy.

1. Performance literacy should not be used in place of script literacy. It is just another avenue for students to work with decontextualized information that is roughly similar to the decontextualized information in print.

2. There is no guarantee that performance literacy will facilitate access to the language structure of script literacy; nevertheless, students are being exposed to the language structure and information at various difficulty levels in the performance literacy mode.

3. There is a great need for empirical research to focus on the decontextualized nature of captured performance literacy information and on the development of skills for working with this type of information.

Recommendations for Future Research

The real goal in the education of students should be the development of literate thought. In the author's opinion, the road to this goal should not be confined to only script literacy because this is a good example of paradigm inflexibility or rigidity. Furthermore, this restriction does not consider the newer models of what it means to be literate, at least from the standpoint of research on both orality and script literacy.

There is still considerable research that needs to be undertaken for this line of thought. Here are a few questions for future research endeavors.

Questions

1. What is literate thought? How is this concept related to the notions of openness, prejudice, bias, and other types of consciousness?
2. What is oral and sign communication (i.e., for deaf and hard-of-hearing students)? What are some examples of oral or sign communication genres?
3. What is oral or sign literacy (used with deaf and hard-of-hearing children)? What are some examples of oral or sign literacy genres?
4. What are some requisites for developing literate thought?
5. What are the contributions of script-literacy to the development of literate thought?
6. What are the contributions of the performance mode to the development of literate thought?
7. What are the contributions of performance literacy to the development of literate thought?
8. Are there differences between performance literacy and script literacy?
9. Are there differences between oral and sign communication (for deaf and hard-of-hearing students)?
10. Are there differences between oral literacy and sign literacy (for deaf and hard-of-hearing students)?
11. Can the focus on script-literacy become an oppressive issue for deaf and hard-of-hearing students?

Table 12-3 provides a summary of major points of the literate thought section.

Table 12-3 Summary of Major Points for the Literate Thought Section

- There is little question that reading and writing skills are important in a scientific technological society such as the United States. Traditionally, there has been the perception that high-level literacy skills are reflective of the ability to think at high levels.

- High-level thinking skills are reflective of literate thought, not high-level literacy skills per se. That is, individuals do not necessarily need to read and write well to think well.

- Literate thought is mode independent; it is not restricted to a particular mode such as print. What is needed is a captured mode of information on which individuals can study and reflect. To proceed to high levels of literate thought, individuals need to become familiar with the metalanguage (specialized vocabulary) of the topics or subjects. As with any other learned activity, it is necessary to acquire and use a bona fide first language at as early an age as possible.

- There is a need for further research on the benefits of performance literacy, which refers to the electronic capture of information presented via the performance modes (i.e., speaking or signing). Performance literacy skills might support the script acquisition process; however, its main value lies in facilitating the development of literate thought.

- If literate thought is mode independent, then the overwhelming reliance on script-literacy for the obtainment of diplomas, degrees, and other prestigious conditions might be considered an oppressive issue for a number of individuals who can develop high levels of literate thought in nonscript-based modes (performance or performance literacy modes) but not in script-literacy modes.

- The main goal of education should be to develop literate thought—the ability to think reflectively, creatively, logically, and rationally.

FINAL REMARKS

This last chapter attempts to provide a few insights into the development of language and script literacy. In addition, a concept that was introduced in Chapter 1, literate thought, was elaborated on. It is quite an understatement to remark that these are complex concepts that are essentially difficult to describe and understand. This is true for all complex concepts although it is possible to operationalize descriptions for research purposes.

One conclusion that can be drawn from the work in the language and communication development of deaf and hard-of-hearing children is that these children cannot be considered as a single population. This is not a trite restatement of the doctrine of individual differences, which does exist and tends to qualify some general developmental patterns. Rather, it is a recognition that the development of language in a deaf or hard-of-hearing child is inextricably related to the form of communication that is used initially and consistently with the child. In addition, language development is also dependent on the representation or completeness of the form and its processing constraints.

Ever since the first edition of this text, the author (and coauthor for earlier editions) argued that there is a persistent need for research on the expression of the communication systems by teachers, clinicians, and parents and on the reception/understanding of such systems by deaf and hard-of-hearing individuals. Despite the varied success of some English signed systems, it is believed that the shortcomings of these systems, especially with respect to phonology, are now clear, albeit controversial.

There is no doubt that educators need to consider seriously the role and challenge of using American Sign Language with some students with severe to profound hearing impairment. The manner in which ASL can be used to teach English as a second language is still not evident or well researched. Scholars have increased the understanding of the manual system of ASL, known popularly as finger spelling; however, researchers have a long way to go to understand how finger spelling can be used to assist deaf children in their acquisition of advanced English literacy skills, especially if such skills are dependent on the application of phonemic awareness. For research to move forward in the ASL/English bilingual/bicultural arena, proponents need to reconsider their interpretations of prevailing views on second language reading and writing. There have been some misinterpretations of extant theory and research on hearing children learning English as a second language.

The last section of this chapter on literate thought should reinforce the fact that language needs to be developed at as early an age as possible. It was argued that literate thought is mode independent; specifically, it is not dependent on the development of script-literacy skills. However, it is dependent on the acquisition of a bona fide language as early as possible. Although the debate on the critical period hypothesis has not been resolved, most scholars seem to be in agreement about the pervasive positive effects of early language acquisition on subsequent developmental activities.

The existence of several possible approaches to language development presents the persons who are primarily responsible for a deaf child's language development with the dilemma of choosing one in the absence of any clear directions from research of the relative effectiveness. In addition, there is growing doubt that the development of an adequate English language level in both the performance and written forms is a feasible goal for some, perhaps a large minority of students with severe to profound impairment. It should still be possible for many of these individuals to develop a high level of literate thought, particularly through the use of American Sign Language.

On the other hand, what has been said in this chapter and in the rest of the book may become obsolete with the advancement of technology involving cochlear implants and other aids (e.g., tactile aids). In the last 10 years, researchers have already seen some of the benefits and have a good glimpse of the potential for the future. Whether cochlear implants will be applicable to most or all individuals with severe to profound hearing impairment is an open question. If this technology is beneficial, then it is believed this will assist in the development of English language and literacy skills. Of course, learning to read and write requires much more than the ability to hear and speak as well as much more than knowledge of the performance form of the language of print.

At the conclusion of the previous editions of this text has been the line: "In any case, it is safe to conclude that there is not, and may never be, a 'true path' to language development for all deaf students." This statement is still applicable. However, with the advancement of technology and the increase in the understanding of literate thought, it is the author's hope that there will be several viable, comparable paths to language development for all deaf and hard-of-hearing students.

A BRIEF SYNTHESIS
COMPREHENSION QUESTIONS

1. The author posed a *How do* question that refers to both the acquisition of the performance form of English (speech and/or sign) and of ASL. What is his response or answer to this question?

2. For the *How well* question, the text attempted to chart and compare the development of English literacy skills in deaf and hard-of-hearing students (including those learning English as a second language) with those of hearing students. What is the author's summary of major points for the *How well* question in this concluding chapter?

3. Discuss briefly the three ways that have been used to enable deaf students to develop a self-controlling communication system (the work of Quigley & Paul, 1994).

4. Describe the meaning and implications of the following phrase: world of vision versus the world of audition. Is this an either-or phenomenon? According to the author, what is the need of future research?

5. What is literate thought? Is this the same as being literate? What are the requisites for literate thought? What evidence exists that literate thought is mode independent? According to the author, is literate thought possible without the ability to read and write adequately? Why or why not?

6. What are some of the major points of the section entitled: "Equity, Diversity, and the Matthew Effects"?

7. What is performance literacy? How is it similar to and different from script literacy?

CHALLENGE QUESTIONS

(Note: Complete answers are not in the text. Additional research is required.)

1. Consider the passage at the beginning of the chapter:

   But what are these fundamentals? One and one only! Language, and then language—spoken, spelled, or written—and the power to read, and the power to understand what is read. Other requirements will then follow more easily and with greater results than now attained. (R. Johnson, 1916, p. 95)

   Are these "fundamentals" similar to the concept of literate thought as discussed in this chapter? Why or why not? How would you reword the passage to reflect the concept of literate thought? (Be sure to end with "Other requirements will then follow more easily and with greater results than now attained"!)

2. Do you agree with the author's conclusions regarding the *How do* and *How well* questions? Why or why not? If not, can you base your response on existing research data that you feel the author may have overlooked or misinterpreted?

3. Given the author's description of literate thought and his argument that it is mode independent, do you believe that it is possible to develop literate thought without having the ability to read and write adequately in this society? Why or why not? Is your belief system supported by theoretical or research data?

4. Is literate thought related to Howard Gardner's theory of multiple intelligences? Why or why not?

FURTHER READINGS

Beveridge, W. (1980). *Seeds of discovery: The logic, illogic, serendipity, and sheer chance of scientific discovery*. New York: Norton.

Medawar, P. (1984). *The limits of science*. New York: Harper & Row.

Guttenplan, S. (1995). *A companion to the philosophy of mind.* Malden, MA: Blackwell.

Peters, J. (1963). *Metaphysics: A systematic survey.* Pittsburgh: Duquesne University Press.

References

Abraham, S., & Stoker, R. (1984). An evaluation of methods used to teach speech to the hearing-impaired using a simulation technique. *Volta Review, 86,* 325–335.

Acoustical Society of America. (1982). *Specification of hearing aid characteristics* (ANSI S3.22–1982). New York: Author.

Adams, M. (1990). *Beginning to read: Thinking and learning about print.* Cambridge, MA: MIT Press.

Adams, M. (1994). Phonics and beginning reading instruction. In F. Lehr & J. Osborn (Eds.), *Reading, language, and literacy: Instruction for the twenty-first century* (pp. 3–23). Hillsdale, NJ: Lawrence Erlbaum.

Adams, M., Foorman, B., Lundberg, I., & Beeler, T. (1998). *Phonemic awareness in young children.* Baltimore: Paul H. Brookes.

Ahn, S. (1996). *A study of incidental vocabulary learning by students with hearing impairment.* Unpublished doctoral dissertation, Ohio State University, Columbus, Ohio.

Aitchison, J. (1994). *Words in the mind: An introduction to the mental lexicon* (2nd ed.). Cambridge, MA: Blackwell.

Akamatsu, C. T. (1982). *The acquisition of fingerspelling in preschool children.* Unpublished doctoral dissertation, University of Rochester, New York.

Akamatsu, C. T., & Armour, V. (1987). Developing written literacy in deaf children through analyzing sign language. *American Annals of the Deaf, 132,* 46–51.

Akamatsu, C. T., & Stewart, D. (1989). The role of fingerspelling in simultaneous communication. *Sign Language Studies, 65,* 361–373.

Akamatsu, C. T., & Stewart, D. (1998). Constructing simultaneous communication: The contributions of natural sign language. *Journal of Deaf Studies and Deaf Education, 3,* 302–319.

Allen, T. (1986). Patterns of academic achievement among hearing impaired students: 1974 and 1983. In A. Schildroth & M. Karchmer (Eds.), *Deaf children in America* (pp. 161–206). Boston: Little, Brown.

Anastasi, A. (1982). *Psychological testing* (5th ed.). New York: Macmillan.

Anderson, D., & Reilly, J. (1997). The puzzle of negation: How children move from communicative to grammatical negation in ASL. *Applied Psycholinguistics, 18,* 411–429.

Anderson, M., Boren, N., Caniglia, J., Howard, W., & Krohn, E. (1980). *Apple Tree.* Beaverton, OR: Dormac.

Anderson, R. (1985). Role of reader's schema in comprehension, learning, and memory. In H. Singer & R. Ruddell (Eds.), *Theoretical models and processes of reading* (3rd ed., pp. 372–384). Newark, DE: International Reading Association.

Anderson, R., & Freebody, P. (1985). Vocabulary knowledge. In H. Singer & R. Ruddell (Eds.), *Theoretical models and processes of reading* (3rd ed., pp. 343–371). Newark, DE: International Reading Association.

Anderson, R., Hiebert, E., Scott, J., & Wilkinson, I. (1985). *Becoming a nation of readers: The report of the commission on reading.* Washington, DC: The National Institute of Education and The Center for the Study of Reading.

Anderson, R., & Pearson, P. D. (1984). A schema-theoretic view of basic processes in reading comprehension. In P. D. Pearson, R. Barr, M. Kamil, & P. Mosenthal (Eds.), *Handbook of reading research* (pp. 255–291). White Plains, NY: Longman.

Andrews, J., & Gonzales, K. (1991). Free writing of deaf children in kindergarten. *Sign Language Studies, 74,* 63–78.

Andrews, J., & Mason, J. (1986). How do deaf children learn about prereading? *American Annals of the Deaf, 131,* 210–217.

Anthony, D. (1966). *Seeing essential English.* Unpublished master's thesis, Eastern Michigan University, Ypsilanti.

Antonacci, P., & Hedley, C. (Eds.). (1994). *Natural approaches to reading and writing*. Norwood, NJ: Ablex.

Au, T. (1988). Language and cognition. In R. Schiefelbusch & L. Lloyd (Eds.), *Language perspectives: Acquisition, retardation, and intervention* (2nd ed., pp. 125–146). Austin, TX: Pro-Ed.

Austin, J. (1962). *How to do things with words*. Oxford, UK: Oxford University Press.

Baars, B. (1986). *The cognitive revolution in psychology*. New York: Guilford.

Babb, R. (1979). *A study of the academic achievement and language acquisition levels of deaf children of hearing parents in an educational environment using signing exact English as the primary mode of manual communication*. Unpublished doctoral dissertation, University of Illinois, Urbana-Champaign.

Baddeley, A. (1990). *Human memory: Theory and practice*. Hillsdale, NJ: Lawrence Erlbaum.

Baetens-Beardsmore, H. (1986). *Bilingualism: Basic principles* (2nd ed.). Clevedon, Avon (England): Multilingual Matters Ltd.

Baker, C., & Cokely, D. (1980). *American Sign Language: A teacher's resource text on grammar and culture*. Silver Spring, MD: T.J. Publishers.

Baker, D. (1989). *Language testing: A critical survey and practical guide*. New York: Edward Arnold.

Baker, K., & de Kanter, A. (1981). *Effectiveness of bilingual education: A review of the literature*. Washington, DC: Department of Education, Office of Planning and Budget.

Baker, L., & Brown, A. (1984). Metacognition skills and reading. In P. D. Pearson, R. Barr, M. Kamil, & P. Mosenthal (Eds.), *Handbook of reading research* (pp. 353–394). White Plains, NY: Longman.

Balota, D., Flores D'Arcais, G., & Rayner, K. (Eds.). (1990). *Comprehension processes in reading*. Hillsdale, NJ: Lawrence Erlbaum.

Balow, B., Fulton, H., & Peploe, E. (1971). Reading comprehension skills among hearing-impaired adolescents. *Volta Review, 73*, 113–119.

Balow, I., & Brill, R. (1975). An evaluation of reading and academic achievement levels of 16 graduating classes of the California School for the Deaf, Riverside. *Volta Review, 77*, 255–266.

Bandura, A. (1997). *Self-efficacy: The exercise of control*. New York: W. H. Freeman & Co.

Barin, L. (1999). *An epidemiological study of the age of identification for children with hearing impairment.* Unpublished doctoral dissertation, Ohio State University, Columbus.

Barry, K. (1899). *The five-slate system. A system of objective language teaching.* Philadelphia: Sherman & Co.

Bartine, D. (1989). *Early English reading theory: Origins of current debates.* Columbia, SC: University of South Carolina Press.

Bartine, D. (1992). *Reading, criticism, and culture: Theory and teaching in the United States and England, 1820–1950.* Columbia, SC: University of South Carolina Press.

Bateman, W. (1990). *Open to question: The art of teaching and learning by inquiry.* San Francisco: Jossey-Bass.

Bates, E. (1976). *Language and context: The acquisition of pragmatics.* San Diego: Academic Press.

Bates, E., Bretherton, I., & Snyder, L. (1988). *From first words to grammar.* New York: Cambridge University Press.

Bates, E., & MacWhinney, B. (1987). Competition, variation, and language learning. In B. MacWhinney (Ed.), *Mechanisms of language acquisition* (pp. 157–194). Hillsdale, NJ: Lawrence Erlbaum.

Beach, R. (1994). Adopting multiple stances in conducting literacy research. In R. Ruddell, M. Ruddell, & H. Singer (Eds.), *Theoretical models and processes of reading* (4th ed., pp. 1203–1219). Newark, DE: International Reading Association.

Bebko, J. (1998). Learning, language, memory and reading: The role of language automatization and its impact on complex cognitive activities. *Journal of Deaf Studies and Deaf Education, 3,* 4–14.

Beck, I., & McKeown, M. (1991). Conditions of vocabulary acquisition. In R. Barr, M. Kamil, P. Mosenthal, & P. D. Pearson (Eds.), *Handbook of reading research* (2nd ed., pp. 789–814). White Plains, NY: Longman.

Becker, W. (1977). Teaching reading and language to the disadvantaged—what we have learned from field research. *Harvard Educational Review, 47,* 518–543.

Beebe, H., Pearson, H., & Koch, M. (1984). The Helen Beebe speech and hearing center. In D. Ling (Ed.), *Early intervention for hearing-impaired children: Oral options* (pp. 15–63). San Diego: College-Hill Press.

Bellugi, U. (1991). The link between hand and brain: Implications from a visual language. In D. Martin (Ed.), *Advances in cognition, education, and deafness* (pp. 11–35). Washington, DC: Gallaudet University Press.

Bellugi, U., Klima, E., & Siple, P. (1974/1975). Remembering in signs. *Cognition*, *3*(2), 93–125.

Bender, R. (1970). *The conquest of deafness: A history of the long struggle to make possible normal living to those handicapped by lack of normal hearing*. Cleveland, OH: Case Western Reserve University Press.

Bereiter, C., & Scardamalia, M. (1983). Levels of inquiry in writing research. In P. Mosenthal, L. Tamor, & S. Walmsley (Eds.), *Research on writing: Principles and methods* (pp. 3–25). White Plains, NY: Longman.

Bereiter, C., & Scardamalia, M. (1987). *The psychology of written composition*. Hillsdale, NJ: Lawrence Erlbaum.

Berent, G. (1996a). The acquisition of English syntax by deaf learners. In W. Ritchie & T. Bhatia (Eds.), *Handbook of second language acquisition* (pp. 469–506). San Diego: Academic Press.

Berent, G. (1996b). Learnability constraints on deaf learners' acquisition of English *wh*- questions. *Journal of Speech and Hearing Research*, *39*, 625–642.

Berent, I., & Perfetti, C. (1995). A rose is a REEZ: The two-cycles model of phonology assembly in reading English. *Psychological Review*, *102*, 146–184.

Berger, K. (1972). *Speechreading: Principles and methods*. Baltimore: National Educational Press.

Berko, J. (1958). The child's learning of English morphology. *Word*, *14*, 150–177.

Bernhardt, E. (1991). *Reading development in a second language*. Norwood, NJ: Ablex.

Berry, M., & Talbot, R. (1966). *Exploratory test for grammar*. Rockford, IL: Berry & Talbot.

Besner, D. (1990). Does the reading system need a lexicon? In D. Balota, G. Flores D'Arcais, & K. Rayner (Eds.), *Comprehension processes in reading* (pp. 73–99). Hillsdale, NJ: Lawrence Erlbaum.

Bialystok, E., & Sharwood-Smith, M. (1985). Interlanguage is not a state of mind: An evaluation of the construct for second-language acquisition. *Applied Linguistics*, *6*, 101–117.

Binnie, C., Jackson, P., & Montgomery, A. (1976). Visual intelligibility of consonants: A lipreading screening test with implications for aural rehabilitation. *Journal of Speech and Hearing Disorders*, *41*, 530–539.

Black, J., O'Reilly, P., & Peck, L. (1963). Self-administered training in lipreading. *Journal of Speech and Hearing Disorders*, *28*, 183–186.

Blackwell, P., Engen, E., Fischgrund, J., & Zarcadoolas, C. (1978). *Sentences and other systems*. Washington, DC: Alexander Graham Bell Association for the Deaf.

Blair, J., Peterson, M., & Viehweg, S. (1985). The effects of mild hearing loss on academic performance of young school-age children. *Volta Review, 87,* 87–93.

Blake, J., & Boysson-Bardies, B. (1992). Patterns in babbling: A cross linguistic study. *Journal of Child Language, 19,* 51–75.

Blanton, R., Nunnally, J., & Odom, P. (1967). Graphemic, phonetic, and associative factors in the verbal behavior of deaf and hearing subjects. *Journal of Speech and Hearing Research, 10,* 225–231.

Bloom, A. (1981). *The linguistic shaping of thought.* Hillsdale, NJ: Lawrence Erlbaum.

Bloom, L. (1970). *Language development: Form and function in emerging grammars.* Cambridge, MA: MIT Press.

Bloom, L. (1973). *One word at a time: The use of single-word utterances before syntax.* The Hague, the Netherlands: Mouton.

Bloom, L., & Lahey, M. (1978). *Language development and language disorders.* New York: John Wiley.

Bloom, L., Lightbown, P., & Hood, L. (Eds.). (1975). Structure and variation in child language. *Monographs of the Society for Research in Child Development, 40*(2), 1–97.

Blumenthal, A. (1970). *Language and psychology: Historical aspects of psycholinguistics.* New York: John Wiley.

Bochner, J., & Albertini, J. (1988). Language varieties in the deaf populations and their acquisition by children and adults. In M. Strong (Ed.), *Language learning and deafness* (pp. 3–48). New York: Cambridge University Press.

Bochner, S., Price, P., & Jones, J. (1997). *Child language development: Learning to talk.* London: Whurr Publishers Ltd.

Bohannon, J. (1993). Theoretical approaches to language acquisition. In J. Berko-Gleason (Ed.), *The development of language* (3rd ed., pp. 239–297). New York: Macmillan.

Bohannon, J., & Warren-Leubecker, A. (1985). Theoretical approaches to language acquisition. In J. Berko-Gleason (Ed.), *The development of language* (pp. 173–226). Columbus, OH: Merrill.

Bonvillian, J. (1999). Sign language development. In M. Barrett (Ed.), *The development of language* (pp. 277–310). Hove, East Sussex, UK: Psychology Press Ltd.

Bonvillian, J., Orlansky, M., & Novack, L. (1983). Developmental milestones: Sign language acquisition and motor development. *Child Development, 54,* 1435–1445.

Boothroyd, A. (1984). Auditory perception of speech contrasts by subjects with sensorineural hearing loss. *Journal of Speech and Hearing Research, 27,* 134–144.

Boothroyd, A. (1986). *Speech acoustics and perception.* Austin, TX: Pro-Ed.

Borg, W., & Gall, M. (1983). *Educational research* (4th ed.). White Plains, NY: Longman.

Bornstein, H. (1982). Towards a theory of use of signed English: From birth through adulthood. *American Annals of the Deaf, 127,* 26–31.

Bornstein, H. (1990). Signed English. In H. Bornstein (Ed.), *Manual communication: Implications for education* (pp. 21–44). Washington, DC: Gallaudet University Press.

Bornstein, H., & Saulnier, K. (1981). Signed English: A brief follow-up to the first evaluation. *American Annals of the Deaf, 126,* 69–72.

Bornstein, H., Saulnier, K., & Hamilton, L. (1980). Signed English: A first evaluation. *American Annals of the Deaf, 125,* 467–481.

Bornstein, H., Saulnier, K., & Hamilton, L. (1983). *The comprehensive signed English dictionary.* Washington, DC: Gallaudet College Press.

Bowerman, M. (1973). Structural relationships in children's utterances: Syntactic or semantic? In T. Moores (Ed.), *Cognitive development and the acquisition of language* (pp. 197–213). San Diego: Academic Press.

Bowerman, M. (1988). Inducing the latent structure of language. In F. Kessell (Ed.), *The development of language and language researchers: Essays in honor of Roger Brown* (pp. 23–49). Hillsdale, NJ: Lawrence Erlbaum.

Boyes-Braem, P. (1973/1990). Acquisition of the handshape in American Sign Language: A preliminary analysis. In V. Volterra & C. Erting (Eds.), *From gesture to language in hearing and deaf children* (pp. 107–127). New York/Berlin: Springer-Verlag.

Bradley-Johnson, S., & Evans, L. (1991). *Psychoeducational assessment of hearing-impaired students.* Austin, TX: Pro-Ed.

Brady, S., & Shankweiler, D. (Eds.). (1991). *Phonological processes in literacy: A tribute to Isabelle Y. Liberman.* Hillsdale, NJ: Lawrence Erlbaum.

Braine, M. (1963a). The ontogeny of English phrase structure: The first phase. *Language, 39,* 1–13.

Braine, M. (1963b). On learning the grammatical order of words. *Psychological Review, 70,* 323–348.

Brasel, K., & Quigley, S. (1977). The influence of certain language and communication environments in early childhood on the development of language in deaf individuals. *Journal of Speech and Hearing Research, 20,* 95–107.

Brown, P., & Brewer, L. (1996). Cognitive processes of deaf and hearing skilled and less skilled readers. *Journal of Deaf Studies and Deaf Education, 1,* 263–270.

Brown, P., & Long, G. (1992). The use of scripted interaction in a cooperative learning context to probe planning and evaluating during writing. *Volta Review, 95,* 411–424.

Brown, R. (1958). *Words and things.* New York: Free Press.

Brown, R. (1973). *A first language: The early stages.* Cambridge, MA: Harvard University.

Brownell, W. (1999). How the ear works: Nature's solutions for listening. *Volta Review, 99,* 9–28.

Brumfit, C. (1984). *Communicative methodology in language teaching.* Cambridge, UK: Cambridge University Press.

Bruner, J. (1975). From communication to language: A psychological perspective. *Cognition, 3,* 255–287.

Budwig, N. (1995). *A developmental-functionalist approach to child language.* Hillsdale, NJ: Lawrence Erlbaum.

Bunge, M., & Ardila, R. (1987). *Philosophy of psychology.* New York/Berlin: Springer-Verlag.

Byrnes, J., & Gelman, S. (1991). Perspectives on thought and language: Traditional and contemporary views. In S. Gelman & J. Byrnes (Eds.), *Perspectives on language and thought: Interrelations in development* (pp. 3–27). New York: Cambridge University Press.

Cairns, H. (1996). *The acquisition of language* (2nd ed.). Austin, TX: Pro-Ed.

Calfee, R. (1994). Critical literacy: Reading and writing for a new millennium. In N. Ellsworth, C. Hedley, & A. Baratta (Eds.), *Literacy: A redefinition* (pp. 19–38). Hillsdale, NJ: Lawrence Erlbaum.

Callanan, M. (1991). Parent-child collaboration in young children's understanding of category hierarchies. In S. Gelman & J. Byrnes (Eds.), *Perspectives on language and thought: Interrelations in development* (pp. 440–484). New York: Cambridge University Press.

Calvert, D. (1986). Speech in perspective. In D. Luterman (Ed.), *Deafness in perspective* (pp. 167–191). San Diego: College-Hill Press.

Calvert, D., & Silverman, S. (1983). *Speech and deafness.* Washington, DC: Alexander Graham Bell Association for the Deaf.

Caniglia, J., Cole, N., Howard, W., Krohn, E., & Rice, M. (1975). *Apple Tree.* Beaverton, OR: Dormac.

Cann, R. (1993). *Formal semantics: An introduction.* New York: Cambridge University Press.

Carney, A. (1994). Understanding speech intelligibility in the hearing impaired. In K. Butler (Ed.), *Hearing impairment and language disorders: Assessment and intervention* (pp. 109–121). Gaithersburg, MD: Aspen.

Carnine, D., Silbert, J., & Kameenui, E. (1990). *Direct instruction reading* (2nd ed.). Columbus, OH: Merrill.

Carroll, J. (1961). *Fundamental considerations in testing for English language proficiency of foreign students.* Washington, DC: Center for Applied Linguistics.

Carroll, J., & Gibson, E. (1986). Infant perception of gestural contrasts: Prerequisites for the acquisition of a visually specified language. *Journal of Child Language, 13,* 31–49.

Carrow, E. (1974). *Carrow elicited language inventory.* Austin, TX: Learning Concepts.

Carver, R. (1974). Two dimensions of tests: Psychometric and edumetric. *American Psychologist, 29,* 512–518.

Case, R. (1996). Changing views of knowledge and their impact on educational research and practice. In D. Olson & N. Torrance (Eds.), *The handbook of education and human development* (pp. 75–99). Cambridge, MA: Blackwell.

Center for Assessment and Demographic Studies. (1991). *Stanford achievement test, eighth edition: Hearing-impaired norms booklet.* Washington, DC: Gallaudet University, Gallaudet Research Institute, Author.

Chafe, W. (1970). *Meaning and the structure of language.* Chicago: University of Chicago Press.

Chalifoux, L. (1991). The implications of congenital deafness for working memory. *American Annals of the Deaf, 136,* 292–299.

Chall, J., Jacobs, V., & Baldwin, L. (1990). *The reading crisis: Why poor children fall behind.* Cambridge, MA: Harvard University Press.

Chaney, C. (1989). I pledge allegiance to the flag: Three studies in word segmentation. *Applied Psycholinguistics, 10,* 261–282.

Chaney, C. (1992). Language development, metalinguistic skills, and print awareness in 3-year-old children. *Applied Psycholinguistics, 13,* 485–514.

Charrow, V. (1975). A psycholinguistic analysis of deaf English. *Sign Language Studies, 7,* 139–150.

Charrow, V., & Fletcher, J. (1974). English as the second language of deaf children. *Developmental Psychology, 10,* 463–470.

Chilson, R. (1985). Effects of cued speech instruction on speechreading skills. *Cued Speech Annual, 1*, 60–68.

Chomsky, N. (1957). *Syntactic structures*. The Hague, the Netherlands: Mouton.

Chomsky, N. (1959). Review of Skinner's *Verbal Behavior. Language, 35*, 26–58.

Chomsky, N. (1965). *Aspects of the theory of syntax*. Cambridge, MA: MIT Press.

Chomsky, N. (1975). *Reflections on language*. New York: Pantheon Books.

Chomsky, N. (1980). *Rules and representations*. New York: Columbia University Press.

Chomsky, N. (1988). *Language and problems of knowledge: The Managua lectures*. Cambridge, MA: MIT Press.

Chomsky, N. (1991). Linguistics and adjacent fields: A personal view. In A. Kasher (Ed.), *The Chomskyan turn* (pp. 3–25). Cambridge, MA: Blackwell.

Clark, E. (1973). What's in a word? On the child's acquisition of semantics in his first language. In T. Moores (Ed.), *Cognitive development and the acquisition of language* (pp. 65–110). San Diego: Academic Press.

Clark, E. (1987). The principle of contrast: A constraint on language acquisition. In B. MacWhinney (Ed.), *Mechanisms of language acquisition* (pp. 1–33). Hillsdale, NJ: Lawrence Erlbaum.

Clark, E. (1991). Acquisitional principles in lexical development. In S. Gelman & J. Byrnes (Eds.), *Perspectives on language and thought: Interrelations in development* (pp. 31–71). New York: Cambridge University Press.

Clark, M. D. (1993). A contextualist/interactionist model and its relationship to deafness research. In M. Marschark & M. D. Clark (Eds.), *Psychological perspectives on deafness* (pp. 353–362). Hillsdale, NJ: Lawrence Erlbaum.

Clarke, B., & Ling, D. (1976). The effects of using cued speech: A follow-up study. *Volta Review, 78*, 23–35.

Clarke School for the Deaf. (1971). *Auditory training*. Northampton, MA: Author.

Clay, M. (1994). Foreword. In R. Ruddell, M. Ruddell, & H. Singer (Eds.), *Theoretical models and processes of reading* (4th ed., pp. ix–xiii). Newark, DE: International Reading Association.

Cokely, D. (1983). When is a pidgin not a pidgin? An alternate analysis of the ASL-English contact situation. *Sign Language Studies, 38*, 1–24.

Cole, E., & Gregory, H. (Eds.). (1986). Auditory learning [Special Issue]. *Volta Review, 88*(5).

Collins-Ahlgren, M. (1974). Teaching English as a second language to young deaf children: A case study. *Journal of Speech and Hearing Disorders, 39*, 486–500.

Commission on Education of the Deaf. (1988). *Toward equality: Education of the deaf, a report to the President and the Congress of the United States, February.* Washington, DC: Government Printing Office.

Conley, J. (1976). Role of idiomatic expressions in the reading of deaf children. *American Annals of the Deaf, 121,* 381–385.

Connor, L. (1986). Oralism in perspective. In D. Luterman (Ed.), *Deafness in perspective* (pp. 117–129). San Diego: College-Hill Press.

Conrad, R. (1979). *The deaf school child.* New York: Harper & Row.

Conway, D. (1990). Semantic relationships in the word meanings of hearing-impaired children. *Volta Review, 92,* 339–349.

Cook, V. (1991). *Second language learning and language teaching.* New York: Edward Arnold.

Cook, V., & Newson, M. (1996). *Chomsky's universal grammar: An introduction* (2nd ed.). Cambridge, MA: Blackwell.

Cooper, J., Heward, W., & Heron, T. (1987). *Applied behavior analysis.* Columbus, OH: Merrill.

Cooper, R. (1967). The ability of deaf and hearing children to apply morphological rules. *Journal of Speech and Hearing Research, 10,* 77–86.

Cooper, R., & Rosenstein, J. (1966). Language acquisition of deaf children. *Volta Review, 68,* 58–67.

Copleston, F. (1985). *Book two: A history of philosophy: Volumes 4, 5, and 6.* Garden City, NY: Image.

Cornett, R. O. (1967). Cued speech. *American Annals of the Deaf, 112,* 3–13.

Cornett, R. O. (1984). Book review: Language and deafness. *Cued Speech News, 17*(3), 5.

Cornett, R. O. (1990). The century-old wisdom of Alexander Graham Bell. *Volta Review, 92,* 145–153.

Cornett, R. O. (1991). A model for ASL/English bilingualism. In S. Polowe-Aldersley, P. Schragle, V. Armour, & J. Polowe (Eds.), *Proceedings of the 55th Biennial Meeting of CAID and the 63rd Annual Meeting of CEASD* (pp. 33–39). New Orleans, LA: Convention of American Instructors of the Deaf.

Corson, H. (1973). *Comparing deaf children of oral deaf parents and deaf parents using manual communication with deaf children of hearing parents on academic, social, and communication functioning.* Unpublished doctoral dissertation, University of Cincinnati, Ohio.

Craig, H., & Gordon, H. (1988). Specialized cognitive function and reading achievement in hearing-impaired adolescents. *Journal of Speech and Hearing Disorders, 53,* 30–41.

Crandall, K. (1978). Inflectional morphemes in the manual English of young hearing impaired children and their mothers. *Journal of Speech and Hearing Research, 21*, 372–386.

Crawford, J., Dancer, J., & Pittenger, J. (1986). Initial performance level on a speechreading task as related to subsequent improvement after short-term training. *Volta Review, 88*, 101–105.

Creaghead, N., & Newman, P. (1985). Articulatory phonetics and phonology. In P. Newman, N. Creaghead, & W. Secord (Eds.), *Assessment and remediation of articulatory and phonological disorders* (pp. 13–39). Columbus, OH: Merrill.

Crittenden, J. (1993). The culture and identity of deafness. In P. Paul & D. Jackson (Eds.), *Toward a psychology of deafness: Theoretical and empirical perspectives* (pp. 215–235). Boston: Allyn & Bacon.

Cromer, R. (1974). The development of language and cognition: The cognition hypothesis. In B. Foss (Ed.), New perspectives in child development (pp. 184–252). New York: Penguin Books.

Cromer, R. (1976). The cognitive hypothesis of language acquisition and its implications for child language deficiency. In D. Morehead & A. Morehead (Eds.), *Normal and deficient child language* (pp. 283–333). Baltimore: University Park Press.

Cromer, R. (1981). Reconceptualizing language acquisition and cognitive development. In R. Schiefelbusch & D. Bricker (Eds.), *Early language: Acquisition and intervention* (pp. 51–137). Baltimore: University Park Press.

Cromer, R. (1988a). Differentiating language and cognition. In R. Schiefelbusch & L. Lloyd (Eds.), *Language perspectives: Acquisition, retardation, and intervention* (2nd ed., pp. 91–124). Austin, TX: Pro-Ed.

Cromer, R. (1988b). The cognition hypothesis revisited. In F. Kessel (Ed.), *The development of language and language researchers: Essays in honor of Roger Brown* (pp. 223–248). Hillsdale, NJ: Lawrence Erlbaum.

Cromer, R. (1994). A case study of dissociations between language and cognition. In H. Tager-Flusberg (Ed.), *Constraints on language acquisition: Studies of atypical children* (pp. 141–153). Hillsdale, NJ: Lawrence Erlbaum.

Cronbach, L. (1960). *Essentials of psychological testing*. New York: Harper & Row.

Crutchfield, P. (1972). Prospects for teaching English Det + N structures to deaf students. *Sign Language Studies, 1*, 8–14.

Cruttenden, A. (1979). *Language in infancy and childhood: A linguistic introduction to language acquisition.* New York: St. Martin's Press.

Crystal, D. (1987). *The Cambridge encyclopedia of language.* New York: Cambridge University Press.

Crystal, D. (1995). *The Cambridge encyclopedia of the English language.* New York: Cambridge University Press.

Crystal, D. (1997). *The Cambridge encyclopedia of language* (2nd ed.). New York: Cambridge University Press.

Culicover, P. (1997). *Principles and parameters: An introduction to syntactic theory.* New York: Oxford University Press.

Cummins, J. (1977). Cognitive factors associated with the attainment of intermediate levels of bilingual skill. *The Modern Language Journal, 61,* 3–12.

Cummins, J. (1978). Educational implications of mother tongue maintenance in minority-language groups. *Canadian Modern Language Review, 34,* 395–416.

Cummins, J. (1979). Linguistic interdependence and the educational development of bilingual children. *Review of Educational Research, 49,* 222–251.

Cummins, J. (1980). The entry and exit fallacy in bilingual education. *NABE Journal, 4,* 25–60.

Cummins, J. (1984). *Bilingualism and special education: Issues in assessment and pedagogy.* San Diego: College-Hill Press.

Cummins, J. (1988). Second language acquisition within bilingual education programs. In L. Beebe (Ed.), *Issues in second language acquisition: Multiple perspectives* (pp. 145–166). New York: Newbury House.

Cummins, J. (1989). A theoretical framework for bilingual special education. *Exceptional Children, 56,* 111–119.

Curme, G. (1947). *English grammar.* New York: Barnes & Noble Books.

Curtis, M. (1987). Vocabulary testing and vocabulary instruction. In M. McKeown & M. Curtis (Eds.), *The nature of vocabulary acquisition* (pp. 37–51). Hillsdale, NJ: Lawrence Erlbaum.

Czerniewska, P. (1992). *Learning about writing: The early years.* Cambridge, MA: Blackwell.

Cziko, G. (1992). The evaluation of bilingual education: From necessity and probability to possibility. *Educational Researcher, 21*(2), 10–15.

Dale, E., & Chall, J. (1948). A formula for predicting readability. *Educational Research Bulletin, 27,* 11–20, 37–54.

Dale, E., & Eicholtz, G. (1960). *Children's knowledge of words.* Columbus, OH: Ohio State University, Bureau of Educational Resources.

Dale, P. (1976). *Language development: Structure and function* (2nd ed.). New York: Holt, Rinehart & Winston.

Dancer, J., Krain, M., Thompson, C., Davis, P., & Glenn, J. (1994). A cross-sectional investigation of speechreading in adults: Effects of age, gender, practice, and education. *Volta Review, 96*, 31–40.

Daneman, M., Nemeth, S., Stainton, M., & Huelsmann, K. (1995). Working memory as a predictor of reading achievement in orally educated hearing-impaired children. *Volta Review, 97*, 225–241.

Davey, B., & King, S. (1990). Acquisition of word meanings from context by deaf readers. *American Annals of the Deaf, 135*, 227–234.

Davies, A. (1990). *Principles of language testing.* Cambridge, MA: Blackwell.

Davies, A., Criper, C., & Howatt, A. (1984). *Interlanguage.* Edinburgh, Scotland: Edinburgh University Press.

Davis, H. (1978). Anatomy and physiology of the auditory system. In H. Davis & S. R. Silverman (Eds.), *Hearing and deafness* (4th ed., pp. 46–83). New York: Holt, Rinehart & Winston.

Davis, J., & Blasdell, R. (1975). Perceptual strategies employed by normal-hearing and hearing-impaired children in the comprehension of sentences containing relative clauses. *Journal of Speech and Hearing Research, 18*, 281–295.

Davis, J., Elfenbein, J., Schum, R., & Bentler, R. (1986). Effects of mild and moderate hearing impairments on language, educational, and psychosocial behavior. *Journal of Speech and Hearing Disorders, 51*, 53–62.

Davis, J., Shepard, N., Stelmachowicz, P., & Gorga, M. (1981). Characteristics of hearing-impaired children in the public schools: Part II—Psychoeducational data. *Journal of Speech and Hearing Disorders, 46*, 130–137.

Deal, R., & Thornton, R. (1985). An exploratory investigation of the comprehension of English through sign English (Siglish) and seeing essential English (SEE I). *Language, Speech, and Hearing Services in Schools, 161*, 267–279.

DeCasper, A., & Fifer, W. (1980). Of human bonding: Newborns prefer their mothers' voices. *Science, 208*, 1174–1176.

Dechant, E. (1991). *Understanding and teaching reading: An interactive model.* Hillsdale, NJ: Lawrence Erlbaum.

De Filippo, C., & Scott, B. (1978). A method for training and evaluating the reception of ongoing speech. *Journal of the Acoustical Society of America, 63*, 1186–1192.

De Filippo, C., & Sims, D. (Eds.). (1988). New reflections on speechreading [Special Issue]. *Volta Review, 90*(5).

Deighton, L. (1959). *Vocabulary development in the classroom.* New York: Teachers College, Columbia University, Bureau of Publications.

de Jong, J., & Verhoeven, L. (1992). Modeling and assessing language proficiency. In L. Verhoeven & J. de Jong (Eds.), *The construct of language proficiency: Applications of psychological models to language assessment* (pp. 3–19). Philadelphia: Benjamins.

Delaney, M., Stuckless, E. R., & Walter, G. (1984). Total communication effects—a longitudinal study of a school for the deaf in transition. *American Annals of the Deaf, 129,* 481–486.

Demopoulos, W. (1989). On applying learnability theory to the rationalism-empiricism controversy. In R. Matthews & W. Demopoulos (Eds.), *Learnability and linguistic theory* (pp. 77–88). Boston: Kluwer Academic Publishers.

Denny, J. P. (1991). Rational thought in oral culture and literate decontextualization. In D. Olson & N. Torrance (Eds.), *Literacy and orality* (pp. 66–89). New York: Cambridge University Press.

de Villiers, J., & de Villiers, P. (1978). *Language acquisition.* Cambridge, MA: Harvard University Press.

de Villiers, P. (1991). English literacy development in deaf children: Directions for research and intervention. In J. Miller (Ed.), *Research on child language disorders: A decade of progress* (pp. 349–378). Austin, TX: Pro-Ed.

de Villiers, P., & Pomerantz, S. (1992). Hearing-impaired students learning new words from written context. *Applied Psycholinguistics, 13,* 409–431.

DiFrancesca, S. (1972). *Academic achievement test results of a national testing program for hearing-impaired students—United States, Spring* (Series D, No. 9). Washington, DC: Gallaudet College, Office of Demographic Studies.

Dixon, K., Pearson, P. D., & Ortony, A. (1980, December). *Some reflections on the use of figurative language in children's textbooks.* Paper presented at the annual meeting of the National Reading Conference, San Diego.

Dodd, B. (1976). The phonological systems of deaf children. *Journal of Speech and Hearing Disorders, 41,* 185–198.

Dodd, B., & Campbell, R. (Eds.). (1987). *Hearing by eye.* Hillsdale, NJ: Lawrence Erlbaum.

Dodd, B., & Hermelin, B. (1977). Phonological coding by prelinguistically deaf children. *Perception and Psychophysics, 21,* 413–417.

Doehring, D., Bonnycastle, D., & Ling, A. (1978). Rapid reading skills of integrated hearing impaired children. *Volta Review, 80*, 399–409.

Dole, J., Duffy, G., Roehler, L., & Pearson, P. D. (1991). Moving from the old to the new: Research on reading comprehension instruction. *Review of Educational Research, 61*, 239–264.

Dolman, D. (1992). Some concerns about using whole language approaches with deaf children. *American Annals of the Deaf, 137*, 278–282.

Dore, J. (1974). A pragmatic description of early language development. *Journal of Psycholinguistic Research, 3*, 343–350.

Dore, J. (1975). Holophrases, speech acts, and language universals. *Journal of Child Language, 2*, 21–40.

Dore, J., Franklin, M., Miller, R., & Ramer, A. (1976). Transitional phenomena in early language acquisition. *Journal of Child Language, 3*, 13–28.

Downing, J. (1979). *Reading and reasoning.* New York/Berlin: Springer-Verlag.

Drasgow, E. (1998). American Sign Language as a pathway to linguistic competence. *Exceptional Children, 64*, 329–342.

Drasgow, E., & Paul, P. (1995). A critical analysis of the use of MCE systems with deaf students: A review of the literature. *ACEHI/ACEDA, 21*(2/3), 80–93.

Duchan, J. (1984). Language assessment: The pragmatic revolution. In R. Naremore (Ed.), *Language science: Recent advances* (pp. 147–180). San Diego: College-Hill.

Dudley-Marling, C., & Searle, D. (1988). Enriching language learning environments for students with learning disabilities. *Journal of Learning Disabilities, 21*, 140–143.

Dunn, C., & Newton, L. (1994). A comprehensive model for speech development in hearing-impaired children. In K. Butler (Ed.), *Hearing impairment and language disorders: Assessment and intervention* (pp. 122–143). Gaithersburg, MD: Aspen.

Durkin, D. (1989). *Teaching them to read* (5th ed.). Boston: Allyn & Bacon.

Eacker, J. (1975). *Problems of philosophy and psychology.* Chicago: Nelson-Hall.

Ehri, L. (1991). Development of the ability to read words. In R. Barr, M. Kamil, P. Mosenthal, & P. D. Pearson (Eds.), *Handbook of reading research* (2nd ed., pp. 383–417). White Plains, NY: Longman.

Ehri, L., & Wilce, L. (1985). Movement into reading: Is the first stage of printed word learning visual or phonetic? *Reading Research Quarterly, 20*, 163–179.

Eimas, P. (1985). The perception of speech in early infancy. *Scientific American, 252*, 46–52.

Eimas, P., Siqueland, E., Jusczyk, P., & Vigorito, J. (1971). Speech perception in infants. *Science, 171*, 303–306.

Elliott, R., & Powers, A. (1988). Preparing teachers to serve the learning disabled hearing impaired. *Volta Review, 90*, 13–18.

Epstein, S. (Ed.). (1999). Medical aspects of hearing loss for the consumer and the professional [Special Issue]. *Volta Review, 99*(5).

Erber, N. (1982). *Auditory training.* Washington, DC: Alexander Graham Bell Association for the Deaf.

Erickson, M. (1987). Deaf readers reading beyond the literal. *American Annals of the Deaf, 132*, 291–294.

Erting, C. (1992). Partnerships for change: Creating new possible worlds for deaf children and their families. *In Conference proceedings: Bilingual considerations in the education of deaf students: ASL and English* (pp. 35–45). Washington, DC: Gallaudet University, College for Continuing Education.

Everhart, V., & Marschark, M. (1988). Linguistic flexibility in signed and written language productions of deaf children. *Journal of Experimental Child Psychology, 46*, 174–193.

Ewoldt, C. (1981). A psycholinguistic description of selected deaf children reading in sign language. *Reading Research Quarterly, 17*, 58–89.

Ewoldt, C. (1996). Deaf bilingualism: A holistic perspective. *Australian Journal of the Education of the Deaf, 2*, 5–9.

Ewoldt, C., & Hammermeister, F. (1986). The language-experience approach to facilitating reading and writing for hearing-impaired students. *American Annals of the Deaf, 131*, 271–274.

Fabbretti, D., Volterra, V., & Pontecorvo, C. (1998). Written language abilities in deaf Italians. *Journal of Deaf Studies and Deaf Education, 3*, 231–244.

Farwell, R. (1976). Speech reading: A research review. *American Annals of the Deaf, 121*, 13–30.

Feldman, C. (1991). Oral metalanguage. In D. Olson & N. Torrance (Eds.), *Literacy and orality* (pp. 47–65). New York: Cambridge University Press.

Feldman, L. (1994). Beyond orthography and phonology: Differences between inflections and derivations. *Journal of Memory and Language, 33*, 442–470.

Felix, S. (1982). *Psycholinguistische Aspekte des Zwitsprachenerwerbs.* Tubingen, Germany: Gunter Narr Verlag.

Ferguson, C., & Farwell, C. (1975). Words and sounds in early language acquisition: English consonants in the first 50 words. *Language, 51*, 419–439.

Fincher-Kiefer, R. (1992). The role of prior knowledge in inferential processing. *Journal of Research in Reading*, 15, 12–27.

Fine, R. (1973). *The development of Freud's thought: From the beginnings (1886–1900) through id psychology (1900–1914) to ego psychology (1914–1939)*. Northvale, NJ: Jason Aronson.

Fischer, S. (1998). Critical periods for language acquisition: Consequences for deaf education. In A. Weisel (Ed.), *Issues unresolved: New perspectives on language and deaf education* (pp. 9–26). Washington, DC: Gallaudet University Press.

Fitzgerald, E. (1929). *Straight language for the deaf: A system of instruction for deaf children*. Staunton, VA: The McClure Company.

Fitzgerald, E. (1949). *Straight language for the deaf: A system of instruction for deaf children*. Washington, DC: Volta Bureau.

Flavell, D. (1985). *Cognitive development* (2nd ed.). Englewood Cliffs, NJ: Prentice Hall.

Fleetwood, E., & Metzger, M. (1998). *Cued language structure: An analysis of cued American English based on linguistic principles*. Silver Spring, MD: Calliope Press.

Fletcher, J., Shaywitz, S., Shankweiler, D., Katz, L., Liberman, I., Stuebing, K., Francis, D., Fowler, A., & Shaywitz, B. (1994). Cognitive profiles of reading disability: Comparisons of discrepancy and low achievement definitions. *Journal of Educational Psychology*, 86, 6–23.

Fletcher, P., & MacWhinney, B. (Ed.). (1995). *The handbook of child language*. Cambridge, MA: Blackwell.

Flexer, C. (1997). Individual and sound-field FM systems: Rationale, description, and use. *Volta Review*, 99, 133–162.

Flower, L., & Hayes, J. (1980). The dynamics of composing: Making plans and juggling constraints. In L. W. Gregg & E. R. Steinberg (Eds.), *Cognitive processes in writing* (pp. 31–50). Hillsdale, NJ: Lawrence Erlbaum.

Fodor, J. (1983). *The modularity of mind: An essay on faculty psychology*. Cambridge, MA: MIT Press.

Folven, R., & Bonvillian, J. (1991). The transition from nonreferential to referential language in children acquiring American Sign Language. *Developmental Psychology*, 27, 806–816.

Fowler, A. (1991). How early phonological development might set the stage for phoneme awareness. In S. Brady & D. Shankweiler (Eds.), *Phonological processes in literacy* (pp. 97–117). Hillsdale, NJ: Lawrence Erlbaum.

French, M. (1999). *Starting with assessment: A developmental approach to deaf children's literacy*. Washington, DC: Gallaudet University, Pre-College National Mission Programs.

French-St. George, M. (1986). What does speech sound like to the hearing-impaired? *Volta Review, 88*, 109–122.

Frishberg, N. (1975). Arbitrariness and iconicity: Historical change in American Sign Language. *Language, 51*, 676–710.

Fruchter, A., Wilbur, R., & Fraser, B. (1984). Comprehension of idioms by hearing-impaired students. *Volta Review, 86*, 7–18.

Furth, H. (1966). *Thinking without language: Psychological implications of deafness*. New York: Free Press.

Fusaro, J., & Slike, S. (1979). The effect of imagery on the ability of hearing-impaired children to identify words. *American Annals of the Deaf, 124*, 829–832.

Gallaudet Research Institute. (1985). *Gallaudet Research Institute Newsletter*. Washington, DC: Author.

Gamez, G. (1979). Reading in a second language: Native language approach vs. direct method. *The Reading Teacher, 32*, 665–670.

Gannon, J. (1981). *Deaf heritage: A narrative history of deaf America*. Silver Spring, MD: National Association of the Deaf.

Gardner, J., & Zorfass, J. (1983). From sign to speech: The language development of a hearing-impaired child. *American Annals of the Deaf, 128*, 20–24.

Gaustad, M. (1986). Longitudinal effects of manual English instruction on deaf children's morphological skills. *Applied Psycholinguistics, 7*, 101–128.

Gee, J., & Goodhart, W. (1985). Nativization, linguistic theory, and deaf language acquisition. *Sign Language Studies, 49*, 291–342.

Gee, J., & Goodhart, W. (1988). American Sign Language and the human biologial capacity for language. In M. Strong (Ed.), *Language learning and deafness* (pp. 49–74). New York: Cambridge University Press.

Geers, A., & Moog, J. (1978). Syntactic maturity of spontaneous speech and elicited imitations of hearing-impaired children. *Journal of Speech and Hearing Disorders, 43*, 380–391.

Geers, A., & Moog, J. (1989). Factors predictive of the development of literacy in profoundly hearing-impaired adolescents. *Volta Review, 91*, 69–86.

Geers, A., & Moog, J. (1994). Effectiveness of cochlear implants and tactile aids for deaf children: The sensory aids study at Central Institute for the Deaf [Special Issue]. *Volta Review, 96*(5).

Gelman, S., & Byrnes, J. (Eds.). (1991). *Perspectives on language and thought: Interrelations in development*. New York: Cambridge University Press.

Genesee, F. (1987). *Learning through two languages: Studies of immersion and bilingual education*. Cambridge, MA: Newbury House.

Gerken, L., Jusczyk, P., & Mandel, D. (1994). When prosody fails to cue syntactic structure: 9-months-olds' sensitivity to phonological versus syntactic phrases. *Cognition, 51*, 237–265.

Geuss, R. (1981). *The idea of a critical theory: Habermas and the Frankfurt school*. New York: Cambridge University Press.

Gibbs, K. (1989). Individual differences in cognitive skills related to reading ability in the deaf. *American Annals of the Deaf, 134*, 214–218.

Gibson, R. (1986). *Critical theory and education*. London: Hodder & Stoughton.

Gilman, L., Davis, J., & Raffin, M. (1980). Use of common morphemes by hearing impaired children exposed to a system of manual English. *Journal of Auditory Research, 20*, 57–69.

Giorcelli, L. (1982). *The comprehension of some aspects of figurative language by deaf and hearing subjects*. Unpublished doctoral dissertation, University of Illinois, Urbana-Champaign.

Glazzard, P. (1982). *Learning activities and teaching ideas for the special child in the regular classroom*. Englewood Cliffs, NJ: Prentice Hall.

Gleason, J. (1993). Studying language development: An overview and a preview. In J. Gleason (Ed.), *The development of language* (3rd ed., pp. 1–37). New York: Macmillan.

Gliedman, J., & Roth, W. (1980). *The unexpected minority: Handicapped children in America*. New York: Harcourt Brace Jovanovich.

Goldberg, D. (1993). Auditory-verbal philosophy: A tutorial. *Volta Review, 95*, 181–186.

Goldberg, D., & Flexer, C. (1991, June). *Where are they now? Survey of auditory-verbal graduates*. Paper presented at the Auditory-Verbal International Conference, Easton, PA.

Goldberg, J., & Bordman, P. (1975). The ESL approach to teaching English to hearing impaired students. *American Annals of the Deaf, 120*, 22–27.

Golinkoff, R., & Hirsch-Pasek, K. (1995). Reinterpreting children's sentence comprehension: Toward a new framework. In B. MacWhinney & P. Fletcher (Eds.), *Handbook of child language* (pp. 430–461). Cambridge, MA: Blackwell.

Goodluck, H. (1991). *Language acquisition: A linguistic introduction*. Cambridge, MA: Blackwell.

Goodman, K. (1976). Reading: A psycholinguistic guessing game. In H. Singer & R. Ruddell (Eds.), *Theoretical models and processes of reading* (2nd ed., pp. 497–508). Newark, DE: International Reading Association.

Goodman, K. (1985). Unity in reading. In H. Singer & R. Ruddell (Eds.), *Theoretical models and processes of reading* (3rd ed., pp. 813–840). Newark, DE: International Reading Association.

Goodman, K. (1994). Reading, writing, and written texts: A transactional sociopsycholinguistic view. In R. Ruddell, M. Ruddell, & H. Singer (Eds.), *Theoretical models and processes of reading* (4th ed., pp. 1093–1130). Newark, DE: International Reading Association.

Gormley, K., & Sarachan-Deily, A. (1987). Evaluating hearing-impaired students' writing: A practical approach. *Volta Review, 89,* 157–170.

Grabe, W. (1988). Reassessing the term "interactive." In P. Carrell, J. Devine, & D. Eskey (Eds.), *Interactive approaches to second language reading* (pp. 56–70). New York: Cambridge University Press.

Grabe, W. (1991). Current developments in second-language reading research. *TESOL Quarterly, 25,* 375–406.

Graesser, A., Millis, K., & Zwaan, R. (1997). Discourse comprehension. *Annual Review of Psychology, 48,* 163–189.

Greenberg, M., & Kusche, C. (1989). Cognitive, personal, and social development of deaf children and adolescents. In M. Wang, M. Reynolds, & H. Walberg (Eds.), *The handbook of special education: Research and practice* (Vol. 3, pp. 95–129). New York: Pergamon.

Greenfield, P., & Smith, J. (1976). *The structure of communication in early language development.* San Diego: Academic Press.

Gregory, J. (1987). An investigation of speechreading with and without cued speech. *American Annals of the Deaf, 132,* 393–398.

Grice, H. (1975). Logic and conversation. In P. Cole & J. Morgan (Eds.), *Speech acts* (pp. 41–58). San Diego: Academic Press.

Griffith, P., & Ripich, D. (1988). Story structure recall in hearing-impaired, learning-disabled, and nondisabled children. *American Annals of the Deaf, 133,* 43–50.

Griswold, E., & Cummings, J. (1974). The expressive vocabulary of preschool deaf children. *American Annals of the Deaf, 119,* 16–28.

Groce, N. (1985). *Everyone here spoke sign language: Hereditary deafness on Martha's Vineyard.* Cambridge, MA: Harvard University Press.

Groht, M. (1958). *Natural language for deaf children.* Washington, DC: The Volta Bureau.

Grosjean, F. (1992). The bilingual and the bicultural person in the hearing and in the deaf world. *Sign Language Studies, 77*, 307–320.

Grosjean, F. (1998). Living with two languages and two cultures. In I. Parasnis (Ed.), *Cultural and language diversity and the Deaf experience* (pp. 20–37). New York: Cambridge University Press.

Grushkin, D. (1998a). Why shouldn't Sam read? Toward a new paradigm for literacy and the deaf. *Journal of Deaf Studies and Deaf Education, 3*, 179–204.

Grushkin, D. (1998b). Lexidactylophobia: The (irrational) fear of fingerspelling. *American Annals of the Deaf, 143*, 404–415.

Gustason, G. (1983). *Teaching and learning signing exact English*. Los Alamitos, CA: Modern Signs Press.

Gustason, G. (1990). Signing exact English. In H. Bornstein (Ed.), *Manual communication: Implications for education* (pp. 108–127). Washington, DC: Gallaudet University Press.

Gustason, G., Pfetzing, D., & Zawolkow, E. (1975). *Signing exact English* (Rev. ed.). Los Alamitos, CA: Modern Signs Press.

Gustason, G., Pfetzing, D., & Zawolkow, E. (1980). *Signing exact English*. Los Alamitos, CA: Modern Signs Press.

Gustason, G., & Zawolkow, E. (1993). *Signing exact English*. Los Alamitos, CA: Modern Signs Press.

Hakuta, K. (1986). *Mirror of language: The debate of bilingualism*. New York: Basic Books.

Hakuta, K., & Mostafapour, E. F. (1998). Perspectives from the history and politics of bilingualism and bilingual education in the United States. In I. Parasnis (Ed.), *Cultural and language diversity and the Deaf experience* (pp. 38–50). New York: Cambridge University Press.

Halliday, M. (1975). *Learning how to mean: Explorations in the development of language*. London: Edward Arnold.

Hamers, J. (1998). Cognitive and language development of bilingual children. In I. Parasnis (Ed.), *Cultural and language diversity and the Deaf experience* (pp. 51–75). New York: Cambridge University Press.

Hamers, J., & Blanc, M. (1982). Towards a social-psychological model of bilingual development. *Journal of Language and Social Psychology, 1*, 29–49.

Hamers, J., & Blanc, M. (1989). *Bilinguality and bilingualism*. Cambridge, UK: Cambridge University Press.

Hanson, V. (1989). Phonology and reading: Evidence from profoundly deaf readers. In D. Shankweiler & I. Lieberman (Eds.), *Phonology and reading disability: Solving the reading puzzle* (pp. 69–89). Ann Arbor, MI: University of Michigan Press.

Hanson, V. (1990). Recall of order information by deaf signers: Phonetic coding in temporal order recall. *Memory and Cognition, 18,* 604–610.

Hanson, V., Liberman, I., & Shankweiler, D. (1984). Linguistic coding by deaf children in relation to beginning reading success. *Journal of Experimental Child Psychology, 37,* 378–393.

Hanson, V., & Lichtenstein, E. (1990). Short-term memory coding by deaf signers: The primary language coding hypothesis reconsidered. *Cognitive Psychology, 22,* 211–224.

Harris, M., & Beech, J. (1998). Implicit phonological awareness and early reading development in prelingually deaf children. *Journal of Deaf Studies and Deaf Education, 3,* 205–216.

Harris, P. (1992). Cognitive prerequisites to language? *British Journal of Psychology, 73,* 187–195.

Harrison, A. (1983). *A language testing handbook.* New York: Macmillan.

Harste, J., Burke, C., & Woodward, V. (1982). Children's language and world: Initial encounters with print. In J. Langer & M. T. Smith-Burke (Eds.), *Reader meets author/bridging the gap* (pp. 105–131). Newark, DE: International Reading Association.

Hatcher, C., & Robbins, N. (1978). *The development of reading skills in hearing-impaired children.* Cedar Falls, IA: University of Northern Iowa. (ERIC Document Reproduction Service No. ED 167 960)

Hayes, P., & Arnold, P. (1992). Is hearing-impaired children's reading delayed or different? *Journal of Research in Reading, 15,* 104–116.

Heath, S. (1982). What no bedtime story means: Narrative skills at home and school. *Language and Society, 2,* 49–76.

Heider, F., & Heider, G. (1940). A comparison of sentence structure of deaf and hearing children. *Psychological Monographs, 52,* 42–103.

Heimlich, J., & Pittelman, S. (1986). *Semantic mapping: Classroom applications.* Newark, DE: International Reading Association.

Hester, M. (1969). Education of the deaf. In J. Griffith (Ed.), *Persons with hearing loss* (pp. 150–165). Springfield, IL: Charles C. Thomas.

Hillocks, G. (1986). *Research on written composition: New directions for teaching.* Urbana, IL: National Conference on Research in English.

Hirsh-Pasek, K. (1986). Beyond the great debate: Fingerspelling as an alternative route to word identification for deaf or dyslexic readers. *The Reading Teacher, 40,* 340–343.

Hirsh-Pasek, K. (1987). The metalinguistics of fingerspelling: An alternative way to increase written vocabulary in congenitally deaf readers. *Reading Research Quarterly, 22,* 455–474.

Hirsh-Pasek, K., & Freyd, P. (1983a, August). *Deaf readers' ability to analyze morphological regularities.* Paper presented at the meeting of the American Psychological Association, Anaheim, CA. (ERIC Document Reproduction Service No. ED 239 425)

Hirsh-Pasek, K., & Freyd, P. (1983b). *What deaf individuals bring to the reading task: A focus on word identification strategies.* (ERIC Document Reproduction Service No. ED 239 424)

Hirsh-Pasek, K., & Freyd, P. (1984). *Vocabulary development: How deaf individuals can learn to use the information given.* (ERIC Document Reproduction Service No. ED 246 404)

Hoffmeister, R., & Wilbur, R. (1980). The acquisition of sign language. In H. Lane & F. Grosjean (Eds.), *Recent perspectives on American Sign Language* (pp. 61–78). Hillsdale, NJ: Lawrence Erlbaum.

Holzman, M. (1983). *The language of children: Development in home and school.* Englewood Cliffs, NJ: Prentice Hall.

Horkheimer, M. (1995). *Critical theory: Selected essays.* New York: Continuum.

Houck, J. (1982). *The effects of idioms on reading comprehension of hearing impaired students* [Abstract]. Unpublished doctoral dissertation, University of Northern Colorado.

Huck, G., & Goldsmith, J. (1995). *Ideology and linguistic theory: Noam Chomsky and the deep structure debates.* New York: Routledge.

Huey, E. (1968). *The psychology and pedagogy of reading.* New York: Macmillan. (Original work published 1908)

Hunt, K. (1965). *Grammatical structures written at three grade levels.* Champaign, IL: National Council of Teachers of English.

Hunt, K. (1970). Syntactic maturity in school children and adults. *Monographs of the Society for Research in Child Development, 35,* 134.

Hutchinson, K. (1990). An analytic distinctive feature approach to auditory training. *Volta Review, 92,* 5–12.

Huttenlocher, J., & Smiley, P. (1987). Early word meanings: The case of object names. *Cognitive Psychology, 19,* 63–89.

Hymes, D. (1974). *Foundations in sociolinguistics: An ethnographic approach.* Philadelphia: University of Pennsylvania Press.

Ingram, D. (1989). *First language acquisition: Method, description, and explanation.* New York: Cambridge University Press.

Iran-Nejad, A., Ortony, A., & Rittenhouse, R. (1981). The comprehension of metaphorical uses of English by deaf children. *Journal of Speech and Hearing Research, 24,* 551–556.

Isenhath, J. (1990). *The linguistics of American Sign Language.* Jefferson, NC: McFarland & Company.

Jackson, D., Paul, P., & Smith, J. (1997). Prior knowledge and reading comprehension ability of deaf and hard-of-hearing adolescents. *Journal of Deaf Studies and Deaf Education, 2,* 172–184.

Jakobson, R. (1968). *Child language aphasia and phonological universals.* The Hague, the Netherlands: Mouton.

Jarvella, R., & Lubinsky, J. (1975). Deaf and hearing children's use of language describing temporal order among events. *Journal of Speech and Hearing Research, 18,* 58–73.

Jeffers, J., & Barley, M. (1971). *Speechreading (lipreading).* Springfield, IL: Charles C. Thomas.

Jensema, C. (1975). *The relationship between academic achievement and the demographic characteristics of hearing-impaired children and youth* (Series R, No. 2). Washington, DC: Gallaudet University, Center for Assessment and Demographic Studies.

Johnson, D., Moe, A., & Baumann, J. (1983). *The Ginn word book for teachers: A basic lexicon.* Lexington, MA: Ginn.

Johnson, D., & Pearson, P. D. (1984). *Teaching reading vocabulary* (2nd ed.). New York: Holt, Rinehart & Winston.

Johnson, R. (1916). What are the fundamentals? *American Annals of the Deaf, 61,* 92–95.

Johnson, R., Liddell, S., & Erting, C. (1989). *Unlocking the curriculum: Principles for achieving access in deaf education* (Working Paper 89-3). Washington, DC: Gallaudet University, Gallaudet Research Institute.

Johnson-Laird, P. (1988). *The computer and the mind: An introduction to cognitive science.* Cambridge, MA: Harvard University Press.

Johnston, J. (1985). Cognitive prerequisites: The evidence from children learning English. In D. Slobin (Ed.), *The crosslingusitic study of language acquisition: Vol. 2. Theoretical issues* (pp. 961–1004). Hillsdale, NJ: Lawrence Erlbaum.

Jones, P. (1979). Negative interference of signed language in written English. *Sign Language Studies, 24,* 273–279.

Jordan, I. K., Gustason, G., & Rosen, R. (1979). An update on communication trends at programs for the deaf. *American Annals of the Deaf, 124,* 350–357.

Jordan, I. K., & Karchmer, M. (1986). Patterns of sign use among hearing-impaired students. In A. Schildroth & M. Karchmer (Eds.), *Deaf children in America* (pp. 125–138). Boston: Little, Brown.

Joyce, B., Weil, M., & Showers, B. (1992). *Models of teaching* (4th ed.). Boston: Allyn & Bacon.

Jusczyk, P., Friederici, A., Wessels, J., Svenkerud, V., & Jusczyk, A. (1993). Infants' sensitivity to the sound patterns of native language words. *Journal of Memory and Language, 32,* 402–420.

Just, M., & Carpenter, P. (1987). *The psychology of reading and language comprehension.* Boston: Allyn & Bacon.

Kantor, R. (1980). The acquisition of classifiers in American Sign Language. *Sign Language Studies, 28,* 193–208.

Kantor, R. (1982). Communicative interaction: Mother modification and child acquisition of American Sign Language. *Sign Language Studies, 36,* 233–282.

Karmiloff-Smith, A. (1989). Quantitative hardware stages that constrain language development. *Human Development, 32,* 272–275.

Kelly, L. (1993). Recall of English function words and inflections by skilled and average deaf readers. *American Annals of the Deaf, 138,* 288–296.

Kelly, L. (1995). Processing of bottom-up and top-down information by skilled and average deaf readers and implications for whole language instruction. *Exceptional Children, 61,* 318–334.

Kelly, L. (1996). The interaction of syntactic competence and vocabulary during reading by deaf students. *Journal of Deaf Studies and Deaf Education, 1,* 75–90.

Kelly, L. (1998). Using silent motion pictures to teach complex syntax to adult deaf readers. *Journal of Deaf Studies and Deaf Education, 3,* 217–230.

Kempson, R. (1977). *Semantic theory.* Cambridge, UK: Cambridge University Press.

King, C. (1981). *An investigation of similarities and differences in the syntactic abilities of deaf and hearing children learning English as a first or second language.* Unpublished doctoral dissertation, University of Illinois, Champaign-Urbana.

King, C. (1984). National survey of language methods used with hearing-impaired students in the United States. *American Annals of the Deaf, 129,* 311–316.

King, C., & Quigley, S. (1985). *Reading and deafness.* San Diego: College-Hill Press.

Kisor, H. (1990). *What's that pig outdoors: A memoir of deafness*. New York: Hill & Wang.

Klima, E., & Bellugi, U. (1979). *The signs of language*. Cambridge, MA: Harvard University Press.

Kluwin, T. (1981). The grammaticality of manual representation of English in classroom settings. *American Annals of the Deaf, 126*, 417–421.

Kluwin, T., Getson, P., & Kluwin, B. (1980). The effects of experience on the discourse comprehension of deaf and hearing adolescents. *Directions, 1*(3), 49.

Kluwin, T., & Kelly, A. (1991). The effectiveness of dialogue journal writing in improving the writing skills of young deaf writers. *American Annals of the Deaf, 136*, 284–291.

Kodman, F. (1963). Educational status of hard-of-hearing children in the classroom. *Journal of Speech and Hearing Disorders, 28*, 297–299.

Krakow, R., & Hanson, V. (1985). Deaf signers and serial recall in the visual modality: Memory for signs, fingerspelling, and print. *Memory and Cognition, 13*, 265–272.

Krashen, S. (1981). *Second language acquisition and second language learning*. New York: Pergamon.

Krashen, S. (1982). *Principles and practices of second language acquisition*. New York: Pergamon.

Krashen, S. (1985). *The input hypothesis: Issues and implications*. White Plains, NY: Longman.

Kretschmer, R. R., & Kretschmer, L. (1978). *Language development and intervention with the hearing impaired*. Baltimore, MD: University Park Press.

Kretschmer, R. R., & Kretschmer, L. (Eds.). (1988). *Communication assessment of hearing-impaired children: From conversation to classroom* [Monograph Supplement]. (ERIC Document Reproduction Service ED 311 656)

Kronenberger, L. (Ed.). (1951). *Alexander Pope: Selected works*. New York: Random House.

Krose, J., Lotz, W., Puffer, C., & Osberger, M. (1986). Language and learning skills of hearing impaired children. *ASHA Monographs, 23*, 66–77.

Kuhn, T. (1970). *The structure of scientific revolutions* (2nd ed.). Chicago: University of Chicago Press.

Kusche, C., & Greenberg, M. (1991). Cortical organization and information processing in deaf children. In D. Martin (Ed.), *Advances in cognition, education, and deafness* (pp. 243–249). Washington, DC: Gallaudet University Press.

Labov, W. (1972). *Sociolinguistic patterns.* Philadelphia: University of Pennsylvania Press.

Laine, C., & Schultz, L. (1985). Composition theory and practice: The paradigm shift. *Volta Review, 87,* 9–20.

Lambert, W. (1972). A social psychology of bilingualism. In W. Lambert (Ed.), *Language, psychology, and culture* (pp. 212–235). Stanford, CA: Stanford University Press.

Lambert, W., & Tucker, G. (1972). *The bilingual education of children: The St. Lambert experiment.* Rowley, MA: Newbury House.

Lamendella, J. (1977). General principles of neurofunctional organization and their manifestation in primary and nonprimary language acquisition. *Language Learning, 27,* 155–196.

Landauer, T., & Dumais, S. (1997). A solution to Plato's problem: The latent semantic analysis theory of acquisition, induction, and representation of knowledge. *Psychological Review, 104,* 211–240.

Lane, H. (1984). *When the mind hears: A history of the deaf.* New York: Random House.

Lane, H. (1988). Is there a "psychology of the deaf"? *Exceptional Children, 55,* 7–19.

Lane, H. (1992). *The mask of benevolence: Disabling the Deaf community.* New York: Vintage.

Lane, H., & Baker, D. (1974). Reading achievement of the deaf: Another look. *Volta Review, 76,* 489–499.

Lane, H., & Grosjean, F. (Eds.). (1980). *Recent perspectives on American Sign Language.* Hillsdale, NJ: Lawrence Erlbaum.

Lane, H., Hoffmeister, R., & Bahan, B. (1996). *A journey into the DEAF-WORLD.* San Diego: DawnSign Press.

Lane, H., & Philip, F. (1984). *The deaf experience: Classics in language and education.* Cambridge, MA: Harvard University Press.

LaSasso, C., & Davey, B. (1987). The relationship between lexical knowledge and reading comprehension for prelingually, profoundly hearing-impaired students. *Volta Review, 89,* 211–220.

LaSasso, C., & Metzger, M. (1998). An alternate route for preparing deaf children for bibi programs: The home language as L1 and cued speech for conveying traditionally-spoken languages. *Journal of Deaf Studies and Deaf Education, 3,* 265–289.

LaSasso, C., & Mobley, R. (1997). National survey of reading instruction for deaf or hard-of-hearing students in the U.S. *Volta Review, 99,* 31–58.

Layton, T., Holmes, D., & Bradley, P. (1979). A description of pedagogically imposed signed semantic-syntactic relationships in deaf children. *Sign Language Studies, 23,* 137–160.

Lee, L. (1966). Developmental sentence types: A method for comparing normal and deviant syntactic development. *Journal of Speech and Hearing Disorders, 31,* 311–330.

Lee, L. (1969). *Northwestern syntax screening test.* Evanston, IL: Northwestern University Press.

Lee, L. (1974). *Developmental sentence analysis.* Evanston, IL: Northwestern University Press.

Lee, L., & Canter, S. (1971). Developmental sentence scoring: A clinical procedure for estimating syntactic development in children's spontaneous speech. *Journal of Speech and Hearing Disorders, 36,* 315–340.

Lemley, P. (1993). *Deaf readers and engagement in the story world: A study of strategies and stances.* Unpublished doctoral dissertation, Ohio State University, Columbus.

Lenneberg, E. (1967). *Biological foundations of language.* New York: John Wiley.

Leverentz, F., & Garman, D. (1987). What was that you said? *Instruction, 96,* 66–77.

Levine, E. (1981). *The ecology of early deafness: Guides to fashioning environments and psychological assessments.* New York: Columbia University Press.

Levitt, H. (1989). Technology and speech training: An affair to remember. *Volta Review, 91,* 1–6.

Lewis, D. (1995). FM systems: A good idea that keeps getting better. *Volta Review, 97,* 183–196.

Leybaert, J. (1993). Reading in the deaf: The roles of phonological codes. In M. Marschark & M. D. Clark (Eds.), *Psychological perspectives on deafness* (pp. 269–309). Hillsdale, NJ: Lawrence Erlbaum.

Leybaert, J., & Charlier, B. (1996). Visual speech in the head: The effect of cued-speech on rhyming, remembering, and spelling. *Journal of Deaf Studies and Deaf Education, 1,* 234–248.

Liberman, I., Shankweiler, D., Fischer, F., & Carter, B. (1974). Explicit syllable and phoneme segmentation in the young child. *Journal of Experimental Child Psychology, 18,* 201–212.

Liberman, I., Shankweiler, D., & Liberman, A. (1989). The alphabetic principle and learning to read. In D. Shankweiler & I. Liberman (Eds.), *Phonology and reading disability: Solving the reading puzzle* (pp. 1–33). Ann Arbor, MI: University of Michigan Press.

Lichtenstein, E. (1983). *The relationships between reading processes and English skills of deaf students.* Unpublished manuscript, National Technical Institute for the Deaf, Rochester, NY.

Lichtenstein, E. (1984). Deaf working memory processes and English language skills. In D. Martin (Ed.), *International symposium on cognition, education, and deafness: Working papers* (Vol. 2, pp. 331–360). Washington, DC: Gallaudet University Press.

Lichtenstein, E. (1985). Deaf working memory processes and English language skills. In D. Martin (Ed.), *Cognition, education, and deafness: Directions for research and instruction* (pp. 111–114). Washington, DC: Gallaudet University Press.

Lichtenstein, E. (1998). The relationships between reading processes and English skills of deaf college students. *Journal of Deaf Studies and Deaf Education, 3,* 80–134.

Liddell, S. (1980). *American Sign Language syntax.* The Hague, the Netherlands: Mouton.

Liddell, S. (1995). Real, surrogate, and token space: Grammatical consequences in ASL. In K. Emmorey & J. Reilly (Eds.), *Language, gesture, and space* (pp. 19–41). Hillsdale, NJ: Lawrence Erlbaum.

Liddell, S., & Johnson, R. (1989). American Sign Language: The phonological base. *Sign Language Studies, 64,* 195–277.

Liedel, J., & Paul, P. (1991). An interactive-interaction bilingual-bicultural program model. In S. Polowe-Aldersley, P. Schragle, V. Armour, & J. Polowe (Eds.), *Conference proceedings of the 1991 CAID/CEASD convention* (pp. 106–109). New Orleans, LA: Convention of American Instructors of the Deaf.

Lightfoot, D. (1999). *The development of language: Acquisition, change, and evolution.* Cambridge, MA: Blackwell.

Lillo-Martin, D., Hanson, V., & Smith, S. (1991). Deaf readers' comprehension of complex syntactic structure. In D. Martin (Ed.), *Advances in cognition, education, and deafness* (pp. 146–151). Washington, DC: Gallaudet University Press.

Lillo-Martin, D., Hanson, V., & Smith, S. (1992). Deaf readers' comprehension of relative clause structure. *Applied Psycholinguistics, 13,* 13–30.

Lindfors, J. (1980). *Children's language and learning*. Englewood Cliffs, NJ: Prentice Hall.

Ling, D. (1976). *Speech and the hearing-impaired child: Theory and practice.* Washington, DC: Alexander Graham Bell Association for the Deaf.

Ling, D. (Ed.). (1984). *Early intervention for hearing-impaired children: Oral options.* San Diego: College-Hill Press.

Ling, D. (1986). Devices and procedures for auditory learning. *Volta Review, 88,* 19–28.

Ling, D. (1989). *Aural habilitation: The foundation of verbal learning in hearing-impaired children* (2nd ed.). Washington, DC: Alexander Graham Bell Association for the Deaf.

Ling, D. (1993). Auditory-verbal options for children with hearing impairment: Helping to pioneer an applied science. *Volta Review, 95,* 187–196.

Ling, D., & Clarke, B. (1975). Cued speech: An evaluative study. *American Annals of the Deaf, 120,* 480–488.

Ling, D., Leckie, D., Pollack, D., Simser, J., & Smith, A. (1981). Syllable reception by hearing impaired children trained from infancy in auditory-oral programs. *Volta Review, 83,* 451–457.

Lipson, M., & Wixson, K. (1997). *Assessment and instruction of reading and writing disability: An interactive approach* (2nd ed.). White Plains, NY: Longman.

Livingston, S. (1989). Revision strategies of deaf student writers. *American Annals of the Deaf, 134,* 21–26.

Livingston, S. (1997). *Rethinking the education of deaf students.* Portsmouth, NH: Heinemann.

Locke, J. (1993). *The child's path to spoken language.* Cambridge, MA: Harvard University Press.

Locke, J., & Locke, V. (1971). Deaf children's phonetic, visual, and dactylic coding in a grapheme recall task. *Journal of Experimental Psychology, 89,* 142–146.

Long, G., Stinson, M., & Braeges, J. (1991). Students' perceptions of communication ease and engagement, how they relate to academic success. *American Annals of the Deaf, 136,* 414–421.

Long, N., Fitzgerald, C., Sutton, K., & Rollins, J. (1983). The auditory-verbal approach: Ellison, a case study. *Volta Review, 85,* 27–30, 35.

Looney, P., & Rose, S. (1979). The acquisition of inflectional suffixes by deaf youngsters using written and fingerspelled modes. *American Annals of the Deaf, 124*, 765–769.

Lou, M. (1988). The history of language use in the education of the Deaf in the United States. In M. Strong (Ed.), *Language learning and deafness* (pp. 75–98). Cambridge, MA: Cambridge University Press.

Lovett, M., Borden, S., DeLuca, T., Lacerenza, L., Benson, N., & Brackstone, D. (1994). Treating the core deficits of developmental dyslexia: Evidence of transfer of learning after phonologically- and strategically-based reading training programs. *Developmental Psychology, 30*, 805–822.

Lucas, C. (Ed.). (1990). *Sign language research*. Washington, DC: Gallaudet University Press.

Lucas, C., & Valli, C. (1992). *Language contact in the American Deaf community*. San Diego: Academic Press.

Lucas, E. (1980). *Semantic and pragmatic language disorders: Assessment and remediation*. Rockville, MD: Aspen Systems.

Luckasson, R., Coulter, D., Polloway, E., Reiss, S., Schalock, R., Snell, M., Spitalnik, D., & Stark, J. (1992). *Mental retardation: Definition, classification and systems of supports*. Washington, DC: American Association of Mental Retardation.

Luckner, J., & Isaacson, S. (1990). Teaching expressive writing to hearing-impaired students. *Journal of Childhood Communication Disorders, 13*, 135–152.

Luetke-Stahlman, B. (1983). Using bilingual instructional models in teaching hearing-impaired students. *American Annals of the Deaf, 128*, 873–877.

Luetke-Stahlman, B. (1984). Classifier recognition by hearing-impaired children in residential and public schools. *Sign Language Studies, 42*, 39–44.

Luetke-Stahlman, B. (1988a). The benefit of oral English-only as compared with signed input to hearing-impaired students. *Volta Review, 90*, 349–361.

Luetke-Stahlman, B. (1988b). Documenting syntactically and semantically incomplete bimodal input to hearing-impaired subjects. *American Annals of the Deaf, 133*, 230–234.

Luetke-Stahlman, B. (1998). *Language issues in deaf education*. Hillsboro, OR: Butte Publications.

Luetke-Stahlman, B. (1999). *Language across the curriculum: When students are deaf or hard of hearing*. Hillsboro, OR: Butte Publications.

Luetke-Stahlman, B., & Luckner, J. (1991). *Effectively educating students with hearing impairments*. White Plains, NY: Longman.

Luetke-Stahlman, B., & Milburn, W. (1996). Seeing essential English. *American Annals of the Deaf, 141*, 29–33.

Luetke-Stahlman, B., & Weiner, F. (1982). Assessing language and/or system preferences of Spanish-deaf preschoolers. *American Annals of the Deaf, 127,* 789–796.

Lyons, J. (1995). *Linguistic semantics: An introduction.* New York: Cambridge University Press.

MacGinitie, W. (1969). Flexibility in dealing with alternative meanings of words. In J. Rosenstein & W. MacGinitie (Eds.), *Verbal behavior of the deaf child: Studies of word meanings and associations* (pp. 45–55). New York: Columbia University, Teachers College Press.

Macnamara, J. (1966). *Bilingualism and primary education: A study of the Irish experience.* Hawthorne, NY: Aldine.

MacSweeney, M., Campbell, R., & Donlan, C. (1996). Varieties of short-term memory coding in deaf teenagers. *Journal of Deaf Studies and Deaf Education, 1,* 249–262.

Marbury, N., & Mackinson-Smyth, J. (1986, April). *ASL and English: A partnership.* Paper presented at the American Sign Language Research and Teaching Conference, Newark, CA.

Markowicz, H. (1980). Myths about American Sign Language. In H. Lane & F. Grosjean (Eds.), *Recent perspectives on American Sign Language* (pp. 1–6). Hillsdale, NJ: Lawrence Erlbaum.

Marmor, G., & Pettito, L. (1979). Simultaneous communication in the classroom: How well is English grammar represented? *Sign Language Studies, 23,* 99–136.

Marr, D. (1982). *Vision.* New York: Freeman.

Marschark, M. (1993). *Psychological development of deaf children.* New York: Oxford University Press.

Marschark, M. (1997). *Raising and educating a deaf child: A comprehensive guide to the choices, controversies, and decisions faced by parents and educators.* New York: Oxford University Press.

Marschark, M., & Everhart, V. (1997). Relations of language and cognition: What do deaf children tell us? In M. Marschark, P. Siple, D. Lillo-Martin, R. Campbell, & V. Everhart (Eds.), *Relations of language and thought: The view from sign language and deaf children* (pp. 3–23). New York: Oxford University Press.

Marschark, M., Mouradian, V., & Halas, M. (1994). Discourse rules in the language processing of deaf and hearing children. *Journal of Experimental Child Psychology, 57,* 89–107.

Marschark, M., Siple, P., Lillo-Martin, D., Campbell, R., & Everhart, V. (1997). *Relations of language and thought: The view from sign language and deaf children.* New York: Oxford University Press.

Marshall, W., & Quigley, S. (1970). *Quantitative and qualitative analysis of syntactic structure in the written language of deaf students.* Urbana, IL: University of Illinois, Institute for Research on Exceptional Children.

Martin, D. (Ed.). (1991). *Advances in cognition, education, and deafness.* Washington, DC: Gallaudet University Press.

Martin, D. (1993). Reasoning skills: A key to literacy for deaf learners. *American Annals of the Deaf, 138,* 82–86.

Marton, W. (1988). *Methods in English language teaching: Frameworks and options.* Englewood Cliffs, NJ: Prentice Hall.

Mason, D., & Ewoldt, E. (1996). Whole language and deaf bilingual-bicultural education—naturally! *American Annals of the Deaf, 141,* 293–298.

Matthews, P. (1991). *Morphology* (2nd ed.). Cambridge, MA: Cambridge University Press.

Matthews, R. (1989). Introduction: Learnability and linguistic theory. In R. Matthews & W. Demopoulos (Eds.), *Learnability and linguistic theory* (pp. 1–17). Boston: Kluwer Academic Publishers.

Mavilya, M., & Mignone, B. (1977). *Educational strategies for the youngest hearing impaired children, 0–5 years of age.* New York: Lexington School for the Deaf.

Maxwell, M. (1983). Language acquisition in a deaf child of deaf parents: Speech, sign variations, and print variations. In K. Nelson (Ed.), *Children's language* (Vol. 4, pp. 283–313). Hillsdale, NJ: Lawrence Erlbaum.

Maxwell, M. (1984). A deaf child's natural development of literacy. *Sign Language Studies, 44,* 191–224.

Maxwell, M. (1987). The acquisition of English bound morphemes in sign form. *Sign Language Studies, 57,* 323–352.

Maxwell, M. (1990). Simultaneous communication: The state of the art and proposals for change. *Sign Language Studies, 69,* 333–390.

Maxwell, M., & Falick, T. (1992). Cohesion and quality in deaf and hearing children's written English. *Sign Language Studies, 77,* 345–372.

Mayberry, R. (1994). The importance of childhood to language acquisition: Evidence from American Sign Language. In J. Goodman & H. Nusbaum (Eds.), *The development of speech perception* (pp. 57–90). Cambridge, MA: MIT Press.

Mayberry, R., & Eichen, E. (1991). The long-lasting advantage of learning sign language in childhood: Another look at the critical period for language acquisition. *Journal of Memory and Language, 30,* 486–512.

Mayberry, R., & Fischer, S. (1989). Looking through phonological shape to sentence meaning: The bottleneck of non-native sign language processing. *Memory and Cognition, 17,* 740–754.

Mayer, C., & Akamatsu, C. T. (1999). Bilingual-bicultural models of literacy education for deaf students: Considering the claims. *Journal of Deaf Studies and Deaf Education, 4,* 1–8.

Mayer, C., & Wells, G. (1996). Can the linguistic interdependence theory support a bilingual-bicultural model of literacy education for deaf students? *Journal of Deaf Studies and Deaf Education, 1,* 93–107.

McAnally, P., Rose, S., & Quigley, S. (1987). *Language learning practices with deaf children.* San Diego: College-Hill Press.

McAnally, P., Rose, S., & Quigley, S. (1994). *Language learning practices with deaf children.* Austin, TX: Pro-Ed.

McCarthey, S., & Raphael, T. (1992). Alternative research perspectives. In J. Irwin & M. Doyle (Eds.), *Reading/writing connections: Learning from research* (pp. 2–30). Newark, DE: International Reading Association.

McCartney, B. (1986). An investigation of the factors contributing to the ability of hearing-impaired children to communicate orally as perceived by oral deaf adults and parents and teachers of the hearing-impaired. *Volta Review, 88,* 133–143.

McClelland, J., Rumelhart, D., & the PDP Research Group. (1986). *Parallel distributed processing: Explorations in the microstructure of cognition: Vol. 2. Psychological and biological models.* Cambridge, MA: MIT Press.

McClure, W. (1969). Historical perspectives in the education of the deaf. In J. Griffith (Ed.), *Persons with hearing loss* (pp. 3–30). Springfield, IL: Charles C. Thomas.

McCormick, L. (1986). Keeping up with language intervention trends. *Teaching Exceptional Children, 18,* 123–129.

McGarr, N. (Ed.). (1989). Research on the use of sensory aids for hearing-impaired people [Special Issue]. *Volta Review, 91*(5).

McGarr, N., & Whitehead, R. (1992). Contemporary issues in phoneme production by hearing-impaired persons: Physiological and acoustic aspects. *Volta Review, 94,* 33–45.

McGill-Franzen, A., & Gormley, K. (1980). The influence of context on deaf readers' understanding of passive sentences. *American Annals of the Deaf, 125*, 937–942.

McIntire, M. (1977). The acquisition of American Sign Language hand configurations. *Sign Language Studies, 16*, 247–266.

McKee, P., Harrison, M., McCowen, A., Lehr, E., & Durr, W. (1966). *Reading for meaning* (4th ed.). Boston: Houghton Mifflin.

McLaughlin, B. (1984). *Second-language acquisition in childhood: Vol. 1. Preschool children* (2nd ed.). Hillsdale, NJ: Lawrence Erlbaum.

McLaughlin, B. (1985). *Second-language acquisition in childhood: Vol. 2. School-age children* (2nd ed.). Hillsdale, NJ: Lawrence Erlbaum.

McLaughlin, B. (1987). *Theories of second-language learning*. Baltimore: Edward Arnold.

Meadow, K. (1968). Early manual communication in relation to the deaf child's intellectual, social, and communicative functioning. *American Annals of the Deaf, 113*, 29–41.

Meadow, K. (1980). *Deafness and child development*. Berkeley, CA: University of California Press.

Medin, D., & Ross, B. (1992). *Cognitive psychology*. New York: Harcourt Brace Jovanovich.

Meier, R. (1987). Elicited imitation of verb agreement in American Sign Language: Iconically or morphologically determined? *Journal of Memory and Language, 26*, 362–376.

Meier, R., & Willerman, R. (1995). Prelinguistic gesture in deaf and hearing infants. In K. Emmorey & J. Reilly (Eds.), *Language, gesture, and space* (pp. 391–409). Hillsdale, NJ: Lawrence Erlbaum.

Menn, L., & Stoel-Gammon, C. (1993). Phonological development: Learning sounds and sound patterns. In J. Berko Gleason (Ed.), *The development of language* (3rd ed., pp. 65–113). New York: Macmillan.

Menyuk, P. (1963). A preliminary evaluation of grammatical capacity in children. *Journal of Verbal Learning and Verbal Behavior, 2*, 429–439.

Menyuk, P. (1968). The role of distinctive features in children's acquisition of phonology. *Journal of Speech and Hearing Research, 11*, 138–146.

Menyuk, P. (1977). *Language and maturation*. Cambridge, MA: MIT Press.

Messerly, C., & Aram, D. (1980). Academic achievement of hearing-impaired students of hearing parents and of hearing-impaired parents: Another look. *Volta Review, 82*, 25–32.

Meyerhoff, W. (1986). *Disorders of hearing*. Austin, TX: Pro-Ed.

Miller, G. (1956). The magic number seven, plus or minus two: Some limits on our capacity for processing information. *Psychological Review, 63*, 81–97.

Miller, G. (1977). *Spontaneous apprentices: Children and language*. New York: Seabury Press.

Miller, J. (1981). *Assessing language production in children*. Baltimore: University Park Press.

Mitchell, D. (1982). *The process of reading: A cognitive analysis of fluent reading and learning to read*. New York: John Wiley.

Miyamoto, R., Svirsky, M., & Robbins, A. (1997). Enhancement of expressive language in prelingually deaf children with cochlear implants. *Acta Oto-Laryngologica, 117*, 154–157.

Modiano, N. (1968). National or mother language in beginning reading: A comparative study. *Research in the Teaching of English, 2*, 32–43.

Moeller, M. (1988). Combining formal and informal strategies for language assessment of hearing-impaired children. In R. R. Kretschmer & L. Kretschmer (Eds.), *Communication assessment of hearing-impaired children: From conversation to classroom* [Monograph Supplement] (pp. 73–99). (ERIC Document Reproduction Service ED 311 656)

Moerk, E. (1983). *The mother of Eve—as a first language teacher*. Norwood, NJ: Ablex.

Mohay, H. (1983). The effects of cued speech on the language development of three deaf children. *Sign Language Studies, 38*, 25–47.

Moog, J., Biedenstein, J., Davidson, L., & Brenner, C. (1994). Instruction for developing speech perception skills. *Volta Review, 96*, 61–73.

Moog, J., & Geers, A. (1979). *Grammatical analysis of elicited language: Simple sentence level*. St. Louis, MO: Central Institute for the Deaf.

Moog, J., & Geers, A. (1980). *Grammatical analysis of elicited language: Complex sentence level*. St. Louis, MO: Central Institute for the Deaf.

Moog, J., & Kozak, V. (1983). *Teacher assessment of grammatical structures*. St. Louis, MO: Central Institute for the Deaf.

Moog, J., Kozak, V., & Geers, A. (1983). *Grammatical analysis of elicited language: Pre-sentence level*. St. Louis, MO: Central Institute for the Deaf.

Moores, D. (1987). *Educating the deaf: Psychology, principles, and practices* (3rd ed.). Boston: Houghton Mifflin.

Moores, D. (1996). *Educating the deaf: Psychology, principles, and practices* (4th ed.). Boston: Houghton Mifflin.

Moores, D., & Meadow-Orlans, K. (Eds.). (1990). *Educational and developmental aspects of deafness.* Washington, DC: Gallaudet University Press.

Moores, D., & Sweet, C. (1990). Factors predictive of school achievement. In D. Moores & K. Meadow-Orlans (Eds.), *Educational and developmental aspects of deafness* (pp. 154–201). Washington, DC: Gallaudet University.

Moores, D., Weiss, K., & Goodwin, M. (1978). Early intervention programs for hearing-impaired children. *American Annals of the Deaf, 123,* 925–936.

Morse, P. (1974). Infant speech perception: A preliminary model and review of the literature. In R. Schiefelbusch & L. L. Lloyd (Eds.), *Language perspective: Acquisition, retardation, and intervention* (pp. 19–53). Baltimore: University Park Press.

Morton, M. (1993). *The critical turn: Studies in Kant, Herder, Wittgenstein, and contemporary theory.* Detroit, MI: Wayne State University Press.

Muma, J. (1971). Language intervention: Ten techniques. *Language, Speech and Hearing Services in Schools, 5,* 7–17.

Muma, J. (1986). *Language acquisition: A functionalistic perspective.* Austin, TX: Pro-Ed.

Muma, J. (1998). *Effective speech-language pathology: A cognitive socialization approach.* Hillsdale, NJ: Lawrence Erlbaum.

Musselman, C., & Akamatsu, C. T. (1999). The interpersonal communication skills of deaf adolescents and their relationship to communication history. *Journal of Deaf Studies and Deaf Education, 4,* 305–320.

Musselman, C., & Szanto, G. (1998). The written language of deaf adolescents: Patterns of performance. *Journal of Deaf Studies and Deaf Education, 3,* 245–257.

Myklebust, H. (1964). *The psychology of deafness* (2nd ed.). New York: Grune & Stratton.

Naglieri, J., & Das, J. (1988). Planning-attention-simultaneous-successive (PASS): A model for assessment. *Journal of School Psychology, 26,* 35–48.

Nagy, W., & Anderson, R. (1984). How many words are there in printed school English? *Reading Research Quarterly, 19,* 304–330.

Nagy, W., & Herman, P. (1987). Breadth and depth of vocabulary knowledge: Implications for acquisition and instruction. In M. McKeown & M. Curtis (Eds.), *The nature of vocabulary acquisition* (pp. 19–35). Hillsdale, NJ: Lawrence Erlbaum.

Nagy, W., Winsor, P., Osborn, J., & O'Flahavan, J. (1994). Structural analysis: Some guidelines for instruction. In F. Lehr & J. Osborn (Eds.), *Reading, lan-*

guage, and literacy: Instruction for the twenty-first century (pp. 45–58). Hillsdale, NJ: Lawrence Erlbaum.

Navarro, R. (1985). The problems of language, education, and society: Who decides. In E. Garcia & R. Padilla (Eds.), *Advances in bilingual education research* (pp. 289–313). Tucson, AZ: University of Arizona Press.

Negin, G. (1987). The effects of syntactic segmentation on the reading comprehension of hearing-impaired students. *Reading Psychology, 8*, 23–31.

Neisser, A. (1983). *The other side of silence: Sign language and the Deaf community in America.* New York: Knopf.

Nelson, K. (1973). Structure and strategy in learning to talk. *Monographs of the Society for Research in Child Development, 38*, 1–2.

Neuroth-Gimbrone, C., & Logiodice, C. (1992). A cooperative bilingual language program for deaf adolescents. *Sign Language Studies, 74*, 79–91.

Nevins, M., & Chute, P. (1996). *Children with cochlear implants in educational settings.* San Diego: Singular Publishing Group.

Newport, E., & Ashbrook, E. (1977). The emergence of semantic relations in American Sign Language. *Papers and Reports on Child Language Development, 13*, 16–21.

Newport, E., & Meier, R. (1985). The acquisition of American Sign Language. In D. Slobin (Ed.), *The cross-linguistic study of language acquisition* (pp. 881–938). Hillsdale, NJ: Lawrence Erlbaum.

Nicholls, G., & Ling, D. (1982). Cued speech and the reception of spoken language. *Journal of Speech and Hearing Research, 25*, 262–269.

NIH Consensus Program Information Service (1995). *Consensus Statement on Cochlear Implants in Adults and Children.* Kensington, MD: National Institutes of Health.

Ninio, A., & Snow, C. (1996). *Pragmatic Development.* Boulder, CO: Westview.

Nolen, S., & Wilbur, R. (1985). The effects of context on deaf students' comprehension of difficult sentences. *American Annals of the Deaf, 130*, 231–235.

Northern, J. (1994). Universal hearing screening for infant hearing impairment: Necessary, beneficial and justifiable. *Audiology Today, 8*, 10–13.

Novelli-Olmstead, T., & Ling, D. (1984). Speech production and speech discrimination by hearing-impaired children. *Volta Review, 86*, 72–80.

Nunes, T., Bryant, P., & Bindman, M. (1997). Spelling and grammar—the necsed move. In C. Perfetti, L. Rieben, & M. Fayol (Eds.), *Learning to spell: Research, theory, and practice across languages* (pp. 151–170). Hillsdale, NJ: Lawrence Erlbaum.

Odom, P., Blanton, R., & McIntire, C. (1970). Coding medium and word recall by deaf and hearing subjects. *Journal of Speech and Hearing Research, 13,* 54–58.

Ogden, P. (1979). *Experiences and attitudes of oral deaf adults regarding oralism.* Unpublished doctoral dissertation, University of Illinois, Urbana-Champaign.

O'Kane, J., & Goldbart, J. (1998). *Communication before speech: Development and assessment* (2nd ed.). London: David Fulton.

Oller, J. (1979). *Language tests at school.* White Plains, NY: Longman.

Oller, J., & Perkins, K. (1978). *Language in education: Testing the tests.* Rowley, MA: Newbury House.

Oller, J., & Perkins, K. (Eds.). (1980). *Research in language testing.* Rowley, MA: Newbury House.

Olmsted, D. (1971). *Out of the mouth of babes.* The Hague, the Netherlands: Mouton.

Olson, D. (1986). The cognitive consequences of literacy. *Canadian Journal of Psychology, 27,* 109–121.

Olson, D. (1989). Literate thought. In C. K. Leong & B. Randhawa (Eds.), *Understanding literacy and cognition* (pp. 3–15). New York: Plenum.

Olson, D. (1991). Literacy and objectivity: The rise of modern science. In D. Olson & N. Torrance (Eds.), *Literacy and orality* (pp. 149–164). New York: Cambridge University Press.

Olson, D. (1994). *The world on paper.* Cambridge, UK: Cambridge University Press.

Olson, D., & Bruner, J. (1996). Folk psychology and folk pedagogy. In D. Olson & N. Torrance (Eds.), *The handbook of education and human development: New models of learning, teaching and schooling* (pp. 9–27). Cambridge, MA: Blackwell.

O'Neill, J., & Oyer, H. (1981). *Visual communication for the hard of hearing: History, research, methods* (2nd ed.). Englewood Cliffs, NJ: Prentice Hall.

O'Neill, M. (1973). *The receptive language competence of deaf children in the use of the base structure rules of transformational generative grammar.* Unpublished doctoral dissertation, University of Pittsburgh, Pennsylvania.

Ong, W. (1982). *Orality and literacy: The technologizing of the word.* London: Methuen.

Orlando, A., & Shulman, B. (1989). Severe-to-profound hearing-impaired children's comprehension of figurative language. *Journal of Childhood Communication Disorders, 12,* 157–165.

Orlansky, M., & Bonvillian, J. (1984). The role of iconicity in early sign language acquisition. *Journal of Speech and Hearing Disorders, 49,* 287–292.

Orlansky, M., & Bonvillian, J. (1985). Sign language acquisition: Language development in children of deaf parents and implications for other populations. *Merrill-Palmer Quarterly, 31,* 127–143.

O'Rourke, J. (1974). *Toward a science of vocabulary development.* The Hague, the Netherlands: Mouton.

O'Rourke, T. J. (1973). *A basic course in manual communication.* Silver Spring, MD: National Association of the Deaf.

Osberger, M. (1990). Audition. *Volta Review, 92,* 34–53.

Otheguy, R., & Otto, R. (1980). The myth of static maintenance in bilingual education. *Modern Language Journal, 64,* 350–356.

Owens, R. (1996). *Language development: An introduction* (4th ed.). Boston: Allyn & Bacon.

Owens, R., Haney, M., Giesow, V., Dooley, L., & Kelly, R. (1983). Language test content: A comparative study. *Language, Speech, and Hearing Services in Schools, 14,* 7–21.

Paap, K., & Noel, R. (1991). Dual-route models of print and sound: Still a good horse race. *Psychological Research, 53,* 13–24.

Padden, C. (1991). The acquisition of fingerspelling by deaf children. In P. Siple & S. Fischer (Eds.), *Theoretical issues in sign language research: Volume 2: Psychology* (pp. 191–210). Chicago: University of Chicago Press.

Padden, C. (1998a). Early bilingual lives of deaf children. In I. Parasnis (Ed.), *Cultural and language diversity and the Deaf experience* (pp. 99–116). New York: Cambridge University Press.

Padden, C. (1998b). From the cultural to the bicultural: The modern Deaf community. In I. Parasnis (Ed.), *Cultural and language diversity and the Deaf experience* (pp. 79–98). New York: Cambridge University Press.

Padden, C., & Humphries, T. (1988). *Deaf in America: Voices from a culture.* Cambridge, MA: Harvard University Press.

Padden, C., & LeMaster, B. (1985). An alphabet on hand: The acquisition of fingerspelling in deaf children. *Sign Language Studies, 47,* 161–172.

Page, S. (1981). *The effect of idiomatic language in passages on the reading comprehension of deaf and hearing students* [Abstract]. Unpublished doctoral dissertation, Ball State University, Indiana.

Parasnis, I. (Ed.). (1998). *Cultural and language diversity and the Deaf experience.* New York: Cambridge University Press.

Paul, P. (1984). *The comprehension of multimeaning words from selected frequency levels by deaf and hearing subjects*. Unpublished doctoral dissertation, University of Illinois, Urbana-Champaign.

Paul, P. (1985). Reading and other language-variant populations. In C. King & S. Quigley, *Reading and deafness* (pp. 251–289). San Diego: College-Hill Press.

Paul, P. (1988). The effects of viewing angle and visibility on speechreading comprehension ability. *Hearsay: The Journal of the Ohio Speech and Hearing Association*, Fall, 100–103.

Paul, P. (1990). Using ASL to teach English literacy skills. *The Deaf American*, 40(1–4), 107–113.

Paul, P. (1991). ASL to English: A bilingual minority-language immersion program for deaf students. In S. Polowe-Aldersley, P. Schragle, V. Armour, & J. Polowe (Eds.), *Conference proceedings of the 1991 CAID/CEASD Convention* (pp. 53–56). New Orleans, LA: Convention of American Instructors of the Deaf.

Paul, P. (1993). Deafness and text-based literacy. *American Annals of the Deaf*, *138*, 72–75.

Paul, P. (1994). Response to "unlocking the curriculum." *Teaching English to Deaf and Second-Language Learners*, *10*, 18–21.

Paul, P. (1996). Reading vocabulary knowledge and deafness. *Journal of Deaf Studies and Deaf Education*, *1*, 3–15.

Paul, P. (1997). Reading for students with hearing impairment: Research review and implications. *Volta Review*, *99*, 73–87.

Paul, P. (1998a). *Literacy and deafness: The development of reading, writing, and literate thought*. Boston: Allyn & Bacon.

Paul, P. (1998b). Endnote: A perspective on the special issue of literacy. *Journal of Deaf Studies and Deaf Education*, *3*, 258–263.

Paul, P. (1999). Review of Cued language structure: An analysis of cued American English based on linguistics principles. *American Annals of the Deaf*, 144, 4–6.

Paul, P., Bernhardt, E., & Gramley, C. (1992). Use of ASL in teaching reading and writing to deaf students: An interactive theoretical perspective. *In Conference proceedings: Bilingual considerations in the education of deaf students: ASL and English* (pp. 75–105). Washington, DC: Gallaudet University, Extension and Summer Programs.

Paul, P., & Drasgow, E. (1998). The great ASL-MCE debate: A rejoinder. *The CAEDHH Journal/La Revue ACESM*, *24*, 5–15.

Paul, P., & Gustafson, G. (1991). Hearing-impaired students' comprehension of high-frequency multimeaning words. *Remedial and Special Education, 12*(4), 52–62.

Paul, P., & Jackson, D. (1993). *Toward a psychology of deafness: Theoretical and empirical perspectives.* Boston: Allyn & Bacon.

Paul, P., & O'Rourke, J. (1988). Multimeaning words and reading comprehension: Implications for special education students. *Remedial and Special Education, 9*(3), 42–52.

Paul, P., & Quigley, S. (1987a). Some effects of early hearing impairment on English language development. In F. Martin (Ed.), *Hearing disorders in children: Pediatric audiology* (pp. 49–80). Austin, TX: Pro-Ed.

Paul, P., & Quigley, S. (1987b). Using American Sign Language to teach English. In P. McAnally, S. Rose, & S. Quigley, *Language learning practices with deaf children* (pp. 139–166). Boston: Little, Brown.

Paul, P., & Quigley, S. (1989). Education and hard-of-hearing students. In H. Hartmann & K. Hartmann (Eds.), *Conference proceedings: Hard-of-hearing pupils in regular schools* (pp. 48–60; 173–184). Berlin, Germany: International Organization of Hard-of-Hearing Students.

Paul, P., & Quigley, S. (1990). *Education and deafness.* White Plains, NY: Longman.

Paul, P., & Quigley, S. (1994). American Sign Language-English bilingual education. In P. McAnally, S. Rose, & S. Quigley, *Language learning practices with deaf children* (pp. 219–253). Austin, TX: Pro-Ed.

Paul, P., Stallman, A., & O'Rourke, J. (1990). *Using three test formats to assess good and poor readers' word knowledge* (Tech. Rep. No. 509). Urbana-Champaign, IL: University of Illinois, Center for the Study of Reading.

Paul, P., & Ward, M. (1996). Inclusion paradigms in conflict. *Theory into Practice, Inclusive Schools: The Continuing Debate, 35,* 4–11.

Payne, J-A. (1982). *A study of the comprehension of verb-particle combinations among deaf and hearing subjects.* Unpublished doctoral dissertation, University of Illinois, Urbana-Champaign.

Payne, J-A., & Quigley, S. (1987). Hearing-impaired children's comprehension of verb-particle combinations. *Volta Review, 89,* 133–143.

Pearson, P. D., & Fielding, L. (1991). Comprehension instruction. In R. Barr, M. Kamil, P. Mosenthal, & P. D. Pearson (Eds.), *Handbook of reading research* (2nd ed., pp. 815–860).

Pearson, P. D., & Johnson, D. (1978). *Teaching reading comprehension*. New York: Holt, Rinehart & Winston.

Pearson, P. D., & Stephens, D. (1994). Learning about literacy: A 30-year journey. In R. Ruddell, M. Ruddell, & H. Singer (Eds.), *Theoretical models and processes of reading* (4th ed., pp. 22–42). Newark, DE: International Reading Association.

Perfetti, C., Beck, I., Bell, L., & Hughes, C. (1987). Phonemic knowledge and learning to read are reciprocal: A longitudinal study of first grade children. *Merrill-Palmer Quarterly, 33*, 283–319.

Petitto, L. (1987). On the autonomy of language and gesture: Evidence from the acquisition of personal pronouns in American Sign Language. *Cognition, 27*, 1–52.

Petitto, L., & Marentette, P. (1991). Babbling in the manual mode: Evidence for the ontogeny of language. *Science*, 251, 1493–1496.

Philip, M. (1992). The learning center. In *Conference proceedings: Bilingual considerations in the education of deaf students: ASL and English* (pp. 46–47). Washington, DC: Gallaudet University.

Phillips, J. (1981). *Piaget's theory: A primer*. New York: Freeman.

Piaget, J. (1952). *The origins of intelligence in children*. New York: International University Press.

Piaget, J. (1968). *Six psychological studies*. New York: Vintage Books.

Piaget, J. (1971). *Psychology and epistemology*. New York: Vintage Books.

Piaget, J. (1977). *The development of thought: Equilibration of cognitive structures*. New York: Viking.

Piaget, J. (1980). *Six psychological studies*. Brighton, UK: Harvester Press.

Piattelli-Palmarini, M. (1980). *Language and learning*. Cambridge, MA: Harvard University Press.

Piattelli-Palmarini, M. (1994). Ever since language and learning: Afterthoughts on the Piaget-Chomsky debate. *Cognition, 50*, 315–346.

Pinker, S. (1984). *Language learnability and language development*. Cambridge, MA: Harvard University Press.

Pinker, S. (1989). *Learnability and cognition: The acquisition of argument structure*. Cambridge, MA: MIT Press.

Pintner, R., & Lev, J. (1939). The intelligence of the hard-of-hearing school child. *Journal of Genetic Psychology, 55*, 31–48.

Pintner, R., & Paterson, D. (1917). The ability of deaf and hearing children to follow printed directions. *American Annals of the Deaf, 62*, 448–472.

Pintner, R., & Reamer, J. (1920). A mental and educational survey of schools for the deaf. *American Annals of the Deaf, 65,* 451–472.

Poizner, H., Klima, E., & Bellugi, U. (1987). *What the hands reveal about the brain.* Cambridge, MA: MIT Press.

Pollack, D. (1984). An acoupedic program. In D. Ling (Ed.), *Early intervention for hearing-impaired children: Oral options* (pp. 181–253). San Diego: College-Hill Press.

Polloway, E., & Smith, T. (1992). *Language instruction for students with disabilities* (2nd ed.). Denver, CO: Love Publishing Company.

Power, D., & Quigley, S. (1973). Deaf children's acquisition of the passive voice. *Journal of Speech and Hearing Research, 16,* 5–11.

Powers, A., Elliott, R., & Funderburg, R. (1987). Learning disabled hearing-impaired students: Are they being identified? *Volta Review, 89,* 99–105.

Prabhu, N. (1990). There is no best method—why? *TESOL Quarterly, 24,* 161–176.

Pressnell, L. (1973). Hearing-impaired children's comprehension and production of syntax in oral language. *Journal of Speech and Hearing Research, 16,* 12–21.

Priest, J. (1991). *Theories of the mind.* Boston: Houghton Mifflin.

Prinz, P. (1998). (Ed.). ASL proficiency and English literacy acquisition: New perspectives [Special Issue]. *Topics in Language Disorders, 18*(4).

Pugh, B. (1955). *Steps in language development for the deaf: Illustrated in the Fitzgerald Key.* Washington, DC: The Volta Bureau.

Pustejovsky, J., & Boguraev, B. (Ed.). (1996). *Lexical semantics.* New York: Oxford University Press.

Quenin, C., & Blood, I. (1989). A national survey of cued speech programs. *Volta Review, 91,* 283–289.

Quigley, S. (1969). *The influence of fingerspelling on the development of language, communication, and educational achievement in deaf children.* Urbana, IL: University of Illinois, Institute for Research on Exceptional Children.

Quigley, S., & Frisina, R. (1961). *Institutionalization and psychoeducational development of deaf children* (CEC Research Monograph). Washington, DC: Council of Exceptional Children.

Quigley, S., & King, C. (1981). *Reading milestones.* Beaverton, OR: Dormac.

Quigley, S., & King, C. (1982). *Reading milestones.* Beaverton, OR: Dormac.

Quigley, S., & King, C. (1983). *Reading milestones.* Beaverton, OR: Dormac.

Quigley, S., & King, C. (1984). *Reading milestones*. Beaverton, OR: Dormac.

Quigley, S., & Kretschmer, R. E. (1982*). The education of deaf children: Issues, theory, and practice*. Austin, TX: Pro-Ed.

Quigley, S., & Paul, P. (1986). A perspective on academic achievement. In D. Luterman (Ed.), *Deafness in perspective* (pp. 55–86). San Diego: College-Hill Press.

Quigley, S., & Paul, P. (1989). English language development. In M. Wang, M. Reynolds, & H. Walberg (Eds.), *The handbook of special education: Research and practice* (Vol. 3, pp. 3–21). New York: Pergamon.

Quigley, S., & Paul, P. (1990). *Language and deafness*. San Diego: Singular Publishing Group. (Original work published in 1984)

Quigley, S., & Paul, P. (1994). Reflections. In P. McAnally, S. Rose, & S. Quigley, *Language learning practices with deaf children* (2nd ed., pp. 255–272). Austin, TX: Pro-Ed.

Quigley, S., Paul, P., McAnally, P., Rose, S., & Payne, J-A. (1990). *The reading bridge: Teacher's guide: Mosaic*. San Diego: Dormac.

Quigley, S., Paul, P., McAnally, P., Rose, S., & Payne, J-A. (1991). *The reading bridge: Teacher's guide: Patterns*. San Diego: Dormac.

Quigley, S., & Power, D. (1979). *TSA syntax program*. Beaverton, OR: Dormac.

Quigley, S., Power, D., & Steinkamp, M. (1977). The language structure of deaf children. *Volta Review, 79*, 73–83.

Quigley, S., Power, D., Steinkamp, M., & Jones, B. (1978). *Test of syntactic abilities*. Beaverton, OR: Dormac.

Quigley, S., Smith, N., & Wilbur, R. (1974). Comprehension of relativized sentences by deaf students. *Journal of Speech and Hearing Research, 17*, 325–341.

Quigley, S., Steinkamp, M., Power, D., & Jones, B. (1978). *Test of syntactic abilities: Guide to administration and interpretation*. Beaverton, OR: Dormac.

Quigley, S., & Thomure, R. (1968). *Some effects of hearing impairment upon school performance*. Urbana, IL: University of Illinois, Institute for Research on Exceptional Children.

Quigley, S., Wilbur, R., & Montanelli, D. (1974). Question formation in the language of deaf students. *Journal of Speech and Hearing Research, 17*, 699–713.

Quigley, S., Wilbur, R., & Montanelli, D. (1976). Complement structures in the language of deaf students. *Journal of Speech and Hearing Research, 19*, 448–457.

Quigley, S., Wilbur, R., Power, D., Montanelli, D., & Steinkamp, M. (1976). *Syntactic structures in the language of deaf children* (Final report). Urbana, IL: University of Illinois, Institute for Child Behavior and Development. (ERIC Document Reproduction Service No. ED 119 447)

Raffin, M. (1976). *The acquisition of inflectional morphemes by deaf children using seeing essential English*. Unpublished doctoral dissertation, University of Iowa, Iowa City.

Raffin, M., Davis, J., & Gilman, L. (1978). Comprehension of inflectional morphemes by deaf children exposed to a visual English sign system. *Journal of Speech and Hearing Research, 21*, 387–400.

Rayner, K., & Pollatsek, A. (1989). *The psychology of reading*. Englewood Cliffs, NJ: Prentice Hall.

Reagan, T. (1985). The deaf as a linguistic minority: Educational considerations. *Harvard Educational Review, 55*, 265–277.

Reagan, T. (1990). Cultural considerations in the education of deaf children. In D. Moores & K. Meadow-Orlans (Eds.), *Educational and developmental aspects of deafness* (pp. 73–84). Washington, DC: Gallaudet University Press.

Regis, E. (1987). *Who got Einstein's office? Eccentricity and genius at the institute for advanced study*. Reading, MA: Addison-Wesley.

Reich, P. (1986). *Language development*. Englewood Cliffs, NJ: Prentice Hall.

Reich, P., & Bick, M. (1977). How visible is visible English? *Sign Language Studies, 14*, 59–72.

Rice, M., & Schiefelbusch, R. (Eds.). (1989). *The teachability of language*. Baltimore: Paul H. Brookes.

Ries, P. (1986). Characteristics of hearing impaired youth in the general population and of students in special education programs for the hearing-impaired. In A. Schildroth & M. Karchmer (Eds.), *Deaf children in America* (pp. 1–31). San Diego: College-Hill Press.

Ritter-Brinton, K. (1996). The great ASL/MCE debate—what it's telling us and what it's costing us. *The CAEDHH Journal/La Revue ACESM, 22*, 24–34.

Ritzer, G. (1991). *Metatheorizing in sociology*. Lexington, MA: Lexington Books.

Ritzer, G. (Ed.). (1992). *Metatheorizing*. Newbury Park, CA: Sage.

Robbins, A. (1994). Guidelines for developing oral communication skills in children with cochlear implants. *Volta Review, 96*, 75–82.

Robbins, N. (1983). The effects of signed text on the reading comprehension of hearing-impaired children. *American Annals of the Deaf, 128*, 40–44.

Robbins, N., & Hatcher, C. (1981). The effects of syntax on the reading comprehension of hearing-impaired children. *Volta Review, 83,* 105–115.

Roberts, S., & Rickards, F. (1994a). A survey of graduates of an Australian integrated auditory/oral preschool. Part I: Amplification, usage, communication practices, and speech intelligibility. *Volta Review, 96,* 185–205.

Roberts, S., & Rickards, F. (1994b). A survey of graduates of an Australian integrated auditory/oral preschool. Part II: Academic achievement, utilization of support services, and friendship patterns. *Volta Review, 96,* 207–236.

Rodda, M., & Grove, C. (1987). *Language, cognition, and deafness.* Hillsdale, NJ: Lawrence Erlbaum.

Rosenblatt, L. (1978). *The reader, the text, the poem: The transactional theory of the literary work.* Carbondale, IL: Southern Illinois University Press.

Rosier, P., & Farella, M. (1976). Bilingual education at Rock Point—some early results. *TESOL Quarterly, 10,* 379–388.

Ross, M. (1986). *Aural habilitation.* Austin, TX: Pro-Ed.

Ross, M. (Ed.). (1990). *Hearing-impaired children in the mainstream.* Monkton, MD: York Press.

Ross, M., Brackett, D., & Maxon, A. (1982). *Hard of hearing children in regular schools.* Englewood Cliffs, NJ: Prentice Hall.

Ross, M., & Calvert, D. (1984). Semantics of deafness revisited: Total communication and the use and misuse of residual hearing. *Audiology, 9,* 127–143.

Rubin, A., & Hansen, J. (1986). Reading and writing: How are the first two R's related? In J. Orasanu (Ed.), *Reading comprehension: From research to practice* (pp. 163–170). Hillsdale, NJ: Lawrence Erlbaum.

Ruddell, R., & Haggard, M. (1985). Oral and written language acquisition and the reading process. In H. Singer & R. Ruddell (Eds.), *Theoretical models and processes of reading* (3rd ed., pp. 63–80). Newark, DE: International Reading Association.

Ruddell, R., Ruddell, M., & Singer, H. (Eds.). (1994). *Theoretical models and processes of reading* (4th ed.). Newark, DE: International Reading Association.

Rumelhart, D. (1977). Toward an interactive model of reading. In S. Dornic (Ed.), *Attention and performance VI* (pp. 573–603). San Diego: Academic Press.

Rumelhart, D. (1994). Toward an interactive model of reading. In R. Ruddell, M. Ruddell, & H. Singer (Eds.), *Theoretical models and processes of reading* (4th ed., pp. 864–894). Newark, DE: International Reading Association.

Rumelhart, D., McClelland, J., & the PDP Research Group. (1986). *Parallel distributed processing: Explorations in the microstructure of cognition: Vol. 1. Foundations.* Cambridge, MA: MIT Press.

Russell, B. (1948). *Human knowledge: Its scope and limits.* New York: Simon & Schuster.

Russell, B. (1972). *A history of Western philosophy.* New York: Simon & Schuster.

Russell, W., Quigley, S., & Power, D. (1976). *Linguistics and deaf children.* Washington, DC: Alexander Graham Bell Association for the Deaf.

Rymer, R. (1992, April 13). Annals of science: A silent childhood-I. *The New Yorker,* 41–81.

Sachs, J. (1993). The emergence of intentional communication. In J. Gleason (Ed.), *The development of language* (3rd ed., pp. 39–64). New York: Macmillan.

Sacks, O. (1989). *Seeing voices: A journey into the world of the deaf.* Berkeley, CA: University of California Press.

Salvia, J., & Ysseldyke, J. (1991). *Assessment* (5th ed.). Boston: Houghton Mifflin.

Samar, V., Parasnis, I., & Berent, G. (1998). Learning disabilities, attention deficit disorders, and deafness. In M. Marschark & M. D. Clark (Eds.), *Psychological perspectives on deafness* (Vol. II) (pp. 199–242). Hillsdale, NJ: Lawrence Erlbaum.

Samar, V., & Sims, D. (1983). Visual evoked response correlates of speechreading performance in normal-hearing adults: A replication and factor analytic extension. *Journal of Speech and Hearing Research, 26,* 2–9.

Samuels, S. J., & Kamil, M. (1984). Models of the reading process. In P. D. Pearson, R. Barr, M. Kamil, & P. Mosenthal (Eds.), *Handbook of reading research* (pp. 185–224). White Plains, NY: Longman.

Sanders, D. (1982). *Aural rehabilitation: A management model* (2nd ed.). Englewood Cliffs, NJ: Prentice Hall.

Sapir, E. (1958). *Selected writings of Edward Sapir in language, culture, and personality* (D. Mandelbaum, Ed.). Berkeley, CA: University of California Press.

Sarachan-Deily, A. (1982). Hearing-impaired and hearing readers' sentence processing errors. *Volta Review, 84,* 81–95.

Sarachan-Deily, A. (1985). Written narratives of deaf and hearing students: Story recall and inference. *Journal of Speech and Hearing Research, 28,* 151–159.

Saur, R., Popp-Stone, M., & Hurley-Lawrence, E. (1987). The classroom participation of mainstreamed hearing-impaired college students. *Volta Review, 89,* 277–286.

Schein, J., & Stewart, D. (1995). *Language in motion: Exploring the nature of sign*. Washington, DC: Gallaudet University.

Schick, B. (1997). The effects of discourse genre on English language complexity in school-age deaf students. *Journal of Deaf Studies and Deaf Education, 2,* 234–251.

Schick, B., & Moeller, M. (1992). What is learnable in manually coded English sign systems? *Applied Psycholinguistics, 13,* 313–340.

Schirmer, B. (1994). *Language and literacy development in children who are deaf*. New York: Maxwell Macmillan International.

Schirmer, B., & Woolsey, M. L. (1997). Effect of teacher questions on the reading comprehension of deaf children. *Journal of Deaf Studies and Deaf Education, 2,* 47–56.

Schlesinger, H., & Meadow, K. (1972). *Sound and sign: Childhood deafness and mental health*. Berkeley, CA: University of California Press.

Schlesinger, I. (1982). *Steps to language: Toward a theory of native language acquisition*. Hillsdale, NJ: Lawrence Erlbaum.

Schmitt, P. (1969). *Deaf children's comprehension and production of sentence transformation and verb tenses*. Unpublished doctoral dissertation, University of Illinois, Urbana-Champaign.

Schulze, B. (1965). An evaluation of vocabulary development by thirty-two deaf children over a three-year period. *American Annals of the Deaf, 110,* 424–435.

Schumann, J. (1978). *The pidginization process: A model for second language acquisition*. Rowley, MA: Newbury House.

Scouten, E. (1967). The Rochester method: An oral multisensory approach for instructing prelingual deaf children. *American Annals of the Deaf, 112,* 50–55.

Searle, J. (1969). *Speech acts*. Cambridge, UK: Cambridge University Press.

Searle, J. (1976). A classification of illocutionary acts. *Language in Society, 5,* 1–23.

Searle, J. (1992). *The rediscovery of the mind*. Cambridge, MA: MIT Press.

Searle, J. (1995). The problem of consciousness. In C. Hedley, P. Antonacci, & M. Rabinowitcz (Eds.), *Thinking and literacy: The mind at work* (pp. 21–30). Hillsdale, NJ: Lawrence Erlbaum.

Searls, E., & Klesius, K. (1984). 99 multiple meaning words for primary students and ways to teach them. *Reading Psychology: An International Quarterly, 5,* 55–63.

Selinker, L. (1972). Interlanguage. *IRAL, 10,* 209–231.

Selinker, L., Swain, M., & Dumas, G. (1975). The interlanguage hypothesis extended to children. *Language Learning, 25*, 139–191.

Shadbolt, N. (1988). Models and methods in cognitive science. In M. McTear (Ed.), *Understanding cognitive science* (pp. 23–45). New York: Halsted Press.

Shelton, R., & Wood, C. (1978). Speech mechanisms and production. In P. Skinner & R. Shelton (Eds.), *Speech, language, and hearing: Normal processes and disorders* (pp. 54–77). Reading, MA: Addison-Wesley.

Shepard, N., Davis, J., Gorga, M., & Stelmachowicz, P. (1981). Characteristics of hearing-impaired children in the public schools: Part I—Demographic data. *Journal of Speech and Hearing Disorders, 46*, 123–129.

Shepherd, D. (1982). Visual-neural correlate of speechreading ability in normal-hearing adults: Reliability. *Journal of Speech and Hearing Research, 25*, 521–527.

Shipley, E., Smith, C., & Gleitman, L. (1969). A study in the acquisition of language; free responses to commands. *Language, 45*, 322–342.

Shore, C. (1995). *Individual differences in language development*. Thousand Oaks, CA: Sage.

Shu, H., Anderson, R., & Zhang, H. (1995). Incidental learning of word meanings while reading: A Chinese and American cross-cultural study. *Reading Research Quarterly, 30*, 76–95.

Siedlecki, T., & Bonvillian, J. (1993). Location, handshape, and movement: Young children's acquisition of the formational aspects of American Sign Language. *Sign Language Studies, 78*, 31–52.

Siedlecki, T., & Bonvillian, J. (1997). Young children's acquisition of the handshape aspect of American Sign Language signs: Parental report findings. *Applied Psycholinguistics, 18*, 17–39.

Silverman, S. R., & Kricos, P. (1990). Speechreading. *Volta Review, 92*, 21–32.

Silverman-Dresner, T., & Guilfoyle, G. (1972). *Vocabulary norms for deaf children: The Lexington school for the deaf education series, Book VII*. Washington, DC: Alexander Graham Bell Association for the Deaf.

Simmons, A. (1963). *Comparison of written and spoken language from deaf and hearing children at five age levels*. Unpublished doctoral dissertation, Washington University, St. Louis, MO.

Simser, J. (1993). Auditory-verbal intervention: Infants and toddlers. *Volta Review, 95*, 217–229.

Siple, P. (Ed.) (1978). *Understanding language through sign language research*. New York: Academic Press.

Skarakis, E., & Prutting, C. (1977). Early communication: Semantic function and communicative intentions in the communications of the preschool child with impaired hearing. *American Annals of the Deaf, 122*, 382–391.

Skinner, B. F. (1957). *Verbal behavior.* Englewood Cliffs, NJ: Prentice Hall.

Slobin, D. (1979). *Psycholinguistics* (2nd ed.). Glenview, IL: Scott, Foresman.

Snow, C., Burns, S., & Griffin, P. (Eds.). (1998). *Preventing reading difficulties in young children.* Washington, DC: National Academy Press.

Snyder, L. (1984). Cognition and language development. In R. Naremore (Ed.), *Language science* (pp. 107–145). San Diego: College-Hill Press.

Spencer, L., Tomblin, J. B., & Gantz, B. (1997). Reading skills in children with multichannel cochlear-implant experience. *Volta Review, 99*, 193–202.

Spiro, R., Vispoel, W., Schmitz, J., Samarapungavan, A., & Boerger, A. (1987). Knowledge acquisition for application: Cognitive flexibility and transfer in complex content domains. In B. Britton & S. Glynn (Eds.), *Executive control processes in reading* (pp. 177–199). Hillsdale, NJ: Lawrence Erlbaum.

Spradlin, K., Dancer, J., & Monfils, B. (1989). Effects of verbal encouragement on self-ratings of lipreading performance. *Volta Review, 91*, 209–216.

Squires, S., & Dancer, J. (1986). Auditory versus visual practice effects in the intelligibility of words in everyday sentences. *Journal of Auditory Research, 26*, 5–10.

Stahl, S., & Fairbanks, M. (1986). The effects of vocabulary instruction: A model-based meta-analysis. *Review of Educational Research, 56*, 72–110.

Stanovich, K. (1980). Toward an interactive-compensatory model of individual differences in the development of reading fluency. *Reading Research Quarterly, 16*, 32–71.

Stanovich, K. (1986). Matthew effects in reading: Some consequences of individual differences in the acquisition of literacy. *Reading Research Quarterly, 21*, 360–407.

Stanovich, K. (1991). Word recognition: Changing perspectives. In R. Barr, M. Kamil, P. Mosenthal, & P. D. Pearson (Eds.), *Handbook of reading research* (2nd ed., pp. 418–452). White Plains, NY: Longman.

Stanovich, K. (1992). Speculations on the causes and consequences of individual differences in early reading acquisition. In P. Gough, L. Ehri, & R. Treiman (Eds.), *Reading acquisition* (pp. 307–342). Hillsdale, NJ: Lawrence Erlbaum.

Steinberg, D. (1982). *Psycholinguistics: Language, mind, and the world.* White Plains, NY: Longman.

Steinberg, D., & Jakobovits, L. (1971). *Semantics: An interdisciplinary reader in philosophy, linguistics, and psychology.* New York: Cambridge University Press.

Stevens, K. (1992). Theoretical aspects of speech production. *Volta Review, 94,* 5–32.

Stevenson, R. (1988). *Models of language development.* Philadelphia: Open University Press.

Stewart, D. (1985). Language dominance in deaf students. *Sign Language Studies, 49,* 375–385.

Stewart, D., & Luetke-Stahlman, B. (1998). *The signing family: What every parent should know about sign communication.* Washington, DC: Gallaudet University Press.

Stoefen-Fisher, J., & Lee, M. (1989). The effectiveness of the graphic representation of signs in developing word identification skills for hearing-impaired beginning readers. *Journal of Special Education, 23,* 151–167.

Stoker, R., & Ling, D. (Eds.). (1992). Speech production in hearing-impaired children and youth: Theory and practice [Special Issue]. *Volta Review, 94*(5).

Stokoe, W. (1960). *Sign language structure: An outline of the visual communication systems of the American deaf. Studies in Linguistics Occasional Papers No. 8.* Washington, DC: Gallaudet University Press.

Stokoe, W., Casterline, D., & Croneberg, C. (1976). *A dictionary of American Sign Language on linguistic principles* (Rev. ed.). Silver Spring, MD: Linstok Press.

Stone, J. (1998). Minority empowerment and the education of Deaf people. In I. Parasnis (Ed.), *Cultural and language diversity and the Deaf experience* (pp. 171–180). New York: Cambridge University Press.

Strassman, B. (1992). Deaf adolescents' metacognitive knowledge about school-related reading. *American Annals of the Deaf, 137,* 326–330.

Strassman, B. (1997). Metacognition and reading in children who are deaf: A review of the research. *Journal of Deaf Studies and Deaf Education, 2*(3), 140–149.

Strassman, B., Kretschmer, R. E., & Bilsky, L. (1987). The instantiation of general terms by deaf adolescents/adults. *Journal of Communication Disorders, 20,* 1–13.

Streng, A. (1972). *Syntax, speech and hearing: Applied linguistics for teachers of children with language and hearing disabilities.* New York: Grune & Stratton.

Strong, M. (1988). A bilingual approach to the education of young deaf children: ASL and English. In M. Strong (Ed.), *Language learning and deafness* (pp. 113–129). New York: Cambridge University Press.

Strong, M., & Charlson, E. (1987). Simultaneous communication: Are teachers attempting an impossible task? *American Annals of the Deaf, 132,* 376–382.

Strong, M., & Prinz, P. (1997). A study of the relationship between American Sign Language and English literacy. *Journal of Deaf Studies and Deaf Education, 2,* 37–46.

Stuckless, E. R. (1991). Reflections on bilingual, bicultural education for deaf children: Some concerns about current advocacy and trends. *American Annals of the Deaf, 136,* 270–272.

Stuckless, E. R., & Birch, J. (1966). The influence of early manual communication on the linguistic development of deaf children. *American Annals of the Deaf, 111,* 452–460, 499–504.

Stuckless, E. R., & Marks, C. (1966). *Assessment of the written language of deaf students.* Pittsburgh: University of Pittsburgh, School of Education.

Stuckless, E. R., & Pollard, G. (1977). Processing of fingerspelling and print by deaf students. *American Annals of the Deaf, 122,* 475–479.

Sulzby, E. (1996). Conventional literacy. In C. Pontecorvo, M. Orsolini, B. Burge, & L. Resnick, (Eds.), *Early test construction in children* (pp. 25–46). Hillsdale, NJ: Lawrence Erlbaum.

Sulzby, E., & Teale, W. (1987). *Young children's storybook reading: Longitudinal study of parent-child interaction and children's independent functioning* (Final Report to the Spencer Foundation). Ann Arbor, MI: University of Michigan.

Supalla, S. (1986). *Manually coded English: The modality question in signed language development.* Unpublished master's thesis, University of Illinois, Urbana-Champaign.

Supalla, S. (1991). Manually coded English: The modality question in signed language development. In P. Siple & S. Fischer (Eds.), *Theoretical issues in sign language research: Volume 2: Psychology* (pp. 85–109). Chicago: University of Chicago Press.

Swain, M., & Lapkin, S. (1982). *Evaluating bilingual education: A Canadian example.* Clevedon, UK: Multilingual Matters, Ltd.

Swisher, M. V. (1984). Signed input of hearing mothers to deaf children. *Language Learning, 9,* 343–356.

Taylor, L. (1969). *A language analysis of the writing of deaf children.* Unpublished doctoral dissertation, Florida State University, Tallahassee.

Taylor, R. (1983). *Metaphysics* (3rd ed.). Englewood Cliffs, NJ: Prentice Hall.

Taylor, T. (1997). *Theorizing language: Analysis, normativity, rhetoric, history.* New York: Pergamon.

Templeton, S., & Bear, D. (Eds.). (1992). *Development of orthographic knowledge and the foundations of literacy: A memorial festschrift for Edmund H. Henderson.* Hillsdale, NJ: Lawrence Erlbaum.

Templin, M. (1950). *The development of reasoning in children with normal and defective hearing.* Minneapolis, MN: University of Minnesota.

The Deaf American. (1990). [Special monograph—Eyes, hands, voices: Communication issues among Deaf people]. *Deaf American, 40*(1–4).

Thies, T., & Trammel, J. (1983). Development and implementation of the auditory skills instructional planning system. In I. Hochberg, H. Levitt, & M. Osberger (Eds.), *Speech of the hearing impaired* (pp. 349–366). Baltimore: University Park Press.

Thompson, M., Biro, P., Vethivelu, S., Pious, C., & Hatfield, N. (1987). *Language assessment of hearing-impaired school age children.* Seattle, WA: University of Washington Press.

Tierney, R. (1994). Dissension, tensions, the models of literacy. In R. Ruddell, M. Ruddell, & H. Singer (Eds.), *Theoretical models and processes of reading* (4th ed., pp. 1162–1182). Newark, DE: International Reading Association.

Tierney, R., Carter, M., & Desai, L. (1991). *Portfolio assessment in the reading-writing classroom.* Norwell, MA: Christopher-Gordon.

Tierney, R., & Leys, M. (1984). *What is the value of connecting reading and writing?* (Reading Education Rep. No. 55). Champaign, IL: University of Illinois, Center for the Study of Reading.

Tierney, R., & Pearson, P. D. (1983). Toward a composing model of reading. *Language Arts, 60,* 568–580.

Tompkins, G. (1990). *Teaching writing: Balancing process and product.* Columbus, OH: Merrill.

Troike, R. (1981). Synthesis of research on bilingual education. *Educational Leadership, 38,* 498–504.

Trybus, R., & Karchmer, M. (1977). School achievement scores of hearing-impaired children: National data on achievement status and growth patterns. *American Annals of the Deaf, 122,* 62–69.

Tyack, D., & Gottesleben, R. (1974). *Language sampling, analysis, and training: A handbook for teachers and clinicians.* Palo Alto, CA: Consulting Psychologist's Press.

Tye-Murray, N., Spencer, L., & Woodworth, G. (1995). Acquisition of speech by children who have prolonged cochlear implant experience. *Journal of Speech and Hearing Research, 38,* 327–337.

Tye-Murray, N., Tyler, R., Lansing, C., & Bertschy, M. (1990). Evaluating the effectiveness of auditory training stimuli using a computerized program. *Volta Review, 92,* 25–30.

Tyler, R., Fryauf-Bertschy, H., Gantz, B., Kelsay, D., & Woodworth, G. (1997). Speech perception in prelingually implanted children after four years. *Advances in Oto-Rhino-Laryngology, 52,* 187–192.

Tzeng, S-J. (1993). *Speech recoding, short-term memory, and reading ability in immature readers with severe to profound hearing impairment. Unpublished doctoral dissertation,* Ohio State University, Columbus.

Van Cleve, J., & Crouch, B. (1989). *A place of their own.* Washington, DC: Gallaudet University Press.

Van Ert Windle, J., & Stout, G. (1984). *Developmental approach to successful listening.* San Diego: College-Hill Press.

van Uden, A. (1977). *A world of language for deaf children, Part 1. Basic principles: A maternal reflective method* (2nd ed.). Lisse, the Netherlands: Swets & Zeitlinger.

Verhoeven, L. (1990). Acquisition of reading in a second language. *Reading Research Quarterly, 25,* 90–114.

Verhoeven, L. (1992). Assessment of bilingual proficiency. In L. Verhoeven & J. de Jong (Eds.), *The construct of language proficiency: Applications of psychological models to language assessment* (pp. 125–136). Philadelphia: Benjamins.

Verhoeven, L., & de Jong, J. (Eds.). (1992). *The construct of language proficiency: Applications of psychological models to language assessment.* Philadelphia: Benjamins.

Vernon, M., & Andrews, J. (1990). *The psychology of deafness: Understanding deaf and hard-of-hearing people.* White Plains, NY: Longman.

Volterra, V., & Erting, C. (Eds.). (1990). *From gesture to language in hearing and deaf children.* Berlin: Springer.

Vygotsky, L. (1962). *Thought and language.* Cambridge, MA: MIT Press.

Vygotsky, L. (1978). *Mind in society: The development of higher psychological processes.* Cambridge, MA: Harvard University Press.

Walter, G. (1978). Lexical abilities of hearing and hearing-impaired children. *American Annals of the Deaf, 123,* 976–982.

Wampler, D. (1972). *Linguistics of visual English*. Santa Rosa, CA: Author.

Washburn, A. (1983). Seeing essential English: The development and use of a sign system over two decades. *Teaching English to Deaf and Second-Language Students, 2*, 26–30.

Weaver, C. (1994). Parallels between new paradigms in science and in reading and literacy theories: An essay review. In R. Ruddell, M. Ruddell, & H. Singer (Eds.), *Theoretical models and processes of reading* (4th ed., pp. 1185–1202). Newark, DE: International Reading Association.

Webster, A. (1986). *Deafness, development, and literacy*. New York: Methuen.

Webster's New Collegiate Dictionary. (1979). Springfield, MA: G. & C. Merriam Company.

Werker, J., & Lalonde, C. (1988). Cross-language speech perception: Initial capabilities and developmental change. *Developmental Psychology, 24*, 672–683.

Whitehead, M. (1990). *Language and literacy in the early years: An approach for education students*. London, UK: Chapman.

Whorf, B. (1956). *Language, thought, and reality*. Cambridge, MA: MIT Press.

Wiig, E., & Semel, E. (1984). *Language assessment and intervention for the learning disabled* (2nd ed.). Columbus, OH: Merrill.

Wilbur, R. (1977). An explanation of deaf children's difficulty with certain syntactic structures in English. *Volta Review, 79*, 85–92.

Wilbur, R. (1987). *American Sign Language: Linguistics and applied dimensions* (2nd ed.). Boston: Little, Brown.

Wilbur, R., Fraser, J., & Fruchter, A. (1981). *Comprehension of idioms by hearing-impaired students*. Paper presented at the American Speech-Language-Hearing Association Convention, Los Angeles.

Wilbur, R., & Goodhart, W. (1985). Comprehension of indefinite pronouns and quantifiers by hearing-impaired children. *Applied Psycholinguistics, 6*, 417–434.

Wilbur, R., Goodhart, W., & Fuller, D. (1989). Comprehension of English modals by hearing-impaired children. *Volta Review, 91*, 5–18.

Williams, C. (1994). The language and literacy worlds of three profoundly deaf preschool children. *Reading Research Quarterly, 29*, 124–155.

Williams, C., & McLean, M. (1996, April). *Response to literature as a pedagogical approach: An investigation of young deaf children's response to picturebook reading*. Paper presented at the annual meeting of the American Educational Research Association in New York.

Wilson, K. (1979). *Inference and language processing in hearing and deaf children.* Unpublished doctoral dissertation, Boston University.

Wilson, M., & Emmorey, K. (1997). Working memory for sign language: A window into the architecture of the working memory system. *Journal of Deaf Studies and Deaf Education, 2,* 121–130.

Wixson, K., Bosky, A., Yochum, M., & Alvermann, D. (1984). An interview for assessing students' perceptions of classroom reading tasks. *Reading Teacher, 37,* 346–352.

Wolff, A., & Harkins, J. (1986). Multihandicapped students. In A. Schildroth & M. Karchmer (Eds.), *Deaf children in America* (pp. 55–81). San Diego: College-Hill Press.

Wong Fillmore, L. (1989). Teachability and second language acquisition. In M. Rice & R. Schiefelbusch (Eds.), *The teachability of language* (pp. 311–332). Baltimore: Paul H. Brookes.

Woodward, J. (1978). Historical bases of American Sign Language. In P. Siple (Ed.), *Understanding language through sign language research* (pp. 333–348). San Diego: Academic Press.

Woodward, J., & Allen, T. (1988). Classroom use of artificial sign systems by teachers. *Sign Language Studies, 61,* 405–418.

Yamashita, C. (1992). *The relationships among prior knowledge, metacognition, and reading comprehension for hearing-impaired students.* Unpublished master's thesis, Ohio State University, Columbus.

Yoshinaga-Itano, C., & Downey, D. (1996). Development of school-aged deaf, hard-of-hearing, and normally hearing students' written language: Introduction. *Volta Review, 98,* 3–8.

Yoshinaga-Itano, C., Snyder, L., & Mayberry, R. (1996). How deaf and normally hearing students convey meaning within and between written sentences. *Volta Review, 98,* 9–38.

Yoshinaga-Itano, C., & Stredler-Brown, A. (1992). Learning to communicate: Babies with hearing impairments make their needs known. *Volta Review, 95,* 107–129.

Zemlin, W. (1968). *Speech and hearing science: Anatomy and physiology.* Englewood Cliffs, NJ: Prentice Hall.

Index